W9-CFV-351

Vertebrate
Endocrinology
FOURTH EDITION

Vertebrate Endocrinology

FOURTH EDITION

David O. Norris

AMSTERDAM • BOSTON • HEIDELBERG • LONDON
NEW YORK • OXFORD • PARIS • SAN DIEGO
SAN FRANCISCO • SINGAPORE • SYDNEY • TOKYO
Academic Press is an imprint of Elsevier

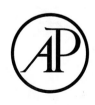

Elsevier Academic Press
30 Corporate Drive, Suite 400, Burlington, MA 01803, USA
525 B Street, Suite 1900, San Diego, CA 92101-4495, USA
84 Theobald's Road, London WC1X 8RR, UK

This book is printed on acid-free paper. ⊗

Copyright © 2007, Elsevier Inc. All rights reserved.

No part of this publication may be reproduced or transmitted in any form or by any means,
electronic or mechanical, including photocopy, recording, or any information
storage and retrieval system, without permission in writing from the publisher.

Permissions may be sought directly from Elsevier's Science & Technology Rights
Department in Oxford, UK: phone: (+44) 1865 843830, fax: (+44) 1865 853333,
E-mail: permissions@elsevier.co.uk. You may also complete your request on-line
via the Elsevier homepage (http://elsevier.com), by selecting "Customer Support"
and then "Obtaining Permissions."

Library of Congress Cataloging-in-Publication Data
Norris, David O.
   Vertebrate endocrinology/author, David O. Norris.—4th ed.
      p.   cm.
   Includes index.
   ISBN-13: 978-0-12-088768-2 (alk. paper)
   ISBN-10: 0-12-088768-1 (alk. paper)
   1.   Vertebrates—Endocrinology.   I.   Title.
   QP187.N67 2007
   596′.0142—dc22

                                                        2006020110

British Library Cataloguing in Publication Data
A catalogue record for this book is available from the British Library.

ISBN 13: 978-0-12-088768-2
ISBN 10: 0-12-088768-1

For all information on all Elsevier Academic Press publications
visit our Web site at www.books.elsevier.com.

Printed in the United States of America
Transferred to Digital Printing, 2011

Working together to grow
libraries in developing countries

www.elsevier.com | www.bookaid.org | www.sabre.org

ELSEVIER   BOOK AID
            International   Sabre Foundation

This book is dedicated to my family (spouse Kay and daughters Sara Engel and Linda Quintana) who have supported me even when I haven't deserved it, and to the hundreds of bright, inquiring students at the University of Colorado that have made the last 40 years of teaching and research in vertebrate endocrinology a thorough delight.

CONTENTS

PREFACE TO THE FOURTH EDITION

Vertebrate Endocrinology has evolved into a 4th edition that has incorporated new information and insights gained by this author during a fourth decade of teaching and research within the field of endocrinology. It represents a virtual rewrite and reorganization with the addition of many new chemical bioregulators as well as new understandings of the synthesis, actions, and metabolism of former bioregulators. Included are new insights into the evolution of these systems. Furthermore, the old distinction of separate regulatory systems (e.g., nervous, endocrine, immune, paracrine) has become so blurred during the past decade that we now must consider an organism to be an integrated playing field for chemical bioregulators produced in a variety of manners by a great variety of tissues and organs with a considerable amount of cross-talk. Perhaps, even the title of this edition should have been altered to simply *The Chemical Bioregulation of Vertebrate Physiology and Behavior* to reflect this change of emphasis from endocrinology *sensu stricto*.

I hope this new edition will continue the tradition of introducing undergraduate and graduate students to the exciting, complicated, and integrative field of "endocrinology" that is more broadly interpreted in this edition as "chemical bioregulation." Whether interested in clinical, evolutionary, and/or environmental aspects of endocrinology, it is my intention that students receive a broad exposure in this book that will enable them to become self-learners by providing a background to the primary literature.

Although tremendous gains in molecular techniques since the 3rd edition have allowed creative scientists to greatly increase our understandings of the intricate interrelatedness among chemical bioregulatory mechanisms and their evolution, perhaps the most important changes have been the recognition and documentation of endocrine disruption by chemicals in the environment. These environmentally endocrine active chemicals (EACs) are capable of disrupting normal life history events including development, sexual differentiation, and post-embryonic functions such as metabolism, stress responses, sexual maturation, reproduction, and behavior. The possible clinical implications of these EACs for present human populations are of immediate concern, and there is mounting evidence of their potential impacts on future generations. Some of these EACs have appeared in the environment simply through careless and/or thoughtless behavior related to our obsessions for "better living through chemistry" and for "economic gain" regardless of the cost to the environment. Other EACs are the consequence of the burgeoning size of the human population, its concentrations into cities, and its reliance on artificially maintained agriculture and animal husbandry. EACs include pesticides, herbicides, antibiotics, fertilizers, and industrial products (e.g., PCBs, dioxins, and plasticizers) as well as ingredients of household products such as detergents, shampoos, and cosmetics. Furthermore, high densities of humans and domestic animals have resulted in the addition of biologically relevant concentrations of reproductively active hormones and pharmaceuticals to aquatic environments through wastewater effluents and application of biosolids to agricultural fields. Of greatest long-term (evolutionary) concern perhaps may be the effects of thyroid inhibitors on central nervous system development and the effects of estrogenic and androgenic EACs on sexual differentiation (sex reversal and intersex production) of embryos and immature animals as well as the induction of estrogen-based cancers and contraception in adults and future generations. The widespread use of pharmaceuticals, especially in the "developed" countries, is resulting in the presence of biologically relevant quantities of these drugs in water supplies and even in drinking water. Among these drugs are estrogenic birth control ingredients, β-blockers used for blood pressure control or cardiac therapy, selective serotonin reuptake inhibitors (SSRIs) such as fluoxetine (i.e., Prozac®), and plasma cholesterol-lowering compounds, to name a few. The widespread contamination of natural environments means that it is no longer possible to study animals under natural conditions. Hence, field studies must rely on reference populations lacking only the bioregulator they wish to study rather than control populations since all animals in nature are exposed to some EACs. And the ultimate impacts of EACs on microorganisms, plants, and invertebrate populations and their implications for natural ecosystems may be even more important than those on vertebrates. It is my hope that students who understand the intricacies and interrelatedness of chemical bioregulatory systems such as described in this text will be best prepared to deal with the threat of environmental EACs in the future. If left unchecked, EACs could lead to the destruction of natural ecosystems as we know them.

ACKNOWLEDGEMENTS

This book is in part a product of my need to teach the excitement of discovery in the biological sciences that was instilled in me by my undergraduate advisor and botany professor at Baldwin-Wallace College, Dr. Donald S. Dean. Were I to attempt to name all of the endocrine people who have contributed directly or indirectly to this edition, I would undoubtedly overlook many of them. I can acknowledge the vast majority, however, by simply referring to the many direct academic descendents and postdoctoral students of my past mentors in vertebrate endocrinology: Aubrey Gorbman, Howard Bern, and Donald Farner as well their many academic sons and daughters, grandsons and grand-daughters, great-grand sons and great-grand-daughters, etc. These descendents continue to add to our understanding of vertebrate endocrinology through teaching and research.

My own understanding of chemical bioregulation has been strongly influenced by my many years of interactions with colleagues Dr. Richard Evan Jones and more recently Dr. Pei-San Tsai, as well as with the many undergraduate and graduate students in vertebrate endocrinology we have trained in our laboratories at the University of Colorado in Boulder. Questions, challenges, and independent interpretations of the literature by these students have strongly affected my thinking about chemical bioregulation over the years to the extent that I can no longer honestly separate their ideas from my own. Among those former graduate students are

Dr. Harriet B. Austin
Dr. James A. Carr
Dr. Laura M. Carruth
Dr. Rubai Ding
Dr. David Duvall
Dr. Kevin T. Fitzgerald
Dr. William A. Gern
Dr. John C. Gill
Dr. Louis P. Guillette, Jr.
Dr. Earl T. Larson

Dr. Kristin Lopez
Dr. Tammy A. Maldonado
Dr. Frank L. Moore
Dr. Mark F. Norman
Dr. James S. Norris
Dr. Toni R. Pak
Dr. Martha K. Pancak
Dr. Scott Panter
Dr. James E. Platt
Dr. Matthew S. Rand
Dr. Greta Rosen
Dr. George Snow
Dr. Richard R. Tokarz
Dr. Alan M. Vajda
Dr. John D. Woodling

1

An Overview of Chemical Bioregulation in Vertebrates

Endocrinology as a scientific subdiscipline within physiology began a little over 100 years ago as the study of certain glands called **endocrine glands**, or glands of "internal secretion" that secreted their products into the blood. These secretions were called **hormones** (*hormon*, to stimulate or excite) because of their effects on distant **target cells**. Each hormone binds to a specific **receptor** molecule located in or on a target cell and the resultant **hormone-receptor complex** causes a measurable change in the target cell. Many mechanisms employed in the vertebrate endocrine system have their counterparts among invertebrate animals as well as in microbial and botanical organisms. Originally a traditional field of specialization that focused on the endocrine glands and their secretions, endocrinology has expanded as a specialty within physiology and now deals with chemical regulation of virtually all biological phenomena in animals at the molecular, cellular, organism, and population levels of organization. The study of chemical regulation or **bioregulation** can be defined to include secretions of the endocrine system, the nervous system, the immune system, and virtually all cells in the body that use chemical messengers to communicate with one another (Figure 1-1). The many secretions involved as chemical messengers then can be called **bioregulators**.

Learning about the intricacies of how the activities of animals are regulated and coordinated by bioregulators is one of the most fascinating and complicated endeavors in biology. Every act that an animal performs either is initiated, modulated, or blocked by bioregulators. Understanding the endocrine systems of invertebrate and vertebrate animals is essential if we are ever to understand how bioregulatory mechanisms and systems evolved in animals and how they operate to maintain the vast array of living animal species. Furthermore,

1

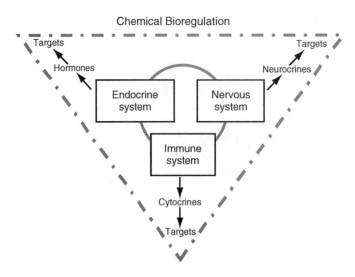

Figure 1-1.   **Chemical bioregulation**. The endocrine system, nervous system, and immune system each secretes its own bioregulators: hormones, neurocrines, and cytocrines, respectively. However, all of these systems influence each other and from a homeostatic viewpoint, we can assume they function as one great bioregulatory system. See color insert, plate 2.

the continued health of each ecosystem depends on continued reproductive success of its component animal species.

Because the nervous system and endocrine system act together to integrate environmental information with bioregulation of physiology and behavior, a subdiscipline called **environmental endocrinology** has emerged within the more traditional approaches to endocrinology. This area of research is focused not only on natural environmental factors such as pheromones, behavior, light (e.g., photoperiod), and temperature, but has expanded to include effects of pesticides, heavy metals, and all manner of organic compounds added to the environment by human activities. These chemicals can alter normal bioregulatory mechanisms by mimicking or inhibiting the work of natural bioregulators. This interference of endocrine bioregulation by environmental pollutants and some natural chemicals is called **endocrine disruption**, and these chemicals are called **endocrine-disrupting chemicals (EDCs)** or **endocrine-active chemicals (EACs)**.

The application of the estrogenic mimic **diethylstilbestrol (DES)** to cattle and to pregnant women was recognized many years ago by John McLachlin and others as a disruption of normal endocrine function that has serious consequences for exposed animals and their offspring. Recent evidence suggests permanent DES exposure of effects can be transmitted. The use of the pesticide **DDT** and **polychlorinated biphenyls (PCBs)** were banned in the USA when it was recognized that they were accumulating in the environment and were affecting the reproductive health of wildlife and humans. However, awareness of the potentially harmful nature of extremely low concentrations of estrogenic (feminizing) pollutants in the environment represents a greater threat than ever before. Louis Guillette in Florida was the first to observe that a natural population of alligators exhibited abnormal sexual development after exposure in nature to low concentrations of DDT and its metabolite **DDE**. Soon, evidence of reproductive disturbances surfaced through the efforts of John Sumpter and numerous colleagues in the UK and Europe as a result of the exposure of fishes to incredibly low concentrations of estrogenic compounds present in wastewater effluents. We have now observed similar effects of wastewater effluents in the USA as well. Knowledge of the intricate workings of the endocrine system is essential to understand how such effects happen and to understand the enormous implications of these observations (see below).

I. The Comparative Vertebrate Approach

Comparative vertebrate endocrinology emphasizes the evolution of bioregulatory systems and the discrete structures and bioregulators that constitute the vertebrate neuroendocrine and endocrine systems. Also of interest is the evolution of vertebrate endocrine glands and secretions from invertebrates. Vertebrate endocrine systems may be studied in a variety of ways. Some comparative endocrinologists may have a basic interest in fishes or reptiles and study their endocrine systems to better understand their ecology and/or evolution. Others may be interested in a specific phenomenon such as aging, learning, or reproduction and employ non-mammalian vertebrates as model systems in which to unravel basic mechanisms and/or evolutionary relationships. Certain procedures may be more readily performed on non-mammals where processes are spread out stepwise over time while in the mammal these steps all occur simultaneously. Comparative approaches may have direct applications for aiding our understanding of these same phenomena in mammals including humans. There are numerous examples of basic research in non-mammalian vertebrates that have had direct applications to human biology. For example, Spiedel made the first observation of neurosecretory neurons in the posterior spinal cord of fishes. Later, Ernst and Berta Scharrer extended this observation to the description of the hypothalamus-pituitary neuroendocrine system. Genetically controlled platyfish strains have provided a system for studying the bioregulation of aging and the reproductive system in relationship to genetic factors. Many species of fishes are used extensively as models for stress, growth, carcinogenesis, aging, and behavioral studies. The toad urinary bladder was an excellent *in-vitro* model for the initial studies of the mechanism of action for the mineralocorticoid hormone, aldosterone. Similarly, the amphibian ovarian follicle has provided an *in-vitro* system for studying the bioregulation of oocyte maturation and the process of ovulation. Studies of non-mammals have been crucial for understanding mechanisms of tissue induction and chemical regulation of gene activity during embryonic development and differentiation. Numerous important hypotheses about development were first tested in amphibians. The discovery by Alberto Houssay that removal of the pituitary gland greatly reduced the severity of the removal of the pancreas in a toad became a model for studying diabetes mellitus using dogs. The origin of the gonadotropin-releasing hormone (GnRH) in neural ectoderm and the subsequent migration of GnRH neurons from the olfactory placode to the hypothalamus were first reported by Linda Muske and Frank Moore in an amphibian. Additional confirmation of the origin of the pituitary was performed using transplantation of normally pigmented toad embryonic cells into albino toad embryos and following their pigmented descendents. Furthermore, ingenious experiments using chicken-quail chimaeras with cytologically distinct cell markers verified the neural origin of a number of endocrine cells. The lizard *Anolis carolinensis* was used by Richard Jones to study hormonal and neural control of the alternating pattern of ovulation by the paired ovaries, a phenomenon that also occurs in humans where it is more difficult to study. Avian systems have been used extensively for studies of development, neurobiology, immunology, cancer, and molecular genetics. F. Anne McNabb has used the quail as a model for the actions of a common pollutant, ammonium perchlorate, on the inhibition of thyroid function. The discovery of pheromones among invertebrates and later studies in non-mammalian vertebrates as well as in mice and voles have led to new understandings in the roles of such secretions controlling mammalian reproductive and maternal behavior. Each of these systems has wide applicability to other vertebrates as well as to the mechanisms of hormone actions.

II. The Origins of Bioregulation

Regulatory chemicals were probably essential for the survival of the first living cells both for coordination of internal events and for cell-to-cell interactions. Secretions that favored survival of the secreting cell no doubt led to further evolution of new chemical bioregulators. Thus, bioregulation probably had its origin in local secretions that affected nearby cells as well as bioregulators that affected internal cellular processes. The evolution of multicellular aggregates and eventually of multicellular organisms allowed further cell-to-cell types of bioregulation but more importantly allowed for the eventual evolution of endocrine and neural bioregulation. The earliest appearance of neurons is noted in the most primitive of multicellular animals, the cnidarian invertebrates (Cnidaria), and these neurons secrete both peptides and non-peptides that function as typical neural and local bioregulators. By definition, true endocrine glands that secrete hormones did not appear until the type of internal transport mechanisms we call blood vascular systems. These bioregulatory systems have been termed **neuroendocrine systems** since they involve both neural and endocrine components. Complex neuroendocrine systems have evolved in annelids (Annelida), mollusks (Mollusca), insects, arachnids, and crustaceans (Arthropoda) as well as in the chordates (including the vertebrates).

III. Categories of Bioregulators

In addition to traditional endocrine regulation, we now recognize several other patterns of chemical bioregulation as illustrated in Figure 1-2. The first of these involves the nervous system. Neurons produce bioregulators called **neurotransmitters** or **neuromodulators** that are secreted into the synapses formed where they make direct connections with their target cells (typically other neurons, muscle cells, or gland cells). Once the neuroregulator is bound to its receptor molecule, it brings about distinct changes in the postsynaptic cell. The parallelisms between endocrine cell and neuron, hormone and neurotransmitter, target cell and postsynaptic cell are obvious. Only the location and chemical composition of the medium through which the bioregulator travels to reach its target cell separate hormones from neurotransmitters.

In the 1950s, Berta and Ernst Scharrer recognized that some neural regulators were released into the blood like hormones. These neural hormones were named **neurosecretions** or **neurohormones** to distinguish them from neurotransmitters, neuromodulators, and the traditional hormones. It seems that it was easier to formulate more definitions than to acknowledge that certain brain regions were also endocrine glands.

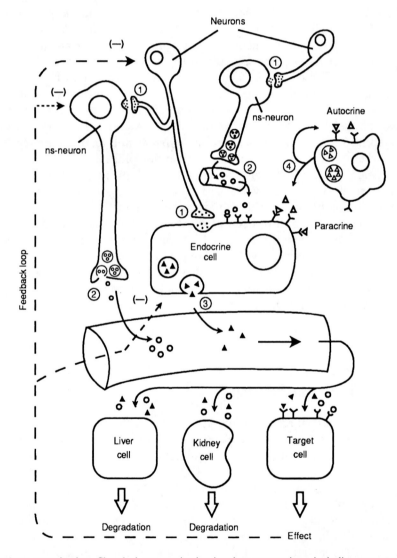

Figure 1-2. **Bioregulator organization.** Chemical communication involves neurocrines, including neurotransmitters or neuromodulators (1), and neurohormones (2), as well as hormones (3) and autocrine/paracrine regulators (4). Target cells may produce feedback (dashed lines) on neuroendocrine or endocrine cells. The liver and kidney serve as major sites for metabolism and excretion of bioregulators. (•, Neurotransmitters, neuromodulators; ○, neurohormone; ▲, hormone; △, cytocrine (autocrine, paracrine.))

Those neurons that secrete neurohormones are sometimes called **neurosecretory neurons** to distinguish them from the others. The term **neurocrine** has been suggested as a general category to include all of these neural regulators (that is, neurotransmitters, neuromodulators, and neurohormones). Although all neurocrines are actually neurosecretions, that latter term has unaccountably been reserved for the neurohormones.

Later, the separation of neural and endocrine systems became even more blurred when it was learned that some established hormones also were produced within the nervous system where they functioned as neurotransmitters or neuromodulators (see Table 1-1). It soon became common knowledge that the neural system had control over certain portions of the endocrine system through direct innervation or via neurohormones. Likewise, hormones were seen to influence markedly not only the development of neural systems but also their activity. Hence, the concept of a neuroendocrine system was established in physiology. Discovery of specific chemicals produced by diverse cellular types and released into extracellular fluids including blood has broadened the concept of chemical bioregulation still further to include cell-to-cell chemical communication that is not mediated via transport in the blood or at a synapse. Additional sources of hormones were discovered to come from traditionally non-endocrine tissues or organs such as the heart, the liver, adipose tissue, and skeletal muscle.

Chemical bioregulators were also discovered that are used for cell-to-cell communication within tissues. Such bioregulators that are secreted into extracellular fluid have been named "local hormones" or **cytocrines**. This category includes locally acting growth factors, mitogenic regulators, embryonic tissue-inducing substances, secretogogues (secretion-enhancing factors), inhibitors, and immune regulators. If cytocrines also affect the emitting cell, they are sometimes termed **autocrines**. When they affect other cell types, they are called **paracrines**. However, both types of local cytocrine secretion into the general extracellular fluids are sometimes loosely termed as paracrine secretion.

Table 1-1. Some Mammalian Neurocrine Regulators[a]

Class of regulator	Example
Nonpeptides	Acetylcholine (ACh)
	Carbon monoxide (CO)
	Dopamine (DA)
	Epinephrine (E)
	γ-Aminobutyric acid (GABA)
	Glutamate
	Nitric oxide (NO)
	Norepinephrine (NE)
	Serotonin (5-HT)
Hypothalamic-releasing peptides	Corticotropin-releasing hormone (CRH)
	Gonadotropin-releasing hormone (GnRH)
	Melanotropin release-inhibiting hormone (MRIH)
	Prolactin-releasing hormone (PRH)
	Prolactin release-inhibiting hormone (PRIH)
	Somatostatin (SS or GHRIH)
	Thyrotropin-releasing hormone (TRH)
Other neuropeptides	Angiotensin II (ANG-II)
	Arginine vasopressin (AVP)
	Atrial natriuretic peptide (ANP)
	Brain natriuretic peptide (BNP)
	Cholecystokinin (CCK$_8$)
	Insulin
	Neuropeptide Y (NPY)
	Neuropeptide YY (PYY)
	Peptide histidine isoleucine (PHI)
	Substance P (SP)
	Vasoactive intestinal peptide (VIP)

[a] Some of these molecules may function only as a neurotransmitter, neuromodulator, neurohormone, or paracrine regulator whereas others may perform multiple roles.

Chemicals released from neurons into the cerebrospinal fluid (CSF) do not quite fit the definition of neurohormone since they are released into a filtrate of blood but they do not quite fit the definition of paracrine secretion, either. For our purposes, we will refer to these bioregulators as neurohormones.

Intracellular chemical messengers that govern intracellular events have been called **intracrines**. These intracrine bioregulators would include chemicals such as the second messengers and transcription factors that are discussed in Chapter 3.

In its broadest sense, the study of bioregulation may include specific chemical messengers released by one organism into its environment that may affect the physiology or behavior of other individuals of that species or even of another species. A good name for these substances might have been "exocrines," but that term had already been assigned to the products of **exocrine glands** that secrete their products into ducts through which they are conveyed to their sites of action in such places as the digestive tract or the surface of the skin. Examples of exocrine glands include salivary glands, sweat glands, mammary glands, and portions of the liver and pancreas. These externally secreted bioregulators have been called "ectohormones" or **semiochemicals** (*semio* = signal). Three subclasses of semiochemicals have been identified on functional bases. **Pheromones** are semiochemicals that act only on other members of the same species. **Primer pheromones** usually initiate a series of physiological events such as gonadal maturation. Signal or **releaser pheromones** trigger immediate behavioral responses such as sexual attraction or copulation. **Allelomones** are interspecific semiochemicals and are further separated into two types. If only the emitter of the semiochemical benefits from the effect on the other species, the allelomone is called an **allomone**. The well-known odor released by skunks is a dramatic example of an allomone that protects the skunk from would-be predators. When only the recipient species benefits, the allelomone may be termed a **kairomone**. The release of the simple metabolite L-lactate in sweat of humans attracts female mosquitoes that obtain a blood meal necessary for their reproduction. L-lactate, then, could be classified as a kairomone, for there is no obvious benefit to the emitter and in fact may harm the emitter.

In summary, intra-organismal bioregulation can be classified as endocrine (hormones), neurocrine (neurotransmitters, neuromodulators, neurohormones), paracrine (cytocrines, autocrines), or intracrine (intracellular regulatory messengers). Semiochemicals (pheromones and allelomones) are specialized for interorganismal communication. A listing of these types of bioregulators and their definitions is provided in Table 1-2.

Most bioregulators are peptides, proteins, or derivatives of amino acids. Some are lipids (e.g., steroids) and still others are nucleotides or nucleotide derivatives. A discussion of the chemical nature of regulators, how they are synthesized, how they produce their effects on targets, and how they are metabolized is the subject of

Table 1-2. Types of Regulators

Agent	Description	Examples
Neurotransmitter	Secreted by neurons into synaptic space	Acetylcholine, dopamine, substance P, GABA
Neuromodulator	Secreted by neurons into synaptic space; modulates sensitivity of postsynaptic cell to other neurotransmitters	Endorphins and various other neuropeptides
Neurohormone	Secreted by neurons into the blood or CSF; may be stored in neurohemal organ prior to release	TRH, CRH, oxytocin, dopamine
Hormone	Secreted by specialized nonneural cells into the blood	Thyroxine, GH, insulin
Cytocrine	Secreted by cells into the surrounding extracellular fluid; these local regulators typically travel short distances to nearby target cells	Somatostatin, norepinephrine
Paracrine	Secreted by cells that affect other cell types	Embryonic inducers, somatostatin, interleukins
Autocrine	Secreted by cells that affect emitting cells	Mitogenic agents, interleukins
Intracrine	Intracellular messengers; typically mediators of other regulators that bind to membrane receptors	cAMP, DAG, IP_3, cGMP, calmodulin, calcium ions
Semiochemical	Secreted into environment	Pheromones, allelomones

See Appendix A for explanation of abbreviations.

Chapter 3. However, before examining these bioregulators more closely, we must consider some more general features of bioregulatory systems.

IV. General Organization of Bioregulatory Systems

As stated above, the endocrine system and the nervous system are the sources for most of the chemical messengers we have defined as bioregulators. Traditionally, the vertebrate neuroendocrine system includes the **brain** and the **pituitary gland** plus the classical endocrine glands they control: **the thyroid gland**, the paired **adrenal glands** and **gonads** (testes and ovaries), and the **liver**. In addition, there are **independent endocrine bioregulators**, that is, those not directly under the influence of the brain and/or pituitary. This would include the **parathyroid glands**, the **thymus**, the **endocrine pancreas**, organs of the **gastrointestinal tract**, the **pineal gland**, and the **kidney**. The major focus of this textbook is on the neuroendocrine systems of mammals and non-mammalian vertebrates. The independent endocrine glands are discussed in special cases (for example, the regulation of calcium homeostasis, in Chapter 14) and when they interact with the bioregulators of the neuroendocrine system such as in the bioregulation of metabolism (Chapters 12 and 13).

The vertebrate bioregulatory system is outlined in Figure 1-3 with emphasis on neuroendocrine bioregulation. The major portion of the brain involved in neuroendocrine bioregulation is called the **hypothalamus**, that portion of the diencephalic region of the mammalian brain directly above the **pituitary gland**. The detailed organization and operation of this system are described in Chapters 4 and 5. Special groups of neurosecretory neurons in the hypothalamus produce a variety of neurohormones. Some of these neurohormones control the secretion by the pituitary gland of peptide and protein hormones called **tropic hormones**. These tropic hormones regulate the endocrine activities of the thyroid gland (which secretes thyroid hormones; see Chapters 6 and 7), the adrenal cortex (which secretes corticosteroids; Chapters 8 and 9), the gonads (which secrete reproductive steroids; Chapters 10 and 11) and the liver (which secretes an essential factor for growth; Chapter 4). Furthermore, some tropic hormones influence more general aspects of growth, metabolism, and reproduction and affect many non-endocrine target tissues. Additional neurohormones (**vasopressin** and **oxytocin**) are stored in part of the pituitary until they are needed (Chapters 4 and 5). Vasopressin influences kidney function and reproductive behavior and oxytocin plays many reproductive roles related to both physiology and behavior.

Table 1-3 is a partial listing of bioregulators that are discussed in this book. In addition to their names and abbreviations, their sources, targets, and general effects on the targets are provided.

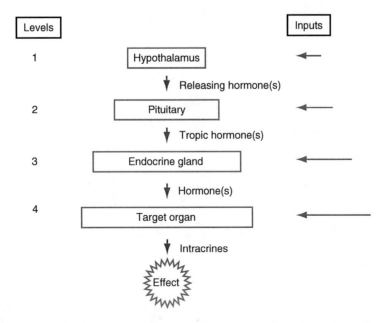

Figure 1-3. **Functional conceptualization of the hypothalamus-pituitary system.** Input from other endogenous or exogenous factors can affect every level of regulation. See text for discussion of the roles of these bioregulators at each level.

Table 1-3. The Mammalian Endocrine System: Major Secretions[a] and Actions

Source[b] and secretions	Target	Action
Anterior pituitary: produces tropic hormones		
Glycoprotein tropic hormones		
Thyrotropin (thyroid-stimulating hormone; TSH)	Thyroid gland	Synthesis and release of thyroid hormones
Luteinizing hormone (lutropin, LH)	Gonads	Androgen synthesis; progesterone synthesis; gamete release
Follicle-stimulating hormone (follitropin, FSH)	Gonads	Gamete formation; estrogen synthesis
Nonglycoprotein tropic hormones		
Growth hormone (somatotropin, GH)	Liver, connective tissues, muscle	Synthesis of IGF, proteins
Prolactin (mammotropin, PRL)	Mammary glands, epididymus	Synthesis of proteins
Corticotropin (adrenocorticostimulating hormone, ACTH)	Adrenal cortex	Synthesis of corticosteroids
Melanotropin (melanocyte- or melanophore-stimulating hormone, MSH)	Melanin-producing cells	Synthesis of melanin
Hypothalamus: neurosecretory nuclei produce neurohormones		
Hypothalamic-releasing hormones		
Thyrotropin-releasing hormone (TRH)	Anterior pituitary	Releases TSH
Gonadotropin-releasing hormone (GnRH)	Anterior pituitary	Releases LH/FSH
Corticotropin-releasing hormone (CRH)	Anterior pituitary	Releases ACTH
Somatostatin (GH-RIH or SST)	Anterior pituitary	Inhibits GH release
Somatocrinin (GHRH)[c]	Anterior pituitary	Releases GH
Prolactin release-inhibiting hormone (PRIH)	Anterior pituitary	Inhibits PRL release
Prolactin-releasing hormone (PRH)[c]	Anterior pituitary	Releases PRL
Melanotropin release-inhibiting hormone (MRIH)[c]	Anterior pituitary	Inhibits MSH release
Melanotropin-releasing hormone (MRH)[c]	Anterior pituitary	Releases MSH
Other neurohormones		
Arginine vasopressin[d] (antidiuretic hormone, AVP)	Kidney	Water reabsorption
	Brain	Drinking behavior
Oxytocin (OXY)	Uterus, vas deferens	Smooth muscle contraction
Endorphins/enkephalins	Pain neurons	Desensitizes neurons
Thyroid gland		
Thyroid hormones		
Thyroxine (T_4) and triiodothyronine (T_3)	Most tissues	Increases metabolism; controls development and differentiation
Calcitonin (thyrocalcitonin, CT)[e]	Bone	Prevents resorption caused by parathyroid hormone
Gonads		
Ovary		
Estrogens (e.g., estradiol)	Primary and secondary sexual structures	Stimulates development
	Brain	Reproductive behavior
Progesterone	Uterus	Stimulates secretion by uterine glands
Inhibin	Anterior pituitary	Blocks FSH release
Testis		
Androgens (e.g., testosterone)	Primary and secondary sexual structures	Stimulates development and secretion
	Brain	Reproductive behavior[f]
Inhibin	Anterior pituitary	Blocks FSH release
Adrenal gland		
Adrenal cortex		
Aldosterone (A)	Kidney	Sodium reabsorption; potassium secretion into urine
Corticosterone (B)/Cortisol (F)	Liver, muscle	Conversion of protein into carbohydrates
Adrenal medulla		
Epinephrine/norepinephrine	Liver, muscle	Glycogen breakdown to glucose

continues

Table 1-3.—*Continued*

Source[b] and secretions	Target	Action
Parathyroid gland		
Parathyroid hormone (parathormone, PTH)	Bone	Bone resorption or growth
	Kidney	Calcium reabsorption and phosphate secretion into urine
Endocrine pancreas		
Insulin	Liver	Glycogen storage
	Muscle	Glucose uptake
	Adipose tissue	Inhibits fat hydrolysis
Glucagon	Liver, adipose tissue	Antiinsulin actions
Pancreatic polypeptide	Liver, muscle?	??
Somatostatin (paracrine substance)	Endocrine pancreas	Blocks release of pancreatic hormones
Gastrointestinal system		
Stomach		
Gastrin	Gastric glands of stomach	Stimulates acid secretion into lumen
Ghrelin	Brain	Stimulates feeding
Small intestine		
Secretin	Exocrine pancreas	Release of basic juice into duodenum
Cholecystokinin (CCK; same as pancreozymin-cholecystokinin, PZCCK)	Exocrine pancreas	Release of enzymes into duodenum
	Gallbladder	Contraction to eject bile into duodenum
Gastrin-releasing peptide	Stomach gastrin cells	Release of gastrin
Glucose-dependent insulinotropic peptide (Gastric inhibitory peptide, GIP)	Endocrine pancreas	Release of insulin
Motilin	Stomach	Stimulates pepsinogen secretion and gastric motility
Somatostatin (paracrine action)	Small intestine	Inhibits release of other regulators
Vasoactive intestinal peptide (VIP)	Visceral blood vessels	Increases blood flow to intestines
Liver		
Insulin-like growth factors (IGF-I, IGF-II)	Many tissues	Mitogenic effects
Synlactin (?)	Mammary gland	Participates in action of PRL on gland
Adipose tissue		
Leptin	Brain	Inhibits feeding
Kidney		
Erythropoietin	Bone marrow	Stimulates RBC formation
Renin	Renin substrate in blood	Produces angiotensin
1,25-dihydroxycholecalciferol (1,25-DHC)[g]	Small intestine	Stimulates calcium absorption
Pineal gland		
Melatonin (neurohormone)	Brain	Controls puberty, thyroid, adrenal, and reproductive rhythms
Immune system		
Thymus		
Thymosins	Lymphocyte-producing tissue	Production of lymphocytes
Macrophages/lymphocytes		
Interleukin 1 (autocrine/cytocrine)	Helper T cell	Activation
Interleukin 2 (autocrine/cytocrine)	Cytotoxic T cell	Activation

[a] In some cases, closely related molecular forms may be present and will be discussed at the appropriate time. One or more alternative names may be used for a regulator and some of these alternates appear within parentheses.

[b] Alternate names are given in parentheses, along with the most common abbreviation.

[c] Exact chemical nature not clear (see Chapter 4 for more details).

[d] Some mammals may rely on a different nonapeptide (e.g., lysine vasopressin or phenypressin; see Chapter 6).

[e] Secretory cells derived from ultimobranchial gland in mammals become incorporated into the thyroid (see Chapter 14).

[f] May require conversion into estrogens within certain brain target cells before effect is observed (see Chapter 11).

[g] Cholecalciferol is made in skin and converted in liver to precursor kidney uses to make 1,25-DHC (see Chapter 14).

V. Cell and Tissue Organization of Bioregulatory Systems

Endocrine and neuroendocrine cells can be identified easily on the basis of their cytological features as specialized secretory cells (Figure 1-4). Peptide-secreting cells have well developed rough endoplasmic reticula and typically contain many protein-filled storage granules or vesicles (see Appendix B for a brief description of cellular structures). Mitochondria of peptide-secreting cells have flat, platelike cristae. The morphology and content of the protein storage granules may be used to differentiate specific types of endocrine cells. For example, the various tropic hormone-secreting cells of the anterior pituitary can be partially identified by the differential sizes of their storage granules or by special immunochemical methods (see Chapters 2 and 4). In contrast, steroid-secreting cells have well-developed smooth endoplasmic reticula, and their mitochondria have tubular cristae (compare steroid- and peptide-secreting cells as shown in Fig. 1-3). Steroids are usually not stored in their cells of origin, but lipid droplets containing cholesterol, the precursor steroid for their synthesis, are commonly observed.

Neurosecretory neurons and regular neurons are not only specialized elongated cells that are readily identifiable but also contain discrete **synaptic vesicles** containing neurocrine products in their axonal tips that characterize them as secretory cells. Neurosecretory neurons tend to be larger than ordinary neurons. Neurons secreting peptides contain larger, dense granules than those secreting nonpeptides such as catecholamines or acetylcholine. For example, the synaptic vesicles for acetylcholine are 30–45 nm in diameter, those for norepinephrine are about 70 nm, whereas peptide-containing vesicles are 100–300 nm.

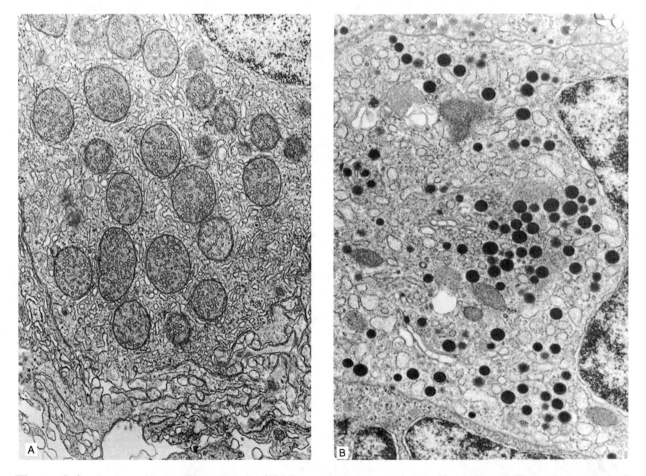

Figure 1-4.   **Cytology of hormone-secreting cells.** (A) Microscopic appearance of a steroid-secreting cell. These adrenocortical cells from juvenile salmon that secrete the steroid cortisol exhibit mitochondria with tubular cristae and an abundance of smooth endoplasmic reticulum. (B) A growth hormone-secreting cell from the coho salmon (*Oncorhynchus kisutch*) showing dense secretory granules, well-developed Golgi apparatus, and mitochondria with platelike cristae. Courtesy of Howard A. Bern and Richard Nishioka, University of California, Berkeley.

In the central nervous system, the cell bodies of neurons are localized in groupings called nuclei and their axons often form specific tracts connecting to other nuclei, blood vessels, or the cerebrospinal fluid, or they may exit from the central nervous system as nerves. In fact, neurosecretory neurons were first characterized as unique because their cell bodies in **neurosecretory nuclei** and axons in **neurosecretory tracts** contained materials that stain with certain dyes, distinguishing these cells from ordinary neurons. However, these general methods usually did not distinguish between different kinds of neurosecretory neurons. Modern immunological techniques now allow us to identify each type of neurosecretory or ordinary neuron with respect to its particular secretions (see Chapter 2).

Another factor that helped in the early identification of endocrine cells was their anatomical relationship to one another in forming discrete tissues. Many endocrine cells are specialized epithelial cells that tend to be clumped in groups that are organized in one of the following ways (see Appendix B for descriptions of epithelia and other tissue types). The most common orientation of secretory cells is to form folded sheets or **cords** of cells as seen in the pituitary gland or the adrenal cortex (Figure 1-5). In a few cases, the cells may

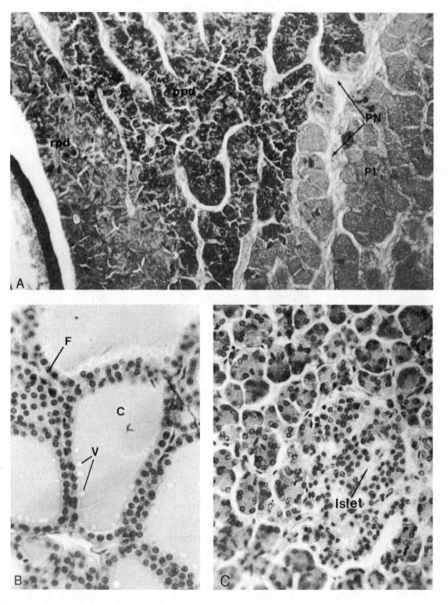

Figure 1-5. Organization of endocrine cells. Most commonly, endocrine cells appear as folded cords of cells. (A) follicles consisting of an epithelium surrounding a fluid-filled lumen. (B) or small clumps of cells or islet. (C) Additionally, endocrine cells may occur singly as is common in the lining of the gastrointestinal tract. (A) is from a teleost pituitary, (B) is from a dog thyroid, (C) is from the rat pancreas.

Table 1-4. Cellular Patterns of Secretion

Secretory pattern	Description	Example
Endocrine	Product secreted into the blood for transport internally to target tissues	Hormones
Exocrine	Product secreted into a duct that opens onto an external or internal surface	Sweat
Exocytosis	Product released from secretory cell via a process essentially the reverse of endocytosis	Peptide hormone release
Merocrine	Product secreted without visible damage to the secretory cell (involves exocytosis)	Thyroxine secretion
Apocrine	Product released by sloughing of "outer" or apical portion of secretory cell	Mammary gland milk
Holocrine	Product released through cell death and lysis	Sebaceous gland secretion
Cytogenous	Release of whole, viable cells	Spermatozoa

form a spherical mass of one cell layer surrounding a fluid-filled space or lumen. This arrangement is termed a **follicle** and occurs in the thyroid gland of all vertebrates and in the pituitaries of some vertebrates. The lumen provides a unique storage site for secretions of the follicular cells. Sometimes, the endocrine cells will be separated into scattered clumps or **islets** of a few cells. Mixed islets containing several secretory cell types are best known in the pancreas where they are called the **islets of Langerhans**.

Many cells that secrete bioregulators are not histologically distinct (i.e., do not form discrete tissues) and were not identified until precise immunochemical techniques were developed. One of the reasons it took so long to identify the sources of gastrointestinal hormones was due to the tendency for these secretory types to occur as **isolated endocrine cells** mixed in with many other cell types in the stomach and intestinal walls (see Chapter 12).

Another critical feature of neuroendocrine organization is the presence of an extensive vascular supply for endocrine cells and neurosecretory neurons. Endocrine glands typically are highly vascularized such that no secretory cell is far from a blood vessel. The axonal endings of many neurosecretory neurons terminate collectively in masses of capillaries to form what is called a **neurohemal organ**. These neurosecretory neurons release their neurohormones into the blood that flows through the neurohemal organ. Some neurosecretory neurons that release their products into the cerebrospinal fluid do not form axonal aggregates at common release sites.

Most regulatory cells employ **merocrine secretion** where secretory products are released by exocytosis with no damage to the cell. In **apocrine secretion**, the apical portion or tip of the cell is sloughed along with stored secretions whereas **holocrine secretion** involves lysis and death of the secretory cell. These latter two patterns are more characteristic of exocrine glands such as the mammary gland (apocrine) or the sebaceous glands of the skin (holocrine). **Cytogenous secretion** is the release of entire cells such as sperm released from testes or ova released from ovaries. These secretory patterns are summarized in Table 1-4.

VI. Homeostasis

Bioregulatory mechanisms are the bases for controlling all physiology and behavior. It is through these mechanisms that homeostatic balance and survival in a harsh and dangerous environment is possible. Although Claude Bernard formulated the concept of homeostasis in the 19th century, it was the American physiologist Walter B. Cannon who in 1929 coined the term **homeostasis** to describe balanced physiological systems operating in the organism to maintain a dynamic equilibrium; that is, a relatively constant steady state maintained within certain tolerable limits. In Cannon's words,

> When we consider the extreme instability of our bodily structure, its readiness for disturbance by the slightest application of external forces and the rapid onset of its decomposition as soon as favoring circumstances are withdrawn, its persistence through many decades seems almost miraculous. The wonder increases when we realize that the system is open, engaging in free exchange with the outer world, and that the structure itself is not permanent but is being continuously broken down by the wear and tear of action, and as continuously built up again by processes of repair...

The constant conditions which are maintained in the body might be termed equilibria. That word, however, has come to have fairly exact meaning as applied to relatively simple physico-chemical states, in closed systems, where known forces are balanced. The coordinated physiological processes which maintain most of the steady states in the organism are so complex and so peculiar to living beings - involving, as they may, the brain and nerves, the heart, lungs, kidneys and spleen, all working cooperatively - that I have suggested a special designation for these states, homeostasis. The word does not imply something immobile, a stagnation. It means a condition - a condition which may vary, but which is relatively constant.

(Walter B. Cannon, 1929, "The Wisdom of the Body")

Cannon's original formulation of the homeostatic mechanism emphasized the maintenance of blood parameters such as osmotic pressure, volume, hydrostatic pressure, and levels of various simple chemicals such as calcium, sodium, and glucose. Cannon's viewpoint can be expanded to include all manner of physiological bioregulation at the level of the organism as well as at the molecular and cellular level.

When attempting to comprehend physiological systems, it is helpful to employ simplified models that simulate the various components of the system in a way that is easy to grasp and at the same time provide insights into how the system works as well as predictions on how it will respond to disturbances. In the following paragraphs, we will consider a very simple model of a basic bioregulatory mechanism operating for all physiological systems and provide some insight on how to use this model to understand complicated, integrated endocrine systems such as those discussed in later chapters.

A. A Homeostatic Reflex Model

In this model, **information (I)** is any stimulus that can provide quantitative or qualitative cues detectable is some way by the system. The basic model is depicted in Figure 1-6. The information is detected by a **receptor (R)** or transducer of some sort that translates (transduces) this information into the language of the bioregulatory system. For example, pressure may cause sodium ions to enter a neuron, depolarizing the cell membrane and inducing an action potential that in turn causes a nerve impulse to be generated. The transduced information is now called **input (I')** and is translocated to an integrating center called the **controller (C)**. The controller uses a preprogrammed set of instructions to compare the input with a **set point** and determines whether any adjustments are warranted. If the controller ascertains adjustments are

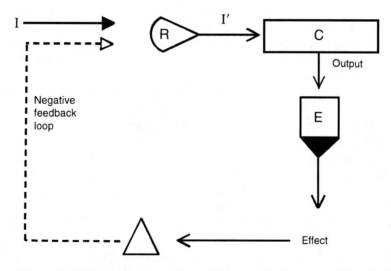

Figure 1-6.   A homeostatic model. This simple homeostatic mechanism could represent a single cell as well as an endocrine or neurocrine unit. The mechanism involves the detection of information (I) by a receptor (R) that converts the information into biologically relevant cues or input (I') and transmits this to the controller (C). The controller compares the input to a programmed set point and makes physiological adjusts as needed by producing output. This output travels by intracellular pathways (intracrines), neural axons (neurocrines), blood (hormones), or even extracellular fluid (autocrines/paracrines) to effectors (E) that in turn cause a change in the system (Δ) that also feeds back via the same or different receptors to alert the controller that a change has occurred. Since this type of feedback drives the system toward the set point, it is called *negative feedback*.

needed to maintain or regain homeostatic balance, it will direct a message called **output (O**; for example, the nerve impulse and release of a neurotransmitter) to one or more **effectors (E**; for example, a post-synaptic muscle cell) which will perform some specific action (**effect, Ef**) which, in turn, will bring about corrective changes in the system (contraction of the muscle cell). The responsiveness of the controller may be influenced by input received from other homeostatic bioregulators (Figure 1-5). These additional inputs may enhance or reduce the output of the controller through altering its sensitivity to other input or by adjusting the set point.

Corrective changes signaled in response to output from the controller will alter the nature of the information originally perceived by the receptors. The controller will be notified immediately by new information detected by receptors if the response has been sufficient and appropriate through a pathway called **feedback**. If the response was insufficient, the controller may increase its output to elevate the effector response. If an overcorrection or **overshoot** has occurred, the controller will alter its output accordingly and may even generate new output to other effectors to bring the system into line with the preprogrammed set point. Therefore, the set point represents the optimal physiological condition. The feedback loop that drives a physiological system toward the preprogrammed set point is called **negative feedback**. Any disturbance, regardless of the direction of the disturbance (i.e., "up" or "down"), causes a homeostatic reflex to be activated to maintain homeostasis.

Consider a controlled temperature room as a physical model of a simple control system similar to what was described for a biological system. The programmable thermostat represents both the receptor and controller components; an air conditioner and a heater are the effectors. Mechanical deformations produced in a bimetal strip (receptor) exposed to the air temperature (information) of the room are transduced into electrical current (input). The controller compares this input with the preprogrammed temperature (set point) and electrically turns on or off (output) the appropriate effector to maintain a constant temperature (homeostasis). The new air temperature will be detected by the same receptor and new input will be sent to the controller that will continue to make adjustments to drive the system toward the set point (negative feedback).

Under some conditions, feedback may drive a system away from the preprogrammed condition. Such a feedback loop is called **positive feedback**, and it drives a system to a different level of activity. Positive feedback is invoked where a rapid change is required, may be associated with an emergency type response, or might be responsible for short-term adaptations to complete a series of changes. The rapid influx of sodium during generation of an action potential, the physiological stress response, certain events during ovulation, and the induction of sexual maturation are all examples of events that employ positive feedback. In general, positive feedback is important for short-term events but is detrimental over longer time periods and can lead to the death of the animal if it persists. In contrast, long-term negative feedback generally is advantageous to survival as it helps maintain homeostatic balance in the face of environmental or internal changes. Negative feedback is the most common type of feedback in physiological systems.

In certain instances, changes in a regulated variable are anticipated through **feedforward regulation** that accelerates homeostatic responses and minimizes fluctuations in the regulated variable. For example, the regulation of internal body temperature involves a classical negative-feedback loop based on the temperature of the blood flowing to the brain. However, changes in body surface temperature before internal temperatures are affected can send additional input to the brain that begins making appropriate adjustments in temperature production and conservation or dissipation of heat to ward off changes in internal body temperature predicted by the input from the skin. Secretions invoked by the digestive system following appearance of glucose in the small intestine result in secretion of insulin from the endocrine pancreas even before blood sugar has become elevated, the normal homeostatic stimulus causing insulin release. These are examples of feedforward regulation.

To apply this homeostatic reflex model to any bioregulatory mechanism, one must ask a series of simple questions. First of all, on what information does the system cue? What are the receptors and where are they located? What sort of input is generated by this stimulus and how is it conducted to the controller? What is the controller and where is it located? What is the set point? What sort of output is generated? What are the effectors and what effects are produced? What change in the system results and how does feedback occur? Is there negative, positive, or feedforward regulation involved?

When examining chemically regulated systems, you will soon discover that complicated responses involve the integration of many different simple homeostatic reflexes. For example, the "controller" for one system may actually be the "effector" of another homeostatic reflex, and there may be pathways that modulate the responsiveness of a controller or effector to other stimuli. An excellent example of the integration of individual reflexes is the **neuroendocrine reflex**.

A typical vertebrate neuroendocrine reflex is represented by the adrenal endocrine axis in Figure 1-7. The liver cell can be considered an effector (target cell) whose activity is regulated by a steroid hormone (e.g., cortisol) from the adrenal cortex. This would make the adrenal cortex the controller, but the adrenal cortex is also an effector for the anterior pituitary that controls its activity through output of a tropic hormone, corticotropin or ACTH. In turn, the anterior pituitary is also an effector for a neurohormone (corticotropin-releasing hormone, CRH) from the hypothalamus (arbitrarily labeled the controller in this diagram). Only the major or primary feedback loop of cortisol is shown, but other feedback loops may be operating in this system (see Chapters 4 and 9). In this neuroendocrine reflex, we have indicated that the hypothalamic controller receives information via the blood (Int-I) but it also can be affected from information accumulated through a variety of receptors associated with other reflexes (Ext-I). Two neural reflex loops are shown, each with its own receptor and controller that might send modulating input to the hypothalamic controller, altering the set point or telling the hypothalamus to ignore the set point altogether. In spite of the apparent complexity of this neuroendocrine reflex as compared to our basic model, one simply asks the same series of questions given above for each level in the system until an understanding is achieved of the integrated whole.

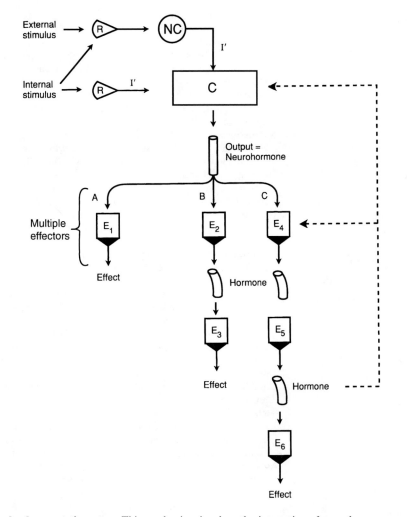

Figure 1-7. **A complex homeostatic system.** This mechanism involves the interaction of neurohormones and hormones to control more complicated events. Note that multiple receptors, multiple effectors, and multiple feedback loops may occur.

VII. Endocrine Disruption of Homeostasis

Traditionally, clinical endocrinology has dealt with disorders of the endocrine system that involve a disruption of homeostasis. Because of the broad actions of hormonal chemical regulators, homeostasis can be profoundly affected by endocrine imbalances. A listing of some well-characterized endocrine disorders is provided in Table 1-5. These disorders are discussed in later chapters after the normal functional aspects of the systems are described.

A recent focus for endocrinologists is the potential for disruption of endocrine functions in natural ecosystems caused by the presence of discarded chemicals in our surroundings, exposures at work, or through daily

Table 1-5. Clinically Relevant Endocrine Disorders[a] (Based on Norman and Litwack, 1997)

Disease	Description
Acromegaly	Inappropriate and continued secretion of growth hormone by a tumor of pituitary cells which leads to soft tissue swelling and hypertrophy of the skeletal extremities (usually in the third or fourth decade).
Addison's disease	Adrenocortical insufficiency resulting from a deficient production of glucocorticoids and/or mineralocorticoids due to a destruction of the adrenal cortex.
Cretinism	Characterized by a permanent neurological and skeletal retardation and results from an inadequate output of thyroid hormone during uterine and neonatal life; may be caused by iodine deficiency, thyroid hypoplasia, genetic enzyme defects, or excessive maternal intake of goitrogens.
Cushing's disease	Hypercortisolism resulting from the presence of small pituitary tumors which secrete ACTH leading to excess production of cortisol by the adrenals.
Cushing's syndrome	The circumstance of glucocorticoid excess without specification of the specific etiology; it may result from endogenous causes but is more commonly iatrogenic (physician-induced).
Diabetes insipidus	A deficient secretion of vasopressin which is manifested clinically as *diabetes insipidus*; it is a disorder characterized by the excretion of an increased volume of dilute urine.
Diabetes mellitus	A disease characterized by a chronic disorder of intermediary metabolism due to a relative lack of insulin which is characterized by hyperglycemia in both the postprandial and fasting state (see also types I and II *diabetes mellitus*).
Diabetes mellitus (insulin-dependent or type I diabetes)	The form of diabetes that usually appears in the second and third decades of life and is characterized by a destruction of the pancreas B cells; this form of the disease is normally treated with daily administration of insulin.
Diabetes mellitus (insulin-independent or type II diabetes)	The form of diabetes often arising after the fourth decade, usually in obese individuals; this form of the disease does not normally require treatment with insulin.
Feminization	Feminization of males, usually as manifested by enlargement of the breasts (gynecomastia) which can be attributed to an increase in estrogen levels relative to the prevailing androgen levels.
Froehlich's syndrome	A condition usually caused by craniopharyngioma (a tumor of the hypothalamus) which results in a combination of obesity and hypogonadism; sometimes termed adiposogenital dystrophy
Galactorrhea	The persistent discharge from the breast of a fluid that resembles milk and that occurs in the absence of parturition or else persists postpartum (4–6 months) after the cessation of nursing.
Gigantism	This condition appears in the first year of life and is characterized by a rapid weight and height gain; affected children usually have a large head and mental retardation; to date no specific endocrine abnormalites have been detected.
Goiter	Goiter may be defined as a thyroid gland that is twice its normal size; endemic goiter is the major thyroid disease throughout the world. Goiter is frequently associated with a dietary iodine deficiency; in instances of sporadic goiter it may occur as a consequence of a congenital defect in thyroid hormone synthesis.
Grave's disease	An autoimmune disease characterized by the presence in serum of a long-acting thyroid stimulator (LATS) that is an antibody for the receptor for TSH. Grave's disease is the most common cause of thyrotoxicosis.
Gynecomastia	Abnormal breast enlargement which may occur in males during puberty.

continues

Table 1-5.—*Continued*

Disease	Description
Hermaphroditism	True hermaphroditism is defined as the presence of both testicular and ovarian tissue in the same individual; pseudohermaphroditism is a discrepancy between gonadal and somatic sex.
Hirsutism	An increase in facial hair in women which is beyond that cosmetically acceptable; this condition may be associated with a number of masculinizing disorders including Cushing's syndrome, congenital adrenal hyperplasia, and polycystic ovary syndrome.
Hyperaldosteronism	An inappropriate secretion of aldosterone. It can occur as a primary adrenal problem (e.g., adrenal tumor) or can be secondary to other metabolic derangements that stimulate its release; it is often characterized by inappropriately high levels of plasma renin.
Hyperparathyroidism	Inappropriately high secretion of PTH leading to hypercalcemia. Frequently associated with the hyperparathyroidism is a metabolic bone disease characterized by excessive bone calcium reabsorption; frequently attributable to an adenoma of the parathyroid gland.
Hypoparathyroidism	Inappropriately low secretion of PTH, leading to hypocalcemia; the disease is either idiopathic or iatrogenically induced.
Klinefelter's syndrome	Typically characterized by male hypogonadism; the presence of extra X chromosomes is likely the fundamental underlying etiological factor. It is characterized by varying degrees of decreased Leydig cell function and seminiferous tubule failure.
Myxedema	Hypothyroidism clinically manifested by the presence of a mucinous edema; the disease may appear at any time throughout life and is attributable to disorders of the thyroid gland or to pituitary insufficiency.
Nelson's syndrome	A pituitary adenoma occurring in 10% of patients with Cushing's disease; afflicted subjects have a severe skin pigmentation.
Osteomalacia	A bone disease in adults characterized by a failure of the skeletal osteoid to calcify; it is usually caused by an absence of adequate access to vitamin D.
Polycystic ovary syndrome (PCOS)	A complex of varying symptoms ranging from amenorrhea to anovulatory bleeding often associated with obesity and hirsutism. The term denotes an absence of ovulation in association with continuous stimulation of the ovary by disproportionately high levels of LH.
Pseudohypoparathyroidism	A familial disorder characterized by hypocalcemia, increased circulating levels of PTH, and a peripheral unresponsiveness to the hormone; afflicted individuals frequently are of short stature, with mental retardation and short metacarpals and/or metatarsals.
Rickets	A failure in the child of the skeletal osteoid to calcify; it is usually caused by an absence of adequate amounts of vitamin D; it is characterized by a bowing of the femur, tibia, and fibulas.
Turner's syndrome	A condition present in females with a 45, XO chromosome pattern (i.e., complete absence of the X chromosome). The XO individual is typically short with a thick neck and trunk and no obvious secondary sex characteristics.
Zollinger-Ellison syndrome	Tumors of the pancreas which result in excessive secretion of gastrin; the afflicted subject has recurrent duodenal ulcers and diarrhea caused by hypersecretion of gastric acid.

[a] This list was abstracted from the United States National Library of Medicine—Medical Subject Headings—Tree Structures—1996, pp. 294–298. U.S. Department of Commerce, Washington, DC, 1996. The diseases were included in the National Library of Medicine table on the basis of frequency of publication of papers about the given disease topics.

contact such as through the use of pharmaceuticals, plastics, certain detergents, personal care products, and food. These EDCs are produced by human activities (i.e., they are anthropogenic), can mimic natural bioregulators or prevent the normal actions of endogenous bioregulators and include a wide variety of compounds of diverse origins (Table 1-6). For example, some of them are pesticides, including insecticides (e.g., DDT, methoprene), herbicides (e.g., atrazine, glyophosate), and fungicides (e.g., vinclozolin). Others are industrial or mining byproducts such as heavy metals, **dioxins**, and PCBs. Estrogenic (feminizing) chemicals such as **phthalates**, **nonylphenols**, and **bisphenyl A (BPA)** leach from a variety of plastics used in food and beverage packaging or dental sealants as well as from cosmetics and personal care products. Derivatives of the

Table 1-6. Classification of Some Known
Endocrine-Disrupting Chemicals (EDCs)

By usage
    Detergents (e.g., alkylphenols)
    Food items (e.g., phytoestrogens)
    Personal care products (e.g., phthalates)
    Pesticides (e.g., DDT, methoxychlor, atrazine, Roundup)
    Pharmaceuticals (e.g., diethylstilbestrol, ethinylestradiol)
    Plasticizers (e.g., phthalates, bisphenol A)
    Phytoestrogens (e.g., genistein)

By chemistry
    Alkylphenol ethoxylates and derivatives (includes nonylphenols)
    Dioxins
    Heavy metals
    Polychlorinated biphenyls (PCBs)
    Perchlorate
    Phthalates
    Steroids

By endocrine-disrupting actions
    Androgenic
    Anti-adrenal
    Anti-androgenic
    Anti-estrogenic
    Anti-thyroid
    Estrogenic

alkylphenolethoxylates used as emulsifiers in detergents and nonylphenols used in sprays also affect endocrine systems. **Phytoestrogens** are endocrine-disrupting steroidal chemicals produced in plants that find their way into animal systems either through diet (e.g., beer, soy products) or as a result of industrial activities (e.g., pulp and paper mill effluents). Humans and livestock excrete natural hormones as well as pharmaceuticals taken for therapeutic purposes that can concentrate in aquatic systems. Pharmaceutical compounds with hormonal activity, such as the birth control steroid **ethynylestradiol** (EE_2), are designed to resist degradation and hence may be more persistent than the excreted natural hormones.

Conventional sewage treatment systems are not designed to remove these EDCs (and may in fact increase their potency). Many of these compounds have been shown in clinical, laboratory, and field studies to be estrogenic (e.g., DDT, 4-nonylphenol, BPA, EE_2), androgenic (e.g., trenbolone), anti-androgenic (e.g., vinclozolin), anti-thyroid (e.g., PCBs, perchlorate), or anti-adrenal (e.g., cadmium). Although most of these compounds end up in biosolid wastes, sufficient estrogenic compounds pass with the processed sewage effluent into freshwater and estuarine environments where feminization of fishes or contraceptive actions have been described. These effects in fishes are being produced by extremely low levels of estrogenic compounds (ng/L concentrations; parts per trillion) that could not be measured in water samples until very recently. These levels are minute compared to the standard safe toxicity levels determined by traditional toxicology; i.e., typically below a mg/L (parts per thousand) or a μg/L (parts per million) is considered a no-observable effect level or NOEL. Apparently, biological receptors can detect natural bioregulators and bioregulator mimics at much greater dilutions than traditional chemistry.

Increased incidences of breast, prostate, and testicular cancer and reduced sperm counts have been reported in human populations in developed countries. Decreases in the proportion of live male to live female births have occurred since the 1990s although the prior ratio was consistent for the past 500 years. Puberty has been occurring at progressively earlier ages in the past 50 years. These are, of course, correlative changes only and the causes of these changes are not established and could be very complex in nature. However, increased incidences of abnormal reproductive development, especially in newborn males, are correlated directly with exposures to estrogenic compounds as are some cases of precocious puberty in girls. The discovery of feminized fishes in wastewater effluent dominated streams and estuaries in Europe, Asia, and North America has been attributed directly to the presence of estrogenic substances of human origin (Figure 1-8). Because EDCs add to or detract from whatever bioregulators are already present, there is theoretically no level for any EDC

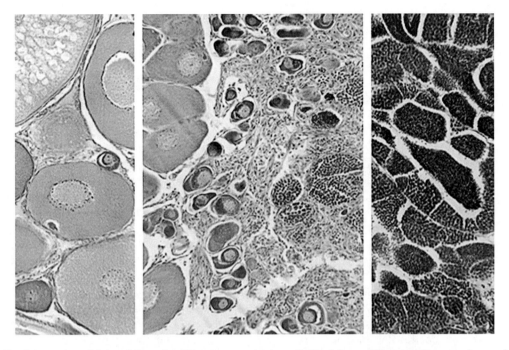

Figure 1-8. **Intersex gonad from white sucker *(Catostomus commersoni)*.** The left panel illustrates the normal ovary from fish at a reference site. The middle panel shows ovarian tissue to the left and spermatogenetic tissue to the right in an intersex gonad of a fish collected downstream of the discharge from a wastewater treatment plant (WWTP). To the right is a section through a normal testis from the reference site. Courtesy of Alan Vajda, University of Colorado. See color insert, plate 1.

that may not have consequences in natural populations. This concept of "no safe level" is in marked contrast to traditional toxicology that could readily define a "safe" level when using death or disease induction as an end point.

EDCs may be additive in producing effects in animals when they all operate through the same mechanism (such as by binding to the same receptor). For example, BPA, nonylphenol, EE_2, and estradiol all bind to the estrogen receptor and produce estrogenic effects if present in sufficient amounts. However, it has been well documented that mixtures of these chemicals are estrogenic even when each is present at a dose that by itself will not produce an estrogenic effect if the total amount of estrogen is sufficient to stimulate enough receptors. Even mixtures of chemicals working through different pathways (e.g., PCBs, dioxins, and BPA) can produce additive effects on reproduction.

Timing of the exposure to EDCs may be critical. The effects of a given EDC might appear during gamete preparation, embryonic or postembryonic development, sexual maturation, or breeding. It might cause a change of sex, reduce survival, prevent normal reproduction, or accelerate senescence. The presence of "normal" levels of estrogenic phthalates in the urine of pregnant women as well as the consumption of vegetarian diets during pregnancy (phytoestrogens?) are correlated with increased incidence of abnormal genitalia in males at birth. Exposure of pregnant women to thyroid inhibitors such as PCBs or perchlorate could alter development of the nervous system and induce mental deficiencies (see Chapter 6). Studies on achievement of children exposed to significant levels of PCBs during development have demonstrated that children of mothers exposed to PCBs through their diet while pregnant performed poorly on intelligence tests as compared to control populations.

Most studies of EDCs have been focused on vertebrates, but many invertebrate species are sensitive to many of the same EDCs. There are surprisingly many parallels in bioregulation with respect to the specific compounds involved and their receptors between the millions of known invertebrates and the relatively small number of vertebrate animals. Already, numerous examples of endocrine disruption have been described in annelids (e.g., earthworms), mollusks (e.g., snails), echinoderms (e.g., sea stars), and arthropods (e.g., insects and crustaceans). No one knows yet the actual impact of EDCs on natural ecosystems, but the potential for devastating effects is there. Recognition of the real and potential consequences of this unique pollution problem has led to recent worldwide attention and considerable controversy. The economic importance of these compounds and potential financial consequences of these disruptive observations versus the health of wildlife and human populations provide a focus for the controversy. Certainly, endocrine disruption and its consequences for the future of life on Earth should be a major focus of comparative and clinical endocrinologists both now and in the future.

VIII. Chordate Evolution

A comparative study of vertebrate bioregulatory systems necessitates some knowledge of the major vertebrate groups, their evolutionary history and relationships to one another. Each group of vertebrates—each species, in fact—is a product of individualistic evolutionary change as well as a product of adaptations to similar environmental problems faced by unrelated groups. The comparative endocrinologist faces the task of sorting out similarities due to convergent evolution of structures and functions as opposed to similarities due to common ancestry. The animals we classify as chordates are all members of the phylum **Chordata** that includes some invertebrate groups as well as the vertebrates.

One needs to be aware that being phylogenetically old does not necessarily mean the organism is primitive as well. Such "living fossils" may have diverged significantly from their ancestors with respect to many characteristics during the same time that new species have evolved. An animal species that has existed for millions of years must be adapted superbly to its environment. Furthermore, even though a species may appear unchanged externally with respect to their fossilized ancestors, we must recognize that physiology and behavior of such animals may be very different from their extinct ancestors. Examination of an endocrine mechanism or the structure of a gene responsible for a given hormone in a phylogenetically old species may shed no light on its specific ancestry

All members of the phylum Chordata, by definition, should exhibit these basic features at some stage in their development: (1) **pharyngeal gill slits**, (2) **a dorsal, hollow nerve cord** (that is, the brain and spinal cord), and (3) a supportive endoskeletal element, the **notochord**, which lies beneath the dorsal nerve cord. Each of these features must be present at some stage in the life cycle to qualify for membership in the Chordata. In addition, most chordates possess a **postanal tail** and an aquatic **tadpole-like larva**. In many fishes and amphibians as well as in reptiles, birds, and mammals, a free-living larval stage *per se* no longer exists, having been reduced to a transitory embryonic sequence.

Earlier classifications of chordates were based largely on anatomical and developmental features, but modern schemes rely more heavily on a wide range of shared characteristics of many kinds and attempt to distinguish among parallel, convergent, and divergent evolution. Older classification systems often relied heavily on anatomical and developmental features whereas contemporary classification schemes focus more on analyses of gene structure.

In the more traditional approaches to classification (see Figure 1-9), the phylum Chordata is subdivided into three subphyla: **Urochordata** (tailed chordates that are called sea squirts, ascidians, or tunicates), **Cephalochordata** (head chordates), and **Vertebrata** (vertebrates). These traditional subphyla are subdivided further into a variable number of Classes, Orders, Families, Genera, and Species. However, in the cladistic approach to classification (i.e., phylogenetic systematics), taxonomic groups are designated by sharing derived characteristics such as the cranium and backbone that characterize all of the vertebrates, or the absence of these features, as is the case for urochordates, cephalochordates, and some jawless fishes. Although the cladistic approach also produces a hierarchy of relationships among groups, it results in different groupings (Figure 1-10) that often transcend the earlier classifications that used categories such as classes and orders. This in turn necessitated coining new names for the newer groupings of organisms that are no longer connected to the historical groupings commonly used in the literature. In the following account, group names are used primarily from the older classification system without designating them as subphyla, classes, orders, etc. since this approach is more consistent with much of the endocrine literature prior to the present decade.

A. The Invertebrate Chordates

1. Urochordates

The all-marine Urochordata is considered to be the most primitive chordate group. A free-swimming aquatic tadpole larva is characteristic. The larva possesses the three basic chordate features, but these are modified

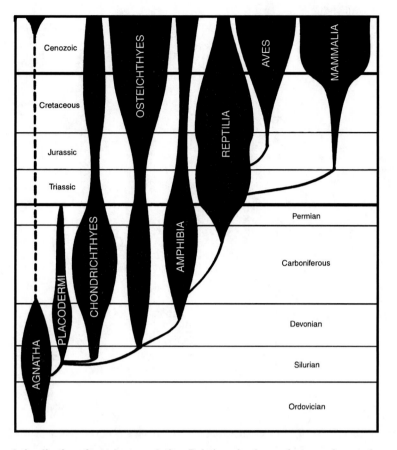

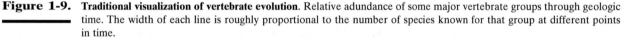

Figure 1-9. **Traditional visualization of vertebrate evolution.** Relative adundance of some major vertebrate groups through geologic time. The width of each line is roughly proportional to the number of species known for that group at different points in time.

or eliminated when the larva undergoes drastic structural modifications during metamorphosis to become a sessile, aquatic adult that is attached firmly to some substrate. The dorsal, hollow nervous system degenerates to a single neural ganglion, the notochord is obliterated, and the animal secretes an exoskeleton or tunic that completely encases the adult (hence one name for the group, the tunicates).

The adult tunicate (sometimes called a sea squirt because of its habit of ejecting a fine stream of water when disturbed by a curious biologist) retains only one obvious chordate characteristic: a gill structure called a **branchial basket**. This apparatus is covered with cilia and has a mucus-secreting structure, the **endostyle**, associated with it. Coordinated ciliary movements cause a current of water to flow into the branchial basket (via the mouth of the larva or the incurrent siphon of the adult) and out via the gill slits (the excurrent siphon of the adult). Mucus secreted by the endostyle traps minute food particles, and the mucus plus trapped food is moved by ciliary action into the gut, where both mucus and trapped food particles are digested. This method for obtaining food is common among many invertebrates including those groups believed to have given rise to the chordates. Organisms possessing such a feeding mechanism are called ciliary-mucus or pharyngeal-filtration feeders.

2. Cephalochordates

The sessile urochordate or tunicate is considered to be an evolutionary dead end, but some ancestral form similar to the larval tunicate may have given rise to the marine Cephalochordata. Certain living tunicates (for example, *Oikopleura*) never undergo metamorphosis to a sessile adult but remain free-living and attain sexual maturity while retaining the larval body form. Prolongation of larval life or retention of larval characteristics in sexually mature animals is termed **paedomorphosis**. If paedomorphosis is brought about by delayed

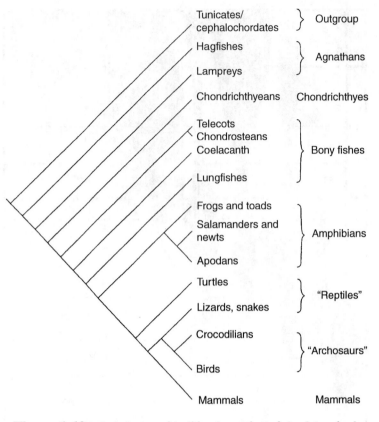

Figure 1-10. A cladogram of traditional groupings of chordate animals.

development of nonreproductive (somatic) tissues, it is called **neoteny**. If it is thought to be a case of precocious gonadal development, it is called **progenesis**. Paedomorphosis has been evoked as an important mechanism in chordate evolution and there are numerous examples of it among extant vertebrates.

The cephalochordates (such as the living amphioxus) have a body plan very similar to larval urochordates, including a branchial basket with a mucus-secreting endostyle and a persistent notochord throughout their life. Furthermore, cephalochordates anatomically resemble the larvae of lampreys (see Figure 1-11). Cephalochordate larvae and adults are ciliary-mucus feeders like the urochordates. Similarities among cephalochordates, urochordates, and larval lampreys support a common evolutionary origin for all three groups, but it is not certain how these groups are related to one another. The ancestral vertebrate may not have been a member of either invertebrate chordate group. Vertebrates have many features not found in either urochordates or cephalochordates; for example, specializations of the head, anterior nervous system, and pharyngeal breathing apparatus that are responsible for the active predaceous life of vertebrates.

B. The Vertebrate Chordates

There are a number of major groups that comprise the vertebrates (Figure 1-10). Two groups of fishes are entirely extinct and the other vertebrate groups all have living members. In addition to possession of the three chordate characteristics, the vertebrates all have **vertebrae**, special cartilaginous or bony structures that surround and protect the spinal cord. Furthermore, there is a special protective case, the **cranium**, that surrounds the enlarged anterior portion of the nervous system, the brain. This latter feature is the basis for another name sometimes applied to vertebrates, the Craniata.

Vertebrates are characterized by a duplication of the entire genome at some early time in their evolution. Among the bony fishes, there appears to have been a second complete duplication of the genome in the teleost fishes that explains the presence of duplicate forms of many chemical regulators and receptors.

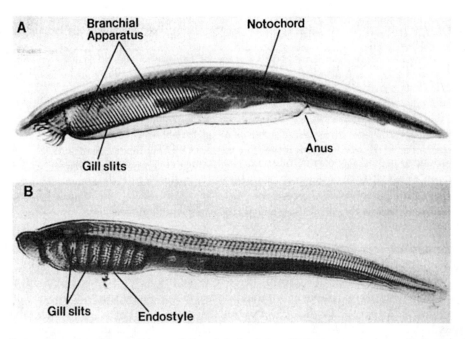

Figure 1-11. Comparision of amphioxus (A), an adult cephalochordate, with the ammocetes larva of a lamprey (B), an agnathan vertebrate. Note the prominent notochord in amphioxus that appears as a clear region in the ammocetes. Gill slits or branchial apparatus is present in both. An endostyle also is present in both but is not clearly visible in amphioxus.

1. Agnathan Fishes

The **Agnatha** consists of ancient, jawless fishes (*a* without + *gnathos*, jaws) believed to have evolved directly from cephalochordates or some cephalochordate-like ancestor. They traditionally are divided into two sub-groups: the extinct **ostracoderms** and the extant **cyclostomes** (*kyklos*, round + *stoma*, mouth) consisting of the lampreys and hagfishes.

The ostracoderms were all small fishes covered with bony plates (armor). They were limited to the ocean bottom where they probably existed primarily as ciliary-mucus feeders. Although the ostracoderms were not sessile like the urochordates, they possibly lived a "sit-and-sift" existence close to the bottom sediments of the oceans. However, recent interpretations of some ostracoderm fossils suggest at least some of them may have been active swimmers and possibly predators.

There are two groups of living cyclostomes, the marine hagfishes, **Myxinoidea**, and the essentially freshwater lampreys, **Petromyzontidae**. Many adult lampreys are parasitic on other vertebrate fishes, but the larvae are ciliary-mucus feeders. The **ammocetes larva** of the lamprey has a branchial basket with an endostyle, and in general, the body form looks much like the cephalochordate, amphioxus (Figure 1-11). Although some biologists suggest these structural similarities imply a close evolutionary relationship, others would argue against such an interpretation. When the ammocetes larva metamorphoses to the adult lamprey, the endostyle differentiates into the thyroid gland of the adult (see Chapter 7).

The Myxinoidea do not have a larval form and have many more primitive features than lampreys. For example, the hagfishes lack vertebrae and probably should not be classified with the vertebrates. Although modern hagfishes may not be much like the first vertebrate, their apparent simplicity may be a degenerate condition rather than a representation of a primitive vertebrate state. Most cladistic analyses place the lampreys closer to the jawed vertebrates than to the hagfishes, indicating that hagfishes and lampreys diverged much earlier from a common ancestor. Consequently, lampreys are probably a better living example of a primitive vertebrate than are hagfishes.

2. Placoderm Fishes

The ostracoderm fishes were ancestors of the first jawed vertebrates, the **placoderms**, a heterogeneous collection of extinct, heavily armored fishes. Hinged jaws developed in the placoderm fishes from modifications of the first gill arch, and this same event can be observed early in embryonic development of all jawed vertebrates. Many zoologists consider development of jaws to be the most significant single event in vertebrate evolution. Certainly it was a significant advancement enabling the placoderm fishes to abandon the bottom-dwelling existence of their ancestors for a pelagic, predatory life style. The fossil record suggests, however, that some placoderms retained the ancestral filter-feeding habit. The placoderms became abundant, attained great size, and sported heavy armor. They were the dominant vertebrates of the Devonian period, but they suddenly declined and disappeared, leaving only a strong fossil record and their apparent descendants. During the Devonian, the placoderms gave rise to two important piscine taxa: the bony fishes, **Osteichthyes**, and the cartilaginous fishes, **Chondrichthyes**. These predatory descendants retained the jaws of their ancestors, but the bony armor was reduced to scales allowing for an emphasis on speed and agility. The demise of the placoderms was probably due in no small part to the success of these more mobile predators.

3. Chondrichthyean Fishes

The chondrichthyeans (*chondros*, cartilage + *ichthy*, fish) have skeletons primarily composed of cartilage or calcified cartilage. Of course, the agnathans also had a cartilaginous skeleton but they lacked jaws. True bone is not present in this group. Since cartilage forms prior to bone in the normal developmental sequence, some zoologists suggest that this group arose from the placoderms via neoteny. Included in the Chondrichthyes are the sharks, rays, and skates (selachians or elasmobranchs) and the ratfishes or chimaeras (holocephalans). The cartilaginous fishes flourished for a time but then declined. Although in recent geological time they are increasing in abundance, they are believed to represent an evolutionary dead end and did not give rise to any other vertebrate group. The cartilaginous fishes have not been as successful as the higher bony fishes (teleosts) in exploiting the aquatic environment (especially fresh water), and they represent a secondary fish fauna today.

4. Osteichthyes: The Bony Fishes

Osteichthyean fishes (*osteon*, bone) have excelled in exploitation of freshwater and marine habitats. These modern bony fishes may have evolved in fresh water and secondarily invaded the marine habitat. It appears that freshwater bony fishes also gave rise to the first terrestrial vertebrates, the amphibians, probably before the exploitation of the marine environment.

The bony fishes can be readily separated into two major subgroupings: the **Actinopterygii** or rayfinned fishes, and the **Sarcopterygii** or lobe-fin fishes. The Actinopterygii (means spiny wings or fins) have distinct rays that support the fins, whereas the Sarcopterygii (fleshy fins) have lobed fins with internal skeletal supports that are homologous to the limb bones of tetrapods.

Early in the evolution of the bony fishes (or possibly in the placoderm group that gave rise to the bony fishes), a pouch developed ventrally off the gut anterior to the stomach, remained connected to the gut by a duct, and evolved into the air bladder. In the actinopterygian fishes, this air bladder was used as a flotation device or swim bladder. Among the sarcopterygians, the air bladder became modified as an accessory breathing device homologous to the lungs of terrestrial vertebrates.

5. Osteichthyes: The Actinopterygii

There are four distinctive groups of actinopterygians that include most of the living bony fishes: Polypteri, Chondrostei, Holostei, and Teleostei. The most ancient ray-finned fishes are the polypterans of which the two living freshwater genera (*Polypterus* and *Calamoichthyes*) are found in Africa. The chondrosteans include sturgeons (for example, *Acipenser* spp.) and spoonbills (*Polyodon*) of Asia and North America. Some zoologists designate the polypterans as the most primitive chondrosteans. The chondrostean fishes all live in fresh water in the northern hemisphere. The living holosteans are restricted to North America, occurring today only in the Mississippi River drainage area. This group consists of the bowfin, *Amia calva*, and several species of gar (*Lepisosteus*).

The teleost fishes (Teleostei) are the most advanced actinopterygians. They exhibit a tremendous adaptive radiation in fresh water and have secondarily invaded the marine habitat where they are the most abundant and successful vertebrate group. The majority of all extant fish species are teleosts with estimates from 20,000 species to as many as 40,000 species. Sometimes the teleosts are divided into the so-called lower teleosts, exemplified by the salmonid fishes, such as trout and salmon, and the higher teleosts, such as the centrarchids (large-mouth bass and bluegill sunfish, etc.). The higher teleosts can be recognized by the strong tendency for the pelvic (ventral) paired fins to move anteriorly to the vicinity of the pectoral (shoulder) paired fins.

6. Osteichthyes: Sarcopterygii

The ancestors of the first four-footed or tetrapod vertebrates were the sarcopterygian fishes. Two groups of sarcopterygian fishes have living representatives: two species of the **Crossopterygii** (fringe fins) and three genera of the **Dipnoi** (*dipnoos*, double breathing; i.e., in air and in water). Both of these groups represent side ventures off the main line of evolution within the Sarcopterygii leading to the tetrapods.

Crossopterygian fishes were known only from their excellent fossil record until 1938 when the first living crossopterygian, *Latimeria chalumnae*, was caught by a fisherman off the coast of Madagascar and attracted the attention of some scientists. Since that time a number of these bizarre, bluish giants have been captured and their anatomy, physiology, behavior, and ecology closely scrutinized by comparative zoologists. In 1998, a second species, *Latimeria menadoensis*, was discovered in Indonesia. Analysis of DNA from *L. menadoensis* confirmed its status as a separate species. *Latimeria*, like other crossopterygian fishes, has internal nares and a lung-like air bladder. It may reach 5 to 6 feet in length and is viviparous (live-bearing).

The Dipnoi consists of three genera of lungfishes (seven species) restricted to tropical regions on three continents: *Protopterus* in Africa, *Lepidosiren* in South America, and *Neoceratodus* in Australia. These fishes are gill breathers that use their lungs as accessory breathing structures. Only *Protopterus* survives breathing air alone. *Protopterus* can secrete a mucus-lined cocoon in which it resides and breathes air during periods of intense drought when its aquatic habitat may disappear altogether. The unusual distribution for these genera of lungfishes relates to the theory of formation of the present continents following the breakup of a "super continent" and a movement or drifting apart of the fragments—that is, continental drift.

Recent molecular studies suggest that lungfishes are most closely related to the amphibians (hence to other terrestrial vertebrates) than are the crossopterygians. Furthermore, the single species of freshwater lungfish, *Neoceratodus fosteri*, found in Australia is considered the most primitive of the living lungfishes and therefore presumed to be closest to the ancestral vertebrates that first invaded the land. Studies of development and physiology of this species by Jean Joss and her colleagues in the outdoor lungfish facility near Sydney suggest that this lungfish may be neotenic.

C. Amphibia

There are three living groups of amphibians: (1) the **Caudata** (Urodela; both *uro* and *cauda* refer to "tail"), which includes salamanders and newts; (2) the **Apoda** (without feet); the limbless caecilians, a tropical group about which little endocrinology is known; (3) the **Anura** (without tail), the tail-less frogs and toads which are the best-studied amphibians in spite of their obvious deviation from the basic tetrapod body plan.

The primitive, large-tailed amphibians or **labyrinthodonts** most probably had their origin from close relatives of the lungfishes that had developed internal nares and lungs for air breathing and had supportive skeletal elements in their fleshy lobed fins. The labyrinthodonts gave rise to the first reptiles as well as to the modern amphibians.

As the name of this group implies (*amphi*, both + *bios*, life), many amphibians lead double lives: one as an aquatic larva and the second as a terrestrial or semi-terrestrial adult. This "typical" life history involves laying eggs in fresh water where they develop into tadpole-like larvae. The larvae remain in fresh water for a period of growth followed by a remarkable hormone-regulated metamorphosis involving drastic structural and biochemical alterations to attain the different adult body form and the physiology and behavior to survive in a desiccating environment. The process of metamorphosis is discussed in Chapter 7. Although numerous species of amphibian have diminished their attachment to the aquatic environment through live bearing or laying eggs on land, a number of species have retained the larval body form (paedomorphosis) and become permanently aquatic.

1. The Archosaurs

Traditional classification separates the reptiles, birds, and mammals into three distinct groupings, but modern phylogenetic analyses suggest that reptiles and birds represent a single clade and that mammals arose from one part of this clade. Indeed, the crocodilians resemble birds very closely in their anatomy, physiology, and biochemistry and together these groups constitute a unique grouping, the living archosaurs.

D. Reptiles

In a sense, it was a mistake for the amphibians to give rise to the reptiles, for the reptiles quickly replaced them as the dominant terrestrial vertebrates. Reptiles owed their success in exploiting the terrestrial environment in part to the evolution of a unique "land egg," which enclosed the aquatic environment for embryonic development within a membrane (the amnion). This **amniote egg** could be laid on land where both egg and "larva" were safe from aquatic predators. The reptilian egg is much more resistant to desiccation than even the "terrestrial" eggs of amphibians. Since the reptiles were no longer tied to water for reproduction, there were fewer restrictions on their movements. The large amniote eggs of reptiles allow young to hatch at a size considerably greater than is possible from the smaller eggs of most oviparous fishes and amphibians.

Birds and mammals have retained many of the features of the reptilian egg, including the amnion and other membranes (the chorion, allantois, and, in some cases, the yolk sac). Bird eggs are little different from reptilian eggs, and embryonic development is very similar. In mammals, these membranes have greatly modified, especially among the placental mammals. Reptiles, birds, and mammals are often referred to collectively as the amniote vertebrates or **amniotes** (that is, they all possess an amnion), whereas fishes and amphibians are termed **anamniotes** (without an amnion as well as the other membranes).

Primitive amphibians gave rise to the **cotylosaurs** or stem reptiles, which early in reptilian evolution diverged into several separate pathways. Only four of these pathways have living representatives. One pathway (the Anapsida) separated early and gave rise to the heavily armored **chelonians**: the turtles, tortoises, and terrapins. The chelonians are anatomically a conservative group, having changed little in appearance over several million years. However, it might be a mistake to assume that their physiology has remained equally conservative. All are oviparous.

A second pathway (Lepidosaura) produced two important groups, the **Squamata** (snakes and lizards) and the more ancient **Rhynchocephalia** that has only one living species, the New Zealand tuatara, *Sphenodon punctatus*. The tuatara is of special interest because it is the only living representative of a very old reptilian group. Live bearing (viviparity) evolved numerous times within the squamates with variations from simple retention and development of the eggs within the oviducts to development of a placenta.

The Archosaura represents a third evolutionary line of which only the crocodilians (crocodiles and alligators) have living reptilian representatives. The extinct dinosaurs were part of this evolutionary line. In addition, one group of archosaurs, the **thecodonts**, gave rise to modern birds (Aves) that are considered to be archosaurs by some.

The final reptilian group, the now-extinct **Synapsidia**, gave rise to the mammals. This reptilian group separated early and gave rise to mammals before the archosaurs gave rise to birds. Apparently, the ability to maintain a relatively constant body temperature developed in the synapsids (specifically in the **therapsid** group of synapsids) independently of its development in the thecodont reptiles, which gave rise to the birds.

E. Birds

Birds are characterized by having feathers, no teeth, a relatively constant body temperature (ranging from 37°–43°C in different species), a four-chambered heart analogous but not homologous to that of mammals, and numerous structural modifications for flight. Their complicated mating rituals and intricate behavioral mechanisms associated with rearing of young have contributed greatly to their success. Although viviparity has developed in all other tetrapod classes (as well as in some fishes), all birds lay eggs. However, birds have been successful at exploiting the terrestrial habitat in such a way as to avoid undue competition with reptiles and mammals, and hence birds exhibit an impressive adaptive radiation.

F. Mammals

The most distinctive and uniform features of mammals are the possession of hair and the mammary glands, for which the group is named. Like birds, they maintain a high internal body temperature but are almost exclusively live bearing. Mammals traditionally have been separated into three distinct subgroups: **Prototheria** (*protos*, first + *thereon*, animal), **Metatheria** (*meta*, middle), and **Eutheria** (*eu*, good).

The **monotremes** are the most primitive group of mammals (Monotremata or Prototheria). This group includes the duckbill platypus (*Ornithorhynchus anatinus*) and the spiny anteaters, *Tachyglossus* spp. All members of this group lay eggs, and they are found only in Australasia.

The Metatheria consists of the **marsupials** (*marsupium* = pouch) or pouched mammals. After a very short intrauterine period, newborn marsupials spend most of their early life in the pouch provided by their mother. The marsupials include the kangaroos, wallabies, and others of Australia, the opossum of North America, and a few rodent-like marsupials still persisting in South America. The fossil record indicates that marsupials were just beginning their adaptive radiation when continental drift began to separate the continents. This explains in part their present skewed distribution, with the vast majority of extant species being found in Australia.

The Eutheria consist of the placental mammals. The insectivores represent the most primitive group of eutherian mammals from which 13 other groups have evolved. The eutherian mammals evolved in the Old World, entered North America from Asia, and eventually migrated southward and invaded South America. Although marsupials once were common elements of the New World, they were replaced almost completely by the eutherians. The geographical isolation of Australia as a result of continental drift allowed the persistence of a great many marsupial species there. The primates are considered (by humans, of course) to be the most highly evolved group of mammals, that group showing the most advanced evolutionary adaptations, the greatest intelligence, and the highest ecological success.

Suggested Reading

General/Mammalian

Baulieu, E.-E., and Kelly, P. A. (1990). "Hormones." Chapman & Hall, New York.

Bern, H. A. (1990). The "new" endocrinology: Its scope and its impact. *Am. Zool.* **30**, 877–885.

Bolander, F. (2004). "Molecular Endocrinology," 3rd Ed. Academic Press, San Diego.

Brabant, G., Prank, K., and Schofl, C. (1992). Pulsatile patterns in hormone secretion. *Trends Endocrinol. Metab.* **3**, 183–190.

Brown, R. E. (1994). "An Introduction to Neuroendocrinology." Cambridge Univ. Press, New York.

DeGroot, L. J., Besser, G. M., Cahill, G. F., Jr., Marshall, J. C., Nelson, D. H., Odell, W. D., Potts, J. T., Jr., Rubenstein, A. H., and Steinberger, E. (1989). "Endocrinology," 2nd Ed., Vols. 1–3. Saunders, Philadelphia, PA.

Gass, G. H., and Kaplan, H. M. (1996). "Handbook of Endocrinology," 2nd Ed. CRC Press, Boca Raton, FL.

Goodson, M. (2003). "Basic Medical Endocrinology," 3rd Ed. Academic Press, San Diego.

Griffin, J. E., and Ojeda, S. R. (1996). "Textbook of Endocrine Physiology," 3rd Ed. Oxford Univ. Press, New York.

Hadley, M. E. (2000). "Endocrinology," 5th Ed. Prentice Hall, Upper Saddle Park, NJ.

Martin, C. (1995). "The Dictionary of Endocrinology and Related Biomedical Sciences." Oxford Univ. Press, New York.

Nelson, R. J. (2005). "An Introduction to Behavioral Endocrinology," 3rd Ed. Sinauer Assoc., Sunderland, MA.

Norman, A. W., and Litwack, G. (1997). "Hormones," 2nd Ed. Academic Press, San Diego.

Pfaff, D. (2002). "Basic Medical Endocrinology." Academic Press, San Diego.

Schulkin, J. (1999). "The Neuroendocrine Regulation of Behavior." Cambridge Univ. Press, UK.

Timiras, P. S., Quay, W. B., and Vernadakis, A. (1995). "Hormones and Aging." CRC Press, Boca Raton, FL.

Comparative

Barrington, E. J. W. (1979). "Hormones and Evolution," Vols. 1 and 2. Academic Press, New York.

Becker, J. B., Breedlove, S. M., and Crews, D. (1992). "Behavioral Endocrinology," MIT Press, Cambridge, MA.

Bentley, P. J. (1998). "Comparative Vertebrate Endocrinology," 3rd Ed. Cambridge Univ. Press, UK.

Chester-Jones, I., Ingleton, P. M., and Phillips, J. G. (1987). "Fundamentals of Comparative Vertebrate Endocrinology," Plenum, New York.

Davey, K. G., Peter, R. E., and Tobe, S. S. (1994). "Perspectives in Comparative Endocrinology," National Research Council of Canada, Ottawa.

Dawson, A. and Chaturvedi, C. M. (2002). "Avian Endocrinology." CRC Press, Boca Raton, FL.

Dawson, A. and Sharp, P. J. (2005). "Functional Avian Endocrinology." Narosa Publishing House, New Dehli.

Diana, J. S. (2004). "Biology and Ecology of Fishes," 2nd Ed. Cooper Publishing Corp., Traverse City, MI.

Epple, A., and Stetson, M. H. (1980). "Avian Endocrinology." Academic Press, New York.

Gorbman, A., and Bern, H. A. (1962). "A Textbook of Comparative Endocrinology." Wiley, New York.

Gorbman, A., Dickhoff, W. W., Vigna, S. R., Clark, N. B., and Ralph, C. L. (1983). "Comparative Endocrinology." Wiley, New York.

Grimmelikhuijzen, C. J. P., Carstensen, K., Darmer, D., Moosler, A., Nothacker, H.-P., Reinscheid, R. K., Schmutzler, C., Vollert, H., McFarlene, I., and Rinehart, K. L. (1992). Coelenterate neuropeptides: Structure, action and biosynthesis. *Am. Zool.* **32**, 1–12.

Heatwole, H. (2005). "Amphibian Biology, Vol. 6: Amphibian Endocrinology." Surrey Beatty & Sons, Chipping Norton, NSW, Australia.

Matsumoto, A., and Ishii, S. (1992). "Atlas of Endocrine Organs: Vertebrates and Invertebrates." Japan Society for Comparative Endocrinology and Springer-Verlag, Berlin.

Matt, K. S. (1993). Neuroendocrine mechanisms of environmental integration. *Am. Zool.* **33**, 266–274.

Nelson, R. J. (1995). "An Introduction to Behavioral Endocrinology." Sinauer, Sunderland, MA.

Pang, P. K. T., and Epple, A. (1980). "Evolution of Vertebrate Endocrine Systems." Texas Tech. Press, Lubbock, TX.

Pang, P. K. T., and Schreibman, M. P. (1986). "Vertebrate Endocrinology: Fundamentals and Biomedical Implications," Morphological Considerations. Academic Press, San Diego.

Ralph, C. L. (1986). "Comparative Endocrinology: Developments and Directions." Alan R. Liss, New York.

Reinecke, M.. Zaccone G., and. Kapoor B. G. (eds.) (2006). "Fish Endocrinology." Oxford and Science Publishers, Enfield, NH.

Robash, M., and Hall, J. C. (1989). The molecular biology of circadian rhythms. *Neuron* **3**, 387–398.

Scanes, C. G., Ottinger, M. A., Kenny, A. D., Balthazart, J., Cronshaw, J., and Chester-Jones, I. (1982). "Aspects of Avian Endocrinology: Practical and Theoretical Implications." Texas Tech. Press, Lubbock, TX.

Schofl, C., Prank, K., Wiersinga, W., and Brabant, G. (1995). Pulsatile hormone secretion: Analysis and biological significance. *Trends Endocrinol. Metab.* **6**, 113–114.

Schreibman, M. P., and Scanes, C. G. (1989). "Development, Maturation, and Senescence of Neuroendocrine Systems: A Comparative Approach." Academic Press, San Diego.

Schreibman, M. P., Scanes, C. G., and Pang, P. K. T. (1993). "The Endocrinology of Growth, Development, and Metabolism in Vertebrates." Academic Press, San Diego.

Sharp, P. J. (1993). "Avian Endocrinology." The Society for Endocrinology, Bristol, UK.

Clinical

Ambrecht, H. J., Coe, R. M., and Wongsurawat, N. (1990). "Endocrine Function and Aging." Springer-Verlag, New York.

Becker, K. L. (1995). "Principles and Practice of Endocrinology and Metabolism," 2nd Ed. Lippincott-Raven, Philadelphia, PA.

Brook, C. G. D. (1995). "Clinical Paediatric Endocrinology," 3rd Ed. Blackwell, Oxford.

Collu, R., Brown, G. M., and Van Loon, G. R. (1988). "Clinical Neuroendocrinology." Blackwell, Oxford.

Grossman, A. (1992). "Clinical Endocrinology." Blackwell, Oxford.

Mazzaferri, E. L., and Samann, N. A. (1993). "Endocrine Tumors." Blackwell, Oxford.

Endocrine Disruption

Anway, M. D. and Skinner, M. K. (2006). Epigenetic transgenerational actions of endocrine disruptors. *Endocrin.* **147**, Suppl. S43–S49.

Blaustein, A. R., and Wake, D. B. (1995). The puzzle of declining amphibian populations. *Sci. Am.* **April**, 52–57.

Crews, D. and McLachlan, J. A. (2006). Epigenetics, evolution, endocrine disruption, health, and disease. *Endocrin.* **147**, Suppl. S4–S10.

Di Giulio, R. T., and Tillitt, D. E. (1999). Reproductive and Developmental Effects of Contaminants in Oviparous Vertebrates. The Society for Environmental Chemistry and Toxicology (SETAC). Pensacola, FL.

Fenton, S. (2006). Endocrine-disrupting compounds and mammary gland development: Early exposure and later life consequences. *Endocrin.* **147**, Suppl. S18–S24.

Gore, A. C., Heindel, J. J., and Zoeller, R. T. (2006). Endocrine disruption for endocrinologists (and others). *Endocrin.* **147**, Suppl. S1–S3.

Grün, F. and Blumberg, B. (2006). Environmental obesogens: Organotins and endocrine disruption via nuclear receptor signaling. *Endocrin.* **147**, Suppl. S50–S55.

Guillette, L. J., Jr. (1995). Endocrine disrupting environmental contaminants and developmental abnormalities in embryos. *Hum. Ecol. Risk Assess.* **1**, 25–36.

Guillette, L. and Crain, D. A. (2000). Environmental Endocrine Disrupters. Taylor and Francis, New York.

Henley, D. V. and Korach, K. S. (2006). Endocrine-disrupting chemicals use distinct mechanisms of action to modulate endocrine system function. *Endocrin.* **147**, Suppl. S25–S32.

Hose, J. E., and Guillette, L. J., Jr. (1995). Defining the role of pollutants in the disruption of reproduction in wildlife. *Environ. Health Perspect.* **103** (Suppl. 4), 87–91.

Kendall, R., Dickerson, R., Geisy, J., and Suk, W. (1998). Principles and Processes for Evaluating Endocrine Disruption in Wildlife. The Society for Environmental Chemistry and Toxicology (SETAC). Pensacola, FL.

Kime, D. (2001). "Endocrine Disruption in Fish." Kulwer Academic Publishers, Dordrecht, The Netherlands.

McLachlan, J. A., Guillette, L. J., and Iguichi, T. (2001). Environmental hormones: The scientific basis of endocrine disruption. *Ann. NY Acad. Sci.* **948**.

Mosconi, G., Carnevali, O., Franzoni, M. F., Cottone, E., Lutz, I., Kloas, W., Yamamoto, K., Kikuyama, K., and Polzonetti-Magni, A. M. (2002). Environmental estrogens and reproductive biology in amphibians. *General and Comp. Endocrin.* **126**, 125–129.

Naz, R.-K. (2005). "Endocrine Disruptors: Effects on Male and Female Reproductive Systems," 2nd Ed. CRC Press, Boca Raton, FL.

Newbold, R. R., Padilla-Banks, E., and Jefferson, W. N. (2006). Adverse effects of the model environmental estrogen diethylstilbestrol are transmitted to subsequent generations. *Endocrin.* **147**, Suppl. S11–S17.

Norris, D. O., and Carr, J. A. (2006). "Endocrine Disruption: Biological Bases for Health Effects in Wildlife and Humans." Oxford Univ. Press, New York.

Petersen, S. L., Krishnan, S., and Hudgens, E. D. (2006). The aryl hydrocarbon receptor pathway and sexual differentiation of neuroendocrine functions. *Endocrin.* **147**, Suppl. S33–S42.

Sharpe, R. M., and Shakkebaek, N. E. (1993). Are oestrogens involved in falling sperm counts and disorders of the male reproductive tract? *Lancet* **341**, 1392–1395.

Sparling, D. W., Linder, G., and Bishop, C. A. (2000). Ecotoxicology of Amphibians and Reptiles. The Society for Environmental Chemistry and Toxicology (SETAC). Pensacola, FL.

Stoka, A. M. (1999). Phylogeny and evolution of chemical communication: An endocrine approach. *J. Mol. Endocrin.* **22**, 207–225.

Welshons, W. V., Nagel, S. C., and vom Saal, F. S. (2006). Large effects from small exposures. III. Endocrine mechanisms mediating effects of bisphenol A at levels of human exposure. *Endocrin.* **147**, Suppl. S56–S69.

Chordate Evolution

Carroll, R. L. (1988). "Vertebrate Paleontology and Evolution." W.H. Freeman and Co., New York.

Kardong, K. (2004). "Vertebrates: Comparative Anatomy, Function, Evolution," 4th Ed. McGraw-Hill Science/Engineering/Math, New York.

Meyer, A. (1995). Molecular evidence on the origin of tetrapods and the relationships of the coelacanth. *Trends Ecol. Evol.* **10**, 111–116.

Musick, J. A., Bruton, M. N., and Balon, E. K. (1991). "The Biology of *Latimeria chalumnae* and Evolution of Coelacanths." Kluwer Academic Publishers, Dordrecht, Germany.

Pough, F. H., Janis, C. M., and Heiser, J. B. (2004). "Vertebrate Life," 7th Ed. Macmillan Publishing Co., New York.

Serials

Annual Review of Medicine
Annual Review of Physiology
Cell Signalling
Endocrine Reviews
Frontiers in Neuroendocrinology
Pharmacological Reviews
Recent Progress in Hormone Research
Trends in Endocrinology and Metabolism
Trends in Neurosciences
Vitamins and Hormones

2

Methods to Study Bioregulation

The basic method of scientific investigation has changed little over the years, but dramatic advances in observational, manipulative, and analytical tools during the last 50 years have resulted in a virtual explosion in our knowledge of animal biology that parallels similar events in chemistry, physics, engineering, and other scientific disciplines. For example, our observational powers have been increased several orders of magnitude by advances in the field of microscopy. Miniature radiotransmitters have made it possible to tag secretive animals such as rattlesnakes and follow their natural migrations without disturbing them. Sensitive techniques in chemistry such as high-performance liquid chromatography and mass spectroscopy can be used to analyze volumes as small as a few microliters that may contain only a few nanograms or even picograms of an important molecule. From a tiny sample, one can determine the chemical structure of a molecule and, if it is a peptide, then construct a gene that will direct the synthesis of large amounts of the peptide. And we can tell when a gene begins to turn on production of a peptide even before we can detect the final peptide product. This tremendous capability of probing the activities of a single cell has created an additional problem for the endocrinologist. How does one distinguish between random noise in the system and changes that have relevance to the organism at the physiological level? The endocrinologist must be able to bridge the gap between molecular information and physiological responses in organismal events such as metabolism or reproduction or link molecular information to clinical disorders.

The advent of computers and associated technology has not only automated and accelerated many of our laboratory procedures but has greatly augmented our ability to analyze complex sets of data. Computers also can be used to simulate natural conditions and to construct models of natural phenomena that we can manipulate and use to predict events in nature.

I. The Scientific Method

The process used by animal biologists to investigate the lives and activities of animals is the **scientific method**. We seek facts called data (singular, *datum*) and organize them into hypotheses, theories, or laws that give these data order and meaning. Many scientists are engaged primarily in the processes of gathering data. These data may be accumulated through careful observation or by use of planned experiments. Creative scientists also take data and try to organize them to form generalizations. From a series of observations, the scientist might formulate a **hypothesis** (Gr. *hypothesis*, supposition) or a predictive statement, a statement of what may be the true explanation of certain phenomena. Until it is tested experimentally, it is only a working hypothesis that must be supported or rejected on the basis of experimental results. If the hypothesis does not hold up to the test, it must be rejected or possibly revised and retested. If supported, the scientist may choose to test it more vigorously or formulate additional hypotheses on the relationships observed.

Hypotheses must be testable through observation or experimentation. The proposal that life on earth originated from outer space would be difficult to test, as would the notion that dinosaurs became extinct because other animals ate their eggs. All scientific generalizations and hypotheses must be tested no matter how "self-evident" or "unlikely" they might appear. Hypotheses or theories that are contradicted by data obtained from valid testing procedures must be modified or discarded. Hence, the scientist must distinguish between what we *believe* to be true, which may be true or false, and what we *know* to be true based on the results of tested hypotheses. In the final analysis, however, science often relies on the human interpretations of known facts, and the scientist must constantly evaluate what she/he knows and what she/he believes.

Testing of any hypothesis involves rigorous attention to details. Unless the test is reliable, the data obtained can neither contradict nor support the hypothesis or theory. Although it is possible to disprove hypotheses, it usually is not possible to prove one with a single observation or experiment. The data obtained may support the hypothesis, but since there are frequently many other ways one might test the hypothesis, it is not yet proven beyond all doubt. Hence the experimental design, the analytical tools employed, and the methods of data analysis are critical to testing hypotheses.

The more ways scientists test a hypothesis, the more confident they become of its validity. When a preponderance of new data supports a generalization, it becomes a **theory** (Gr. *theoria*, speculation). Continued testing of the theory never stops. Every theory must be reexamined and modified if necessary as new data are accumulated. However, be aware that a scientific theory is not just an educated guess, as "theory" is often used by the nonscientist or as is suggested by the ancient origin of the word. A scientific theory is an established concept based on accumulated data. Once a theory is accepted with certainty, it becomes a **law** or **principle**. Some people refer to it as **dogma**. However, even principles are still subjected to retesting and revision of their parts when new data are not explained by the reigning theory or dogma.

A. Controlled Experimental Testing

Science has accepted ways in which hypotheses or theories may be tested through observation or experimentation. There are techniques for making observations or for designing experiments and evaluating the result so that prejudice (bias) on the part of either investigator or subject is eliminated. Procedures are rigidly followed to control for inadvertent biases produced by the methodologies used, and an attempt is made to control other factors that might influence the results. This must be done so that scientists can be confident that the outcome of an experiment is a consequence of certain manipulations only. A **variable** is an event or condition that is subject to change. The scientist may allow or cause one or more variables to change while keeping all others constant. The changed or manipulated variable is the **independent variable** and those variables that are altered as a result of manipulating the independent variable are called **dependent variables**. One group of organisms serves as the **experimental group** subjected to the changed independent variable. The independent variable is unchanged for a second group known as the **control group**. In the simplest situations, there is only one independent variable but multi-variables are commonly examined in endocrine research.

One type of experimental control is a complete match to the manipulated animal minus only the factor being tested. If one group of rats is receiving injections of a drug or hormone dissolved in a solvent (called a **vehicle**), the appropriate control would be a second group of similar rats (matched for age, body weight, sex, history, etc.) receiving injections of an equivalent amount of vehicle without the drug or hormone (to control for effects of administering the injection). If a researcher wishes to investigate the effects of removal of some body organ, the appropriate control would not be an unoperated animal, because the anesthesia or the surgical procedure could influence the result. A more appropriate control would be a **sham-operated** animal, one that was also anesthetized and surgically disturbed but in which the gland in question was left intact. Looking at drug treatments of surgically altered animals requires a more complicated design (see Table 2-1).

One of the consistent flaws in experimental studies is the omission of **initial controls**. Frequently, scientists will collect or purchase animals and set up a controlled laboratory experiment with appropriate experimental and control (sham-operated, vehicle-injected, etc.) groups. At the conclusion of the experiment, they measure a dependent variable and determine whether it is different in the two test groups. However, because they didn't know where the two groups of animals were at the beginning of the experiment with respect to the dependent variable, the interpretation of the results may be limited (see Figure 2-1). For example, if animals in the experimental group A have significantly larger grumbacks after two weeks in the laboratory than those of the control group B, are they larger because (a) the treatment stimulated grumback development in Group A, or because (b) the treatment prevented regression of the grumback in Group A but allowed it to regress in Group B. If we knew the grumback size at the start of the experiment, we could easily decide between these alternatives.

Appropriate controls are often more difficult to establish in human subjects either because of moral and ethical issues or because of complicating psychological factors. It is well known, for example, that subjects expecting certain responses to treatments may respond differently from other subjects told to anticipate different responses. Consequently, in studies of the effects of a drug on the performance of long-distance runners, some subjects receive the real drug and the others are given an inactive substitute or a **placebo** (L., "I will please") administered in the same manner to control for psychological factors. In a **double-blind study**, neither the subjects nor the people administering the drug or placebo know which subjects are receiving which treatment. Another type of control is to switch treatments after a suitable period of observation, without telling the subjects, and then observing the subjects for a second period. These approaches also can be useful when working with nonhumans.

It is much easier to control experimental variables under laboratory conditions, especially in cellular or tissue culture, than in nature. **Control sites** for field research actually do not exist because of the myriad of environmental factors that the investigator cannot control at two locations and which will not be the same. For

Table 2-1. Comparison of Adequate and Inadequate Controls[a]

Treatment 1	Treatment 2		Treatment 3	Treatment 4
	Adequate control	Inadequate control		
One independent variable: Surgery				
Surgically altered animal	Sham-operated animal	Unaltered animal		
One independent variable: Injection				
Animal injected with chemical regulator in vehicle (a vehicle is some medium)	Animal injected with vehicle only	Uninjected animal		
Two independent variables: Surgery and injection				
Surgery plus chemical regulator in vehicle	Sham operated plus chemical in vehicle		Surgery plus vehicle only	Sham operated plus vehicle only

[a] A simple experiment involving only one independent variable (either surgery or injection) and a more complicated experiment involving both independent variables. Why are some attempts to establish control groups labeled as inadequate? Note that although two treatment groups are all that is necessary when manipulating a single variable, four are needed for two variables. How many experimental groups would be needed if three independent variables were examined simultaneously ($hint: 2^1 = 2$)?

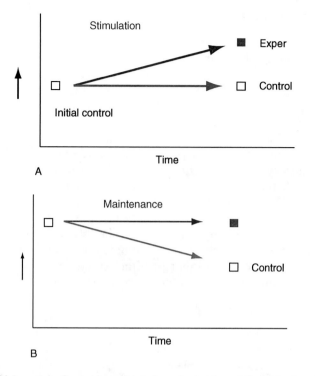

Figure 2-1. **Importance of initial controls**. Comparison of data for animals taken at the beginning of the experiment (initial controls) allows one to determine whether the experimental treatment stimulated the animals (A) or simply maintained the initial conditions (B) while the "controls" declined.

example, close examination of a site contaminated with cadmium and comparing it to a site without measurable cadmium may reveal not only subtle differences in natural variables (such as photoperiod, temperature, food items) but also the presence of unique chemicals at the "control" site not present at the "experimental" site. Consequently, we call the comparison site a **reference site** rather than a control site, acknowledging our awareness that they are not identical.

B. Representative Sampling

An important method used by the biologist is the examination of a **representative sample**. It is rarely feasible to test all potential subjects in a population or all the individuals of one kind of animal, so the scientist must establish a representative sample to test. Again, care must be exercised to ensure that the subjects have not been identified with any biases that might influence the results and therefore might not reflect characteristics of the entire population. The size of the representative sample will be influenced by the availability of animals, expected variability in factors being measured, statistical test criteria, previous experience of the investigator, and so forth.

Since scientists work with what they discern to be representative samples, they need a reliable method of analyzing experimental results and comparing appropriate control groups to see if their results are valid and representative. At the end of an experiment, changes in dependent variables of the experimental group are compared to the same variables in the control group. The branch of mathematics called **statistics** is the scientific tabulation and treatment of data. Statistical treatments provide tests for determining if the results are highly reproducible—that is, what is the probability that the differences observed in a dependent variable between experimental and control group are significant.

Reports of experimental data must be examined carefully not only to see if statistical analyses were performed but whether the appropriate statistical test was performed. Thus, it is essential that all researchers have a background in statistical methods not only for analyzing data but also for designing experiments. The design of a study must reflect knowledge of what appropriate statistical tests are to be applied. Many published studies are difficult to interpret because of errors in experimental design and/or in the application of inappropriate statistical tests.

C. The Dose-Response Relationship

Biological systems are very sensitive to the quantity of available chemical regulators, and small changes in concentration may have profound effects on physiology and behavior. This influence of concentration on physiology and behavior is summarized in the **dose-response relationship**. We can use a graph to illustrate this by comparing the physiological or behavioral response (dependent variable) on the *y*-axis with the dose of regulator (independent variable) on the *x*-axis (Figure 2-2). Typically, there is a minimally effective dose necessary to produce any response. This is often called the **threshold dose**. Smaller doses producing no response are called **subthreshold doses**. Some systems show an **all-or-none response**, meaning that the effect, if produced at all, occurs at the maximal intensity and adding more regulator will not give a greater response (Figure 2-2a). However, in most systems, increasing the dose produces a greater response up to some maximal or **optimal level** beyond which further increases in regulator actually produce a reduction in the optimal response (Figure 2-2b). This reduction may be due to interfering effects of the regulator on other systems or may be simply a toxic action that decreases the ability of the system to respond. The lowest dose that produces a maximal response is called the **optimal dose**. Generally speaking, the natural physiological range for the normal regulator in the animal is between the threshold dose and the optimal dose. Notice that if you ran an experiment with only one dose of a hormone and measured a certain response, you could be using a physiological dose or a supramaximal dose. When designing an experiment that involves treatment with any

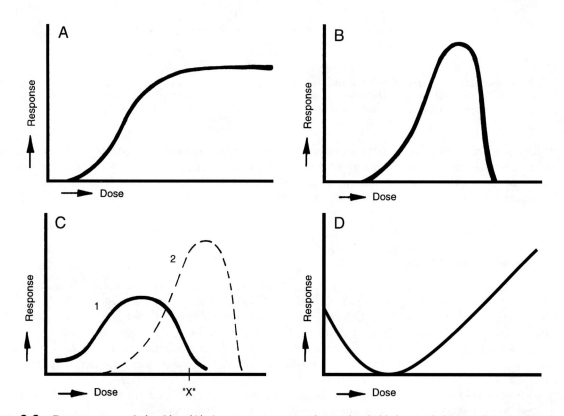

Figure 2-2. **Dose-response relationships**. (A) A system may respond to a threshold dose and then continue to show increased response with increasing dose until the process reaches a maximum. Additional bioregulator then produces no increased response over a wide range. (B) Relationship with optimal response to an "optimal" dose. A dose too low to produce a response is consider subthreshold. Doses above the "optimal" dose produce diminished responses and may indicate a toxicity to the tissue or animal. Alternatively, the bioregulator may reach a threshold that triggers accelerated removal of the bioregulator and hence a reduction in response at higher doses. Such doses often are considered to be "pharmacological" although any level of a regulator that exceeds natural levels also could be termed "pharmacological." Notice that when observing the response of a single dose you might not know whether you were above the optimal dose or below it. Consequently, when the data are not readily available, multiple doses should be employed to determine a useful dose-response relationship. (C) Species-specific or tissue-specific dose responses. An "optimal" dose for one tissue or one animal might be either subthreshold or pharmacological for another. (D) J-shaped or u-shaped dose-response curves are common in biological systems when dealing with very low doses.

regulator or other chemical such as antagonistic or agonistic drugs, it is essential to ascertain either from the literature or experimentally what the appropriate dose should be. Excessive doses may produce toxic effects via different pathways that influence your interpretation of the data.

When testing actions of a chemical substance on physiology and behavior, it is often difficult to separate direct actions from unanticipated actions on other tissues which might influence the results. Some drugs useful for studying one system in fact may produce toxic side effects of a **paradoxical nature** on other tissues. For example, the drug thiourea is an effective inhibitor of thyroid gland function. However, the response of the liver to thiourea produces effects opposite to those caused by surgical thyroidectomy, making interpretation of the effects of thiourea on the whole animal open to question.

The graphic illustration of the relationship between the concentration of a chemical substance and its action is called a **dose-response curve**. Comparison of the dose-response relationship in different tissues, in different individuals, or in different species may give very different results (Figure 2-2c). Consequently, one has to be very careful when using data based on one species for an experiment with another species or when extrapolating from doses observed in cell or tissue culture to the intact animal.

Dose-response data for biological systems often exhibit a J-shaped pattern (Figure 2-2d). In this case, doses below "threshold" may be stimulatory. Whereas simple *in-vitro* systems may not show this phenomenon, intact organism commonly do. The explanation lies in the complex interactions between different thresholds for different tissues of an intact organism to respond to a bioregulator as well as changes in the ability of the animal to metabolize the bioregulator. This phenomenon is called **hormesis** (see "Suggested Readings" at end of this chapter). Hormesis may have serious implications for clinical situations, for experimental studies, and in environmentally induced endocrine disruption.

D. Occam's Razor and Morgan's Canon

There is an old principle of logic called **Occam's razor** which should be invoked when interpreting data. Occam's razor states that if several explanations are compatible with the evidence, the simplest one should be considered the most probable one. Experience tells us that complicated explanations may not be necessary to explain a phenomenon when a simple one will do. A modification of Occam's razor called **Morgan's canon** was formulated in the late 1800s with respect to interpreting animal behavior. Morgan's canon says that when considering at what level a behavior might be controlled by the nervous system we should invoke the lowest level (that is, the least complicated) that will work. These are important principles to keep in mind as you continue your studies of physiology. This is not meant to imply that more complicated explanations are always incorrect but to emphasize that we don't have to make them more complicated than necessary.

E. Biological Rhythms

The release of hormones and other chemical regulators often occurs in bursts (**phasic secretion**) rather than at a continuous and constant rate (**tonic secretion**). Many of these bursts exhibit distinct, predictable diurnal, monthly, or seasonally cyclic patterns of secretion that are termed **biological rhythms** (Figure 2-3). For example, maximal level of testosterone in the blood of human males normally occurs between 2 and 6 a.m. The monthly fluctuation for estradiol and progesterone levels in human female blood plasma recurs with precise regularity. A predictable increase of androgens in the blood of the Italian frog *Rana esculenta* occurs every spring, signaling the onset of the spring breeding season. As one might expect, not only can hormone levels vary predictably, but the sensitivity of target cells may show diurnal or seasonal fluctuations. For example, the responsiveness of the pigeon crop to the stimulatory actions of the tropic hormone prolactin varies with time of day. Furthermore, the metabolic responses of killifish to a given dosage of prolactin varies with the season of the year in which the fish are treated.

The existence of biological rhythms suggests caution when interpreting data. Failure of a regulator to produce an effect when applied at 11:00 a.m. on September 15th may not mean that this regulator has no action in this animal but that the animal is not responsive to this dose at this time. If we had tried a different time of day or another time of the month or season of the year, we might have had different results. If the regulator had produced an effect, we still could not conclude that we would always see that effect.

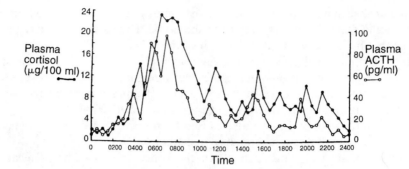

Figure 2-3.   **Diurnal pattern of plasma corticotropin (ACTH) and cortisol**. More ACTH produced in the pituitary gland is released in the early morning than at other times of day. Since ACTH stimulates the adrenal cortex to secrete cortisol, the latter shows a matching rhythm in blood concentration trailing that of ACTH. From G. P. Vinson (1993). "The Adrenal Cortex." Prentice Hall, Inc., Upper Saddle River, NJ.

The discovery of biological rhythms has opened many new areas of research and has opened old data to new interpretations. Today, experimental designs more frequently consider the times for treatment and the repeating of experiments with diurnal or seasonal treatments. Increasingly, experiments are conducted to understand what internal and/or external factors are responsibile for regulating these rhythms.

II. Methods of Endocrine Analysis

In recent years, the development and application of new techniques have caused a revolution in endocrinological studies resulting in many new and exciting discoveries. Some of these developments as well as older techniques are discussed briefly here.

A. Extirpation-Observation and Replacement-Observation

Early studies of hormone actions were limited to gross manipulations and observations because there were no precise ways to estimate levels of chemical regulators. Putative regulators were identified by first removing a gland or other organ (**extirpation**) and observing the effects of removal on the organism. Then an attempt was made to replace the lost tissue through transplants or grafts or by administering extracts of the tissue (**replacement**). If continued observations verified that the symptoms caused by extirpation were relieved by the replacement therapy, evidence for the existence of a chemical regulator was established.

A related early technique that evolved from the classical approaches involved the use of a **bioassay system**, a system employing animals or animal parts that could provide a quantitative or at least a qualitative estimate of the presence of a regulator in a tissue extract. Such bioassays made it possible not only to determine if a chemical fraction of a gland had the biological activity that represented the sought-after regulator but the quantitative assays could provide an estimate of how much of the regulator was present. Through their use, bioassays made it possible to obtain seasonal data on fluctuations in chemical regulator levels. Furthermore, they could be used to isolate chemical regulators and eventually to obtain highly purified preparations. Bioassays made it possible to identify and test suspected agonists and antagonists, too, and bioassays were used to validate the methods now used to estimate regulator levels in tissues and body fluids.

Hormones and other chemical regulators operate at minute concentrations, typically in the ranges of μg, ng, or even pg/ml of blood or extracellular fluids. This means 10^6, 10^9, or 10^{12} g/ml, or 1 millionth, 1 billionth, or 1 trillionth of a gram. These natural levels are often refered to as "physiological" and should be considered when designing experiments to observe the actions of a regulator. Treatment levels that produce circulating levels in excess of natural or optimal levels are termed **"pharmacological" doses** (commonly in the mg range). Interpretations of such pharmacological studies may be complicated with respect to understanding natural functions of regulators. Large doses greatly increase the probability of paradoxical or toxic side effects.

Until the advent of sensitive biochemical procedures that allowed us to measure actual hormone levels, endocrinology was limited to extirpation-replacement—"inject 'em and inspect 'em"—or crude estimates based on bioassays. Many of these studies emphasized pharmacological doses that produced excessive and possibly unnatural responses. Some of the molecular approaches that have led to a revolution in our understanding of the nature of chemical regulation and produced an unprecedented explosion in data generation are described below.

B. Imaging

Visualization has been an integral part of endocrine assessment since the beginning. Initial observations of entire organisms soon led to examination of tissues through **light microscopy** and eventually of cells by **transmission electron microscopy (TEM)**. Development of the **fluorescence light microscope** allowed for localization within cells or tissue of naturally fluorescing compounds or compounds labeled by addition of a molecule that fluoresces when viewed by ultraviolet light. The ability to reconstruct tissues three-dimensionally was later aided by development of the **scanning electron microscope (SEM)** and most recently by **confocal microscopy** that allows the scientist to view individual cells through relatively thick blocks of tissue such as brain slices.

Whole-body scanning techniques or **tomography** produce images of entire organs or organisms that can be viewed with the aid of a computer. Specific whole-body scanning techniques include **computer axial tomography (CAT scans)**, **magnetic resonance tomography (MRT)**, and **positron emission tomography (PET scans)**. CAT scans rely on X-rays to construct two-dimensional slices that can be converted to a three-dimensional image by a computer. MRT was originally called nuclear magnetic resonance imaging (NMRI), but "nuclear" was dropped to avoid an association by patients with radiation, which is not involved in this procedure. This form of tomography relies on the bipolar nature of water molecules. Because one end of the water molecule is positively charged with respect to the opposite end that is negatively charged, water molecules can be aligned in a magnetic field. Although the precise nature of this process requires a discussion of quantum mechanics, suffice it to say that this behavior by the water molecules can be used by a computer to provide a three-dimensional image.

PET scans do employ the use of common metabolic molecules that are labeled with short-lived radioisotopes (e.g., ^{11}C, ^{13}N, ^{15}O, ^{18}F) that produce minimal radiation exposure to the subject. With a PET scan, it is possible to measure the uptake of labeled glucose or other molecules by brain cells and allow the investigator or clinician to determine regions of increased or decreased activity. They can be useful in locating a rapidly developing tumor, for example, that might exhibit heightened metabolic activity.

C. Radioimmunoassay

Once purified molecules became available for experimentation, a number of techniques developed that allowed endocrinologists to routinely measure regulator levels in body fluids, localize specific molecules in a particular cell or part of a cell, and monitor these parameters under a multitude of experimental conditions. The first major technical breakthrough was the development of the **radioimmunoassay (RIA)** by Rosalind Yalow and Solomon Berson. While studying the occurrence of insulin resistance in patients with diabetes mellitus, these investigators noted that these people had antibodies to insulin in their blood. In part because they had difficulty in convincing the scientific community of the validity of their observations, Yalow and Berson went ahead and showed that addition of excess insulin could displace radioactively labeled insulin from these antibodies. This demonstration together with their fully developed mathematical treatment of these interactions provided the foundations for RIA, a technique that quickly revolutionized the entire field of endocrinology. Today, many RIAs are used routinely to measure all sorts of chemical regulators in nanogram and even picogram quantities, a feat never possible with bioassay systems. Because of his early death at age 54, Berson did not share the Nobel Prize awarded to Yalow in 1977 in recognition of the importance of their contribution to the entire field of physiology and medicine.

Development of any RIA relies on the availability of a pure source of regulator that can be used to induce formation of highly specific antibodies against it. Secondly, one must be able to radioactively tag or label a quantity of the regulator. It is assumed that the antibody cannot distinguish between an unlabeled or "cold" molecule of the regulator and a labeled or "hot" one and will bind each ligand with equal affinity. A scientist simply sets up a balanced and carefully controlled competition between cold and hot regulators for the binding sites on antibody molecules. The competition is designed with a constant amount of antibody and constant amount of hot ligand in the reaction mixture. When no cold ligand is present, the amount of hot ligand bound to the antibody at the end of a prescribed period of time is defined as 100% binding. Then, additional mixtures are prepared with increasing quantities of cold ligand. As the quantity of cold ligand increases, the competition for antibody binding sites increases in favor of the cold ligand so that less and less hot ligand is bound. Consequently, the percentage of hot ligand bound decreases with the addition of increasing amounts of cold ligand. Then, the antibody-ligand complexes are precipitated, leaving the unbound hot and cold ligands in the supernatant. By measuring the radioactivity of either the precipitate or the supernatant, the percentage of bound or unbound (also called "free") hot ligand (the dependent variable) can be plotted against the known concentrations of cold ligand added (the independent variable; see Figure 2-4). Radiation detection equipment (scintillation counter or gamma counter) is used to measure

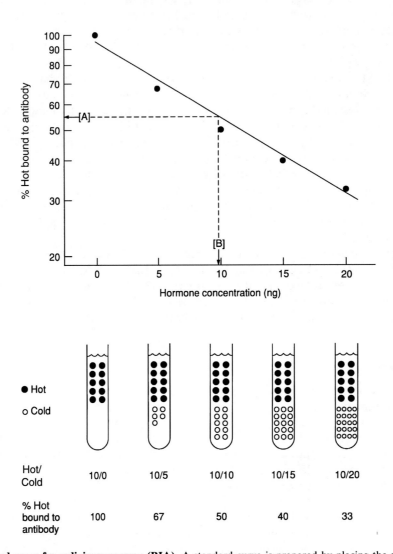

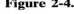

Figure 2-4.   Standard curve for radioimmunoassay (RIA). A standard curve is prepared by placing the same amount of antibody and radiolabeled (hot) hormone into every test tube and adding a different known amount of unlabeled (cold) hormone to each tube so that cold and hot hormone will compete for the same binding sites on the antibody. The greater the amount of cold hormone added, the lower will be the amount of radioactivity bound to the antibody. The antibody with its bound load of hot and cold hormone is precipitated from the solution and either the radioactivity of the supernatant or of the precipitate is counted. Thus, one can plot the percentage of hot hormone bound to the antibody against the amount of cold hormone in the solution to produce a standard relationship or what is called a standard curve. If an additional tube is prepared with the same amounts of antibody and hot hormone but with an unknown amount of cold hormone (such as might be present in a blood sample), one can determine the percentage of hot hormone bound [A] and extrapolate from the standard curve to estimate how much cold hormone [B] was present in the blood sample.

the amount of free or bound radioactivity. The plot of percent bound in Figure 2-4 constitutes a standard curve from which the quantity of cold ligand in a sample of unknown quantity (the "unknown") can be estimated. A similar competition is set up with the same quantity of antibody and hot ligand plus a sample of the unknown solution in which we wish to determine the level of cold ligand. By determining the percent bound for the unknown sample (y-axis), the quantity of cold ligand can be estimated by extrapolating to the x-axis.

At first, this technique proved useful only for peptides, but soon it became possible to trick antibody-synthesizing cells to make specific antibodies against all manner of chemical substances. Hence, we can measure thyroid hormones and steroids with the same ease that we measure insulin or thyrotropin (TSH).

D. High-Performance Liquid Chromatography/Spectroscopy

Chemists, while searching for techniques to improve the ability to separate closely related molecules from one another, developed a sophisticated separation system known as **high-performance liquid chromatography**, or **HPLC**. This technique is a modification of column chromatography that operates under high pressures and relies on differential solubility of molecules in the solvents employed to wash the columns and the affinities of these same molecules for the substances of which the columns are made. A mixture of molecules in a particular solvent is applied to the column and the solvent collected in aliquots as it comes off at the bottom. If properly designed, all of one type of molecule will come off in the same aliquot. What aliquot contains a given type of molecule depends on the affinity of each type for the column vs. the solvent. Special spectroscopic detectors allow investigators to identify individual molecules and quantify them in various mixtures. Such an approach allows investigators to quantitatively determine all of the steroids and steroid metabolites or all of the biogenic amine neurotransmitters and their metabolites in a given sample simultaneously (see Figure 2-5). With RIA, a separate analysis must be done for each molecule you expect to find.

Mass spectroscopy techniques following chromatographic separation have further refined analytical chemistry such that it is possible to measure multiple chemicals very accurately in a single sample when present at extremely low concentrations (e.g., ng/L or parts per trillion). These approaches are now being applied to measure bioregulators as well as endocrine-disrupting chemicals (EDCs) in blood and other body fluids

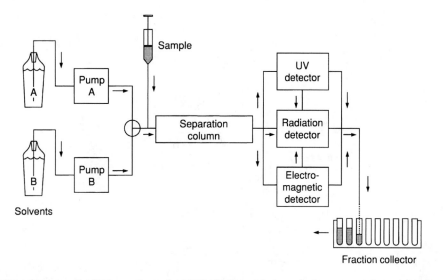

Figure 2-5. **High-performance liquid chromatography (HPLC).** A sample is applied to a separation column in a particular solvent. Additional solvents can be mixed and pumped through the separation column and depending on the affinity of the sample components for the column and the solvents, the sample components will leave the column at different times and pass through some kind of detector. Some compounds, such as steroids, are best detected and quantified by their absorbance of ultraviolet light (uv) whereas others (e.g., catecholamines) can be quantified using electrochemical detectors. HPLC can be coupled to radiation detectors for identifying a labeled molecule or specific metabolic products of a radioactive precursor, and the radiation detector may be used in tandem with either uv or electrochemical detectors. Various fractions from the column may be recovered by using a fraction collecting device.

as well as in environmental aquatic samples. Thus a complete steroid profile can be obtained from a single blood sample, or all of the chemical impurities of interest can be detected at extreme dilution in a large water sample.

E. Immunohistochemistry

Another analytical use for antibodies is to localize particular regulators, synthesizing enzymes, or degrading enzymes in tissues, cells, or parts of cells. This approach, called **immunohistochemistry** (or immunocytochemistry), employs an antibody made in one species, say a mouse, against the specific molecule (antigen) you wish to localize in the brain of a song sparrow. There are several variations of this technique based on a simple procedure (see Figure 2-6). First, you make the mouse antibody that would be a mouse gamma-globulin protein and apply that to sections of the tissue placed on a microscope slide. Theoretically, the antibody will bind only to cells that contain the antigen. In another species, you make an antibody against mouse gamma-globulin and conjugate that with an enzyme known as a peroxidase. This is also applied to the tissue sections. This second antibody will bind to the gamma-globulin which has bound previously to the song sparrow antigen. Next you add a substrate for the peroxidase enzyme that results in a colored product that will be localized in the cell containing the antigen-gamma-globulin anti-gamma-globulin-peroxidase complex. This complex can then be viewed with the microscope (Figure 2-7).

There are other variations on this basic technique using different enzyme-substrate markers that allow one to examine more than one antigen in a single section. **Immunofluorescence** is a modification that attaches a compound to the antigamma-globulin that will fluoresce under certain wavelengths of light (usually ultraviolet) instead of the peroxidase enzyme.

Another related approach is the **enzyme-linked immunoabsorbant assay (ELISA)** that is used to detect the presence of a specific molecule. Molecules of a specific regulator are coated onto walls of special microtiter plates (used commonly in immunological studies) and are used to compete with free molecules in plasma or a tissue extract for a specific antibody. The peroxidase-antiperoxidase method is then used to reveal the immobilized hormone-antibody complexes.

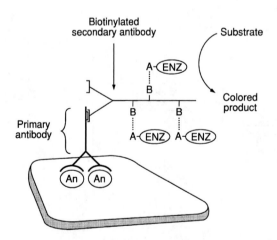

Figure 2-6. **Immunocytochemistry**. This method requires a pure source of antigen to make a specific antibody (primary antibody) in a mouse (or rabbit, etc.). Although the primary antibody usually is applied to sections of cells or tissues, this method also can be used on whole blocks of tissue. A secondary antibody is made against mouse immunoglobulins (for example, in a goat) to amplify the location of the primary antibody that is bound *in situ* to the antigen. The secondary antibody can be complexed to either an enzyme, a fluorescing compound, or a radioactive marker for detecting the exact location of the antigen in a cell or tissue. This approach can be used for detecting presence or absence of an antigen or to determine the number of reactive cells, etc. It also can be coupled with other techniques to estimate the intensity of the reaction and relate that to the quantity of antigen present.

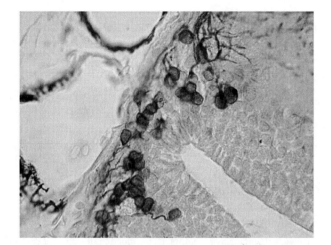

Figure 2-7. **Immunocytochemistry at light microscopic level.** The dark reaction product staining the neurons in this section of brain of the tiger salamander represents immunoreactive antigen that cross-reacts with a primary antibody for tyrosine hydroxylase, the rate-limiting enzyme for catecholamine sysnthesis. Photo courtesy of Anne Marie Scholl.

F. Techniques for Determining the Number and Characteristics of Receptors

For a protein to be a receptor for a chemical regulator, it must have certain properties. Because of the small number of regulator molecules usually present, a receptor must have a high **affinity** for the regulator; that is, a strong tendency to bind the regulator. Secondly, the receptor should have high **specificity** for the regulator and little tendency to bind other molecules. A third feature of receptors is their low **capacity**. This means that all available receptor sites are occupied at relatively low concentrations of regulator; that is, the receptor is said to be **saturated**. Finally, the distribution of a putative receptor should correspond to the known target tissues for the regulator and should be correlated with some biological effect.

Many regulators may "stick" to proteins other than their specific receptors, especially in cell or tissue homogenates where the process of disrupting the normal cell architecture may unmask potential binding sites normally not available to the regulator. Thus, it is important to distinguish **specific binding** (high-affinity, low-capacity proteins) from **nonspecific binding** (low-affinity, high-capacity binding proteins). These nonspecific binding sites do not saturate unless huge doses of regulator are applied. To distinguish between specific and nonspecific binding, we take advantage of the availability of radioactively labeled regulators to determine total binding capacity of a cell or tissue homogenate. Then, by adding an excess of unlabeled regulator to another sample also containing the labeled regulator, a competition is set up for the small number of high-affinity, low-capacity sites (the true receptors) causing labeled regulator to be displaced from only the specific binding sites. Because the nonspecific binding sites have such a high capacity, there is little competition occurring there. This competition is done using a range of unlabeled concentrations, and the difference between total binding (homogenate sample without unlabeled excess) and the nonspecific binding (homogenate with unlabeled excess) provides an estimate of specific binding (Figure 2-8). However, since specific binding is a function of both the affinity of the receptors as well as the number of receptors, simply demonstrating specific binding cannot be used for comparative purposes. Therefore, investigators compare the kinetics of the regulator-receptor binding, much like you would do for studies of substrate-enzyme interactions, to provide an estimate of both the affinity of a receptor for the specific regulator in question as well as an estimate of the number of receptors present. The most commonly used procedure for kinetic studies is the **Scatchard analysis**, a relationship first employed by G. Scatchard in 1949. The analysis of the experimentally derived data is similar to that done for enzymatic kinetics. Although this method involves certain assumptions and necessitates careful, repeatable laboratory procedures, it provides information on affinity (slope of the line), receptor number (*y*-axis intercept), and purity of the preparation (straight line vs. curvilinear plot).

A substance bound by a receptor can generally be termed a **ligand**. The chemical kinetics you have studied for reversible enzyme-substrate interactions are appropriate for describing ligand-receptor

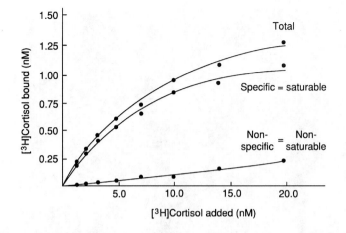

Figure 2-8. **"Specific" and "nonspecific" binding by receptors.** Determination of saturable (receptor or "specific") and nonsaturable (nonreceptor or "nonspecific") binding of cortisol to a liver cytosolic preparation using ^{3}H-cortisol as the ligand. Nonsaturable binding is not affected much by the amount of ligand since it has a high capacity. This is determined by adding a large excess of unlabeled cortisol in an attempt to displace the saturable receptors (specific binding) while not affecting the nonsaturable (nonspecific) binding. The difference between the binding observed with and without the excess of unlabeled ligand is defined as the saturable or specific binding. After Chakraborti and M. Weisbart (1987). High-affinity cortisol receptor in the liver of the brook trout, *Salvelinus fontinalis. Can J. Zool.* **65,** 2498–2503.

interactions. Normally, a ligand [L] binds reversibly with its receptor [R] to form a **ligand-receptor complex** [LR].

$$[L] \quad + \quad [R] \quad \leftrightharpoons \quad [LR]$$
free ligand   unoccupied receptor   bound ligand = occupied receptor.

The affinity or association of the ligand for the receptor is described by an **association rate constant**, k_1, and the tendency for LR to dissociate to L + R is described by the **dissociation rate constant**, k_2. At equilibrium,

$$k_1[L][R] = k_2[LR].$$

This can be expressed as

$$\frac{[L][R]}{[LR]} = \frac{k_2}{k_1} = K_d,$$

where K_d represents the dissociation constant. The reciprocal of the dissociation constant is the association constant K_a, and

$$K_d = \frac{1}{K_a}.$$

Therefore,

$$K_a = \frac{[LR]}{[L][R]}.$$

From this equation, you can see that the K_a is equal to the ratio of bound to free ligand.

If a fixed number of target cells (in other words, a fixed number of receptors) is incubated in replicates with increasing concentrations of ligand in each replicate, the number of occupied receptors also will increase until all of the available receptors are complexed to ligand (saturation or 100% bound). At saturation, the number of bound ligand molecules equals the number of available receptors while the ratio of bound ligand to free ligand approaches zero. If we plot the bound/free ratio for each replicate incubation against the bound concentration of ligand, the resulting straight line will intercept the *y*-axis

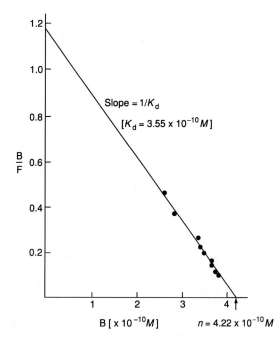

Figure 2-9. **Scatchard plotting method for receptor determination.** The Scatchard plot is described in the text. From F. F. Bolander (1989). "Molecular Endocrinology." Academic Press, Inc.

of our graph at a point that defines the total number of receptors or the receptor capacity. This graph (Figure 2-9) is called a **Scatchard plot**. The slope of the line on the Scatchard plot is equal to the negative value of the K_a (or $-1/K_d$). Thus, by determining only the bound ligand and the ratio of bound ligand to free ligand, where the number of receptors is kept constant and only the concentration of free ligand varies, allows one to extrapolate the number of receptors and the association constant for that particular receptor.

Most Scatchard plots, however, do not yield a straight line but rather a downward curving line. The most common explanation for repeated observations of this sort is that one is dealing with a heterogenous mixture of high-affinity and low-affinity sites. Special mathematical methods are available to separate these binding sites and allow differentiation of the numbers of high- and low-affinity sites.

III. Molecular Biology and Bioregulation

In the past few years, the field of genomics has elucidated the entire genomes of certain species including humans and the zebrafish and has contributed immensely to the arsenal of molecular techniques available to the clinical and experimental endocrinologist for investigating bioregulation. More recently, efforts focused on the study of proteins, proteomics, are providing new tools to evaluate cellular events. Whereas the human genome, for example, contains only about 22,000 different genes, there are about 400,000 resulting proteins and peptides that occur from alternative splicing of RNAs and post-translational processing of resulting proteins (see Chapter 3) indicating that knowledge based on genomics alone cannot explain the complexity of organisms. Genomic and proteomic tools are revolutionizing our understanding of bioregulation as well as how we approach the study of bioregulation.

A. Genetic and Genomic Approaches in Endocrinology

Use of the **polymerase chain reaction (PCR)** is another amplifying technique that allows the investigator to increase a small quantity of DNA to amounts that can be analyzed readily. PCR can be used to create cDNA probes, to detect mRNA synthesis even before new peptides or proteins are measurable, to screen for mutations of specific genes, and to amplify a specific mRNA using reverse transcription (making DNA from RNA instead of making RNA from DNA) coupled with PCR to amplify the product. cDNA probes can be prepared that bind to specific mRNAs and ascertain when a certain gene is turned on in a given cell. (cDNA is "copy" DNA made from RNA using a reverse transcription process.) The application of PCR technology to amplification of mRNAs provides a new way to measure even weakly stimulated gene activity following application of a bioregulator.

The presence of computerized banks of gene sequences for some or all of the genes in a given genome has proven extremely useful in identifying genes of interest to endocrinologists in other organisms. These approaches have helped discover related genes in other species as well as related gene products. Genomics has provided the identity of many receptor molecules (initially called orphan receptors) that eventually led to the discovery of their natural ligands and new insights into bioregulation. Being able to analyze entire gene sequences rather than just the amino acid sequence of the active peptide that represents only a fragment of the entire gene has enabled comparative endocrinologists to construct much more meaningful phylogenetic trees and thus gain a better grasp on evolutionary relationships.

Transgenic animals are lines of animals produced by inserting multiple copies of a specific gene or genes into a fertilized egg or early embryo. These genes may be responsible for producing a specific hormone such as the growth hormone (GH). Insertion of GH genes into mice resulted in production of an exceptionally large phenotype, and this trait was passed on to their offspring. In other cases, investigators may insert genes complexed to "reporter" genes that code for some very unique protein and are linked to a known hormone-responsive element. This reporter gene will only function once the appropriate transcription factor is present. Insertion of a gene for making the enzyme **luciferase** is a popular reporter gene as is the gene for making **green fluorescent protein (GFP)**.

Genetic engineering techniques have allowed us to develop sensitive assays for the determination of minute quantities of hormones. For example, the use of yeast cells transfected with genes for the human estrogen receptor (called the YES-assay) has provided a sensitive assay for detecting estrogenic compounds in solutions such as wastewater effluents or river water (see Appendix D). The YES assay can identify the presence of estrogenic chemicals even when conventional chemical methods such as RIAs were unable to detect them.

Knockout (KO) animals in which a nonfunctional gene replaces the normal gene have proven very useful. Not only do they demonstrate the roles such genes normally play, but they can provide model animals for studying disease states or for other molecular studies. Hence βERKO mice are mice homozygous for a gene defective at producing the β-form of the estrogen receptor (ER).

B. Proteomics

Proteomics includes a variety of approaches from protein separation, identification, and quantification to sequence and structural analyses of these molecules. Furthermore, proteomics is concerned with protein-to-protein interactions at the molecular and cellular levels as well as with post-translational processing of these essential gene products. One branch of proteomics is attempting to map the actual locations of proteins and their interactions within whole cells, information which is of central importance to endocrinologists focused on the molecular and cellular aspects of bioregulation. Among the many analytical approaches employed in proteomics research are X-ray crystallography and tomography, MRT, and a myriad of new approaches to study protein-DNA interactions.

IV. Animal Models

One of the most useful approaches in physiology research at all levels has been the development of specific species for use by many investigators studying a common problem. Some of these species have been breed artificially for generations specifically for research purposes (for example, laboratory mice and rats) and still other organisms have been genetically engineered to express or not express particular traits. Natural and genetically modified animal models for studying clinical disorders have provided considerable insight for understanding of the onset and progression of endocrine-related disorders such as diabetes, obesity, and Alzheimer's disease. Often times, non-mammalian species have proven useful models for experimental research. Examples include the frog amphibian bladder for molecular investigations of the role of aldosterone in regulating sodium transport, the nematode worm *C. elegans* in aging studies, the development of specific bioassays for hormones employing specific species such as the pigeon crop sac assay for prolactin (see Appendix D) or the fathead minnow, *Pimephales promelas*, as an indicator for estrogen in wastewater treatment plant effluents and polluted rivers.

V. Statistics

Regardless of the approaches used, proper statistical processing of experimental data is critical for establishing a database upon which to draw scientific conclusions and formulate new, testable hypotheses. Understanding what statistical test is appropriate and what is required for its application should be an integral part of every experimental design. Thus, knowledge of basic statistical procedures is essential before attempting to design experiments to test any hypothesis. Data collected may consist of a series of precise measurements or numerical scales based on subjective evaluations of such things as color reactions, behaviors, physical appearance, etc. under experimental and control conditions. The nature of the data and the number of variables examined dictate what statistical tests can be used. Use of initial controls, positive or negative controls, etc. as discussed previously will also influence the choice of analysis for the data collected. A working knowledge of statistics is essential for proper conduct of endocrine research.

Suggested Reading

Books

Beesley, J. E. (1993). "Immuncytochemistry: A Practical Approach." IRL Press at Oxford Univ. Press, Oxford.

dePablo, F., and Scanes, C. G. (1993). "Handbook of Endocrine Research Techniques." Academic Press, San Diego.

The Endocrine Society (1996). "Introduction to Molecular and Celluluar Research," Syllabus. The Endocrine Society Press, Bethesda, MD.

Martin, B. M. (1994). "Tissue Culture Techniques: An Introduction." Birkhauser, Basel.

Articles

Barsano, C. P., and Baumann, G. (1989). Editorial: Simple algebraic and graphic methods for the apportionment of hormone (and receptor) into bound and free fractions in binding equilibria; or how to calculate bound and free hormone. *Endocrin.* **124**, 1101–1106.

Calabrese, E. J., and Baldwin, L. A. (1999). Reevaluation of the fundamental dose-response relationship. *Bioscience* **49**, 725–732.

Eidne, K. A. (1991). The polymerase chain reaction and its uses in endocrinology. *Trends Endocrinol. Metab.* **2**, 169–175.

Ekins, R. (1990). Measurement of free hormones in blood. *Endocr. Rev.* **11**, 5–46.

Findling, J. W., Engeland, W. C., and Raff, H. (1990). The use of immunoradiometric assay for the measurement of ACTH in human plasma. *Trends Endocr. Metab.* **1**, 283–287.

Nilson, J. H., Keri, R. A., and Reed, D. K. (1995). Transgenic mice provide multiple paradigms for studies in molecular endocrinology. In "Molecular Endocrinology: Basic Concepts and Clinical Implications" (B. D. Weintraub, ed.), pp. 77–94. Raven, New York.

Orchinik, M., and Propper, C. (2006). Hormone action on receptors. In D. O. Norris and J. A. Carr (eds) "Endocrine Disruption: Biological Bases for Health Effects in Wildlife and Humans," pp. 28–57. Oxford University Press, Oxford.

Segre, G. V. (1990). Advances in techniques for measurement of parathyroid hormone: Current applications in clinical medicine and directions for future research. *Trends Endocrinol. Metab.* **1**, 243–247.

Shizuru, J. A., and Sarventnick, N. (1991). Transgenic mice for the study of diabetes mellitus. *Trends Endocr. Metab.* **2**, 97–104.

Stewart, T. A. (1994). Models of human endocrine disorders in transgenic rodents. *Trends Endocr. Metab.* **5**, 136–141.

Weiss, J., and Jameson, J. L. (1993). Perfused pituitary cells as a model for studies of gonadotropin biosynthesis and secretion. *Trends Endocr. Metab.* **4**, 265–270.

3

Synthesis, Metabolism, and Actions of Bioregulators

The chemical properties of each bioregulatory molecule are keys to understanding much of its physiology. They prescribe not only how a bioregulator is synthesized but also how it is secreted and transported to its target site, where its receptors are located, how it produces its effects on a specific target, and how it is metabolized or inactivated. Most bioregulators, such as monoamines, small peptides, polypeptides, or proteins,

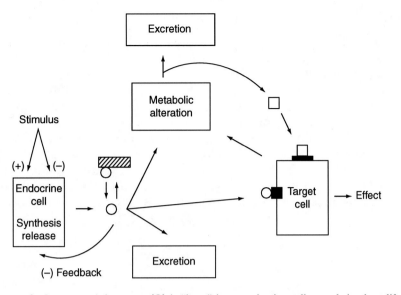

Figure 3-1. **Life history of a hormone.** A hormone (O) is "born" in an endocrine cell, spends its short life "free" in the blood or bound to binding proteins (▨). It may be metabolized and/or excreted ("die") before or after it binds to a target cell receptor (■) where it causes changes that result in its characteristic effect. In some cases, the hormone is secreted in an inactive form and must be metabolized to an active form (□) before it can bind to its receptor and produce an effect.

are at home in aqueous media. In sharp contrast, steroids, thyroid hormones, and eicosanoids have low solubility in aqueous media and, unlike peptides, readily pass through cell membranes. These hydrophobic bioregulators have markedly different synthetic pathways and processes of secretion, transport, and action on target cells. A bioregulator has a distinct life history, as illustrated in Figure 3-1 for a typical hormone. It is born (synthesis), may have an immature stage that is later modified to the active form, has a life (action), and dies (metabolism and/or excretion). Because the features of each group of bioregulators are uniquely tied to their chemical composition, each major type is discussed separately: (1) amino acids, amines, peptides, and proteins, (2) steroids, (3) thyroid hormones, (4) eicosanoids, and (5) other kinds of bioregulatory molecules.

I. Amino Acids, Amines, Peptides, and Proteins

Most neurotransmitters, neuromodulators, neurohormones, and classical hormones as well as many bioregulators common to interstitial fluids are composed of linear sequences of amino acids linked together by peptide bonds (see Table 3-1). These peptides vary in length from the tripeptide known as thyrotropin-releasing hormone (TRH) to large molecules of 200 or more amino acids (e.g., growth hormone, GH). Some common bioregulators are single amino acids (e.g., the neurotransmitter glutamate) or modified amino acids such as the catecholamines, indoleamines, and thyroid hormones.

Table 3-1. Amino Acid Composition of Some Peptide Regulators

Name	Primary role	Structure
Thyrotropin-releasing hormone[a]	Neurohormone	Pyro-E-H-P-CONH$_2$
Substance P[b]	Neuromodulator	NH$_2$-R-P-K-P-Q-Q-F-F-G-L-M-CONH$_2$
Glucagon	Hormone	NH$_2$-H-S-Q-G-T-F-T-S-D-Y-S-K-Y-L-D-S-R-R-A-Q-D-F-V-Q-W-L-M-N-T-COOH

See Appendix C for explanation of amino acid designations.
[a]Amino (pyro) and carboxyl (amide) ends are modified.
[b]Substance P is amidated at the carboxy end.

A. Catecholamines

A **catechol** is an unsaturated six-carbon ring (phenolic group) with two hydroxyl groups attached to adjacent carbons (dihydroxyphenol; see Figure 3-2). Attachment of the catechol ring to a side chain with an amine group characterizes a **catecholamine**. Catecholamines are synthesized in the following manner (see Figure 3-3). Addition of a phenolic group to the three-carbon amino acid alanine results in formation of another amino acid, phenylalanine. Combining one hydroxyl to the opposite end of the phenolic group converts phenylalanine into the amino acid tyrosine (also called hydroxyphenylalanine). Addition of one more hydroxyl to the phenolic ring followed by removal of the carboxyl group from the alanine portion yields a catecholamine.

Three important catecholamines are synthesized from tyrosine by neurons and cells of the adrenal medulla (Figure 3-3). The addition of an OH– group to tyrosine by the enzyme **tyrosine hydroxylase** yields **dihydroxyphenylalanine (DOPA)**. Next, the carboxyl group is removed by the enzyme **DOPA decarboxylase** to form the catecholamine **dopamine (DA)**, a common neurotransmitter in the central nervous system. In some

Figure 3-2. A catechol.

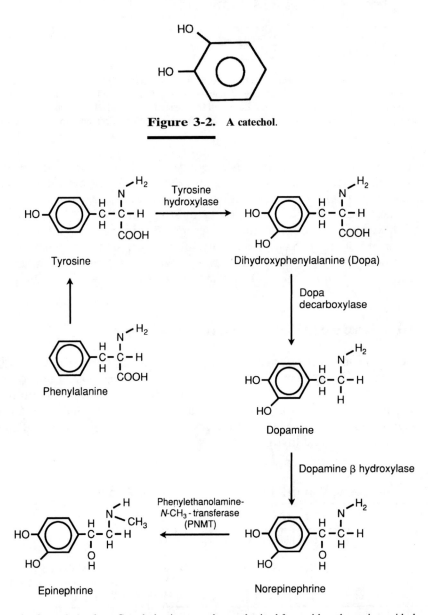

Figure 3-3. **Synthesis of catecholamines.** Catecholamines may be synthesized from either the amino acid phenylalanine or tyrosine. The rate-limiting enzyme for this pathway is tyrosine hydroxylase. Depending upon which enzymes are active in a cell, the final secretory product may be dopamine, norepinephrine, or epinephrine.

neurons, an additional enzyme, **dopamine β-hydroxylase**, converts DA to the catecholamine neurotransmitter **norepinephrine (NE)** by addition of an OH– group to the former alanine side chain. NE also is called phenylethanolamine. In still other neurons, NE is further altered by addition of a methyl group to the amine group to make the catecholamine neurotransmitter **epinephrine (E)**. This last conversion is catalyzed by the enzyme **phenylethanolamine N-methyltransferase (PNMT)**. Tyrosine hydroxylase immunoreactivity is often used as a histochemical marker to locate catecholamine-secreting cells, although it doesn't indicate whether the final secretory product of that cell is DA, NE, or E.

Catecholamines are more than just neurotransmitters. DA, NE, and E can all be released into the circulation where they exhibit endocrine functions. The hypothalamus releases DA that acts as a neurohormone to inhibit release of prolactin from the pituitary gland (see Chapter 4). The adrenal medulla, a modified sympathetic ganglion, secretes NE and E into the blood in response to neural signals directed via sympathetic nerve pathways from the hypothalamus (see Chapter 8). Although traditionally recognized as hormones, these adrenal medullary secretions also could be called neurohormones. Finally, in the central nervous system, there is evidence that NE is acting as a paracrine bioregulator, too.

Release of catecholamine neurotransmitters is followed by their partial reuptake and recycling and/or degradation by the secreting neuron to free the postsynaptic receptors and turn off the postsynaptic cell. The intraneuronal enzyme complex called **monoamine oxidase (MAO)** is responsible for degrading catecholamines. Local neuroglial cells also may participate in the degradation of these neurotransmitters. A second enzyme, **catechol-O-methyl transferase (COMT)** in the nervous system, is important in the degrading of catecholamines by neuroglial cells. A summary of brain catecholamine metabolism and structures of their metabolites are provided in Figure 3-4. NE and E in the peripheral circulation are metabolized by liver MAO and aldehyde oxidase to produce slightly different metabolites than those found in the brain (Figure 3-5).

Numerous agonists (mimics) and antagonists (inhibitors of receptor binding) for catecholamines have been developed as well as inhibitors of MAO and COMT. Other drugs have been developed that block release of the catecholamines. A partial listing of these compounds is provided in Table 3-2. The development of specific

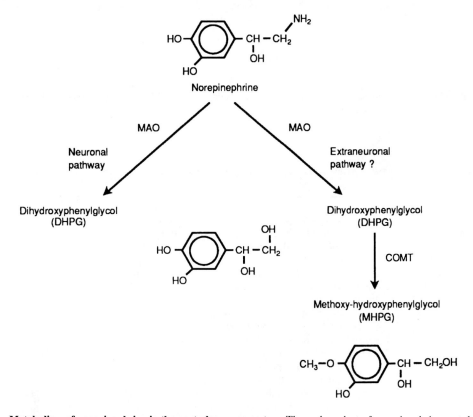

Figure 3-4. **Metabolism of norepinephrine in the central nervous system.** The end product of norepinephrine metabolism in neurons is thought to be DHPG whereas in glial cells (extraneuronal pathway) the major product is MHPG. MAO = monoamine oxidase; COMT = catecholamine-O-methyltransferase.

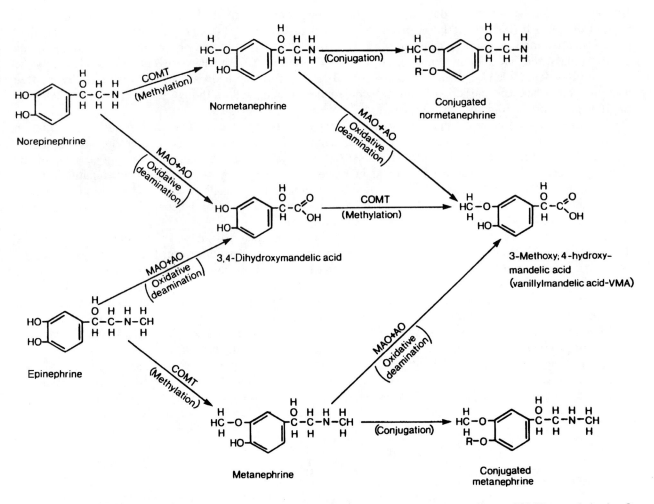

Figure 3-5. **Peripheral metabolism of norepinephrine and epinephrine.** AO = amine oxidase; COMT = catecholamine-O-methyltransferase; MAO = monoamine oxidase.

Table 3-2. Some Pharmacological Compounds That Alter Catecholamine Activity

Compound	Action
Propranolol	Antagonist that binds competitively to β_1- and β_2-adrenergic receptors and prevents actions of epinephrine or norepinephrine; consequently, propranolol is called a β-blocker
Phentolamine	An α-antagonist that competively blocks norepinephrine action
Haloperidol	Antagonist that binds competitively to dopaminergic receptors and blocks effects of dopamine on its target cells
Isoproterenol	General β-agonist that mimics both epinephrine and norepinephrine
Dobutamine	A relative selective β_1-agonist that is an effective heart stimulant
Ephedrine	An agonist that binds to α- and β-adrenergic receptors
Amphetamine	Potent agonist of α- and β-adrenergic receptors that binds especially well to central nervous system receptors but poorly to peripheral receptors
Reserpine	Blocks reuptake of catecholamines by presynaptic neurons
Pyrogallol	Blocks the enzyme catechol O-methyltransferase (COMT), an enzyme necessary for metabolism of catecholamines
Harmaline	Inhibitor of monoamine oxidase (MAO), an important enzyme for degradation of catecholamines

agonists and antagonists of neurotransmitters has allowed the investigation of the roles of catecholamine neurotransmitters in the regulation of endocrine function by the brain.

B. Indoleamines

Synthesis of the indoleamines is outlined in Figure 3-6. The amino acid tryptophan is hydroxylated by the enzyme tryptophan hydroxylase to yield 5-hydroxytryptophan. This metabolite is converted by L-aromatic amino acid decarboxylase to the neurotransmitter 5-hydroxytryptamine or **serotonin (5-HT)**. A form of MAO degrades serotonin to inactive **5-hydroxyindoleacetic acid (5-HIAA)**. In the pineal gland, the enzyme **N-acetyltransferase (NAT)** alters serotonin to an N-acetylated form that in turn is altered by **hydroxyindole-O-methyltransferase (HIOMT)** to the pineal neurohormone, **melatonin** or N-acetyl-5-methoxytryptamine (see Chapter 4). NAT is considered to be the rate-limiting enzyme for melatonin synthesis.

Melatonin is secreted primarily during the dark (**scotophase**) and appears to be important in regulating cyclical functions as well as having negative influences on thyroid and reproductive functions. Daytime levels (**photophase**) are very low. For example, cessation of melatonin secretion in children can lead to precocial sexual development (see Chapter 10). Some agonists and antagonists of serotonin and melatonin functions are provided in Table 3-2.

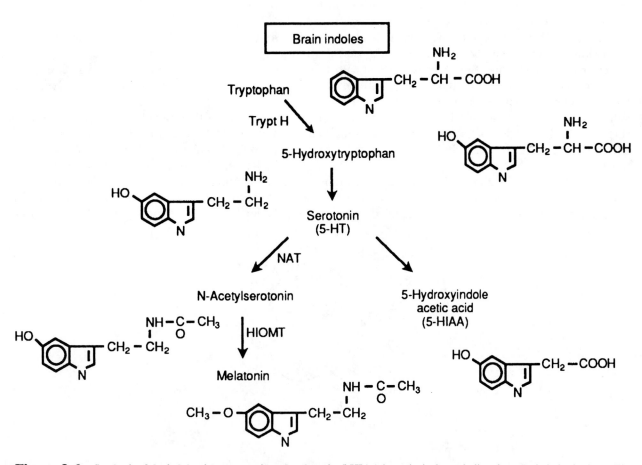

Figure 3-6. **Synthesis of the indolamines: serotonin and melatonin.** 5-HIAA is a principal metabolite of serotonin in brain tissue. The rate-limiting enzyme for melatonin synthesis is N-acetyltransferase (NAT). TryptH = tryptophan hydroxylase; HIOMT, hydroxyindole-O-methyltransferase.

Table 3-3. Some Pharmacological Compounds That Alter Indoleamine Activity

Compound	Action
Methysergide	Antagonist of serotonin at receptor sites
LSD	Antagonist of serotonin at receptor sites
Fenfluramine	Blocks reuptake of serotonin by presynaptic neurons
Harmaline	Inhibitor of monoamine oxidase (MAO), an important enzyme for degradation of indoleamines

C. Peptides

Similar to most peptides and proteins destined for export from the cell, peptide and protein bioregulators are synthesized at the ribosome-studded rough endoplasmic reticulum (RER) in the cytoplasm according to directions encoded in nuclear genes composed of deoxyribonucleic acid (DNA). Genes are responsible for the production of structural (e.g., microtubule proteins) and functional proteins (e.g., enzymes, antibodies, etc.). A molecule of ribonucleic acid (RNA) is transcribed from the molecule of DNA by an enzyme called **RNA-polymerase**. This enzyme attaches to the promoter region of the DNA. Following transcription of the RNA, intervening sequences corresponding to the nucleotides making up the **introns** of the parent DNA are excised from the RNA and the remaining pieces (representing **exons** in the DNA) are spliced together to form the messenger RNA (mRNA) that leaves the nucleus and travels to the ribosome of the RER for translation into an amino acid sequence (i.e., a polypeptide). Alternative processing of the original RNA transcript sometimes results in **splice variants** of mRNA that can result in translation of different forms of the peptide originally coded in the nuclear DNA.

RNA polymerase does not always have ready access to promoter sites on the DNA, and one or more **transcription factors** may be necessary to expose the promoter to RNA polymerase. Transcription factors are cytoplasmic proteins that typically migrate into the nucleus, bind to the bioregulatory sites on a gene, and enhance transcription of that gene. Although a variety of transcription factors have been identified, the predominant ones consist of special peptides complexed to zinc ions (Zn^{2+}). The interaction of certain amino acid residues with Zn^{2+} causes the peptide to develop special loops that have been called **zinc fingers** (Figure 3-7). Interaction of the zinc fingers with the major grooves of DNA unmasks the promoter site and allows transcription to occur. Steroid and thyroid receptors that directly affect gene transcription have zinc fingers that are highly specific for binding only to certain gene promoters. For example, the estrogen receptor has a sequence of 80 amino acids that forms two zinc fingers for binding to a particular DNA sequence allowing only a specific promoter site to be exposed for transcription. Once the steroid has bound to the receptor and dimerized with another occupied receptor, the complex becomes a **ligand-activated transcription**

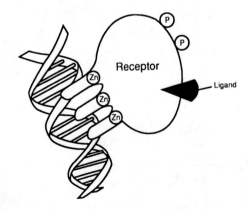

Figure 3-7. **Zinc fingers.** Certain sequences of amino acids can fold around zinc ions (Zn) to form projections called "zinc fingers." These zinc fingers are associated with the DNA-binding domains of steroid receptors and facilitate binding to specific sites on the DNA. Only a monomer is depicted here. P = phosphate.

factor that can now interact with DNA to initiate transcription. Additional proteins may complex with the ligand-activated transcription factor, facilitating its interaction with DNA.

1. Translation and Post-Translational Events

An mRNA directs the translation of its nucleotide sequence into a linear sequence of amino acids. For products destined for export from the cell, this sequence of amino acids is called a **prepropeptide** (Figure 3-8). There is a special sequence of amino acids located at the amino terminal end of the prepropeptides that is termed the **signal peptide**. The newly synthesized signal peptide sequence is synthesized first and recognized quickly by a special particle called a **signal recognition particle**. Attachment of the signal recognition particle to the translation complex halts further translation. The signal recognition particle also recognizes a specific **docking protein**, a special receptor embedded in the RER membrane. Thus, the prepropeptide is attached to the RER membrane, the signal recognition particle detaches, and translation is resumed on membrane-bound ribosomes of the RER. While the hydrophobic signal peptide is firmly attached to the membrane, the remainder of the prepropeptide, called the **propeptide**, is synthesized and intruded through the membrane into the cisterna of the RER. Once in the cisterna, the propeptide can migrate to vesicle-forming regions of the RER and be packaged into vesicles for translocation to the Golgi apparatus. The signal peptide does not enter the RER.

Additional post-translational processing of the propeptide may occur within the RER, in the Golgi apparatus, or possibly in the storage granules prior to release from the cell. Typically, enzymes will remove a portion or portions of the propeptide to produce the final peptide or peptides destined for export. Endocrinologists refer to the precursor forms of a peptide hormone as a **preprohormone** (prepropeptide) and a **prohormone** (propeptide). For example, the prohormone for the pancreatic hormone insulin consists of a long polypeptide folded through the formation of disulfide bonds between cysteine residues located in different parts of the chain. A special enzyme, a prohormone **convertase**, cleaves off a connecting sequence known as the **C-peptide**, leaving what appears to be two separate peptides (A-peptide and B-peptide) joined together by disulfide bonds. This resulting molecule is known as insulin (see Figure 3-9). Both the C-peptide and insulin are released from the cell although no peripheral function is known for the C-peptide. Enzymatic cleavage may occur at several sites along the prohormone as is the case for the tripeptide, TRH (Figure 3-10). This results in production of five identical TRH tripeptides from each prohormone molecule, thus amplifying the amount of neurohormone synthesized.

For certain peptide products, other compounds such as carbohydrates or lipids may be added as well. Post-translational processing may involve additions to the basic prohormone as well as deletions. For example, some peptides are amidated or acetylated. Such changes increase their resistance to degradation and/or improves their binding to receptors. In the synthesis of glycoprotein hormones (GTHs and TSH) in the anterior pituitary, carbohydrates are complexed to two separate propeptides which are then joined together to yield the biologically active hormones. In other cases, there is no post-translational processing, and the translated peptide enters the RER ready for export.

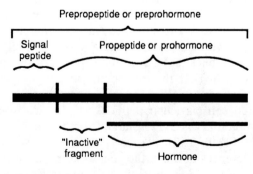

Figure 3-8. **Synthesis of export proteins.** The product of mRNA at the ribosome is the preprohormone. The signal peptide is necessary to transport the prohormone into the cisterna of the endoplasmic reticulum. The prohormone is later cleaved to produce an "inactive fragment" and the definitive hormone. Typically, both the inactive fragment and the hormone will be released from the cell. Sometimes the entire prohormone may be released as well.

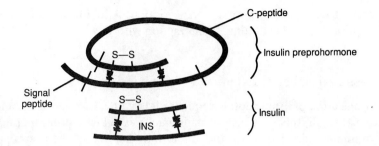

Figure 3-9. **Insulin synthesis.** The hormone insulin is synthesized from the preprohormones by first removing the signal peptide, folding the single peptide chain of the prohormone, and cleaving it in two places to yield a connecting C-peptide fragment and the hormone insulin that now appears to be made of two separate polypeptide chains. Some proinsulin is secreted along with the C-peptide and insulin.

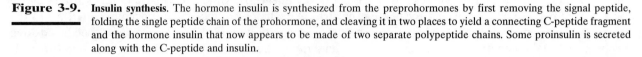
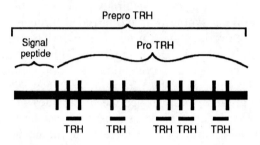

Figure 3-10. **Synthesis of thyrotropin-releasing hormone, TRH.** Five copies of the TRH tripeptide are produced by multiple cleavages of each prohormone.

Another variation in post-translational processing can produce more than one biologically active species from the same preprohormone depending on what processing enzymes are involved in different cell types. For example, a prohormone called **proopiomelanocortin (POMC)** is cleaved to produce the pituitary tropic **hormone corticotropin (ACTH)** in a particular cell type in the pars distalis region of the pituitary whereas different processing enzymes in pars intermedia cells of the pituitary release **melanotropin (α-MSH)** from proopiomelanocortin (see Chapter 4 for details about proopiomelanocortin and other enzymatic products).

2. Homologies in Peptide and Protein Structure

Analysis of bioregulatory peptides and proteins shows that it is possible to group molecules with common amino acid sequences into families of related peptides. In many cases, the genes responsible for directing the synthesis of structurally related or homologous peptides are also similar structurally with respect to their nucleotide sequences that ultimately code for these peptides and proteins. Some examples of homologous families are provided in Table 3-4 and Figure 3-11. Many argue that the peptides or proteins that represent a single family had, in an evolutionary sense, a common ancestral gene that, through duplications and subsequent independent, random mutations, evolved via natural selection into a family of closely related genes. In the case of the glycoprotein pituitary hormones that are each composed of two peptide subunits (α and β), there has been little change in the gene coding for the α-subunit, but the β-subunit shows considerable variation related to the different functions that have evolved for these hormones (see Chapter 4 for more details).

Smaller variations may exist between particular peptides or proteins isolated from different species. For example, the primary structure of pituitary ACTH isolated from humans differs by only one amino acid from those produced in sheep and pigs (Figure 3-12). Because ACTH is cleaved from a much larger prohormone, one should expect many more differences between the genes that produce ACTH in these species.

The sequence of amino acids gives rise to the primary structure of a peptide or protein. The secondary and tertiary structures that are based largely on the primary structure also may be similar, resulting in considerable overlap in their three-dimensional structures. This may cause overlap with respect to the receptors that bind these similar molecules. Such an overlap in binding may yield confusing experimental results, especially when

Table 3-4. Families of Peptide Chemical Regulators

Family member	No. of AA residues	No. AA common to molecule 1 or other homologous feature
Neurohypophysial octapeptides		
1. Arginine vasopressin	9	9
2. Lysine vasopressin	9	8
3. Arginine vasotocin	9	8
4. Mesotocin	9	7
5. Oxytocin	9	7
6. Phenypressin	9	8
Glucagon-secretin family		
1. PACAP-27	27	27
2. Secretin	27	11
3. PHI/PHM	27	14
4. VIP	28	19
5. Glucagon	29	10
6. GLP-1	30	
7. GLP-2	35	
8. GIP	42	6
9. GHRH (GRH, GRF)	44	8
10. PACAP-related peptide (PRP)	48	
Insulin-like peptides		
1. Insulin ($\alpha + \beta$ chain)	51	51
2. Relaxin ($\alpha + \beta$ chain)	54	Insulin-like
3. IGF-1 (single chain)	70	24 like insulin
4. IGF-2 (single chain)	67	29 like insulin
Endothelins		
1. Endothelin 1	21	21
2. Endothelin 2	21	18
3. Endothelin 3	21	15
4. Sarafotoxin S6b	21	14
CRH-like peptides		
1. hCRH	41	41
2. oCRH	41	34
2. Sauvagine	39	18
3. Urotensin I (carp)	41	22
POMC-related peptides		
hACTH-like		
1. ACTH 39	39	39
2. α-MSH	13	1–13 of ACTH
3. CLIP	22	18–39 of ACTH
hLPH-like		
1. β-LPH	89	
2. γ-LPH	56	1–56 of γ-LPH
3. β-endorphin	31	59–89 of γ-LPH
4. DynorphinA	16	1–4 like β-endorphin
5. met-Enkephalin	5	59–63 of β-endorphin & 1–5 of dynorphin

See text for explanation of abbreviations.

large doses of a bioregulator are applied. In such cases, the applied bioregulator normally may not compete effectively for binding to receptors of a chemically related bioregulator. However, by adding excessive amounts, sufficient binding to a related receptor may produce actions that are not physiologically associated with that particular bioregulator.

3. Transport of Peptide Bioregulators to Target Cells

Completed peptide and protein bioregulators along with peptide fragments separated during post-translational processing are packaged into secretory vesicles or granules at the Golgi apparatus and are retained or stored

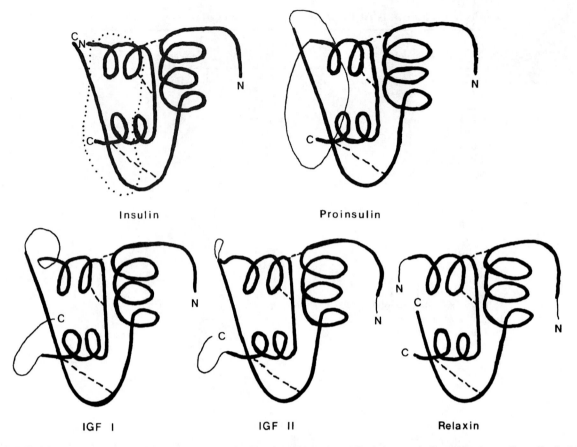

Insulin   Proinsulin

IGF I   IGF II   Relaxin

Figure 3-11. **Structural homologies in the insulin family of peptides.** A and B chains are indicated by heavy lines. Dashed lines represent the disulfide bonds between A and B chains. The C-peptide or extensions of the molecule homologous to parts of the insulin C-peptide are represented by the thin lines. From F. F. Bolander (1989). "Molecular Endocrinology," p. 265, Academic Press, Inc.

	5	10	15	20	25	30	35	39
Human	S-Y-S-M-E-H-F-R-W-G-K-P-V-G-K-K-R-R-P-V-L-V-Y-P-N-G-A-E-R-E-S-A-E-A-F-P-L-E-F
Bovine						E	S	
Ovine						Q	S	
Porcine						E	L	

Figure 3-12. **Amino acid sequences for some mammalian corticotropins (ACTHs).** The amino acid sequences are shown for human, cow, sheep, and pig ACTH. Only the differences (substitutions) with respect to human ACTH are shown. Amino acid abbreviations are provided in Appendix A.

in the cytoplasm until released from the cell through exocytosis into the interstitial fluids or blood. Bioregulators released into interstitial fluids (i.e., cytocrines, autocrines, neurotransmitters, neuromodulators) rely on diffusion and any movement of the interstitial fluid that might occur to allow them to reach their target sites more rapidly. In the blood, bioregulatory peptides may complex to specific plasma proteins that enhance their transportability in the blood, slow their rate of metabolism by blood peptidases, and may even facilitate interactions with target cells.

The time for removal or rate of disappearance of any bioregulator from the blood through degradation, excretion, or removal by target cells is termed its **biological half-life**. This usually is determined by following the rate of removal of radioactively labeled molecules from the blood. The time required to remove or clear half of the labeled dose from the blood is the half-life. In general terms, a larger peptide will have a longer biological

Table 3-5. Families of Human Protein Chemical Regulators

Family	Members	Molecular weight	Common features
Pituitary/placental glycoproteins	1. hTSH	32,000	α Subunit of 89 AA, β subunit, 112 AA
	2. hFSH	32,000	α Subunit of 89 AA, β subunit, 115 AA
	3. hLH	32,000	α Subunit of 89 AA, β subunit, 115 AA
	4. hCG	38,000	like LH in structure and action
Nonglycoprotein pituitary/placental hormones	1. hGH	22,650	191 AA
	2. hProlactin	23,510	198 AA
	3. hPL (hCS)	22,000	191 AA
TGF-β superfamily	1. TGF-β1		Composed of α and β subunits
	2. Bone morphogenic proteins (BMPs)		Composed of α and β subunits
	3. Müllerian-inhibiting substance (MIS)		Composed of α and β subunits
	4. Inhibins		Composed of α and β subunits
	5. Activins		Composed of α and β subunits

half-life than a smaller peptide (see Table 3-5). Notable exceptions are the smallest peptides such as TRH that are modified during post-translational processing in a manner that slows their enzymatic degradation while in the blood. A number of hormones possess special modifications or activities that prolong their presence in the blood (see below).

D. Receptors for Amine and Peptide Bioregulators

Although amino acids, amines, peptides, and proteins are soluble in blood plasma and interstitial fluids, they cannot readily pass through cell membranes that are composed largely of phospholipids and cholesterol. Instead, they bind to **receptor proteins** embedded in the target cell membrane. A **target cell** for a peptide bioregulator is a cell possessing receptor proteins in its external membrane that specifically bind the bioregulator. A molecule that binds to a binding site on a receptor is termed a **ligand**. Receptor binding of a ligand employs a specific key-and-lock mechanism like that of an enzyme and its substrate. Binding of the ligand is followed by observable changes in the target cell that are characteristic for each ligand-receptor complex. These changes could involve (1) opening or closing of ion channels affecting membrane potentials and/or secretion, (2) activating or inactivating of an enzyme, (3) initiating a series of reactions or cascading events, and/or (4) activating transcription factors that alter gene activity. Changes caused by such mechanisms could affect development and differentiation, cellular biochemistry and morphology, as well as general aspects of physiology and behavior.

A receptor molecule consists of several functional regions or **domains**. One of these domains has a three-dimensional **binding site** for the bioregulator that recognizes the shape of this bioregulator and will not bind any other molecule unless it closely or exactly conforms to that shape (Figure 3-13). This relationship is like the lock-and-key fit so often described for an enzyme (the receptor, in this case) and its substrate (the bioregulator). Once a ligand is bound to a receptor, the receptor changes from **unoccupied receptor** to **occupied receptor**. A responsive target cell typically has thousands of receptors for a specific ligand. Many non-target cells may express a low number of receptors for the same ligand but are unresponsive for reasons discussed below.

There are several classes of membrane receptor types, each of which is specific for different ligands or groups of closely related ligands. Since a portion of these receptors passes through the membrane, they can be described as **transmembrane receptors**. Some receptors have innate enzymatic activity following binding of a ligand whereas others may produce their effects secondarily through other kinds of proteins.

Receptors are often characterized by the types of cellular activity they produce. **Insulin, growth hormone (GH)**, and **insulin-like growth factor-I (IGF-I)** as well as **epidermal growth factor (EGF), colony-stimulating factor (CSF)**, and **platelet-derived growth factor (PDGF)** have receptors possessing **tyrosine kinase** enzymatic activity. Tyrosine kinases are a general class of enzymes that phosphorylate tyrosine residues in proteins. A number of receptors have been characterized as having innate protein kinase activity with the ability to

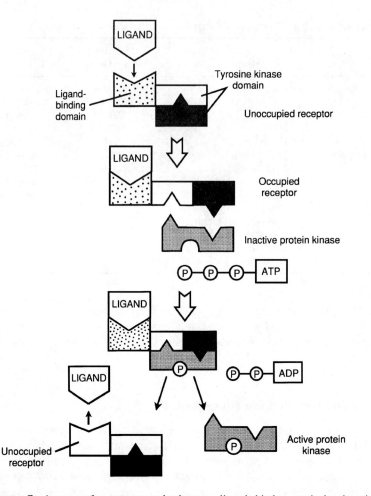

Figure 3-13. **Ligand-receptor fit.** As occurs for enzymes and substrates, ligands bind to particular domains on receptor molecules and typically cause conformational changes in the receptor that are important for initiating a response in a target cell. This hypothetical illustration imagines a ligand that binds to a receptor with tyrosine kinase activity. Once occupied, the receptor changes shape and now interacts with ATP and a protein kinase. The protein kinase is activated by phosphorylation and now can produce other effects in the cell. The receptor releases its ligand for degradation and returns to its unoccupied state. Alternatively, the ligand-receptor complex may be internalized prior to release of ligand and/or degrading of the receptor.

phosphorylate tyrosine in other proteins. There are also kinases that phosphorylate other amino acids, such as serine or threonine kinases.

Receptor tyrosine kinases have several molecular domains. The **extracellular domain** is responsible for binding a specific ligand and is represented by the α-subunit. This domain is unique for each type of receptor and the ligand it binds preferentially. The **transmembrane domain** crosses the plasma membrane once to connect the extracellular domain to the β-subunit that houses the **intracellular** or **tyrosine kinase domain**. The receptor also contains one or more **regulatory domains**, and there is also a **juxtamembrane region** that separates the intracellular domain from the plasma membrane and the transmembrane domain.

Receptor tyrosine kinases for growth factors form dimers after binding their ligand, and experimental studies show that formation of dimers is necessary to fully activate the tyrosine kinase domain. The receptor tyrosine kinases for insulin and insulin-like growth factors apparently are effectively dimerized prior to addition of ligand. Typically, both tyrosine kinase receptors bind a ligand before forming dimers. In the case of GH, one molecule of GH binds to two receptors that activate two kinases. This complex is called a **Janus kinase**, named for the two-faced Greek god who guarded gates.

Numerous studies have shown that occupied membrane receptors eventually are internalized through formation of endosomes. The activity of these receptors on the membranes of endosomes may be important

Table 3-6. Biological Half-Life of Some Mammalian Hormones

Hormone	Size[a]	Species	Approximate half-life (min)
TRH	3	Mice	2
		Human	5
OXY	9	Rat	2
		Human	3
AVP	9	Rat	3–4
α-MSH	13	Dog	2
GnRH	10	Pig	12
		Dog	5
		Human	2–5
Gastrin	17	Human	7–8
ACTH	39	Rat	1–4
		Pig	5–7
		Human	5–29
Glucagon	29	Human	5–10
β-Endorphin	31	Human	15
Calcitonin	32	Rat	2
		Human	3
		Pig	2–5
CCK	33	Human	2
Insulin	51	Pig	6
		Human	3–4
Proinsulin	82	Pig	20
		Human	18–25
GH	200	Human	20–30
PRL	198	Rabbit	16
		Cow	29
LH	32,000[b]	Human	136
FSH	32,000[b]	Human	220
Cortisol	300[b]	Human	90
Aldosterone	300[b]	Human	35
T_4	777[b]	Human	7 days
T_3	651[b]	Human	24 hr

[a] Number of amino acids or [b] molecular weight; except for glycoproteins, the number of amino acids × 100 gives an approximate estimate of molecular weight of any peptide (120 × is more accurate but not as easy to calculate).

in maintaining sustained effects of a ligand following internalization of the ligand-receptor complex. However, studies employing mutant forms of insulin and EGF receptors that fail to undergo internalization when occupied show that internalization is not a requisite for transduction of the external signal into the cell. Once occupied, these mutant receptors exhibit tyrosine kinase activity followed by the typical intracellular events normally associated with that ligand.

The receptor tyrosine kinases undergo rapid autophosphorylation that makes them capable of interacting with other proteins. Phosphorylation of tyrosine residues facilitates binding of other proteins to the receptor tyrosine kinase. There is evidence for interactions of receptor tyrosine kinase with intracellular serine and threonine protein kinases that may carry the message to other intracellular sites.

Molecules in the secretin-glucagon family of peptides, which includes **vasoactive intestinal peptide (VIP)**, **pituitary adenylate cyclase-activating polypeptide (PACAP)**, **glucagon**, and **secretin** all have similar sequences of amino acids and often bind to the same receptor proteins. **Growth hormone (GH)** and **prolactin (PRL)** from the pituitary have similar molecular structures as do their receptors. Similarly, there may be more than one kind of receptor for a given ligand, of which each differs slightly in its composition and binding characteristics. Thus, different tissues may contain different receptor forms for the same ligand (Table 3-7).

An important group of receptors are the **G-protein coupled receptors**. These G-proteins are embedded within the cell membrane and were so-named because they can bind and hydrolyze the nucleotide **guanosine triphosphate**, or **GTP**. The transmembrane domain of these G-protein coupled receptors traverses the cell

Table 3-7. Receptor Types

Enzyme-linked receptors (one transmembrane unit)
    Tyrosine kinase activity
      EGF family
      Insulin family
      PDGF family
      NGF family
    Serine kinase activity
      TGFβ
      Activin
      AMH/MIS
    Guanylate cyclases
      cGMP generating
Serpentine (7 transmembrane units; G-protein linked) receptors
    β-Type receptors (increase Ca^{2+}; increase cAMP)
      β-Adrenergic (βAR)
      αAR
      Dopamine receptor
      Serotonin receptors
    Muscarinic type (increase Ca^{2+}; decrease cAMP)
    Neurokinin type
    Non-neurokinin type
      Calcitonin receptor
Fibronectin-like receptors
    Class 1: Cytokine family
      Erythropoietin receptor
      Interleukin-1 receptor
    Class 2: TNF/IFN family
      TNF receptor
      Interferon (IFN) receptor
      Ubiquitin receptor
Nuclear receptor superfamily
See Table 3-13

membrane seven times (see Figure 3-14). Because of this snake-like traversing of the membrane, these receptors are sometimes reffered to as **serpentine receptors**. G-proteins are critical for the action of bioregulators employing this mechanism that generate formation of "second messengers" in the cytosol of the target cells that mediate the ligand's actions (see below).

1. Multiple Receptor Subtypes

Each bioregulator must have a specific receptor associated with its target cell in order to produce a localized and specific effect. However, there may be more than one kind of receptor for a given bioregulator resulting in different tissue-specific responses to the same bioregulator. Receptor variants or subtypes may be the product of gene duplications or may be due to splice variants formed during their synthesis. Cell membrane receptors are often complexes of several proteins, each the product of different genes. As we learn more about bioregulator actions, we note that there are small differences in cell membrane receptors for a given bioregulator in different tissues that influence binding and may even be connected to different intracellular mechanisms. Typically, because of variances in the molecular composition of receptors, there is differential sensitivity of receptors to agonists or antagonists (see Box 3A). This differential sensitivity often becomes incorporated into the name of the receptor type. For example, there are two types of **cholinergic receptors** for the neurotransmitter **acetylcholine** in heart muscle and skeletal muscle. The cholinergic receptors of heart muscle cells are stimulated by a substance obtained from certain mushrooms called **muscarinic acid** but those of skeletal muscle are not. In turn, skeletal muscle cholinergic receptors are activated by **nicotine** whereas heart muscle receptors are not. Consequently, we refer to the heart receptors as **muscarinic cholinergic receptors** and those of skeletal muscle as **nicotinic cholinergic receptors**. **V$_2$ receptors** for arginine vasopressin are linked

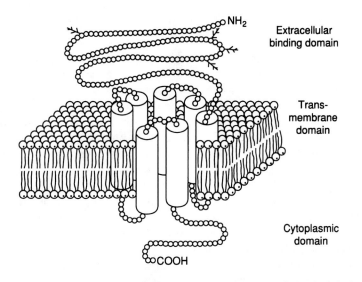

Figure 3-14. **Representation of a serpentine transmembrane receptor**. The extracellular domain is responsible for binding the specific ligand. The transmembrane domain traverses the membrane seven times before ending in the cytoplasmic domain that is coupled with a G-protein. The type of G-protein is dependent upon the type of receptor. Occupied receptors often form dimers prior to activation of G-proteins and production of second messengers. Based on numerous sources.

to a different cellular mechanisms of action than are **V₁ receptors**, and arginine vasopressin produces markedly different intracellular events in different tissues depending on the type of receptor present.

Receptors for the catecholamine neurotransmitters NE and E are designated as **α-receptors** or **β-receptors**. These receptors involve several proteins each and exist in a variety of subforms (for example, β1 and β2). NE has a higher affinity for the α-receptors whereas as E binds well to either α- or β-receptors. Biochemists have synthesized specific agonists and antagonists for each adrenergic receptor and its subtypes. Thus there can be multiple ligands (keys) with differing specificities for receptors (locks) as illustrated in Box Table 3A-1. Dopamine **D₁-receptors** are distinct from **D₂-receptors** and also are characterized by binding different synthetic agonists and antagonists.

The mechanisms of action for these multiple receptor types may be very different with one type operating through one mechanism and another type through a different mechanism of action. However, the biological meaning of variance in receptor types is not always so obvious. In some cases, we may be looking at evolving receptors moving toward greater selectivity and tissue specificity for ligands. Consequently, we may not be able to assign an "adaptive value" at this time, leading to confusion about what their roles might be. Nevertheless, from the pharmacological point of view, this diversity in receptor types has provided mechanisms through which we can experimentally investigate how bioregulators interact with cells and produce their dramatic effects and has provided avenues for specific drug therapies of clinical disorders.

E. The Second Messenger Concept

Following binding of the bioregulator to its receptor, a new set of events is initiated in the target cell which are specific to that bioregulator and its receptor. How is this orchestrated? Generally speaking, the bioregulator can be considered the **first messenger** carrying a signal from the secreting cell to a target cell. The first messenger binds to its receptor and may initiate the synthesis of cytosolic **second messenger** molecules that carry the bioregulatory signal into the interior of the cell. The message of relatively few molecules of first messenger is thereby amplified as many second messenger molecules are produced for each first messenger bound to a receptor and for as long as the receptor is occupied by the ligand (Figure 3-15). The need for this amplification at least in part relates to the short half-life of second messengers. It is critical that there be enough membrane receptors and second messengers available to amplify the message sufficiently to bring about specific internal changes in the target cell.

Box 3A.   Agonists and Antagonists

The development of agonists and antagonists for various bioregulatory ligands has been instrumental in experimental studies of the mechanism of action of ligands but also for clinical studies and development of drug therapies for various endocrine disorders. Agonists bind to the natural receptor for a particular ligand and mimic its action. A strong agonist may bind even better than the natural ligand (i.e., it may have a higher affinity for the receptor) as opposed to a weak agonist. Similarly, an antagonist also binds to the same receptor but does not activate it. Strong antagonists may bind so tightly to the receptor that they prevent binding of the natural ligand. The discovery that some agonists or antagonists were more effective in certain target tissues than in others led to the discover of multiple receptor types.

One of the first ligands to be recognized as having multiple receptor types was epinephrine. First we discovered two receptor types, the α-adrenergic receptor and the β-adrenergic receptor. Soon, subtypes of each receptor were discovered (α_1, α_2, β_1, etc.). The binding of epinephrine and its agonists to different adrenergic receptor (AR) subtypes in an array is similar to the keying of locks in a building used by multiple groups of people (Table 3A-1). Like a master key, epinephrine binds to and activates all adrenergic receptor subtypes. Phenylephrine is like a submaster key that opens all of the α-sublocks but none of the β-sublocks.

Various endocrine-disrupting chemicals (EDCs) present as environmental pollutants may produce their effects through different receptor subtypes. Thus, knowledge of receptor specificity is important when evaluating their effects. For example, phytoestrogens bind principally to ERβ receptors whereas estrogenic phthalates bind to ERα. Because these receptor subtypes appear in different tissues in the body, it would influence where you should look for possible effects.

Table 3A-1.   Relationship between a Ligand and Its Receptor Subtypes

Keys	Locks	Ligands	Receptor subtypes
Master key	Opens all locks	Epinephrine	Binds to all ARs
Submaster key α	Opens all α locks	Phenylephrine	Binds to all αARs
Submaster key β	Opens all β locks	Isoproteronol	Binds to all βARs
Key α 1	Opens α1 locks	Clonidine	Binds to α_1ARs
Key α 2	Opens α2 locks	Prazosin*	Binds to α_2ARs
Key β 1	Opens β1 locks	ICI 89,406*	Binds to β_1ARs
Key β 2	Opens β2 locks	Salbutamol	Binds to β_2ARs

* Antagonist (related key) that fits into a specific AR subtype binding site (lock) and blocks access to any agonist but doesn't activate receptor (doesn't open the lock).

In the 1960s, Earl Sutherland and his coworkers discovered the first second messenger, **cyclic adenosine monophosphate (cAMP)**, while attempting to elucidate the mechanism of action for E on glycogen breakdown in skeletal muscle and liver cells. E has its actions on muscle and liver cells by first binding to what we know now as a cell membrane-bound G-protein coupled receptor. Sutherland was awarded a Nobel Prize for this pioneering work in 1972. Much later, the discovery of the membrane-bound intermediate G-protein operating between the first and second messengers led to a Nobel Prize in 1994 for Alfred Gilman and Martin Robdell. Although the G-protein logically could be called a second messenger, this latter term has been retained for the type of cytosolic messenger originally described by Sutherland's group. Several types of second messenger systems have been discovered that involve the interaction of an occupied receptor with a specific G-protein and results in the production of second messengers.

Activated G-proteins may interact directly with a **signal-generating enzyme** adjacent to or located in the membrane but on the cytosolic side. When a signal-generating enzyme is activated, it catalyzes the synthesis of a second messenger from a specific substrate. The second messenger then initiates intracellular events normally associated with the actions of the first messenger on that cell. Thus, through the second messenger system, a

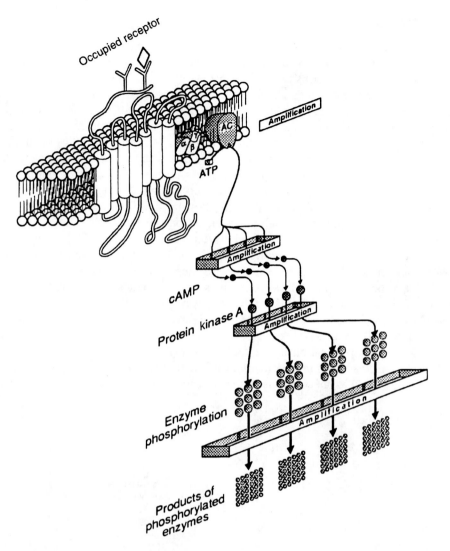

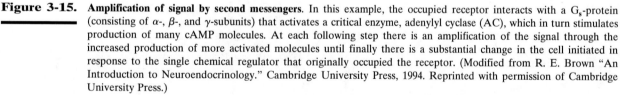

Figure 3-15. **Amplification of signal by second messengers.** In this example, the occupied receptor interacts with a G_s-protein (consisting of α-, β-, and γ-subunits) that activates a critical enzyme, adenylyl cyclase (AC), which in turn stimulates production of many cAMP molecules. At each following step there is an amplification of the signal through the increased production of more activated molecules until finally there is a substantial change in the cell initiated in response to the single chemical regulator that originally occupied the receptor. (Modified from R. E. Brown "An Introduction to Neuroendocrinology." Cambridge University Press, 1994. Reprinted with permission of Cambridge University Press.)

small amount of bioregulator can be amplified to hundreds of active molecules that bring about specific changes in a target cell. Because the ligand-receptor complex is not located at a fixed site in the membrane, it can migrate within the membrane and contact more than one G-protein, thus possibly amplifying its effect even further.

G-proteins may also interact with **ion channels** in the cell membrane. Opening of a calcium channel can influence entrance or exit of calcium ions (Ca^{2+}) that, if a sufficient number of channels are affected, may in turn alter intracellular or membrane events. Hence, an ion such as Ca^{2+} that enters the cell and causes specific changes, such as activation of an enzyme, following binding of a bioregulator to its receptor also can be called a second messenger. Other types of receptors can influence Ca^{2+} influx by mechanisms that do not involve G-proteins.

Second messengers also may alter cytoplasmic phosphorylating systems. This may result in additional effects including activation of transcription factors resulting in delayed effects on protein synthesis, altered functioning of enzymes, etc. Such generalized effects may even mimic some events activated by other bioregulators that are capable of altering phosphorylating systems (see discussion of kinase cascade ahead).

1. The Cyclic AMP Second Messenger System

Seconds after epinephrine binds to the target cell, a unique compound is synthesized. The new molecule is **cAMP**, the end product of the hydrolysis of the energy-rich molecule **adenosine triphosphate (ATP)**. In this novel form of AMP, the phosphate forms two bonds instead of one to the adenine base (Figure 3-16). cAMP is formed by a cell membrane-associated, signal-generating enzyme called **adenylyl cyclase**. Different forms of adenylyl cyclase are known that may be stimulated, inhibited, or unaffected by calcium ions. Epinephrine-occupied receptor interacts with a particular G-protein called G_s-**protein** that in turn interacts with adenylyl cyclase and generates many molecules of cAMP (amplification). Additional studies show that administration of cAMP can mimic all the actions of E, supporting its role as a true intracellular messenger.

When the receptor is unoccupied, the adenylyl cyclase is inactive and GDP is bound to the G_s-protein. The G_s-protein consists of three peptide subunits: α-, β-, and γ-subunits (Figure 3-17). The occupied receptor interacts with the β- and γ-subunits of the G_s-protein allowing the dissociation of GDP and the binding of GTP to the α-subunit of G_s-protein. The α-subunit then dissociates from the β- and γ-units to interact with the catalytic portion of the adenylyl cyclase and generate cAMP. Intrinsic GTPase-degrading activity of the α-subunit converts the GTP back to GDP, reducing its stimulatory effect on the catalytic domain of adenylyl cyclase. The α-subunit then returns to its association with the other G_s-subunits.

The specific cellular response to cAMP as a second messenger depends on the cell type involved. Once generated in a liver or skeletal muscle cell, cAMP can repeatedly combine with **protein kinase A (PKA)**, a cytosolic enzyme that phosphorylates the inactive enzyme **phosphorylase kinase** which in turn coverts **phosphorylase-b** into its active form, **phosphorylase-a**. Active phosphorylase-a triggers the enzymatic breakdown of glycogen to provide glucose for energy production in the target cell (see Figure 3-18). In an adipose or fat cell, the cAMP-activated PKA activates a **hormone-dependent lipase** that results in hydrolysis of fats. cAMP also may produce effects via other cellular mechanisms associated with the same or different first messengers. For

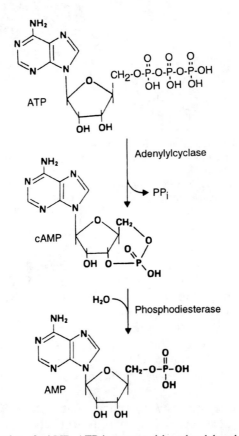

Figure 3-16. **Formation and degradation of cAMP.** ATP is converted by adenylyl cyclase to cAMP. One of several phosphodiesterases (see Table 3-8) inactivates cAMP by converting it to ordinary AMP.

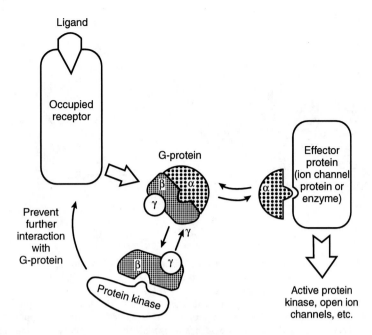

Figure 3-17. **G-proteins consist of three subunits.** The α-subunit which has innate GTP-binding and hydrolyzing capacity can separate from the other subunits following interaction with an appropriate, occupied receptor. The free α-subunit interacts with a membrane channel protein or an enzyme that generates a second messenger. Once the GTP has been hydrolyzed, the subunits recombine. The complex of free β- and γ-subunits may interact with the occupied receptor and prevent its interaction with intact G-proteins as reported for the β-adrenergic receptor (see text).

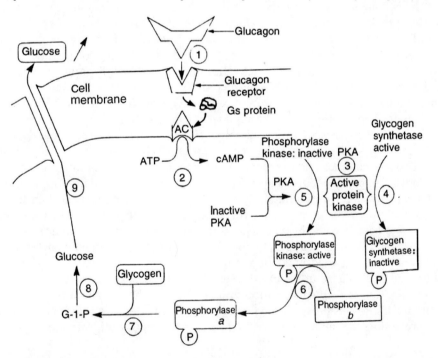

Figure 3-18. **Actions of cAMP within target cell.** After binding to its cell membrane receptor (1), the peptide hormone glucagon produces multiple effects in liver cells by first stimulating production of cAMP (2) which activates protein kinase A, PKA (3). PKA phosphorylates the enzyme glycogen synthetase converting it from an active to an inactive form (4) thus reducing glycogen synthesis. Phosphorylation of the enzyme phosphorylase kinase (5) converts inactive enzyme phosphorylase-*b* through an additional phosphorylation to its active form (6) and causes hydrolysis of glycogen to release glucose-1-phosphate, G-1-P (7) which in liver can be hydrolyzed to free glucose and free phosphate (8). Free glucose leaves the cell via mediated transport (9). AC = adenylyl cyclase. [Modified from Norman and Litwack (1997). "Hormones," 2nd Ed., p. 8, Academic Press, Inc., San Diego.]

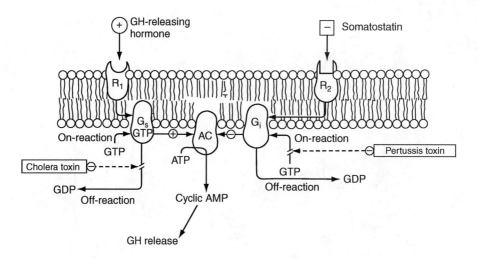

Figure 3-19. **G-protein inteactions and inhibition of cellular reactions.** Growth hormone (GH)-releasing hormone binds to its receptor (R_1) and activates the G_s-protein that turns on adenylyl cyclase (AC) to synthesize cAMP from ATP. cAMP acts as a second messenger to mediate release of GH. Somatostatin (SST), after binding to the R_2 receptor, works through an inhibitory G_i-protein to prevent the activation of AC. Thus, in the presence of SST, it is difficult to stimulate GH release except through addition of exogenous cAMP. A similar mechanism operates in the antagonism of norepinephrine by acetylcholine in cardiac muscle. [Modified from Frohman and Jansson (1986). Growth hormone-releasing hormone. *Endocrine Rev.* **7**, 223–253. © The Endocrine Society.]

example, in cardiac muscle cells, cAMP binds to calcium channels, allowing an influx of Ca^{2+} that prolongs depolarization of the cell membrane and influences the degree of cardiac muscle contraction.

In addition to the cytoplasmic bioregulatory elements associated with cAMP, a **cAMP regulatory element binding protein (CREB)** has been isolated from the nucleus and identified as a transcription factor that can regulate gene transcription. This could explain some of the delayed effects of peptide hormones on protein synthesis observed following initial enzymatic activation through cAMP. Bioregulatory elements like CREB as well as other transcription factors could be considered "third messengers" that mediate nuclear events.

Cell membranes often contain another G-protein called a **G_i-protein** that can inhibit the cAMP mechanism in the following manner. Apparently, certain bioregulators can bind to a receptor that employs the G_i-protein which, like the G_s-protein, consists of three subunits. The G_i-protein also has a unique α-subunit but its β- and γ-subunits are very similar to those of the G_s-protein. The G_i-protein α-subunit interacts with the G_s protein-adenylyl cyclase complex and prevents cAMP generation. Several bioregulators that antagonize the actions of cAMP-dependent peptide bioregulators are known to operate through a G_i-protein (see Figure 3-19).

Several drugs have proven very useful for studying cAMP second messenger mechanisms. Adenylyl cyclase can be activated directly by a diterpene called **forskolin**, obtained from an Indian medicinal herb, *Coleus forskohli*. This plant had been used with some success for centuries in India to treat heart disease, respiratory ailments, convulsions, and insomnia. **Cholera toxin** obtained from the pathogenic bacteria blocks the GTPase activity of the α-subunit of the G_s-protein. It is this action in the digestive tract of a the cholera patient that leads to continuous diarrhea, resulting in excessive dehydration and, eventually, death. Another bacterial product, **pertussis toxin**, causes ADP-ribosylation of a cysteine on the α-subunit of the inhibitory G_i-protein, reducing its affinity for GTP. This prevents the G_i α-subunit from interacting normally, causing a slight rise in cAMP levels and preventing the action of bioregulators that normally work through the G_i-protein.

2. Inositol Trisphosphate and Diacylglycerol as Second Messengers

Some receptors interact with yet another G-protein, the **G_q-protein**, that activates an additional signal-generating enzyme complex called **phospholipase C (PLC)**. The substrate for PLC is **phosphatidylinositol bisphosphate (PIP$_2$)** which is cleaved to produce *two* second messengers, **inositol trisphosphate (IP$_3$)** and **diacylglycerol (DAG)**, each of which has independent actions. The neurotransmitter acetylcholine produces its effects through a G_q-protein, as does the peptide vasopressin in some of its target cells.

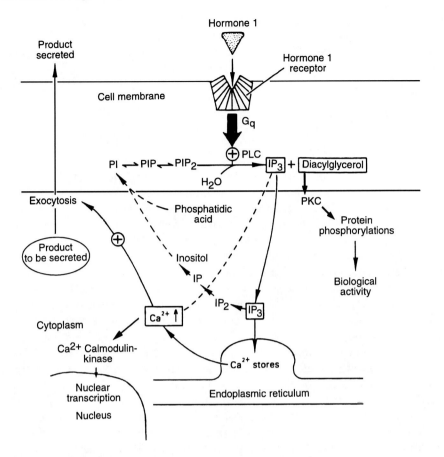

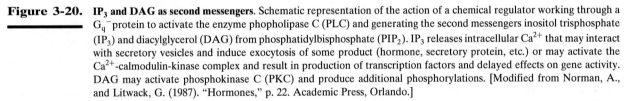

Figure 3-20. **IP$_3$ and DAG as second messengers.** Schematic representation of the action of a chemical regulator working through a G$_q^-$protein to activate the enzyme phopholipase C (PLC) and generating the second messengers inositol trisphosphate (IP$_3$) and diacylglycerol (DAG) from phosphatidylbisphosphate (PIP$_2$). IP$_3$ releases intracellular Ca^{2+} that may interact with secretory vesicles and induce exocytosis of some product (hormone, secretory protein, etc.) or may activate the Ca^{2+}-calmodulin-kinase complex and result in production of transcription factors and delayed effects on gene activity. DAG may activate phosphokinase C (PKC) and produce additional phosphorylations. [Modified from Norman, A., and Litwack, G. (1987). "Hormones," p. 22. Academic Press, Orlando.]

IP$_3$ interacts with IP$_3$-receptors on the external membrane of the endoplasmic reticulum to release stored Ca^{+2} into the cytosolic compartment of the cell. In muscle cells, these ions bind to special proteins that affect contraction. In other cells, the resulting increase in intracellular Ca^{+2} usually involves a cytoplasmic calcium-binding peptide called **calmodulin** (Figure 3-20). Calmodulin can produce a variety of cellular effects depending on the cell Type involved. It can activate certain enzymes and also can increase the rate of degradation of cAMP, thus antagonizing the actions of any first messenger that operates through cAMP as a second messenger. Activated calmodulin actually combines with and activates the major enzyme necessary for cAMP degradation, thus diminishing the effectiveness of cAMP as a second messenger (see ahead).

DAG and Ca^{2+} apparently activate the enzyme **protein kinase C (PKC)** which in turn may activate other cytoplasmic enzymes. Furthermore, DAG may serve as a substrate for production of arachidonic acid, a precursor for the synthesis of eicosanoids, a unique collection of lipid bioregulators (see ahead).

3. cGMP as a Second Messenger

The role of **cyclic guanosine monophosphate (cGMP)** as a second messenger has not been studied to the same extent as the cAMP system but is similar to the cAMP mechanisms in many ways. The signal-generating enzyme **guanylyl cyclase** is activated by a small family of peptide bioregulators that includes **atrial natriuretic**

peptide (ANP). Guanylyl cyclase appears to be an integral part of the receptors for these peptides and, following binding of the appropriate ligand, produces cGMP from GTP.

One of the actions of testosterone on the penis is activation of an enzyme, **nitric oxide synthetase (NOS)**. This enzyme is responsible for production of **nitric oxide (NO)** that in turn elevates cGMP levels and contributes to induction of the erectile response by the penis. Oxytocin also elevates cGMP through activation of NO production.

4. Calcium Flux as an Intracellular Messenger

Recent studies of hormone action have discovered a common theme involving Ca^{2+} cycling across the cell membrane as a potential mechanism for sustaining a cellular response even hours after the initial binding of the hormone. This has led to development of a model system by Howard Rasmussen and his colleagues using mammalian adrenal cortical cells to study the involvement of Ca^{2+} in the action of certain bioregulators. Initial observations of the action of the octapeptide angiotensin II (ANG-II) on the sustained release of the mineralocorticoid hormone aldosterone found only a transient rise in cytosolic Ca^{2+} following binding of ANG-II to cells of the adrenal cortex, yet a prolonged release of aldosterone was observed (Figure 3-20). However, it was noted that there was an increase in Ca^{2+} influx as well as efflux. They discovered that this Ca^{2+} cycling was caused by a calcium-calmodulin-dependent protein kinase. Furthermore, not only does this enzyme phosphorylate and activate the Ca^{2+} pump, it also behaves as a plasma membrane-associated transducer that converts the Ca^{2+} cycling message into a sustained cellular event: release of aldosterone.

When a ligand-receptor complex interacts with the enzyme PLC, the substrate PIP_2 is converted to IP_3 and DAG. The IP_3 interacts with the endoplasmic reticulum causing a transient increase in intracellular Ca^{2+} (Figure 3-20). These Ca^{2+} bind to calmodulin, resulting in the activation of PKC which in the presence of DAG becomes associated with the plasma membrane and stimulates its Ca^{2+} pump. As long as DAG remains in the plasma membrane, the PKC remains there as well. All of these events lead to a submembrane increase in Ca^{2+} that is believed to facilitate the phosphorylating activities of PKC and to bring about a prolonged response.

Aldosterone is responsible for directing reabsorption of Na^+ from the urine by kidney cells and returning Na^+ to the blood (see Chapter 8). An appropriate ratio of Na^+ to K^+ in blood and extracellular fluids is essential for maintaining normal plasma membrane potentials on cells. Inappropriate release of aldosterone could lead to death caused by neural and muscular dysfunction. This is prevented by the sensitivity of the Ca^{2+} channels in adrenocortical cells to circulating levels of K^+. High K^+ hyperpolarizes the plasma membrane of the adrenal cell and its voltage-sensitive Ca^{2+} pumps so that ANG-II cannot produce sustained Ca^{2+} cycling. Likewise, lowered K^+ partially depolarizes the Ca^{2+} channels and makes them more responsive to ANG-II.

A similar mechanism involving Ca^{+2} cycling across the plasma membrane has been described for the regulation of insulin release from the pancreatic B-cell (see Chapter 13). Opening of Ca^{2+} channels is facilitated by high circulating levels of glucose so that more insulin is released to bring about a decrease in blood glucose.

F. Turning Off the Response to Bioregulators

Once a bioregulator binds to its receptors, the target cell is stimulated to produce second messengers until the occupied receptor becomes unoccupied again. In order to terminate the action on the target cell, the bioregulator must be separated from its receptor and the second messengers also must be inactivated. Several mechanisms have evolved in cells to turn off the response of the target cell once it has been stimulated. Different mechanisms turn off the response at the receptor and at the second messenger level.

1. Fate of Membrane-Bound Ligands

The earliest clues to the fate of first messenger ligands came from studies of the action of acetylcholine and NE on their target cells. In the case of acetylcholine, an enzyme called **acetylcholinesterase (AChE)** located in the postsynaptic cell membrane was found to degrade acetylcholine to acetic acid and choline, freeing the receptors from ligand until more acetylcholine was released from the presynaptic cell. Other studies showed that the neurotransmitter NE was either retaken up by the presynaptic neuron where it was recycled or it was taken up by nearby glial cells which degraded it intracellularly. However, the fate of peptide ligands soon was shown to follow a unique pathway.

The first reports of finding peptide bioregulators inside target cells was assumed to be an artifact of the methods employed to demonstrate their presence since it was believed then that they did not enter cells but bound only to the cell membrane. We now know that subsequent to occupation and activation of receptors, occupied receptors with their ligands migrate along the surface of the cell membrane to specialized regions or pits that are involved in formation of internalized vesicles called **endosomes** (or phagosomes). These pits are membrane regions where specific proteins (e.g., **clathrin, calveolin**, or **dynamin**) have accumulated (Figure 3-21). Endosome formation results from endocytosis, and each endosome consists of a small sphere of cell membrane with occupied receptors having the ligand-binding side extending into its lumen. A variety of internal **Rab proteins** are involved in distribution of endosomes within the cell depending on their eventual fate. They may contact lysosomes containing hydrolytic enzymes that fuse with the endosomes to form **endolysosomes** (or phagolysosomes). The hydrolytic enzymes may degrade both the receptors and the ligands. In other cases, endosomes or portions of an endosome may be directed back toward the cell membrane and the associated receptors without their ligands may be recycled back to the cell surface.

The discovery of this internalization of occupied receptors partially explains the phenomenon of **down-regulation** of receptors observed in most bioregulatory systems following arrival of the ligand at its target. Down-regulation refers to the observed reduction in receptor number that typically occurs as evidenced by reduced sensitivity of the target cell following the initial stimulation by the bioregulator. A later increase in receptors or an **up-regulation** of receptors may follow ligand-stimulated protein synthesis. Thus, up- and down-regulation can be considered mechanisms for altering the dynamic range of a hormone-sensitive system. In many developmental systems, the first contact of a ligand with the target cell may result in up-regulation of receptors and accelerated binding and subsequent actions of the ligand on the target cell. Once the target cell

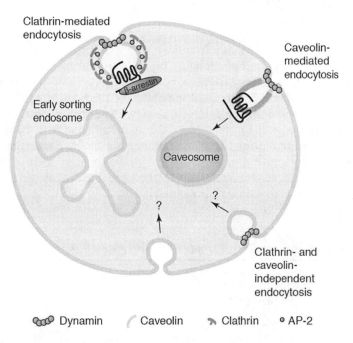

Figure 3-21. Down-regulation of occupied receptors. Occupied receptors migrate along the cell membrane to locations where endosomes form. These sites may be associated with the special proteins such as clathrin or caveolin as well as dynamin. Clathrin- and caveolin-independent endocytosis may occur where only dynamin is present. Fusion of endosomes with lysosomes to form endolysosomes results in degradation of both ligand and most or all of the receptors. Formation of small vesicles containing some receptors allows for possible recycling of receptors directly to the cell surface or indirectly via the Golgi apparatus. (Reprinted from Gaborik, Z., and Hunyady, L. Intracellular trafficking of hormone receptors. *Trends in Endocrin. and Metabolism* **15**, 286–293, 1994. Elsevier Publishers.) See color insert, plate 4.

has responded, down-regulation occurs frequently so that the cell cannot be restimulated until after a period of recovery and reestablishment of a sufficient receptor population in the cell membrane.

2. Receptor and G-Protein Interaction

Phosphorylation of the β-adrenergic receptor prevents it from interacting with the G_s-protein. Once activated, the β-subunit and γ-subunit complex of the G_s-protein can activate a protein kinase called **β-adrenergic receptor kinase (βark)** which then allows a cytosolic protein, **β-arrestin**, to bind to the phosphorylated receptor. In this state, the occupied receptor is unable to continue its interaction with the G_s-protein.

3. Fate of Second Messengers

Just as it is important to remove the first messengers to allow a cell to stop responding to a bioregulator, so second messengers also must be degraded. Specific enzymes are present in the cytosol to degrade second messengers. The best known of these enzymes are the **phosphodiesterases** that degrade cyclic nucleotides (see Table 3-8). One such phosphodiesterase has a high affinity for cAMP and rapidly destroys it. Binding of cAMP to PKA and activation of a specific metabolic pathway in a target cell is thus a dynamic event governed by the generation of cAMP and its rate of degradation by a particular phosphodiesterase. Certain drugs called **methylxanthines** are potent inhibitors of phosphodiesterase and can be used to potentiate the actions of a bioregulator by prolonging the half-life of cAMP. One of these drugs, **caffeine**, is used commonly in experimental studies. Another drug, **theophylline**, is administered to augment the natural action of epinephrine in order to alleviate asthmatic symptoms in humans.

IP_3 is reduced progressively to inositol by **phosphomonoesterases**. These esterases are inhibited by lithium ions. The successful treatment of certain mental illnesses with lithium may be related to its enhancing actions on IP_3 effects.

4. Inactivation in the Blood and/or Excretion of Bioregulators

In addition to the inactivation of peptide bioregulators by their target cells, many of the smaller peptides are degraded rapidly by peptidase enzymes that are present in the blood. These peptidases attack one end of the peptide and remove amino acids one at a time until the ability of the peptide to be recognized by its receptor is diminished, usually progressively, and then lost. Eventually, the entire peptide is demolished. Even larger peptides may be partially degraded while in the blood. Consequently, many peptides of differing numbers of amino acids derived from a secreted bioregulator may be present in the circulation at the same time, all or only some of which may be fully active. For example, the first 34 amino acids of the parathyroid hormone has full biological activity as do larger fragments up to the parent bioregulator of 84 amino acids whereas fragments smaller than the first 34 have little or no activity.

Table 3-8. Classification of Mammalian Phosphodiesterases (PDEs)[a]

Class	Unique features of the PDE	Factors that increase PDE activity
1. Calcium-calmodulin-activated PDE (5 forms described)	Higher affinity for cGMP	GnRH, muscarinic cholinergic agonists
2. cGMP-activated PDE	Have allosteric cGMP-binding site	ANP
3. cGMP-inhibited PDE (3 forms described)	cGMP increases can inhibit cAMP action	Insulin, glucagon, dexamethasone[b]
4. cAMP-specific PDE	cAMP is the intracellular moderator	FSH, PGE, TSH, β-adrenergic agonists
5. cGMP-specific PDE (3 forms described)	Found in retina of eye; employs special G-protein called transducin	Light

[a] See text for abbreviations.
[b] Dexamethasone is a very potent synthetic glucocorticoid.

G. Effects of Membrane-Bound Bioregulators on Nuclear Transcription

In addition to the early actions on target cells by bioregulators that employ membrane-bound receptors, delayed effects on protein synthesis were well known long before we could explain how this effect might be mediated. The physical distance separating the cell membrane from the nucleus is very small by our standards, only about 20 to 30 μm, but this is a huge separation on a molecular scale.

Studies of protein kinase actions have led to the recent development of one hypothesis to link the cell membrane to nuclear events. It is called the **kinase cascade hypothesis** and has evolved from studies of cell division regulation. Cell biologists in many laboratories working on the actions of **mitogens** (factors that stimulate of cell division) or growth factors provided the first connections. Mitogens, such as EGF and many hormones, can cause hyperplasia of target cells (e.g., the effects of IGFs on cartilage and the effect of TSH on goiter formation in the thyroid). New evidence suggests that mitogens induce a cascade of protein kinase-dependent intracellular events not unlike those described for second messenger systems (Figure 3-22). The EGF receptor is one of a family of membrane receptors that when occupied forms a dimer with tyrosine kinase activity. The occupied receptor dimer phosphorylates itself, allowing it to interact with an intracellular heterodimer consisting of two component proteins: **growth factor receptor-binding protein (GRB2)** and the product of a gene first named the **son of sevenless (SOS)** for its role in regulating eye development in fruit flies. Once the heterodimer is activated by occupied EGF receptor, the SOS component interacts with a specific GTP-binding protein (G-protein) called **Ras**, previously identified as a common relay protein for cell growth factors. Ras then exchanges its GDP for a GTP and now binds to a cytoplasmic protein kinase called **Raf-1 protein** which in turn phosphorylates another kinase termed **MEK**. Once activated, MEK phosphorylates a cytoplasmic complex of enzymes known as **mitogen-activated protein kinases (MAPK)**. Among the many proteins phosphorylated by these MAPKs are certain transcription factors (TF) which are translocated to the nucleus where they bind to DNA and ultimately stimulate cell division.

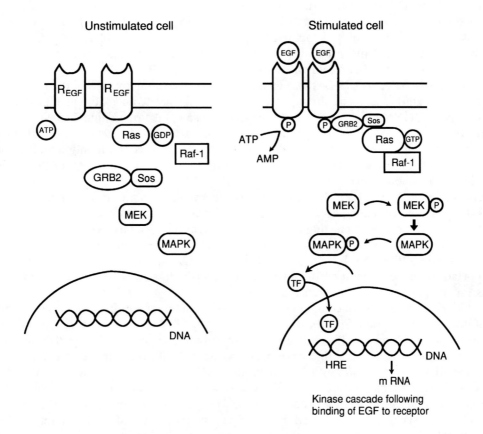

Figure 3-22. The kinase cascade induced by epidermal growth factor (EGF). Occupied receptors interact with a series of protein kinases resulting in production of transcription factors (TF) that as "third messengers" enter the nucleus and alter transcription. See text for explanation of abbreviations.

The kinase cascade hypothesis as outlined here is oversimplified. Evidence suggests there may be additional branches that allow alternative routes for the final activation of the MAPKs. For example, occupied insulin receptors can activate this mitogenic pathway but apparently employ two unique intracellular proteins that interface with the kinase cascade. Nevertheless, the kinase cascade hypothesis provided the first comprehensive explanation of how interactions with a cell membrane receptor can result in nuclear stimulation.

Additional evidence suggests roles for bioregulators that activate PKC and stimulate transcription by employing members of the **Jun-Fos** family of transcription factors. PKA activated by cAMP apparently employs a different family of transcription factors. These observations imply a general role for protein kinases in all the actions of membrane-bound occupied receptors.

1. Cross-Talk

No bioregulator works in a physiological vacuum but rather does its thing amid a complex landscape of simultaneous events. Some bioregulators are known to act cooperatively or antagonistically through effects at their release sites or through interactions at the cell membrane of the target cell. The discovery that many different bioregulators produce their effects through common molecular pathways such as the kinase cascade or via similar second messengers or transcription factors has led to a concept called **cross-talk** that provides another explanation for how different bioregulators can influence cellular processes cooperatively or antagonistically. The possibility of cross-talk emphasizes the importance of not assuming all observations of a bioregulator's action are due only to that bioregulator acting through its own receptor (Figure 3-23).

II. Steroid Bioregulators

The chemical term "**steroid**" refers to a variety of lipoidal compounds, all of which possess the basic structure of four carbon rings known as the cyclopentanoperhydrophenanthrene ring or **steroid nucleus** (Figure 3-24). There are many naturally occurring steroids including cholesterol, 1,25-dihydroxycholecalciferol, the adrenocortical steroids or corticosteroids, and the gonadal sex steroids: androgens, estrogens, and progestogens. The most commonly occurring steroids of these categories are listed in Table 3-9.

1,25-Dihydroxycholecalciferol (1,25-DHC) regulates calcium absorption by cells of the intestinal epithelium. It is synthesized through the sequential cooperation of the skin, liver, and kidney. 1,25-DHC is especially important for growing children and pregnant women to increase uptake of adequate calcium for normal bone development and growth. The initial step in its synthesis depends on the actions of sunlight on skin. An intermediate of 1,25-DHC called **vitamin D** (the "sunshine vitamin") is commonly added to milk in many north temperate countries to ensure an adequate supply of 1,25-DHC for absorption of the calcium provided in milk. Cod liver oil is another rich source of vitamin D.

Androgens (Figures 3-25, 3-26) are defined as compounds that stimulate development of male characteristics; that is, they are masculinizing agents. In males, the primary source for circulating androgens, such as **testosterone**, is the testis, where **luteinizing hormone (LH)** from the pituitary gland stimulates their synthesis and release into the blood. Other important androgens are **dihydrotestosterone (DHT), androstenedione**, and **dehydroepiandrosterone (DHEA)**. In females, the adrenal cortex and the ovaries also synthesize androgens that play important roles (see Chapter 10). During pregnancy, the fetal adrenal becomes an important source of androgens for the placenta (see Chapters 8 and 10).

Estrogens (Figures 3-25, 3-26) are compounds capable of stimulating cornification in epidermal cells lining the vagina of castrate female rats. Cornification involves production of the structural fibrous protein keratin which is the major protein found in skin and hair. A more common test used today for demonstrating estrogen activity involves the use of yeast cells that have been transfected with the estrogen receptor gene. Although traditionally labeled as "female hormones," estrogens are synthesized in males and play important roles just as androgens do in females (see Chapter 10). Estrogens, such as **estradiol**, also stimulate proliferation and vascularization of the uterine mucosa or endometrium. They are converted from androgens by the enzyme **aromatase**. Aromatase synthesis is stimulated by FSH from the pituitary. Additional, important estrogens are **estrone** and **estriol**.

A **progestogen** (Figures 3-25, 3-27) is a compound that maintains pregnancy (i.e., they are progestational) or the secretory condition of the uterine endometrium during the luteal phase of the ovarian cycle. Progestogens

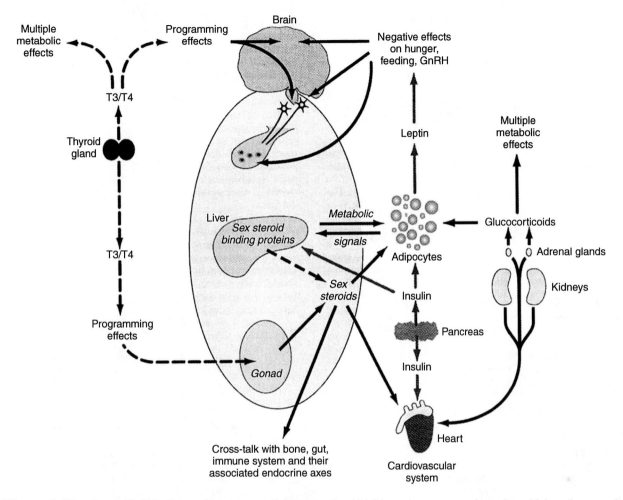

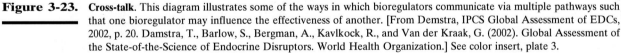

Figure 3-23. **Cross-talk.** This diagram illustrates some of the ways in which bioregulators communicate via multiple pathways such that one bioregulator may influence the effectiveness of another. [From Demstra, IPCS Global Assessment of EDCs, 2002, p. 20. Damstra, T., Barlow, S., Bergman, A., Kavlkock, R., and Van der Kraak, G. (2002). Global Assessment of the State-of-the-Science of Endocrine Disruptors. World Health Organization.] See color insert, plate 3.

(= progestins) such as **pregnenolone, progesterone**, **17α-hydroxypregnenolone**, and **17α-hydroxyprogesterone**, are produced by all steroidogenic tissues as intermediates in the synthesis of most of the other steroid hormones. The role of progesterone as a mammalian reproductive hormone, however, is also well established (see Chapter 10).

There are two subcategories of **corticosteroids** (Figures 3-25, 3-27), glucocorticoids and mineralocorticoids. **Glucocorticoids**, such as **cortisol** and **corticosterone**, can influence protein and carbohydrate metabolism under certain conditions, and their major physiological role appears to be an influence on peripheral utilization of glucose (see Chapters 8, 12). **Mineralocorticoids**, such as **aldosterone**, affect sodium and potassium transport mechanisms in nephrons of the kidney (see Chapter 8). It must be emphasized that these two terms become rather confusing when applied to non-mammalian vertebrates, because a given molecule that possesses gluco-corticoid activity in mammals may have mineralocorticoid activity in non-mammals. Cortisol, for example, is a glucocorticoid in humans, but it also is a mineralocorticoid in teleost fishes (see Chapter 9). Corticoids are synthesized by the outer portions of the adrenal gland (the adrenal cortex) or its homologue in non-mammals (often called **interrenal tissue**) following stimulation by pituitary ACTH (see Chapters 8 and 9). It should be obvious that these definitions for the various categories of steroid hormones are functionally derived.

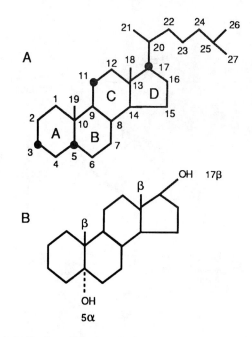

Figure 3-24. **The steroid nucleus.** (A) There are 17 carbons in the nucleus with two additional carbons (18, 19) attached to carbons 13 and 10, respectively. The four rings of the nucleus are labeled A, B, C, and D. The side chain of carbons 20 to 27 is attached to the steroid nucleus at carbon 17 in the β-configuration and is indicated as a solid line. Some of the asymmetric carbons of the nucleus are designated as enlarged dots where the lines representing the covalent bonds intersect. (B) Atoms attached to an asymmetric carbon in the α-configuration are designated with a dashed line. Those attached in the β-configuration (including carbons 18 and 19) are indicated with a solid line.

Table 3-9. Some Common Steroids

Class	Example	Number of Carbons	Site(s) of synthesis
Progestogens	Progesterone	21	Adrenal cortex
			Male: testis
			Female: ovary, adipose tissue
Glucocorticoids	Cortisol	21	Adrenal cortex: zona fasciculata
	Corticosterone	21	Adrenal cortex: zona fasciculata
Mineralocorticoids	Aldosterone	21	Adrenal cortex: zona glomerulosa
Androgens	Testosterone	19	Male: testis
			Female: ovary, adrenal cortex
	Dihydroepiandrosterone (DHEA)	19	Adrenal cortex: zona reticularis
Estrogens	Estradiol	18	Ovary, testis
Vitamin D	Cholecalciferol	25	Skin (in presence of UV light)
	25-Hydroxycholecalciferol	25	Liver (made from cholecalciferol)
	1,25-Dihydroxycholecalciferol	25	Kidney (made from 25-hydroxycholecalciferol)
Cholesterol	Cholesterol	27	Liver, gonads, adrenal cortex

Although naturally occurring steroids that exhibit a particular hormonal activity in vertebrates (estrogenic, androgenic, etc.) are structurally similar to one another (Figures 3-25, 3-26, 3-27), many structurally unrelated compounds may have similar hormonal activity when tested and could be classified accordingly (see Figure 3-27). **Diethylstilbestrol (DES)** is a powerful synthetic estrogen that readily binds to estrogen receptors, but it is not a steroid (Figure 3-28). Additionally, plant sterols (phytoestrogens), components of detergents (alkylphenoethoxylates and their derivatives such as nonylphenols), compounds leached from plastics (e.g., bisphenol A, nonylphenol, phthalates), certain pesticides (e.g., DDT, atrazine), as well as a number of polychlorinated chemicals from industrial production (dioxins, PCBs) are known to bind to estrogen receptors and mimic the naturally occurring estrogens (see discussion of endocrine-disrupting chemicals, Chapter 1).

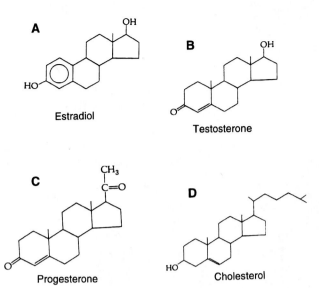

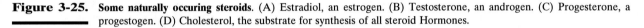

Figure 3-25. **Some naturally occuring steroids**. (A) Estradiol, an estrogen. (B) Testosterone, an androgen. (C) Progesterone, a progestogen. (D) Cholesterol, the substrate for synthesis of all steroid Hormones.

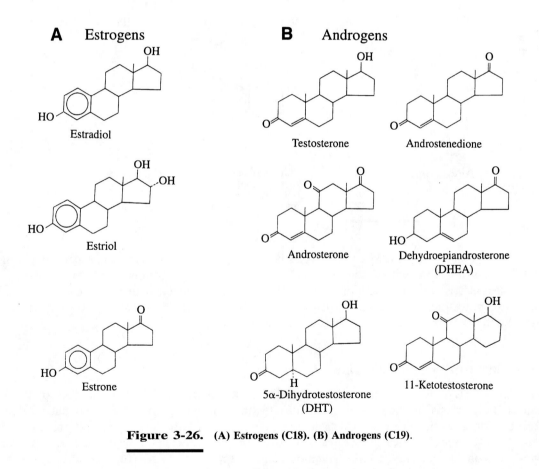

Figure 3-26. **(A) Estrogens (C18). (B) Androgens (C19)**.

Although we have long known that the brain is a target for steroids and that some of these steroids may be converted by neural enyzmes to more active forms for binding to receptors, we must now include the brain as a steroid-synthesizing tissue. These steroids that have been dubbed **neurosteroids** to emphasize their site of origin and distinguish them from steroids modified by neural cells after their accumulation from the

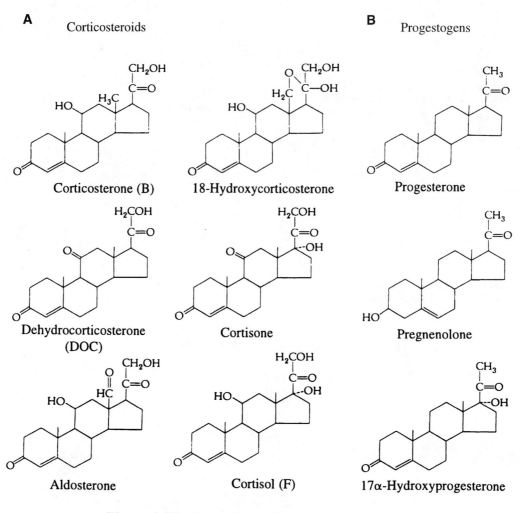

Figure 3-27.   Some corticosteroids (A) and progestogens (B).

blood or cerebrospinal fluid. In recent years, it has been demonstrated that steroids, especially pregnenolone and DHEA, are synthesized within neuroglial cells of the central and peripheral nervous systems and play important roles such as in the myelination process. Numerous steroidogeneic enzymes have been identified in neural cells except for those involved in corticosteroid synthesis. Neurosteroids are believed to function locally (paracrines) and probably do not appear in the general circulation.

A. Steroid Structure and Nomenclature

The literature on steroid hormones is very confusing to the uninitiated in part because of the inclusion of chemical designations in their names and also by the multiplicity of trivial and chemical names in the literature for a single molecule. Cortisol, for example, in addition to being designated by two different imposing chemical names ($11\beta,17\alpha,21$-trihydroxypregn-4-ene-3,20-dione, $11\beta,17\alpha,21$-trihydroxy-Δ^4-pregnene-3,20-dione), has three trivial or common names (cortisol, 17-hydroxycorticosterone, and hydrocortisone). Furthermore, cortisol was known as Reichstein's compound M and Kendall's compound F before its chemical structure was elucidated. The common abbreviation for cortisol has become "F" for Kendall's unknown fraction.

In order to use the established literature, it is necessary to become familiar with the various trivial names as well as to understand the bases for the chemical names. A working knowledge of the chemical nomenclature

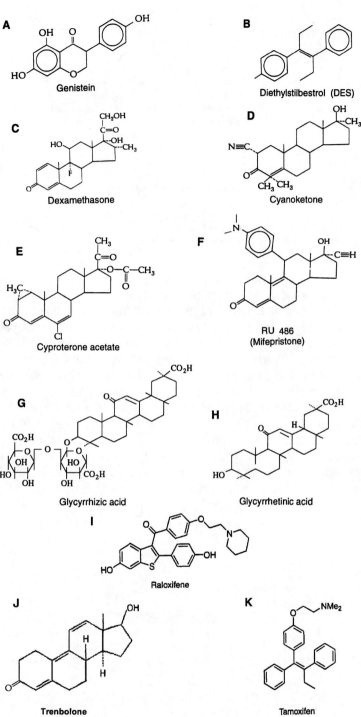

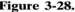

Figure 3-28. **Some synthetic steroids and nonsteroids with steroid-like activity**. (A) Genistein is a phytoestrogen found in clover, soy, and other plants. (B) Diethylstilbestrol is a potent estrogen. (C) Dexamethasone is a synthetic glucocorticoid that is more potent than any of the naturally occuring ones. (D) Cyanoketone is a steroid that inhibits the enzyme that normally converts the steroid pregnenolone to progesterone. (E) Cyproterone acetate is an anti-androgen and blocks androgen binding to receptors. (F) Mifepristine or RU 486 is an antiprogesterone and an antiglucocorticoid. (G) Glycyrrhizic acid and (H) Glycyrrhetinic acid are found in licorice and have weak corticosteroid activity. (I) Raloxifene, a synthetic anti-estrogen. (J) Trenbolone, a synthetic androgen. (K) Tamoxifen, a synthetic anti-androgen.

Table 3-10. Summary of Special Designations in
Steroid Nomenclature

Designation	Explanation
Δ	Location of double bond
-ene	One double bond in steroid nucleus
-diene	Two double bonds in steroid nucleus
-triene	Three double bonds in steroid nucleus
hydroxy-	Hydroxyl (OH) substituted for hydrogen on nucleus
-ol	Hydroxyl (OH) substituted for hydrogen on nucleus
oxo-	Ketone (=O) substituted for hydrogen on nucleus
keto-	Ketone (=O) substituted for hydrogen on nucleus
-one	Ketone (=O) substituted for hydrogen on nucleus
α	Atom or atoms attached to a given carbon of the steroid nucleus projects away from viewer
β	Atom or atoms attached to a given carbon of the steroid nucleus projects toward viewer
Arabic number	Indicates location of substitution or double bond

for steroids is not really necessary for the treatments provided in this textbook, although those students interested in details of synthesis and metabolism of steroids will find knowledge of the chemical nomenclature invaluable. Furthermore, a glance at the chemical structure of a steroid also tells you a great deal about its biological role. Table 3-10 summarizes special designations used in nomenclature of steroids.

The steroid nucleus contains 17 carbons, each designated by a number and arranged into four rings (Figure 3-24). Steroids are named chemically by relating each steroid to a saturated hypothetical parent hydrocarbon compound (i.e., one that has no double bonds present) and modifying this name with one or more prefixes and no more than one suffix to designate the specific compound (Figure 3-29). These hypothetical parent compounds are **estrane** (18 carbons or C_{18}), **androstane** (C_{19}), **pregnane** (C_{21}), and **cholestrane** (C_{27}). Naturally occurring estrogens (all C_{18} compounds) and androgens (C_{19} compounds) possess the basic carbon skeleton of estrane and androstane, respectively, whereas the names for corticoids and progestogens, (both C_{21} compounds) are related to pregnane for naming purposes. Cholestrane is employed for naming cholesterol and other derivatives including bile salts and the vitamin D compounds that are all C_{27} steroids.

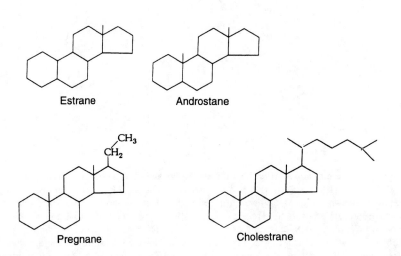

Figure 3-29. **Hypothetical steroids employed in steroid nomenclature**. These compounds do not exist and are used only for the purposes of constructing the chemical names for the four major groups of steroid hormones.

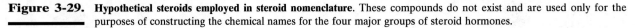

1. Presence of Double Bonds in the Steroid Nucleus

The position of double bonds between carbon atoms within the steroid nucleus was formerly designated by the Greek letter delta (Δ), followed by the superscripted number of the lowest-numbered steroid carbon with which the bond is involved. Thus, Δ^4 would indicate a double bond between carbons 4 and 5 in the steroid nucleus. Currently, a separate scheme employs the term **ene** to refer to one double bond, **diene** for two double bonds, and **triene** for three double bonds in the nucleus, and the location of each bond is indicated by the number of the carbon preceding the location of the double bond (e.g., 4-pregnene refers to a double bond in pregnane between carbons 4 and 5). Nevertheless, much of our steroid-related terminology still employs the older Δ terminology.

2. Common Substitutions to the Steroid Nucleus

Substituted groups applied to the steroid skeleton are designated according to the number of the carbon atom in the steroid skeleton to which they are attached. For example, **17-hydroxy** refers to a hydroxyl group (–OH) attached to carbon number 17. Hydroxyl groups are usually indicated as prefixes on the chemical name unless they are the only substitution on the steroid nucleus in which case the hydroxyl group is designated by the suffix **-ol**. Ketone groups (=O) substituted on the steroid nucleus are indicated by the prefix **oxo-** or **keto-** or by the suffix **-one**; thus, **-3,20-dione** would refer to two ketone groups attached at positions 3 and 20, respectively, as would **3,20-dioxo-**. In naming steroids with both hydroxyl and keto groups, the latter takes priority as the suffix (-one) over the hydroxyl (-ol).

3. Stereoisomerism

One carbon atom is capable of forming four covalent bonds with other atoms. Only two of these bonds are used when a given carbon is incorporated into the steroid nucleus and bound to two other carbon atoms. Because of the necessary bonding angles dictated by the tetrahedral shape of the carbon atom, a steroid does not exist in a flat plane as most diagrams of their chemical structures would suggest. The remaining two sites for each carbon atom incorporated into the steroid nucleus can form covalent bonds with hydrogens, oxygens, or other carbon atoms. Depending on how and where the carbon atom appears in the nucleus, it may be able to bind hydrogen or oxygen to either side. One of these bonds will project toward the viewer when examining the steroid as depicted in Figure 3-24, and the other will project away from the viewer, that is, into the page. Such carbon atoms are referred to as **asymmetric carbons**. There are asymmetric carbons at positions 3, 5, 11, 16, 17 of the steroid nucleus as well as for carbon 20 in the side chain. These numbers appear in their chemical names and sometimes carry over to the trivial names because they form important bonds with ketone or hydroxyl groups.

Two three-dimensional isomers (**stereoisomers**) can be formed by substituting one hydrogen on a given asymmetric carbon with, for example, a hydroxyl group. The chemical formulas would be the same (i.e., the same number of C, H, and O atoms), but the three-dimensional structure of each stereoisomer would differ according to whether the added –OH group projected out from or into the page. A spatial designation of α is used if the substituted group projects away from the viewer, and β is used if the group projects toward the viewer. In estrogens, which have an aromatic A-ring in the steroid nucleus, the carbon at position 3 can be neither α or β. In C_{21} steroids, carbon 20 is connected in the β-configuration to carbon 17. Any other attachment to carbon 17 of a C_{21} steroid must be in the α-position, and it is not necessary to indicate this in the chemical name.

In two-dimensional diagrams, the α-position is indicated by a slashed or dotted line, whereas the β-position is designated with a solid line connecting the substituted group to its carbon (Figure 3-24). Hydrogen atoms usually are not designated, but their presence is implied. Estradiol occurs in two isomeric forms, **17β-estradiol** and **17α-estradiol**. Notice how the trivial name "estradiol" has been embellished with details derived from its chemical name (diol refers to 2 OH groups, one of which is on carbon 17, an asymmetric carbon, and in either the α- or β-conformation). The complete chemical names for these two estradiol molecules are 1,3,5-estratriene-3,17α-diol and 1,3,5-estratriene-3,17β-diol. It was generally accepted that 17β-estradiol was the important estrogen of vertebrates and that 17α-estradiol had little or no estrogenic activity. However, studies

Table 3-11. Some Vertebrate Steroid Hormones

Category	Trivial name	Chemical name
Androgens	Testosterone	17β-Hydroxy-4-androsten-3-one
	Androstenedione	4-Androstene-3,17-dione
	Dehydroepiandrosterone	3β-Hydroxy-5-androsten-17-one
Corticoids	Aldosterone	11β,21-Dihydroxy-3,20-dioxo-4-pregnen-18-o1
	Cortisol	11β,17,21-Trihydroxy-4-pregnene-3,20-dione
	Corticosterone	11β,21-Dihydroxy-4-pregnene-3,20-dione
	11-Deoxycorticosterone	21-Hydroxy-4-pregnene-3,20-dione
Estrogens	Estradiol-17β	1,3,5(10)-Estratriene-3, 17β-diol
	Estrone	3-Hydroxy-1,3,5(10)-estratrien-17-one
	Estriol	1,3,5(10)-Estratriene-3,16α,17β-triol
Progestogens	Pregnenolone	3β-Hydroxy-5-pregnen-20-one
	Progesterone	4-Pregnene-3,20-dione

in both fishes and mammals have demonstrated the effectiveness of 17α-estradiol in binding to and activating estrogen receptors even though they don't bind to plasma-binding proteins. Furthermore, studies in mammals have verified the synthesis of 17α-estradiol in the brain of castrate and adrenalectomized rats. Much remains to be learned about the possible roles of 17α-estradiol, however, and we will continue to consider 17β-estradiol to be the major estrogen of vertebrates. Henceforth, we shall use "estradiol" alone to designate 17β-estradiol.

The chemical structures of several steroids are diagrammed in Figures 3-26 and 3-27, with both chemical and trivial names for some of these steroids indicated in Table 3-11. Can you determine the bases for the chemical name assigned to each steroid?

B. Steroid Synthesis

All vertebrate steroid bioregulators are synthesized from **cholesterol**, a C_{27} steroid (Figure 3-25). Cholesterol is synthesized from acetate (acetyl-coenzyme A) produced via glycolysis or via fatty acid oxidation. The synthesis of the steroid nucleus from acetate units is termed **steroidogenesis**, although often this term is used by endocrinologists for only the synthesis of steroid hormones from cholesterol. Steroidogenesis begins with an involved series of enzymatically catalyzed reactions that convert acetate into cholesterol. Following synthesis of a relatively long hydrocarbon chain, a complex cyclization step results in closure of the carbon skeleton into the steroid nucleus. Cholesterol synthesized in this manner may be used directly in the biosynthesis of the various steroid hormones but cannot be degraded back toward acetate. Excess cholesterol is converted by the liver into bile salts for excretion.

Most cholesterol is synthesized in the liver and is released into the blood as lipid droplets coated with protein (for details, see Chapter 12). Adrenal cortex, ovaries, and testes also can synthesize cholesterol but more commonly utilize lipoprotein complexes absorbed from the gut or synthesized in the liver as sources of cholesterol (see Chapter 12).

Cholesterol and the steroid hormones are synthesized primarily in the liver (cholesterol), the gonads (estrogens, androgens, progesterone), the placenta (estrogens, progesterone), the adrenal cortex (corticosteroids, androgens), and the brain (neurosteroids). In addition, stromal cells present in adipose tissue may be important in estrogen synthesis, especially in postmenopausal women and in aging men. Vitamin D compounds are made by the cooperative activities of the skin, liver, and kidney. The pathway for forming 1,25-DHC differs markedly from that for the gonadal and adrenal steroids and will be described separately.

1. Key Enzymes in Gonadal and Adrenal Steroid Biosynthesis

Identification of certain key synthetic enzymes and quantification of their activity levels are often used as indicators of the biosynthesis of steroid hormones. More than one scheme has been proposed for naming these enzymes (see Table 3-12), and some enzymes may have several different names. The newest methods involve applying a specific name for the gene that is written in italics (e.g., *CYP19*). Each gene is responsible for an

Table 3-12. Names for Key Steroidogenic Enzymes

Gene based	Enzyme name	P450 abbreviation
CYP21	C_{21}-Hydroxylase	$P450_{C21}$
CYP11A	Cholesterol side-chain cleavage, 20–22 Desmolase	$P450_{SCC}$
CYP17	17α-Hydroxylase, 17,20-Lyase	$P450_{C17}$
CYP19	Aromatase	$P450_{ARO}$
CYP11B1	11β-Hydroxylase	$P450_{C11}$
CYP11B2	Aldosterone synthetase	$P450_{ALDO}$
CYP1A1	Aryl hydrocarbon hydroxylase	$P450_{1A1}$

enzyme's production and either a name related to the gene name but without italics (e.g., CYP19) or a more descriptive name (e.g., **$P450_{aro}$** or aromatase) is used for the enzyme. The more descriptive names will be used here to simplify connecting each enzyme to its action and location within the cell. Many of these enzymes are members of a class of membrane-bound enzymes known as the **P450 cytochromes** familiar to physiologists for their role in oxidative phosphorylation. Others are cytosolic proteins.

The initial removal of the cholesterol side chain is accomplished by the **side-chain cleaving enzyme** associated with the inner mitochondrial membrane, **$P450_{scc}$** (CYP11A). Although steroidogenesis begins in steroidogenic tissue most commonly with cholesterol obtained from the blood, it cannot be considered the rate-limiting enzyme because it always appears to be present in sufficient amounts to initiate steroidogenesis (see Table 3-12).

One key step following side-chain hydrolysis is the conversion of pregnenolone to progesterone, which involves moving the double bond from the B ring to the A ring (change from Δ^5 to Δ^4) and converting the β–OH group on carbon 3 to a ketone (=O; see Figures 3-30 and 3-31). In steroidogenic tissue, catalytic activity of the cytosolic enzyme Δ^5, **3β-hydroxysteroid dehydrogenase (3β-HSD)** can be approximated histochemically in frozen sections, thus providing a crude measure of steroid hormone synthesis. Estimation of the rate of steroid hormone synthesis also infers a measure of the rate of release, because steroid hormones are not stored to any appreciable degree in steroidogenic cells and apparently are released into the circulation as they are synthesized. 3β-HSD also is a good immunochemical marker for cells that are capable of steroidogenesis.

The enzyme 3β-HSD can work on a variety of steroid substrates. If 3β-HSD acts early in the sequence by converting Δ^5-pregnenolone to Δ^4-progesterone, the subsequent enzymatic transformations of progesterone are referred to as the **Δ^4-pathway**. When pregnenolone is not converted to Δ^4-progesterone, it is metabolized along the **Δ^5-pathway**. 3β-HSD may act at other points in the Δ^5-pathway and convert other intermediates into components of the Δ^4-pathway; for example, DHEA to androstenedione (see Figure 3-31). Δ^4 Androgens are more active in binding and activating androgen receptors that are Δ^5 androgens. Both of these molecules are C_{19} compounds. The significance of the Δ^4- and Δ^5-pathways in adrenal, testicular, and ovarian steroid syntheses is discussed in Chapters 8 and 10. Pregnenolone and progesterone can be converted to DHEA and androstenedione, respectively, by the enzyme **C_{17}-hydroxylase** ($P450_{c17}$ = CYP17).

The drug **cyanoketone** is known to competitively inhibit the activity of 3β-HSD because of the structural similarity of cyanoketone (Figure 3-28) to pregnenolone (Figures 3-27) and its ability to block access of pregnenolone to the enzyme's binding site. Cyanoketone effectively blocks gonadal steroid biosynthesis and reduces circulating levels of all gonadal steroids. It also prevents synthesis of corticosteroids by adrenal cells. Reduction in circulating steroids reduces negative feedback and causes stimulation of pituitary gonadotropes (cells that synthesize the gonadotropins, FSH and LH). Reduced levels of glucocorticoids activate pituitary corticotropes that secrete ACTH that stimulates glucocorticoid synthesis.

The basic androgen of most vertebrates is **testosterone**. It is synthesized from androstenedione by the enzyme **17β-hydroxysteroid dehydrogenase (17β-HSD)**. The enzyme **5α-reductase** converts testosterone into DHT, an important androgen for development of the penis and scrotum in males. Furthermore, testosterone is converted by the enzyme aromatase ($P450_{aro}$ = CYP19) that results in loss of one carbon and aromatization of the A ring to yield estradiol, a C_{18} estrogen (Figure 3-32). This same enzyme converts androstenedione into estrone that can be converted enzymatically into estradiol as well. The presence of aromatase activity in a cell or tissue is an indicator of the ability to transform androgens into estrogens. $P450_{aro}$ plays an important role in fetal development as levels of this enzyme are high in fetal liver of rats and humans. Although lacking in the human fetal brain, it is present in the fetal mouse brain. $P450_{aro}$ activity is present in the steroidogenic

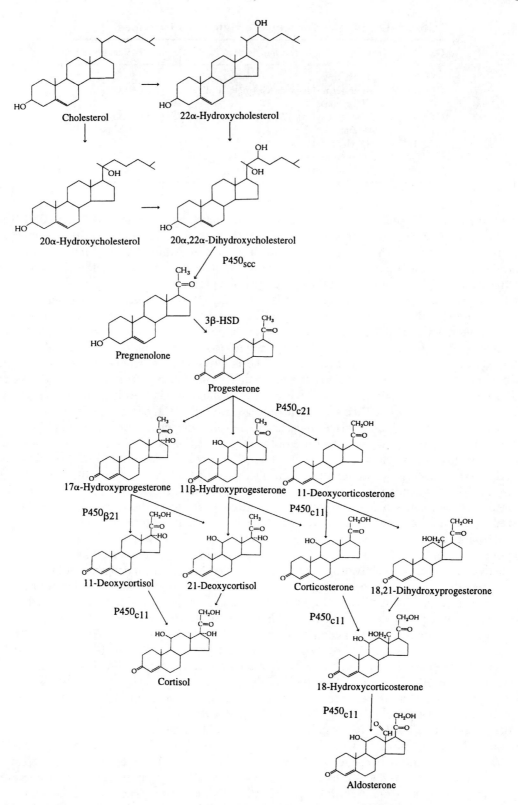

Figure 3-30. **Progesterone and corticosteroid synthesis.** Cortisol, corticosterone, and aldosterone are the major secretory products with hormonal activity. Identification of the key P450 enzymes indicated can be found in the text (Table 3-12).

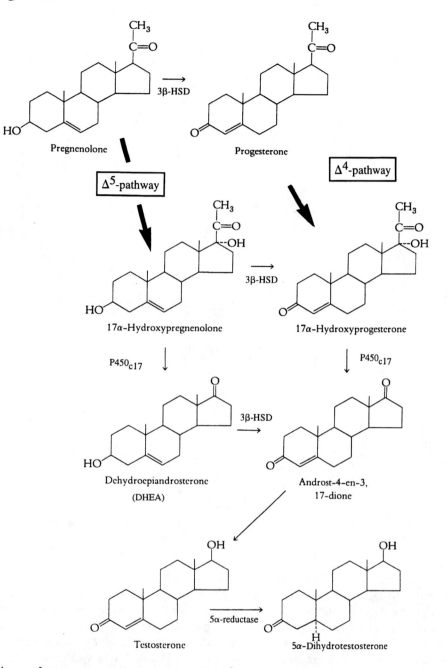

Figure 3-31. Δ^4- and Δ^5-Pathways for androgen synthesis. The Δ^5-pathway typically occurs in the adrenal cortex and usually stops with the production of DHEA or DHEAS. In ovaries of some species, this pathway may lead to testosterone and eventually to estrogen synthesis. Testes employ the Δ^4-pathway.

cells of the adult rat testeis, too. Aromatase activity occurs in adult vertebrate adipose tissue, and certain brain cells where it converts androgens into estrogens. Testosterone, like estradiol, occurs in both α and β forms. α-Testosterone can be converted to 17α-estradiol by P450$_{aro}$. Furthermore, 17α-estradiol can be formed from estrone.

Although DHT is considered to be a non-aromatizable androgen, it can be modified, at least in some mammals, by enzymes to **5α-androstane-3β,17β-diol (3β-diol)** that binds and activates one form of the estrogen receptor found in brain and prostate gland (see ERβ). 3β-diol is chemically an androgen, but it can produce distinct effects via an estrogen receptor in these tissues.

The enzyme **C_{21}-hydroxylase (P450$_{c21}$ = CYP21)** converts either progesterone or 17α-hydroxyprogesterone into **11-deoxycorticosterone** or **11-deoxycortisol**, respectively, in adrenalcorticosteroidogenic tissue. This tissue

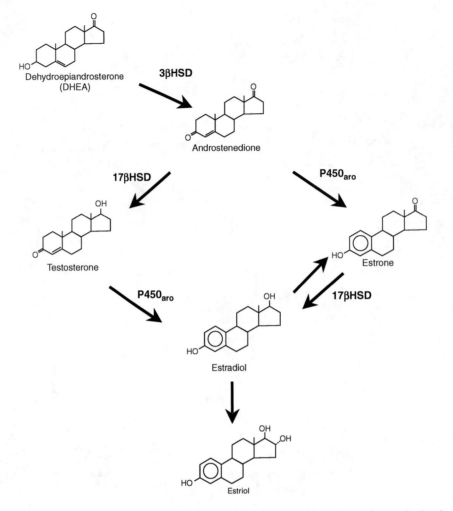

Figure 3-32. **Synthesis of estrogens from testosterone.** Estrogen synthesis requires either prior synthesis of an androgen or an external source of androgen.

also contains another mitochondrial enzyme, **11β-hydroxylase** (**P450$_{11\beta}$** = P450$_{c11}$ or CYP11B1), that applies a third hydroxyl group to these different precursors to form either corticosterone or cortisol, respectively. The activity of this enzyme can be estimated with procedures similar to those described for 3β-HSD. The drug **metyrapone** selectively inhibits 11β-hydroxylase, thus blocking steroidogenesis in adrenocortical cells. Like the case described for cyanoketone, metyrapone has been used successfully to distinguish the corticotropic cells in the pituitary of many vertebrates from gonadotropes. **Aldosterone synthetase** (**P450$_{aldo}$** = CYP11B2) is necessary to convert corticosterone into the mineralocorticoid aldosterone.

2. Cytological Aspects of Gonadal and Adrenal Steroid Biosynthesis

Biosynthesis of steroid hormones is, cytologically speaking, a very complex affair involving cytosolic, mitochondrial, and smooth endoplasmic reticulum (SER) enzymes. The importance of the latter is demonstrated by observations that a major cytological feature of steroidogenic cells is the abundance of SER.

The synthesis of the corticosteroid cortisol illustrates one sequence of cellular events in steroid hormone biosynthesis. Some of these steps are common to the synthesis of other steroids, too. Pregnenolone is synthesized from cholesterol by the action P450$_{scc}$ located at the inner membrane of mitochondria. The alteration of pregnenolone to progesterone, however, necessitates that pregnenolone travel for this conversion step to the SER where 3βHSD is located. The addition of hydroxyl groups by other enzymes acting at the 17 and 21 positions (P450$_{c17}$, P450$_{C21}$) also occurs in the SER, resulting in 11-deoxycortisol. This compound returns to the mitochondria where the 11β-hydrolylase (P450$_{11β}$) is located that converts 11-deoxycortisol to cortisol or 11-deoxycorticosterone to corticosterone. Progesterone conversion to androgens and estrogens also requires reentry of progesterone into the mitochondria.

For many years, it was assumed that cholesterol entered the mitochondrion by simple diffusion. Recent discoveries have identified a **steroidogenic acute regulating protein (StAR)** that facilitates the transfer of cholesterol from the outer mitochondrial membrane to the inner membrane where P450$_{SCC}$ is located. Patients unable to convert cholesterol to corticosteroids but who have demonstrable P450$_{SCC}$ provided the clue to the existence of the StAR protein. These observations suggest that other movements of steroids in and out of cellular organelles also may depend on specific steroid-protein interactions. Because the levels of StAR protein determines the ability of a cell to convert cholesterol to pregnenolone, one might consider this to be the rate-limiting step in steroidogenesis although the StAR protein is not an enzyme.

3. Biosynthesis of 1,25-DHC

The common name "vitamin D" often is applied loosely to all of the intermediates between cholesterol and 1,25-DHC. In the presence of ultraviolet light, cholesterol is modified in the skin to **cholecalciferol** which is also a C$_{27}$ steroid (see Figure 3-33); hence the designation of vitamin D as the "sunshine vitamin." Cholecalciferol is

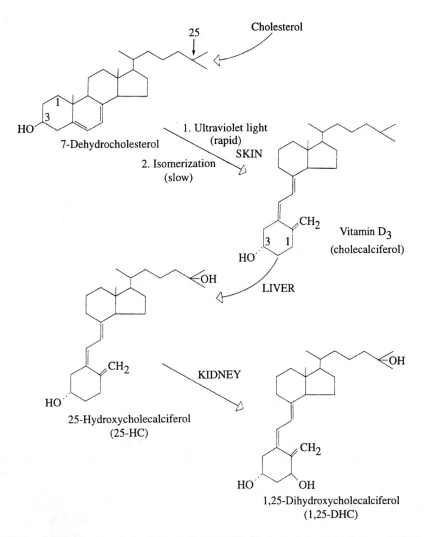

Figure 3-33. **Synthesis of 1,25-dihydroxycholecalciferol (1,25-DHC).** Cholesterol is changed sequentially by the skin, liver, and kidney. Note the rearrangement of the A-ring as a consequence of opening up the B-ring. The kidney also converts a small amount of 25-HC to 24,25-DHC that has much weaker biological activity than 1,25-DHC.

released into the blood from which it is removed by the liver, converted into **25-hydroxycholecalciferol** by the addition of one –OH group, and returned to the blood. Next, the kidney removes 25-hydroxycholecalciferol from the blood and adds an additional –OH to produce 1,25-DHC and releases it into the blood. 1,25-DHC enters certain cells of the intestinal mucosa where it stimulates synthesis of special proteins responsible for calcium uptake from the intestinal contents and transport into the blood.

4. Biosynthesis of Gonadal and Adrenal Steroids

The first series of steps in the biosynthesis of these steroid hormones involves **side-chain hydrolysis** that removes most of the hydrocarbon side chain of cholesterol to yield a C_{21} intermediate, **pregnenolone**. In the gonads, pregnenolone primarily is converted to progesterone (also C_{21}) that may be secreted as a hormone or altered further to C_{19} androgens that in turn may be modified to C_{18} estrogens. In the adrenal, pregnenolone is converted to progesterone and used directly to form corticosteroids (C_{21}) and some androgens.

A summary of basic pathways for C_{18}-, C_{19}-, and C_{21}-steroid hormone biosynthesis is provided in Figures 3-30, 3-31, and 3-32. After these schemes are examined in some detail, it should not be surprising to learn that many steroidogenic tissues produce more than one class of steroid molecule. The mere presence of a given steroid in a tissue or the ability of a tissue to synthesize a particular steroid does not distinguish between a precursor role of that steroid for synthesis of another steroid and the possibility that the given steroid is secreted into the blood as a hormone. Furthermore, the administration of certain steroids to an animal might lead to their use as substrates for conversion to other steroids. Thus, the observed effect might be due to this conversion product and not to innate activity of the applied steroids. For example, androgens may be converted to estrogens by a number of tissues. This also suggests that cholesterol administration may not be a good control for administration of an androgen or an estrogen because under certain circumstances, that cholesterol could be used to make more androgen and/or estrogen in the control animal even though cholesterol itself does not bind to androgen or estrogen receptors and produce effects.

C. Transport of Steroid Hormones in Blood

Steroids are nonpolar compounds and consequently are not very soluble in aqueous solutions such as blood. Furthermore, free steroids readily diffuse or are transported through cellular membranes and rapidly disappear from the blood as a result of the activities of the liver and kidneys. The association of circulating steroids with plasma proteins results in their being retained at higher concentrations for longer times in the circulation. These **plasma binding proteins** reduce removal of active steroid hormones by the liver or kidney and their excretion via the urine. Thus, relatively high titers of steroid hormones can be maintained in the circulation, providing maximal local titers of dissociated free steroid and increasing the probability of their entering appropriate target tissues. As mentioned earlier, plasma binding proteins may facilitate the entrance of steroids into their target cells.

D. Mechanisms of Steroid Action

The original model for steroid hormone action was proposed for estrogens by Elwood Jensen in the early 1970s. Although the model has undergone considerable revision since that time, such as the location of unoccupied receptors, the basic features are still valid. The unoccupied receptors for estrogens primarily are found in the nucleus of target cells. The location of unoccupied androgen receptors may be either cytosolic or nuclear depending on the target tissue. The location of unoccupied progesterone receptors is not confirmed and there is evidence of both cytological and nuclear sites. In contrast, corticosteroid receptors appear to be exclusively cytoplasmic and are translocated to the nucleus following binding of the appropriate ligand.

Initially, all steroids were thought to produce their cellular effects through similar mechanisms (Figure 3-34, 3-35). Once these steroids enter their target cells, they diffuse into the cytosol or nucleus where they bind to specific protein receptors. These nuclear receptor proteins are complexed to various **chaperone proteins** that are involved with maintaining the three-dimensional shape of the receptor prior to binding with the ligand. In the nucleus, occupied adrenal and gonadal steroid receptors form homodimers and behave like

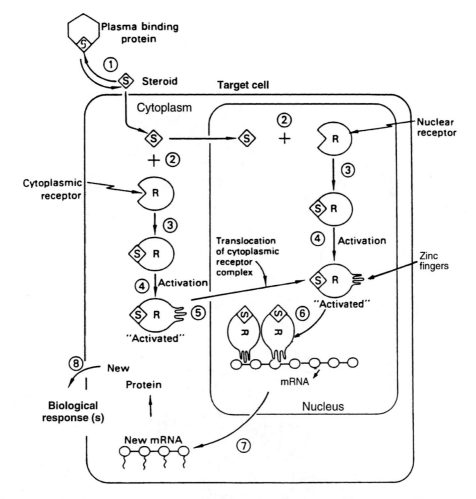

Figure 3-34. **Action of steroids via cytosolic and nuclear receptors.** Free steroid (S) dissociates from plasma binding proteins (1) enters the cell and either binds to a cytosolic or a nuclear receptor, R (2,3). The occupied receptors typically are activated (4) and dimerize (not shown). Cytosolic receptors are translocated to the nucleus (5) and occupied receptor dimers bind via zinc fingers to hormone response elements (HREs) on the DNA (6), facilitating transcription. mRNA leaves the nucleus (7) and directs new protein synthesis associated with the steroid's specific action on that target cell (8). [Modified from A. Norman and G. Litwack (1997). "Hormones," Academic Press, Inc., San Diego, p. 40.]

transcription factors (i.e., ligand-activated transcription factors), bind to specific sites on DNA called **hormone response elements (HREs),** and initiate new mRNA synthesis. **Nuclear adapter proteins** may aid binding of occupied receptor to HREs, influence interactions with RNA polymerase, and facilitate transcription. A different suite of nuclear adapter proteins may be involved with different steroid receptors. The adapter proteins also may vary in different tissues for the same steroid resulting in activation of different HREs. Furthermore, occupied receptors of a specific ligand may have to compete with other species of occupied receptors for the same nuclear adapter proteins.

Once a gene is activated in the target cell, it may direct the synthesis of structural proteins or functional proteins such as peptide bioregulators or enzymes. Enzymes may be responsible for the production of intracrine bioregulators in the target cell that can produce a variety of effects (Figure 3-36).

It generally is accepted that once a steroid receptor is occupied, it is phosphorylated and forms a dimer and that a second phosphorylation occurs after the dimer binds to the HRE (Figure 3-35). Estrogens, androgens, progestogens, and corticosteroids always form homodimers whereas other steroids such as Vitamin D_3 (1,25-DHC) and bile acids form heterodimers with other receptors (Figure 3-37). The resultant transcription and synthesis of new proteins by the target cells bring about the events classically associated with the actions of these hormones. Typically, there is a considerable delay (hours) between contact of the steroid bioregulator with its target cell and the manifestation of its effects rather than almost immediate changes as described

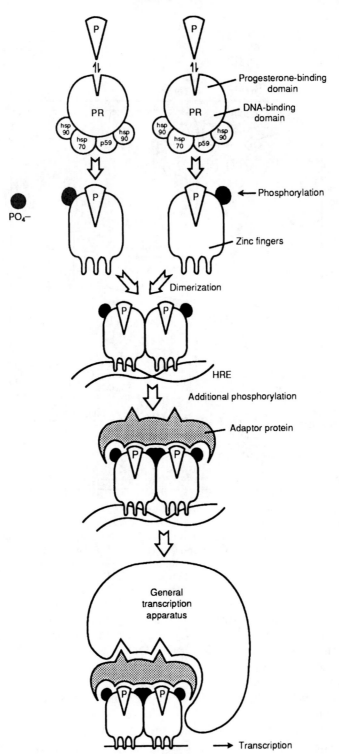

Figure 3-35. **Heatshock proteins and the progesterone receptor.** Unoccupied progesterone receptor is associated with several molecular chaperones including several heatshock proteins (see also Table 3-13). Once occupied, the receptors are phosphorylated, lose some of their heatshock proteins, translocate to the nucleus, and form homodimers. Following binding of the receptor dimer to the HRE site on nuclear DNA, a second phosphorylation occurs and an adapter protein complex is recruited that facilitates interaction with the general transcription apparatus. RNA polymerase activity and hence transcription is thereby modulated. [Based on D. P. McDonnell (1995). Unraveling the human progesterone receptor signal transduction pathway. Insights into antiprogestin action. *Trends in Endocrin. and Metabolism* **6**, 133–138.]

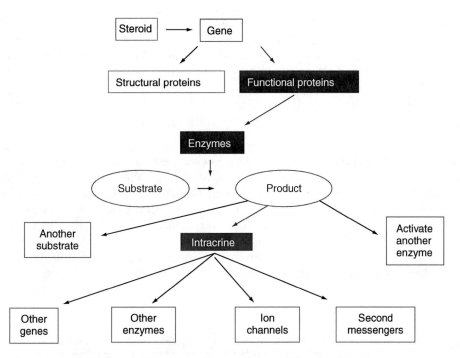

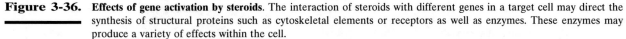

Figure 3-36. **Effects of gene activation by steroids.** The interaction of steroids with different genes in a target cell may direct the synthesis of structural proteins such as cytoskeletal elements or receptors as well as enzymes. These enzymes may produce a variety of effects within the cell.

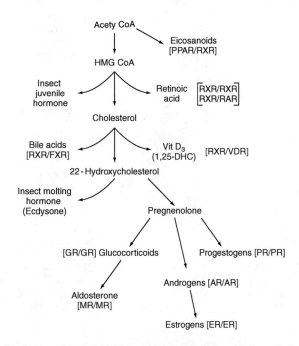

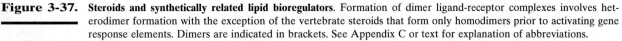

Figure 3-37. **Steroids and synthetically related lipid bioregulators.** Formation of dimer ligand-receptor complexes involves heterodimer formation with the exception of the vertebrate steroids that form only homodimers prior to activating gene response elements. Dimers are indicated in brackets. See Appendix C or text for explanation of abbreviations.

earlier for membrane receptors acting through second messenger systems. Most actions of steroids then are on the time scale of the delayed effects seen with second messenger systems.

In some androgen-specific target cells, testosterone is first altered chemically in the cytoplasm before it migrates to the nucleus and binds to a receptor. Testosterone may be converted by 5α-reductase to DHT in certain target cells (e.g., in brain, prostate) or by aromatase to estradiol (e.g., in brain). Thus, unoccupied nuclear receptors in these cells are not specific for testosterone but for one of its metabolites. In contrast, cortisol, which can bind to either cortisol or aldosterone receptors is altered to the metabolite cortisone when it enters aldosterone target cells and is unable to bind to mineralocorticoid receptors (see Chapter 8).

1. Steroid Receptors and the Nuclear Receptor Superfamily

Regardless of whether unoccupied intracellular steroid receptors are present in the cytosol or the nucleus, all belong to a superfamily of nuclear receptors. This **nuclear receptor superfamily** includes more than 300 receptors, most of which have been identified from gene sequences. Many of these receptors have no known natural ligand and these molecules initially were termed **orphan receptors**. Some authorities subdivide the nuclear receptors into as many as six subfamilies based on common structural features (Table 3-13). One subfamily includes all of the steroid receptors except those for the C_{27} steroids (hydroxycholesterol, bile acids, and vitamin D). The **steroid nuclear receptor subfamily** can be separated into two subgroupings: the glucocorticoid-like receptors (includes receptors for androgens, progestogens, and mineralocorticoids) and the estrogen-like receptors (estrogen receptors as well as estrogen-related receptors). Some researchers include a third grouping here that includes the vitamin D receptor as well as some non-steroid receptors.

Table 3-13. Some Nuclear Receptor Superfamily Members

Endocrine receptors	Abbreviation(s)	Endocrine ligands
Mineralocorticoid	MR (GR type 1)	Mineralocorticoids
Glucocorticoid	GR (GR type 2)	Glucocorticoids
Progesterone	PR	Progesterone
Androgen	AR	Androgens
Estrogen	ERα, β	Estrogens
Retinoic acid	RARα, β, γ	Retinoic acids (RAs)
Thyroid	TRα, β	Thyroid hormones (T_3 & T_4)
Vitamin D	VDR	Vit D_3, LCA

Adopted orphans		**Endogenous & exogenous ligands**
Retinoid X	RXRα, β, γ	9-cis-RA, DHA
Peroxisomal Proliferator-activated	PPARα, Δ, γ	Fatty acids
Liver X	LXR	Oxysterols
Farnesoid X	FXR	Bile acids
Pregnane X	PXR	Xenobiotics
Constitutive androstane	CAR	Xenobiotics

Orphans[1]		**Endogenous ligands uncertain**
Estrogen-related receptor	ERRα, β, γ	Synthetic steroids
	HNF-4α, γ	Fatty acids?
	RORα, β, γ	Fatty acids, sterols?
Steroidogenic factor 1	SF-1	Phospholipids?
	LRH-1	Phospholipids?
	GCNF	?
	PNR	?
	TLX	?
	TR2,4	?
	NGFI-Bα, β, γ	?
	COUP-TFα, β, γ?	?
	RVRα, β	?
	DAX-1	?
	SHP	?

[1] Many of these may function as simple transcription factors without ligands.

The ancestral vertebrate steroid receptor is believed to have been similar to the **estrogen-related receptor (ERR)** present in the primitive lamprey. The ERR gene is considered to be the source from which the **estrogen receptor (ER)** gene evolved. Following a duplication of the ER gene, one copy of the ER gene gave rise to the gene that produces the **progesterone receptor (PR)**. Following duplication of the PR gene, it gave rise to the **androgen receptor (AR)** gene and later to the **glucocorticoid receptor (GR)** and **mineralocorticoid receptor (MR)** genes. Meanwhile, the ER gene duplicated and diverged into two distinct forms we find in mammals, ERα and ERβ. These receptors exhibit different tissue distributions and have different affinities for various estrogenic molecules. No significant variants have been identified for the other steroid receptors.

E. Reproductive Steroid Action

Of the reproductive steroid receptors, ERs have been studied most extensively. Two forms of ER are known for mammals: ERα and ERβ. The ERα was discovered first and is the most widely distributed ER in the body. The ERβ is absent from the liver but is the only ER in the gastrointestinal tract. Furthermore, the ERα is less selective in its acceptance of ligands and is the target for most estrogenic endocrine-disrupting chemicals such as nonylphenols, phthalates, and bisphenol A as well as for estrogenic pharmaceuticals such as ethinylestradiol (EE_2) and DES as well as the antiestrogen **tamoxifen**. The antiestrogen raloxifene antagonizes ERβ. Various drugs that affect estrogen receptors are termed **selective estrogen receptor modulators**, or **SERMs**.

1. Cortiosteroid Action

Two classes of corticosteroid receptors have been described that are located in the cytosol of target cells and form homodimers when occupied. The MR binds aldosterone and glucocorticoids and the GR binds only cortisol or corticosterone. Since the MR binds both aldosterone and the two glucocorticoids, an alternative scheme exists for naming these receptors. Since both receptor types bind glucocorticoids, they also have been called **type 1 glucocorticoid receptor** ($GR_1 = MR$) and **type 2 glucocorticoid receptor** ($GR_2 = GR$). The first scheme (MR, GR) is used here for simplicity, but keep in mind that the MR also can bind glucocorticoids as this will prove to be of physiological importance later. In target cells that are involved in the regulation of mineral balance, a special form of the enzyme **11β-hydroxysteroid dehydrogenase** converts cortisol that enters the cytosol into cortisone which does not bind effectively to the MR. Thus, these cells will respond only to aldosterone even when plasma cortisol levels are elevated.

Recent studies show that GR, like other steroid receptors, is actually a complex of several proteins. One protein, the receptor proper, binds the glucocorticoid. This molecule also contains a domain for binding to the HRE once it is occupied. When unoccupied, the receptor protein is associated with several **heatshock proteins** (e.g., hsp56, hsp 70, and hsp90; Figure 3-35). Heatshock proteins were first described in the fruit fly *Drosophila* and named because they were synthesized in greater amounts following a sudden increase in temperature (i.e., heatshock). This name has persisted although sometimes they are called "stress proteins" when associated with corticosteroid receptors (see Chapter 8). These heatshock proteins are part of a group of proteins known as **molecular chaperones** because they also are involved in the folding process following translation of proteins.

Various molecular chaperones are associated with all of the steroid receptors (Table 3-13), and they are not unique to corticosteroids. Hsp90 is found weakly associated with estrogen receptors and is not associated with 1,25-DHC receptors. Both of these receptors are considered to reside only in the nucleus. In all cases, association of heatshock proteins with the receptor prevents the steroid-receptor complex from binding with DNA, but binding of the specific ligand causes dissociation of hsp90 from the receptor and allows the ligand-receptor complex to migrate and bind to DNA. The roles for the various auxiliary proteins are not completely understood but some may be involved in translocation of occupied corticosteroid receptor into the nucleus. In the case of the occupied glucocorticoid receptor, this complex has been termed a **transportosome** because certain components actually are involved in migration of the ligand-receptor complex into the nucleus.

Box 3B.   An Ancient "Orphan" Nuclear Receptor

The gene responsible for the synthesis of the cytoplasmic aryl hydrocarbon receptor (ahR) is one of the oldest genes known to direct the synthesis of a member of the nuclear receptor family. The ahR gene has been identified in a nematode worm indicating it existed at least 500 MYBP. The ahR gene contains a region known as the Per-ARNT-Sim region and exhibits sequence homologies with Per and Sim (genes identified in the fruit fly *Drosophila*) as well as ARNT, the aryl hydrocarbon nuclear translocator protein.

The ahR is an orphan receptor, having no known endogenous ligand. However, it can bind a number of polyaromatic hydrocarbons. It has the highest affinity for a dioxin known as 2,3,7,8-tetrachlorodibenzo-p-dioxin (TCDD). Dioxins are toxic products of combustion that are naturally produced by forest fires and volcano activity, but they also are produced by human activities through many industrial practices involving combustion of organic materials. Once the ahR has bound a ligand, it sheds heatshock chaparone protein (hsp90), and the occupied ahR enters the nucleus where it forms a heterodimer with ARNT protein. The ahR-ARNT complex binds to specific response elements on a number of CYP genes such as *CYP1A1*. These genes direct the synthesis of enzymes that aid cells to detoxify dioxins as well as other contaminants including pesticides and drugs. Studies conducted in both mammals and fishes demonstrate that glucocorticoid levels often observed in stressed animals are sufficient to potentiate the actions of the ahR. Furthermore, numerous laboratory studies have linked dioxin binding by the ahR to alterations in steroid action and/or metabolism, probably through cross-talk as well as through effects on the production of metabolizing enzymes (see Box 3C).

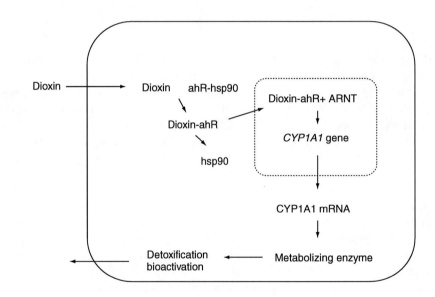

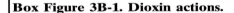

Box Figure 3B-1. Dioxin actions.   Dioxins bind to the arylhydrocarbon receptor (ahR). The ligand-receptor complex enters the nucleus and dimerizes with the aryl hydrocarbon nuclear translocator protein (ARNT) and activates the *CYP1A1* gene. This gene produces a metabolizing enzyme that destroys a variety of potential toxicants including dioxins.

2. 1,25-DHC Actions

C_{27}-steroid bioregulators exhibit similar actions to those described for reproductive and adrenal steroids. A major exception is the formation of heterodimers prior to binding to an HRE. Occupied 1,25-DHC receptors dimerize with PPAR, another member of the steroid nuclear receptor family.

F. Membrane Receptors for Steroids

Numerous steroid actions are very rapid such as the effects of corticosteroids on behavior of progesterone on oocyte maturation. Researchers began to suspect that not all steroid-target interactions involve intracellular receptors and that steroids might have immediate membrane-mediated effects in some target cells such as those described for peptide regulators. Evidence of membrane receptors for corticosteroids in the amphibian brain and for progesterone in the amphibian oocyte has been known for some time, but only recently have the first cell membrane-bound steroid receptors been isolated and characterized. In 1991, Miles Orchinik and Frank Moore of Oregon State University isolated what appears to be a cell membrane-bound corticosterone receptor from the newt brain. Since then, David Crews and his associates at the University of Texas have reported that a large proportion of the estrogen receptors located in the rat brain are surface membrane receptors, too. Presumably, these membrane steroid receptors operate through second messenger systems to alter ion channels or produce other rapid effects in their target cells.

G. Metabolism and Excretion of Steroid Hormones

Steroid hormones are dissociated from their receptors and metabolized by the target cell or the liver which possess enzymes capable of altering the specific steroids and rendering them biologically inactive and water-soluble. The liver performs the major task of steroid inactivation by removing free steroids from the circulation. Metabolism of steroids typically involves reduction or removal of side chains or attached groups or both, as well as combining with other molecules (conjugation) such as glucose to form a a **glucuronide** or conjugation with **sulfate** (Figure 3-38). The relative emphasis on sulfate or glucuronide varies depending on the steroid and/or the species involved. For example, in humans, estradiol is excreted primarily as the glucuronide derivative. The conjugates are water-soluble and when released into the blood will no longer bind effectively to serum proteins or enter cells and bind to receptors. Consequently, they are filtered from the blood by the kidney and readily appear in the urine. Some of the steroids are metabolized, added to the bile, and excreted via the intestinal route.

Steroids also are metabolized via oxidative pathways as well as by reductions. These oxidized metabolites originally were not identified because they occurred in a fraction of urine usually discarded when researchers were isolating urinary steroids for analysis. Oxidized steroid metabolites may represent a substantial portion of the total metabolites for a given steroid. For example, it is estimated that from 12 to 36% of circulating cortisol in humans is converted to oxidized **corotic acids** (cortolic and cortolonic acids; Figure 3-38).

Androgens of both adrenal and gonadal origin are found in the urine primarily as sulfates and can be measured chemically as **17-ketosteroids**. In addition, some androgens are found as conjugates with glucuronic acid. Estrogens may be excreted as either glucuronides or sulfates such as estriol glucosiduronate or estrone sulfate. **Catechol estrogens** are also common excretory products (Figure 3-38; compare to catechol amines). Higher production of one catechol estrogen is associated with breast cancer induction. Progestogens are excreted mainly as glucuronides of pregnanediol or pregnanetriol. However, pregnanediol may be formed from corticosteroid metabolism (that is, from deoxycorticosterone) as well as from progesterone. Pregnanetriol is formed principally from 17α-hydroxyprogesterone, but small amounts also may be produced from 11-deoxycortisol and 17α-hydroxypregnenolone. The corticosteroids are primarily excreted as C_{21} **17-hydroxy-corticosteroids** after conjugation with glucuronic acid.

Under some conditions, membrane-bound **sulfatase** enzymes can remove the sulfate and liberate free steroids that then can enter the cell. Sulfatase activity is very high in the placenta where the sulfated androgen, **DHEA sulfate (DHEAS)**, produced in the fetal adrenal, is desulfated and converted to estrogen. A female fetus is thus protected from the potentially masculinizing actions of this fetal androgen by sulfation. There also are known cases where sulfated steroids can bind to cellular membrane proteins. For example, pregnenolone sulfate produced by certain brain cells is known to bind to and suppress the GABA receptor on nearby neurons. The ability of bacteria associated with wastewater treatment plants (WWTP) to remove both sulfates and glucuronides from steroid metabolites results in the reactivation of excreted steroids that may then find their way into the aquatic systems via WWTP effluents. Estrogenic compounds in WWTP effluents have been associated with feminization of male fishes in rivers throughout the world.

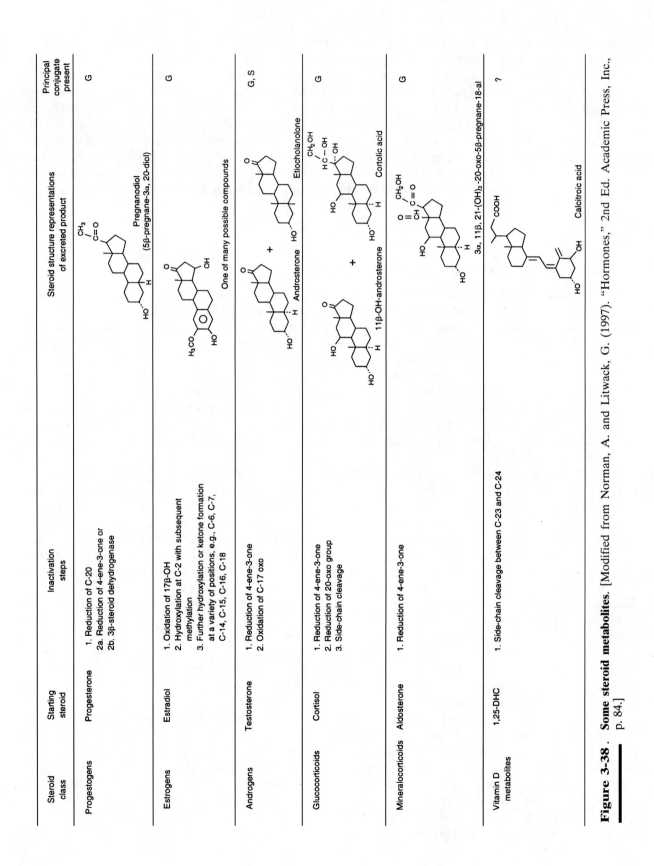

Steroid class	Starting steroid	Inactivation steps	Steroid structure representations of excreted product	Principal conjugate present
Progestogens	Progesterone	1. Reduction of C-20 2a. Reduction of 4-ene-3-one or 2b. 3β-steroid dehydrogenase	Pregnanediol (5β-pregnane-3α, 20-diol)	G
Estrogens	Estradiol	1. Oxidation of 17β-OH 2. Hydroxylation at C-2 with subsequent methylation 3. Further hydroxylation or ketone formation at a variety of positions, e.g., C-6, C-7, C-14, C-15, C-16, C-18	One of many possible compounds	G
Androgens	Testosterone	1. Reduction of 4-ene-3-one 2. Oxidation of C-17 oxo	Etiocholanolone + Androsterone	G, S
Glucocorticoids	Cortisol	1. Reduction of 4-ene-3-one 2. Reduction of 20-oxo group 3. Side-chain cleavage	Cortolic acid + 11β-OH-androsterone	G
Mineralocorticoids	Aldosterone	1. Reduction of 4-ene-3-one	3α, 11β, 21-(OH)₃ -20-oxo-5β-pregnane-18-al	G
Vitamin D metabolites	1,25-DHC	1. Side-chain cleavage between C-23 and C-24	Calcitroic acid	?

Figure 3-38. **Some steroid metabolites.** [Modified from Norman, A. and Litwack, G. (1997). "Hormones," 2nd Ed. Academic Press, Inc., p. 84.]

Box 3C.   Steroid-Metabolizing Enzymes

Steroids are metabolized by a group of generalized enzymes that can operate on a wide variety of substrates including drugs and contaminants from the environment. Many of these enzymes can be induced by the presence of a suitable substrate (Table 3C-1). These enzymes are classified as Phase I (activational) enzymes or as Phase II (conjugation) enzymes. Activation usually involves addition of a hydroxyl group that may result in a more reactive molecule. Conjugation occurs by addition of glucuronate, glutathione, or sulfate, and typically makes the molecule more soluble in water and allows it to be excreted more readily. Phase II reactions may directly follow a Phase I reaction for a given substrate.

Phase I reactions are carried out primarily by cytochrome P450 monooxygenases although numerous other enzymes may participate in Phase I reactions. These monooxygenases are produced by the CYP gene family. They generally are membrane-bound hemoproteins associated with the smooth endoplasmic reticulum. In addition to their involvement in metabolizing steroid hormones prior to their excretion, these same enzymes can metabolize a wide variety of drugs and pollutants including caffeine, pesticides, PCBs, and phthalates.

Table 3C-1. Metabolizing Enzymes

Some Substrates Capable of Inducing CYP Gene Expression in Mammals

Gene family	Mammalian subfamily	Substrate examples
CYP1	1A, 1B	PAHs,[1] pesticides, natural estrogens, arachidonic acid, caffeine, indoles, flavenoids
CYP2	2A-2G, 2J	Various drugs, steroids, pesticides, caffeine, alcohol
CYP3	3A	Various drugs, steroids, PAHs, pesticides, caffeine
CYP4	4A, 4B, 4F	PCBs,[2] phthalates, arachidonic acid, lauric acid

[1] PAH = polynuclear aromatic hydrocarbons.

[2] PCB = polychlorinated biphenyls; includes dioxins; aroclors are commercial mixtures of PCBs.
  Based on Celander, M. 1999. Impact of stress in animal toxicology. In P. H. M. Balm (ed.) "Stress Physiology in Animals." CRC Press, Boca Raton, FL, pp. 246–278.
  Phase II reactions are catalyzed by a great variety of enzymes including glucuronosyl transferease, glutathione transferases, and sulfotransferases, transaminases, esterases, etc. These enzymes participate with Phase I enzymes to help cells eliminate the products of Phase I activations.

A number of chemical methods formerly were employed to identify and quantify various steroid metabolites in urine, but these approaches have given way to radioimmunoassay techniques, ELISAs, and sophisticated chromatographic separation and identification by mass spectroscopy techniques (see Chapter 2).

III. Thyroid Hormones

Thyroid hormones are important developmental and metabolic bioregulators synthesized in the follicular cells of the thyroid gland under the influence of pituitary thyrotropin (TSH). Details of this process in association with the structure of thyroid follicular cells are provided in Chapter 6 and only a general overview of the chemical events is given here. The original molecule isolated from the thyroid gland by Edward C. Kendall in 1915 was believed for many years to be the active thyroid hormone and was named **thyroxine**. It was known to contain four iodide atoms attached to a unique compound called a **thyronine**. The chemical name for thyroxine is **3,5,3′, 5′-tetraiodothyronine** (Figure 3-39). Because of the presence of four iodide atoms per molecule (tetraiodo), the abbreviation for thyroxine became T_4. In 1952, J. Gross and Rosalind Pitt-Rivers discovered a second form of thyroid hormone lacking one of the iodides found in T_4. This molecule was named **3,5,3′-triiodothyronine** or **triiodothyronine** and the abbreviation became T_3. Many endocrinologists now consider T_3 to be the biologically active form of thyroid hormone and that T_4 is a precursor. Although T_4 is not a propeptide,

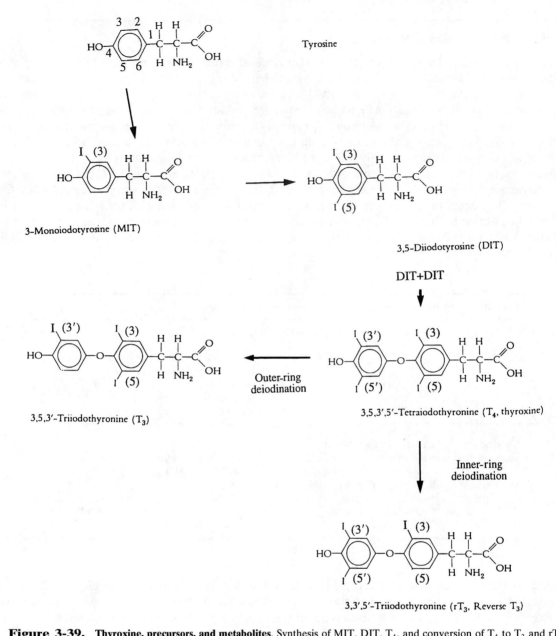

Figure 3-39. Thyroxine, precursors, and metabolites. Synthesis of MIT, DIT, T_4, and conversion of T_4 to T_3 and rT_3.

it may be termed a prohormone for T_3. This point is considered further in Chapter 6, and we will refer to both of them here simply as thyroid hormones since both can bind and activate thyroid hormone receptors.

A. Structure and Synthesis of Thyroid Hormones

The thyroid hormones are derived from two molecules of iodinated tyrosine. Tyrosine is first incorporated into a large globular protein called **thyroglobulin (Tgb)** and then iodinated by an enzyme, **thyroid peroxidase (TPO)**. An iodinated tyrosine has two iodides attached at positions 3 and 5 of the phenolic ring, respectively. This molecule is called **3,5-diiodotyrosine**, or **DIT**. Two DITs are joined by TPO through removal of the phenolic ring of one DIT and the attachment of it to the hydroxyl group extending from the phenolic group of the other DIT. The resulting chemical structure (Figure 3-39) is a thyronine with four iodides attached.

The carbons of the recently added phenolic ring are designated by a prime (′) symbol that appears in the chemical name of the resultant thyronine, T_4. When thyroglobulin containing T_4 molecules is hydrolyzed in the thyroid cell, T_4 is released and then enters the blood. In most cases, T_4 is the major circulating thyronine and is converted peripherally to T_3 by removing one iodide from the outer ring (see below). A small proportion of the circulating T_3 is a result of deiodination of T_4 by a thyroid deiodinase prior to release from the thyroid gland.

Thyroid hormones are hydrophobic and hence poorly soluble in water but, like steroids, highly capable of readily passing through cell membranes. There is also a specific transport mechanism to enhance thyroid hormone movement across cell membranes.

B. Transport of Thyroid Hormones in the Blood

Most of the circulating thyroid hormones (about 99%) are bound reversibly to plasma proteins. Binding to plasma protein by thyroid hormones is considered helpful for their transport in the blood, because T_3 and T_4 are somewhat hydrophobic and are not highly soluble in blood. When thyroid hormone molecules leave the blood and enter a target cell, additional hormone dissociates from the transport proteins, instantly replenishing the pool of free hormones. Thus, the binding proteins provide a ready reservoir of thyroid hormones in the circulation that are ready for immediate usage. The relationship of bound and free hormone to their actions and pathological roles is controversial, and measurement of both total hormone and free hormone often are determined (see Chapter 6).

Several different serum proteins are capable of binding and transporting thyroid hormones. In humans, for example, about 75% of the bound hormones are linked to the α_2-globulins and 15 and 10%, respectively, are bound to prealbumin (also called **transthyretin**) and albumin. Only a very small fraction (<1%) are transported free in the blood. Free thyroid hormones are thought to cross cell membranes readily by both diffusion and by carrier-mediated transport mechanisms, and they are rapidly removed from the blood by target tissues or metabolized directly by the liver and kidneys.

C. Mechanism of Thyroid Hormone Action

The molecular mechanism of action for thyroid hormones appears to be similar to that described above for estrogens. Thyroid hormones enter target cells where they migrate to the nucleus and bind to specific nuclear receptor proteins. Following the binding to nuclear receptors, occupied thyroid hormone receptors form dimers and initiate nuclear gene transcription resulting in synthesis of new proteins.

Nuclear receptors for thyroid hormones have been isolated and characterized. Typically, they have greater affinity for T_3 than for T_4, supporting the hypothesis that conversion of T_4 to T_3 is requisite for thyroid hormone action. Target cells for thyroid hormones are equipped with a specific deiodinase enzyme to accomplish this conversion. Mitochondrial receptor proteins also have been demonstrated, and these mitochondrial receptors are associated with observed effects on mitochondrial protein synthesis and oxidative metabolism in target cells (see Chapter 6).

The interactions of thyroid hormones and nuclear DNA have proven to be even more complicated than what we described earlier for steroids. At least two major isoforms of nuclear **thyroid receptor proteins (TRs)** have been demonstrated in humans, mice, and rats, suggesting there may be a separate functional role for each type. In the rat, two forms, TRα-1 and TRβ-1, are found in all tissues, whereas another form, TRβ-2, is limited to the pituitary, hypothalamus, and other brain areas. Thyroid receptors belong to the same superfamily of nuclear receptor types that includes the steroid receptors and retinoic acid receptors (see Table 3-13).

Occupied TRs bind to **thyroid-responsive elements (TREs)** in or near specific genes in target cell nuclei but may do this in a variety of ways. Monomers of occupied receptor may bind directly to TREs but they do not produce much transcription by the thyroid-responsive gene. Similarly, occupied TR homodimers bind for such a short time that they also produce little transcription. However, formation of a unique heterodimer provides maximal stimulation of transcription. An occupied TR monomer may form a heterodimer with the **retinoic acid receptor (RAR)** or the orphan **retinoid X receptor (RXR)**.

D. Metabolism of Thyroid Hormones

Thyroxine has several metabolic fates after being released from the thyroid gland. Approximately 33 to 40% is converted to T_3 by 5'-deiodination in the liver. This is accomplished by a special deiodinase enzyme called **5'-deiodinase** (also called Type 1 deiodinase) and represents the source for most of the circulating T_3 in many species. About 15 to 20% of the circulating T_4 is deaminated and decarboxylated in the liver to form **tetraiodothyroacetate (TETRAC)**, which is very soluble in water, has no physiological activity, and is excreted rapidly in urine or bile (Figure 3-40). T_3 also may be converted similarly to form **triiodothyroacetate (TRIAC)** or the latter can be formed by deiodination of TETRAC. Some glucuronide conjugates of T_4 and to a lesser extent of T_3 also may be formed. All of these metabolized molecules are more soluble in water, cannot bind effectively to plasma binding proteins or receptors, and are quickly eliminated via the bile or urine.

In recent years, it was discovered that approximately one-half of the circulating T_4 is eventually converted by deiodination to a unique form of T_3 with the structure of 3,3',5'-triiodothyronine or **reverse T_3, rT_3** (Figure 3-39). This conversion is accomplished by enzymatic 5-deiodination (by a **5-deiodinase** or Type 2 deiodinase) which removes an iodide from the internal phenolic ring of a thyronine. Reverse T_3 has no biological activity, and it is degraded more rapidly than normal T_3. As a result of its rapid clearance, rT_3 levels in the blood are rather low and hence escaped detection for many years. However, increases or decreases in circulating T_3 levels are always accompanied by reciprocal changes in rT_3 levels. The liver may continue to deiodinate T_3 and rT_3, removing the remaining iodides to produce **3,3'-diiodothyronine (T_2)**, and then **monoiodothyronines**.

IV. Eicosanoids

The **eicosanoids** are small lipids derived from a common precursor, **arachidonic acid**. This group includes the prostaglandins, the leukotrienes, and the thromboxanes. In the early 1930s, Maurice Goldblatt in England and U.S. von Euler in Sweden independently discovered **prostaglandins (PGs)**. Elucidation of these important bioregulatory compounds and their synthetic pathways resulted in the awarding of the 1982 Nobel Prize in Physiology or Medicine to three principal prostaglandin researchers: Sune Bergstrom, Bengt Samuellson, and John Vane.

Prostaglandins were named on the belief that their source in men was the prostate gland. Since then, they have been found in most tissues of both men and women. The PGs have many diverse actions including stimulation of smooth muscle contraction in the intestine and uterus, vasodilation (but may cause vasoconstriction in certain vessels), and modulation of central nervous system function. They also stimulate synthesis of corticosteroids, testosterone, and a variety of specific enzymes. One PG ($PGF_{2\alpha}$) is believed to be the uterine luteolytic substance in certain mammalian species (see Chapter 10). Prostaglandins also reduce progesterone synthesis by the corpus luteum, induce ovulation and lactation in rodents, and may be involved in the induction of labor. Furthermore, they may induce inflammation and fever. The anti-inflammatory and antipyretic (fever-decreasing) action of aspirin is due to its inhibition of PG synthesis. **Prostacyclin (PGI_2)**, another form of prostaglandin, is a potent inhibitor of blood platelet aggregation and inhibits blood clotting.

Researchers discovered the **thromboxanes** during studies on prostaglandin metabolism and action. Thromboxane A_2 causes translocation of free calcium ions to bring about changes associated with the shape of blood platelets. It is this change in platelet shape that allows platelets to aggregate and facilitate clotting. Other thromboxanes may be released from the platelet, causing local constriction of vascular smooth muscle. This paracrine effect might enhance clotting by reducing the diameter of the arterioles and slowing blood flow through the capillary beds of damaged tissues.

Leukotrienes are synthesized and released by white blood cells in response to injury. They contribute to inflammatory or allergic responses by causing contraction of vascular smooth muscle and by increasing vascular permeability. Increased levels of leukotrienes have been associated with allergic reactions, asthma, cystic fibrosis, septic shock, and a number of other disorders.

A. Chemical Structure of Eicosanoids

Prostaglandins are all related structurally to **prostanoic acid**, and they can be separated into four classes (E, F, A, and B) on the basis of structural differences (Figure 3-41). Bergstrom succeeded in elucidating the

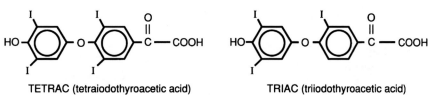

TETRAC (tetraiodothyroacetic acid)   TRIAC (triiodothyroacetic acid)

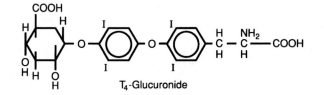

T$_4$-Glucuronide

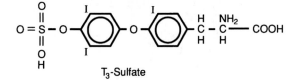

T$_3$-Sulfate

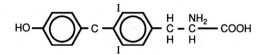

3,5-T$_2$ (3,5-Diiodothyronine)

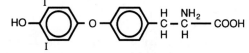

3′,5′-T$_2$ (3′,5′-Diiodothyronine)

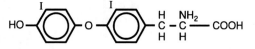

3,3′-T$_2$ (3,3′-Diiodothyronine)

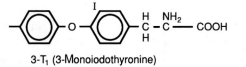

3-T$_1$ (3-Monoiodothyronine)

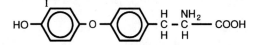

3′-T$_1$ (3′-Monoiodothyronine)

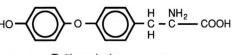

T$_0$ (thyronine)

Figure 3-40. **Additional thyroid hormone metabolites**. See text for explanation.

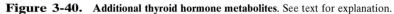

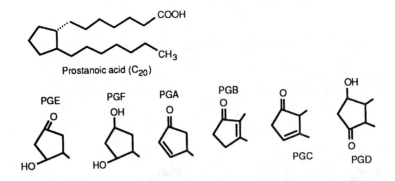

Figure 3-41. **Prostaglandin structures.** The basic chemical formula for the prostaglandins is that of prostanoic acid. These C_{20}-lipids are divided into classes (A, B, F, etc.) based on substitutions to the five-membered carbon ring. Modifications of the side chains results in different forms within a class, each designated by a subscript; e.g., $PGF_{2\alpha}$, PGE_1.

structures for 16 PGs in 1956. The most commonly occurring PGs are PGE_1, PGE_2, and $PGF_{2\alpha}$. Prostacyclin (PGI_2) represents a unique class of prostaglandins called PGI. The leukotrienes consist of at least 15 related compounds occurring in five structural classes, A, B, C, D, and E (Figure 3-41). Thromboxanes are very short-lived molecules, some of which also are depicted in Figure 3-42.

B. Biosynthesis and Actions of Eicosanoids

Arachidonic acid is synthesized from linolenic acid or diacylglycerol (DAG). Once formed, arachidonic acid can be converted to any of the eicosanoids (Figure 3-42). **Cyclooxygenase** is an enzyme that transforms arachidonic acid into endoperoxides which are used to synthesize prostaglandins, prostacyclin, or thromboxanes. Drugs such as **aspirin** and **indomethacin** inhibit cyclooxygenase and block the syntheses of prostaglandins and thromboxanes. Certain flavenoids obtained from plants also block cyclooxygenase. A separate enzyme, **5-lipoxygenase**, forms the leucotrienes from arachidonic acid. This enzyme is not inhibited by aspirin or indomethacin but can be inhibited by specific lipoxygenase inhibitors as well as by plant flavenoids.

Eicosanoids produce their effects by binding to the **(PPAR)** receptor. PPAR is also a member of the same superfamily of nuclear receptors that includes steroids and thyroid hormones and is in the same subgrouping as the thyroid receptors. Occupied PPAR form heterodimers with RXR prior to binding to gene response elements.

V. Other Important Bioregulators

In this section, we will briefly describe a number of bioregulators and their chemistry to serve as background information for later discussions. Some limited information about their synthesis and metabolism is also provided. Although these bioregulators typically are not classified as hormones, they do influence the activity of a variety of endocrine systems that are discussed in this book.

A. Acetylcholine

Acetylcholine (ACh) was first demonstrated as a major neurotransmitter in the peripheral nervous system and only much later was its role in the brain clarified. Synthesis of ACh from its precursors, choline and acetate, is accomplished by an enzyme called **choline acetyl-transferase (CAT)**. After release into the synaptic space, ACh is degraded back to choline and acetate by **acetylcholinesterase (AChE)** associated with the postsynaptic cell membrane. The presynaptic cells may take up free choline for use in the resynthesis of ACh. The distribution of CAT immunoreactivity in the brain corresponds to the distribution of ACh receptors. In contrast, the distribution of AChE is much wider than that of either CAT or ACh receptors and therefore is an unreliable indicator of cholinergic synapses.

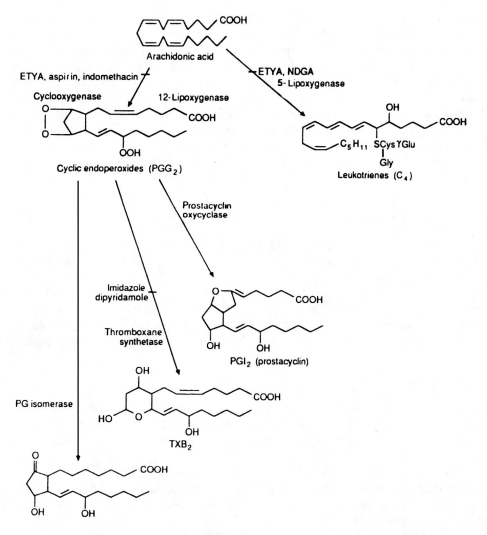

Figure 3-42. **Eicosanoid synthesis.** The precursor for all eicosanoids, arachidonic acid, can be synthesized from diacylglycerol (DAG) which has dual roles as second messenger and eicosanoid precursor. Indomethecin, aspirin, and ETYA (eicosatetraynoic acid) inhibit the enzyme cyclooxygenase and block prostaglandin and thromboxane synthesis. ETYA and NDGA (nordihydroguaiaretic acid) block the enzyme 5-lipoxygenase and prevent leukotriene synthesis. EYTA is a modified form of arachidonic acid that competes for any enzyme that normally uses arachidonic acid as its substrate. [Modified from F. F. Bolander (1989). "Molecular Endocrinology." Academic Press, Inc.]

B. Gamma-Aminobutyric Acid (GABA)

The inhibitory neurotransmitter **gamma (γ)-aminobutyric acid (GABA)** is formed mainly from the amino acid glutamate by the enzyme **glutamate decarboxylase (GAD)**. Glutamate may be synthesized from either glutamine or 2-oxoglutarate. GABA, an important central nervous system neurotransmitter, is inactivated by conversion to succinate or γ-hydroxybutyric acid. It may have a role as a neurohormone, too (see Chapter 4). Glutamate also is known to be a neurotransmitter.

C. Interleukins

Certain white blood cells, such as lymphocytes and macrophages, secrete proteins called **interleukins** that operate in autocrine and paracrine fashion within the vascular system and several lymphatic tissues. There are more than a dozen recognized interleukins. For example, once a macrophage has identified a cell infected with a virus, it obtains and transfers the viral antigen complexed with a protein to a lymphocyte known as a helper

T-cell. The macrophage also secretes **interleukin-1 (IL-1)** that further activates the helper T-cell. **Interleukin-2 (IL-2)** is a mitogen secreted by the helper T-cell following its activation by IL-1 which stimulates another lymphocyte type called a B-cell to divide and form plasma cells (antibody-synthesizing cells) and memory cells (responsible for long-term immunity). In autocrine fashion, IL-2 stimulates proliferation of the helper T-cells, too. IL-6 is known to interact with the adrenal system resulting in the release of cortisol (see Chapter 8).

Helper T-cells also produce **γ-interferon** which can transform macrophages and cause them to attack viral-infected cells more vigorously. The interleukins, interferons, and other factors secreted by cells involved with the immune response also are known as **cytokines**. Recently, cytokines have been shown to be involved in other cellular processes. For example, they have been implicated in the endocrine mechanisms controlling release of certain pituitary hormones (see Chapters 4 and 8). Here they are included in the category of bioregulator called cytocrines (see Chapter 1).

D. Miscellaneous Brain Neuropeptides

In recent years, numerous peptides that play important roles as neurotransmitters and neuromodulators have been identified in the brain. Some of these peptides also may function as neurohormones. Foremost among these are the **endorphins**, **dynorphins** and **enkephalins** that play important analgesic (pain-killing) roles. Other important peptides include substance P, VIP, galanin, neuropeptide Y (NPY), neuropeptide YY (PYY), peptide-histidine-isoleucine (PHI), neurotensin, cholecystokinin (CCK), angiotensin II (ANG-II), and calcitonin gene-related peptide (CGRP). The possible roles for many of these neuropeptides will be discussed in Chapter 4 in association with the regulation of pituitary gland functions and in some other systems.

E. Gaseous Bioregulators

Among the most surprising discoveries was the recognition of two well-known toxic gases as physiologically relevant bioregulators: nitric oxide (NO) and **carbon monoxide (CO)**. Failure to recognize them earlier in part is due to their ability to pass readily through cell membranes and the absence of discrete receptors on the cell membranes of target cells.

The first discovery establishing such bioregulatory substances was the identification of NO as the hypothesized **endothelium-derived relaxing factor (EDRF)** of endothelial cells lining blood arterioles. EDRF or NO diffuses into adjacent vascular smooth muscles cells to cause relaxation and allow dilation of the arterioles. These endothelial cells contain the enzyme, nitric oxide synthetase (NOS), which produces NO from the amino acid arginine. NOS has a heme group similar to that of hemoglobin acting as an electron acceptor in this reaction. Once formed, the NO quickly exits and enters adjacent smooth muscle cells where it interacts with intracellular enzymes. Because of its gaseous nature, NO can readily exit from cells and the body and special degrading systems may not be necessary. It readily can be converted to nitrites and nitrates. Soon after its discovery, NO released from certain pelvic nerves was identified as the causative factor producing penile erection through local effects on the vasculature of the penis. There also appear to be links between the ability of brain neurons to synthesize NO and the cellular basis for learning and memory.

Although best known for its role as an insidious poison, carbon monoxide may prove to be a physiological bioregulator, too. In 1987, CO was reported to cause dilation of blood vessels. The enzyme **heme oxygenase**, which breaks down heme, produces CO, and this enzyme is found in many cell types including neurons in certain brain regions. Preliminary studies suggest that CO readily enters smooth muscle cells, interacts with and activates the enzyme guanylyl cyclase, and produces a rise in cGMP. Elevated cGMP in turn promotes relaxation. NO also activates guanylyl cyclase in certain cells as discussed earlier. As scientists look more carefully at these and other potential gaseous bioregulators, we may learn many new things about chemical regulation.

VI. Summary

Neurotransmitters, neurohormones, and hormones may occur as peptides, proteins, modified amino acids (indoleamines, catecholamines, thyroid hormones), or lipids (steroids, eicosanoids). Peptides and proteins neurohormones and hormones are synthesized as preprohormones and are modified post-translationally to prohormones and then cleaved again to the final product. These processes usually occur intracellularly.

Additional post-translational modifications may occur as well (e.g., addition of carbohydrates, dimer formation, amidation, acetylation). Peptides are transported free in the blood or bound to plasma proteins. Most of the steroids (including androgens, estrogens, progesterone, corticosteroids, and 1,25-DHC) and thyroid hormones as well as many amines are transported primarily bound to specific plasma proteins in equilibrium with a small quantity of free hormones. Peptides, proteins, indoleamines, catecholamines, thyroid hormones, and many other bioregulators are formed from one or more amino acids. The amino acid arginine is also the substrate for synthesis of the gaseous bioregulator, nitric oxide. Steroid hormones are all derived from cholesterol, and the eicosanoids have a common precursor, arachidonic acid.

Peptide, protein, and amine bioregulators bind to receptors located on the cell surface and typically produce their actions through production of second messengers. Some of these hormones work through mechanisms that employ a variety of G-proteins that influence levels of second messengers such as cAMP, cGMP, IP_3, and DAG which in turn may affect the activity of specific protein kinases or permeability of the cell membrane. Other receptor complexes may exhibit protein kinase activities themselves and produce their effects through phosphorylation of specific proteins or by activation of phosphorylation cascades. Initial effects of these bioregulators usually alter membrane transport in (uptake) or out (secretion) of the cell or activate intracellular enzyme systems. Many of these membrane ligands also produce a delayed effect on protein synthesis through activation of cytosolic transcription factors. Cell surface receptors may cause in flux of Ca^{2+} that also functions as a second messenger.

Steroids and thyroid hormones enter the cytoplasm where they may bind to what are called nuclear receptors although they are sometimes located in the cytosol. Occupied receptors for these hormones typically form homo- or heterodimers and act as ligand-activated transcription factors, binding to HREs and affecting nuclear mRNA production and subsequent protein synthesis. In a few cases, certain steroids may be ligands for receptors located in the cell membrane. Some steroids and T_4 may be modified by intracellular enzymes that allow them to bind to receptors.

Bioregulators are metabolized in a variety of ways to inactivate them so that activated cells can recover. Metabolism may involve inactivation by enzymes associated with the cell surface or by intracellular enzymes in the target cells or nearby cells. Reuptake of amines by presynaptic neurons or adjacent cells is another method for inactivating the target cell. Steroids and thyroid hormones are often metabolized by addition of special components (e.g., sulfate, glucuronides) that increase their solubility in water and accelerate their excretion via the urine. Sensitivity of target cells also can be influenced by increases (up-regulation) or decreases (down-regulation) in receptor number.

Suggested Reading

Books

Bolander, F. F. (2004). "Molecular Endocrinology," 3rd Ed. Academic Press, San Diego.
Sherwood, N. M., and Hew, C. L. (1994). "Fish Physiology XIII. Molecular Endocrinology of Fish." Academic Press, San Diego.
Weintraub, B. D. (1995). "Molecular Endocrinology: Basic Concepts and Clinical Implications." Raven, New York.

Articles

Arimura, A. (1992). Receptors for pituitary adenylate cyclase-activating polypeptide: Comparison with vasoactive intestinal peptide receptors. *Trends Endocr. Metab.* **3**, 288–294.
Baker, M. E. (2003). Evolution of adrenal and sex steroid action in vertebrates: A ligand-based mechanism for complexity. *Bioessays* **25**, 396–400.
Balla, T., and Catt, K. J. (1994). Phosphoinositides and calcium signaling: New aspects and diverse functions in cell regulation. *Trends Endocr. Metab.* **5**, 250–255.
Bar-Sagi, D. (1994). The Sos (Son of sevenless) protein. *Trends Endocr. Metab.* **5**, 165–169.
Baulieu, E.-E. (1991). The antisteroid RU 486: Its cellular and molecular mode of action. *Trends Endocrinol. Metab.* **2**, 233–239.
Blaustein, J. D., Olster, D. H., and Tetel, M. J. (1993). Heterogenous regulation of steroid hormone receptors in the brain. *Am. Zool.* **33**, 219–228.
Cadena, R. L., and Gill, G. N. (1992). Receptor tyrosine kinases. *FASEB J.* **6**, 2332–2337.
Cheung, J., and Smith, D. F. 2000. Molecular chaparone interactions with steroid receptors: An update. *Molecular Endocr.* **14**, 939–946.

Combarnous, Y. (1992). Molecular basis of the specificity of binding of glycoprotein hormones to their receptors. *Endocr. Rev.* **13**, 670–691.

Conti, M. (2000). Phosphodiesterases and cyclic nucleotide signaling in endocrine cells. *Molecular Endocr.* **14**, 1317–1327.

Conti, M., Jin, S.-L. C., Monaco, L., Repaske, D. R., and Swinnin, J. V. (1991). Hormonal regulation of cyclic nucleotide phosphosdiesterase. *Endocr. Rev.* **12**, 218–234.

DeVivo, M., and Iyengar, R. (1994). G protein pathways: Signal processing by effectors. *Mol. Cell. Endocr.* **100**, 65–70.

Delftos, L. J. (1991). Chromogranin A: Its role in endocrine function and as an endocrine and neuroendocrine tumor marker. *Endocr. Rev.* **12**, 181–188.

Edwards, D. P. (2005). Regulation of signal transduction pathways by estrogen and progesterone. *Ann. Rev. Physiol.* **67**, 335–376.

Ergul, A. and Puett, D. (1999). Hormone receptors, overview. In Knobil ed., "Encyclopedia of Reproduction," Vol 2. Academic Press, San Diego, pp. 654–662.

Escriva, H., Delaunay, F., and Laudet, V. (2000). Ligand binding and nuclear receptor evolution. *Bioessays* **22**, 717–727.

Ferrara, N., Houck, K., Jakeman, L., and Leung, D. W. (1992). Molecular and biological properties of the vascular endothelial growth factor family of proteins. *Endocr. Rev.* **13**, 18–32.

Freedman, L. P. (1999). Multimeric coactivator complexes for steroid/nuclear receptors. *Trends Endocr. Metab.* **10**, 403–407.

Gaborik, Z., and Hunyady, L. (2004). Intracellular trafficking of hormone receptors. *Trends Endocr. Metab.* **15**, 286–293.

Giguere, V. (2002). To ERR in the estrogen pathway. *Trends Endocr. Metab.* **13**, 220–225.

Guengerich, F. P. (1993). Cytochrome P450 enzymes. *Am. Sci.* **81**, 440–447.

Guiochon-Mantel, A., and Milgrom, E. (1993). Cytoplasmic-nuclear trafficking of steroid hormone receptors. *Trends Endocr. Metab.* **4**, 322–328.

Hammond, G. L. (1990). Molecular properties of corticosteroid binding globulin and the sex-steroid binding proteins. *Endocr. Rev.* **11**, 65–79.

Hermanson, O., Glass, C. K., and Rosenfeld, M. G. (2002). Nuclear receptor coregulators: Multiple modes of modification. *Trends Endocr. Metab.* **13**, 55–60.

Hobkirk, R. (1993). Steroid sulfation: Current concepts. *Trends Endocr. Metab.* **4**, 69–74.

Hoyle, C. H. V. (1998). Neuropeptide families: Evolutionary perspectives. *Regulatory Peptides* **73**, 1–33.

Ihle, J. N. (1994). Signaling by the cytokine receptor superfamily: Just another kinase story. *Trends Endocr. Metab.* **5**, 137–143.

Ing, N. H., and O'Malley, B. W. (1995). The steroid hormone receptor: Molecular mechanisms of action. In "Molecular Endocrinology: Basic Concepts and Clinical Implications" (B. D. Weintraub, Ed.), pp. 195–215. Raven, New York.

Kelly, P. A., Djiane, J., and Edery, M. (1992). Different forms of the prolactin receptor: Insights into the mechanism of prolactin action. *Trends Endocr. Metab.* **3**, 54–59.

Kitamura, T., Ogorochi, T., and Miyajima, A. (1994). Multimeric cytokine receptors. *Trends Endocr. Metab.* **5**, 8–14.

Lazar, M. A. (1993). Thyroid hormone receptors: Multiple forms, multiple possibilities. *Endocr. Rev.* **14**, 184–193.

Lin, D., Sugawara, T., Straus, J. F., III, Clark, B. J., Stocco, D. M., Saenger, P., Rogol, A., and Miller, W. L. (1995). Role of steroidogenic acute regulatory protein in adrenal and gonadal steroidogenesis. *Science* **267**, 1828–1831.

Linder, M. E., and Gilman, A. G. (1992). G proteins. *Sci. Am.* **253**(7), 56–65.

Maggi, A., Ciana, P., Belcredito, S., and Vegeto, E. (2004). Estrogens in the nervous system: Mechanisms and nonreproductive functions. *Ann. Rev. Physiol.* **66**, 291–313.

Malbon, C. C., Rapiejko, P. J., and Watkins, D. C. (1988). Permissive hormone regulation of hormone-sensitive effector systems. *Trends Pharmacol. Sci.* **9**, 33–36.

Mayer, E. A., and Baldi, J. P. (1991). Can regulatory peptides be regarded as words in a biological language? *Am. J. Physiol.* **261**, G171–G184.

McDonald, D. P. (1995). Unraveling the human progesterone receptor signal transduction pathway: Insights into antiprogestin action. *Trends Endocr. Metab.* **6**, 133–138.

Mellon, S. H., and Griffin, L. D. (2002). Neurosteroids: Biochemistry and clinical significance. *Trends Endocr. Metab.* **13**, 35–43.

Miller, W. L. (1988). Molecular biology of steroid hormone synthesis. *Endocr. Rev.* **9**, 295–318.

Naor, Z., Benard, O., and Seger, R. (2000). Activation of MAPK cascades by G-protein-coupled receptors: The case of gonadotropin-releasing hormone receptor. *Trends Endocr. Metab.* **11**, 91–99.

Nettles, K. W., and Greene, G. L. (2005). Ligand control of coregulator recruitment to nuclear receptors. *Ann. Rev. Physiol.* **67**, 309–333.

Orti, E., Bodwell, J. E., and Munck, A. (1992). Phosphorylation of steroid hormone receptors. *Endocr. Rev.* **13**, 105–128.

Pestell, R. G., and Jameson, J. L. (1995). Transcriptional regulation of endocrine genes by second messenger signalling pathways. In "Molecular Endocrinology: Basic Concepts and Clinical Implications" (B. D. Weintraub, Ed.), pp. 59–76. Raven, New York.

Privalsky, M. L. (2004). The role of corepressors in transcriptional regulation by nuclear hormone receptors. *Ann. Rev. Physiol.* **66**, 315–360.

Putney, J. W., Jr., and Bird, G. St. J. (1993). The inositol phosphate-calcium signaling system in nonexciteable cells. *Endocr. Rev.* **14**, 610–631.

Putney, J. W., Jr., and Bird, St. J. G. (1994). Calcium mobilization by inositol phosphates and other intracellular messengers. *Trends Endocr. Metab.* **5**, 256–260.

Re, R. N. (2003). The intracrine hypothesis and intracellular peptide hormone action. *Bioessays* **25**, 401–409.

Rhodes, D., and Klug, A. (1993). Zinc fingers. *Sci. Am.* **254**(2), 56–65.

Rittmaster, R. S. (1993). Androgen conjugates: Physiology and clinical significance. *Endocr. Rev.* **14**, 121–132.

Robel, P., and Baulieu, E.-E. (1994). Neurosteroids: Biosynthesis and function. *Trends Endocr. Metab.* **5**, 1–8.

Roseler, W. J., Park, E. A., Klemm, D. J., Liu, J., Gurney, A. L., Vandenbark, G. R., and Hanson, R. W. (1990). Modulation of hormone response elements by promoter environment. *Trends Endocr. Metab.* **1**, 347–351.

Rosner, W. (1990). The functions of corticosteroid binding globulin and sex hormone-binding globulin: Recent advances. *Endocr. Rev.* **11**, 80–91.

Saunders, P. T. K. (2005). Does estrogen receptor β play a significant role in human reproduction? *Trends Endocr. Metab.* **16**, 222–227.

Scammell, J. G. (1993). Granins: Markers of the regulated secretory pathway. *Trends Endocr. Metab.* **4**, 14–18.

Segre, G. V., and Goldring, S. R. (1993). Receptors for secretin, calcitonin, parathyroid hormone (PTH)/PTH-related peptide, vasoactive intestinal peptide, glucagonlike peptide I, growth hormone-releasing hormone and glucagon belong to a newly discovered G-protein-linked receptor family. *Trends Endocr. Metab.* **4**, 309–314.

Simpson, E. R., Mahendroo, M. S., Means, G. D., Kilgore, M. W., Hinshelwood, M. M., Graham-Lawrence, S., Amarneh, B., Ito, Y., Fisher, C. R., Michael, M. D., Mendelson, C. R., and Bulun, S. E. (1994). Aromatase cytochrome P450, the enzyme responsible for estrogen biosynthesis. *Endocr. Rev.* **15**, 342–355.

Spiegel, A. M., Shenker, A., Simonds, W. F., and Weinstein, L. S. (1995). G protein dysfunction in disease. *In* "Molecular Endocrinology: Basic Concepts and Clinical Implications" (B. D. Weintraub, Ed.), pp. 297–318. Raven, New York.

Thornton, J. W. (2001). Evolution of vertebrate steroid receptors from an ancestral estrogen receptor by ligand exploitation and serial genome expansion. *Proc. NSA* **98**, 5671–5676.

Turgeon, J. L., and Waring, D. W. (1992). Functional cross-talk between receptors for peptide and steroid hormones. *Trends Endocr. Metab.* **3**, 360–365.

Vassart, G., Parmentier, M., Libert, F., and Dumont, J. (1991). Molecular genetics of the thyrotropin receptor. *Trends Endocr. Metab.* **2**, 151–156.

Visser, T. J., de Herder, W. W., Rooda, S. J. E. R., Rutgers, M., and van Buuren, J. C. J. (1990). The role of sulfation in thyroid hormone metabolism. *Trends Endocr. Metab.* **1**, 211–218.

Walker, E. A., and Stewart, P. M. (2003). 11β-hydroxysteroid dehydrogenase: Unexpected connections. *Trends Endocr. Metab.* **14**, 334–339.

Williams, G. R., and Brent, G. A. (1995). Thyroid hormone response elements. *In* "Molecular Endocrinology: Basic Concepts and Clinical Implications." (B. D. Weintraub, Ed.), pp. 217–239. Raven, New York.

Yen, P. M., and Chin, W. W. (1994). New advances in understanding the molecular mechanisms of thyroid hormone action. *Trends Endocr. Metab.* **5**, 65–72.

Zoeller, R. T. (1993). Molecular mechanisms of signal integration in hypothalamic neurons. *Am. Zool.* **33**, 244–254.

4

Organization of the Mammalian Hypothalamus-Pituitary Axes

The **pituitary gland** or **hypophysis** was initially called the "master gland" because its hormones were shown to control many diverse systems that are essential for survival and reproduction. The later discovery of the complex control of the pituitary by the **hypothalamus** of the brain transferred our attention to the brain as being the "master gland," and the pituitary became just another component of this major system for homeostatic regulation (see Figure 4-1). An overview of this system was provided in Chapter 1. Basically, neurosecretory (NS) neurons in the hypothalamus secrete **hypothalamic-releasing hormones** (Table 4-1) that travel to the pituitary gland where they regulate secretion of the pituitary **tropic hormones** (Table 4-2). These tropic hormones target certain peripheral endocrine glands (e.g., the thyroid gland) that in turn release their hormones (e.g., thyroid hormones) into the blood. These target gland hormones affect specific non-endocrine targets of their own and feedback on the hypothalamus and/or the pituitary.

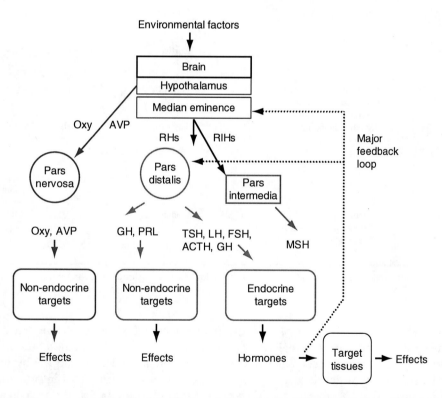

Figure 4-1. **The vertebrate neuroendocrine system.** The hypothalamus secretes RHs and RIHs, stores them in the median eminence, and releases them to the pars distalis and pars intermedia where they regulate release of tropic hormones. The activity of the hypothalamus is influenced by a variety of exogenous environmental factors via the central nervous system. The tropic hormones affect some non-endocrine targets but most have endocrine targets that in turn release hormones that have specific effects on target cells and feedback at the hypothalamus or adenohypophysis (pars distalis). The hypothalamus also secretes the nonapeptides oxytocin (Oxy) and vasopressin (AVP) that are stored in the pars nervosa and released into the blood through which they travel to non-endocrine targets. Only one type of long feedback is shown, but short (tropic hormone feedback) and ultrashort (neuropeptides) may also influence hypothalamic function.

Table 4-1. Major (Primary) and Secondary
Releasing and Release Inhibiting Hormones

	Primary	Secondary
TSH	(+) TRH	VIP (+), CRH (+)
FSH/LH	(+) GnRH	Galanin (+ LH only), NPY (+)
ACTH	(+) CRH	AVP (⌐ response to CRH)
PRL	(−) DA (PRIH)	(−) GAP
	(+) TRH/VIP	(+) PrRH
GH	(−) SST (GH-RIH)	(+) GRH = GHRH; TRH
MSH	(−) DA	

Table 4-2. Synonyms, Abbreviations, Cellular Source, Targets, and Actions for Mammalian Tropic Hormones

Name	Abbreviation[a]	Synonyms	Other abbreviations	Cellular source	One target	One action on target
Prolactin	PRL	Mammotropin, luteotropin, luteotropic hormone	LTH	Lactotrope	Mammary gland	Stimulates milk synthesis
Growth hormone	GH	Somatotropin, somatotropic hormone	STH	Somatotrope	Muscle	Stimulates incorporation of amino acids into protein
Corticotropin	ACTH	Adrenocorticotropic hormone, adrenocorticotropin		Corticotrope	Adrenal cortex	Stimulates synthesis and secretion of corticosteroids
Lipotropin	LPH	None		Corticotrope?	Adipose tissue?	Stimulates hydrolysis of fats to free fatty acids and glycerol
Melanotropin	MSH	Intermedin, melanocyte- or melanophore-stimulating hormone		Pars intermedia	Melanocyte, etc.	Stimulates synthesis of melanin pigment
Thyrotropin	TSH	Thyroid-stimulating hormone		Thyrotrope	Thyroid gland	Stimulates synthesis of thyroid hormone
Follicle-stimulating hormone	FSH	Follitropin		Gonadotrope	Gonad	Stimulates follicular development in females and spermatogenesis in males; estrogen in females
Luteinizing hormone	LH	Interstitial cell-stimulating hormone, lutropin	ICSH	Gonadotrope	Gonad	Stimulates androgen and progesterone synthesis in females and androgen secretion in males

[a] The names in the first column and the abbreviations in the second column are used throughout the text.

The embryonic vertebrate brain develops as four major regions: the **telencephalon** (most anterior), **diencephalon, mesencephalon**, and **rhombencephalon** (most posterior). The telecephalon and diencephalon comprise the **forebrain** while the mesencephalon and rhombencephalon become the **midbrain** and **hindbrain**, respectively. During subsequent development, each of these regions differentiates into major components of the adult brain (Figure 4-2). The telencephalon becomes the **olfactory bulbs**, the **olfactory lobes**, and the **cerebral hemispheres**. The diencephalon differentiates into three regions: the dorsal **epithalamus**, the central **thalamus**, and the ventral **hypothalamus**. Most of the diencephalon becomes the thalamus, a major relay station between higher and lower portions of the brain. The floor or ventral portion of the diencephalon becomes the hypothalamus, containing various NS nuclei, which are sources for the neurohormones involved with regulation of pituitary function. The epithalamus is derived from the roof of the diencephalon and gives rise to the endocrine **epiphysial complex** that includes the **pineal gland**. The mesencephalon gives rise primarily to the **optic tectum**, and the rhombencephalon differentiates into the **cerebellum** and **medulla**.

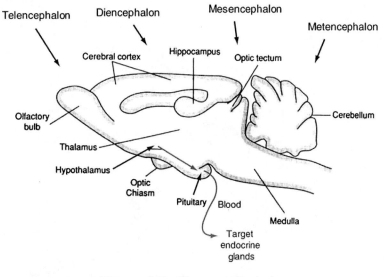

Figure 4-2. The mammalian brain.

There are several distinct axes involving the hypothalamus, a portion of the pituitary gland, and a specific target endocrine gland. Each axis represents a neuroendocrine link between the nervous system and the endocrine system and is a thoroughly integrated system with the hypothalamic NS neurons receiving innervations from non-neurosecretory or ordinary neurons (e.g., adrenergic, cholinergic, serotonergic, and/or peptidergic neurons). Both these ordinary neurons and the NS neurons are responsive to effects of hormones present in the blood or cerebrospinal fluid (CSF). Each **hypothalamus-pituitary (HP) axis** consists of the neurosecretory (NS) neurons within NS nuclei of the hypothalamic region of the brain, specific cell types in the pituitary that secrete tropic hormones, and the endocrine glands directly controlled by these tropic hormones. In this chapter, we focus on four of these axes: the **hypothalamus-pituitary-thyroid (HPT) axis**, the **hypothalamus-pituitary-gonad (HPG) axis**, the **hypothalamus-pituitary-adrenal (HPA) axis**, and the **hypothalamus-pituitary-hepatic** or liver **(HPH) axis**. In addition to these four major axes, we also will consider several pituitary hormones as well as some hypothalamic neurohormones released directly into the general circulation to non-endocrine targets.

Only the mammalian HP axes will be discussed here; non-mammalian vertebrates will be discussed in Chapter 5. Although in an evolutionary sense such a discussion should begin with agnathan fishes and proceed through the other fishes to tetrapods, the mammalian system is better understood and provides the nomenclature with respect to structures, hormones, and functions that later were applied to non-mammalian systems. In fact, the entire field of endocrinology has developed in similar fashion from mammalian investigations, largely of a clinical orientation and motivation, and then applied to wild mammals as well as to non-mammalian vertebrates.

I. The Mammalian Pituitary

The pituitary or hypophysis of adult mammals is located ventral to the brain just posterior to the optic chiasm, and it remains attached to the hypothalamus by a stalk-like connection (Figure 4-3). It is separable into two regions, the **adenohypophysis** and the neurohemal **neurohypophysis**. The anatomical terminology used here for all vertebrate pituitaries is based on Green (1951) and Purves (1961).

The pituitary gland (hypophysis) is located directly beneath the third ventricle of the brain. The third ventricle is a cavity continuous with the other ventricles of the brain and the central canal of the spinal cord. It is filled with cerebrospinal fluid (CSF). Studies in the early 1800s determined that the pituitary developed through an apparent fusion of a ventral growth or evagination from the diencephalon, the **infundibulum**, with an ectodermal sac known as **Rathke's pouch** (Figure 4-4). The latter developed as an inward pocketing or

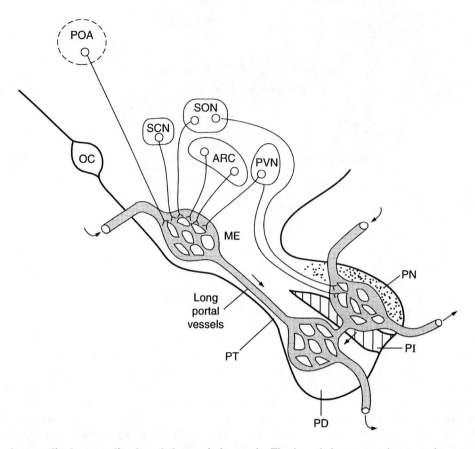

Figure 4-3. **A generalized mammalian hypothalamus-pituitary axis.** The hypothalamus contains several neurosecretory centers including the preoptic area (POA), suprachiasmatic nucleus (SCN), arcuate (ARC) nucleus, supraoptic nucleus (SON), and paraventricular nucleus (PVN). The median eminence (ME) and pars nervosa (PN) are separate neurohemal areas. The ME is connected by hypothalamic portal blood vessels that pass through the pars tuberalis (PT) to the pars distalis (PD) where releasing hormones from the hypothalamus stimulate tropic hormone release. The pars nervosa stores nonapeptides and has a separate blood supply. OC = optic chiasm, PI = pars intermedia.

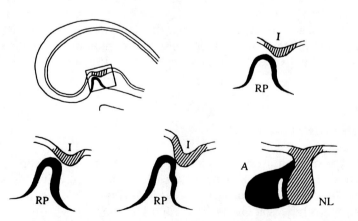

Figure 4-4. **Pituitary gland development.** Early understanding of development of the stomatodeal epidermis into the adenohypophysis (A) from Rathke's pouch (RP) and the neurohypophysis (NL) from the neural infundibulum (I). The pars intermedia developed at the point of contact between I and RP. (Reprinted by permission from Dubois, P. M. and El Amraouri, A. Embryology of the pituitary gland. *Trends Endocr. Metab.* **6**, 1–7. Copyright 1995 by Elsevier Science Inc.)

invagination off the anterior roof of the oral cavity called the stomodeum. Hence it was concluded that cells forming the adenohypophysis arose from non-neural ectoderm. However, numerous recent studies primarily employing amphibian and bird embryos have shown that the secretory cells of the adenohypophysis and the neurosecretory neurons of the hypothalamus have a common origin from the neural ridge of the embryo (neuroectoderm; Figure 4-5) and migrate during development to the tissues that ultimately form the hypophysis and hypothalamus. Evidence also suggests that the hormone-secreting cells of the pituitary are of neural origin (see Box 4A). The neurosecretory cells that control reproduction have their origins in a portion of the neural ridge that gives rise to the nasal placodes (olfactory system), and these neurons migrate along the olfactory nerve eventually to take up residence in the hypothalamus (see below).

The adenohypophysis is an epithelial glandular structure (*adeno*, gland) and can be subdivided into three anatomical regions or pars (bodies): the **pars anterior** or **pars distalis**, the **pars tuberalis**, and the **pars intermedia**. Pars distalis is used more commonly than pars anterior. Each region of the adenohypophysis is distinguished by cytological features as well as by anatomical relationships to the neurohypophysis. Two subregions can be identified in the neurohypophysis: the more anterior **pars eminens** or **median eminence** and the **pars nervosa**. (Note: the term "pars eminens" is rarely used today.) These neurohemal regions consist mostly of aminergic and

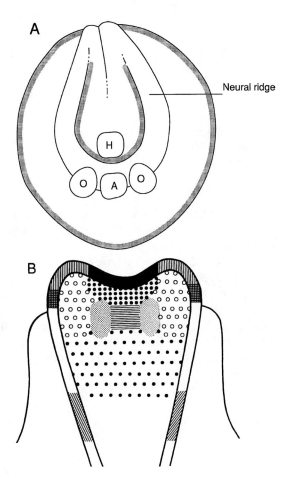

Figure 4-5. **Neural origin of the pituitary gland.** Anterior neural ridge origin for endocrine cells of hypothalamus and adenohypophysis. (A) Neurula of anuran amphibian embryo showing close proximity of origins for hypothalamus (H), adenohypophysis (A), and olfactory placodes (O). GnRH cells of the anterior hypothalamus have their origin from cells that migrate later from the olfactory placodes through the forebrain. Based on communications from K. Kawamura and S. Kikuyama. (B) Similar development in the avian embryo. ■■■, adenohypophysis; ▄▀▄, hypothalamus; ▤▤▤, neurohypophysis; ▦▦▦, optic vesicles; ⌐o⌐, telencephalon; ▗▖, diencephalon; ▥▥▥, ectoderm of nasal cavity; ▦▦▦, olfactory placode; ▧▧▧, mesencephalic neural crest. (Reprinted by permission of the publisher from DuBois, P. M., and El Amraoui, A. Embryology of the pituitary gland. *Trends Endocrinol. Metab.* **6**, 1–7. Copyright 1995 by Elsevier Science Inc.)

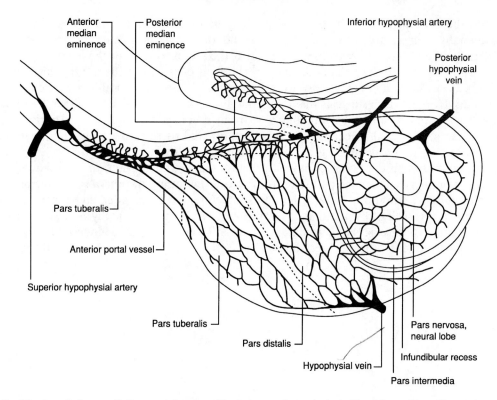

Figure 4-6. **The hypothalamus-pituitary portal system**. The long portal vessels drain blood from the median eminence primarily to the pars distalis. Note that some vessels connect the vasculature of the pars distalis with that of the pars intermedia. [From Matsumoto, A., and Ishii, S. (1992). "Atlas of Endocrine Organs." Springer-Verlag, Berlin.]

peptidergic axonal endings mixed with blood capillaries and what are probably modified neuroglial cells called **pituicytes**. An extensive vascular portal system, the **hypothalamo-hypophysial portal system**, develops between the median eminence of the neurohypophysis and the pars distalis of the adenohypophysis (Figure 4-6). This portal system carries blood from the median eminence directly to the epithelial cells of the pars distalis. The capillaries of the pars nervosa connect directly with the general venous drainage system, and there are no associated portal vessels. Although there are other portal systems in the body, endocrinologists often use "portal system" to refer only to this one.

The portal system forms a neurovascular link between the hypothalamus and the pituitary gland as described in the pioneering anatomical studies of Wislocki. Blood containing hypothalamic-releasing hormones flows from the median eminence to the pars anterior, and the venous drainage from the latter carries pituitary tropic hormones into the general circulation. Additional data suggest that, due to the low blood pressure in this system, there may be significant blood flow from the adenohypophysis to the hypothalamus as well. This **retrograde flow** may prove to be important for feedback actions of pituitary hormones on the hypothalamus.

Sympathetic fibers innervate pituitary blood vessels and influence blood flow through the portal system. In addition, peptidergic fibers containing a variety of neuropeptides have been demonstrated to innervate these vessels, although their significance is unknown.

A. Subdivisions of the Adenohypophysis

The adenohypophysis of most mammals consists of three subdivisions: pars tuberalis, pars intermedia, and pars distalis. The **pars tuberalis** consists of a thin layer of cells projecting rostrally (anteriorly and dorsally) from the adenohypophysis. It is in contact with the median eminence of the neurohypophysis, and the portal vessels of the portal system pass near or through the pars tuberalis *en route* to the capillary beds of the pars distalis.

Box 4A.   APUD Cells and Paraneurons

Among the vertebrates, extensive analyses of the embryonic origins of endocrine glands have provided a partial understanding of the evolution of vertebrate neuroendocrine systems. It was once thought that neurosecretory cells and the neurohemal portion of the pituitary were derived from embryonic neural ectoderm, whereas the portion of the pituitary that secretes tropic hormones was derived from non-neural ectoderm. The liver, thyroid, parathyroids, thymus, and gastrointestinal endocrine cells were believed to come from embryonic endoderm. The gonads and kidneys clearly develop from embryonic mesoderm (see Appendix B for a brief description of embryonic tissues). Endocrinologists believed that the fundamental differences among these groups of glands reflected their embryological origins until sophisticated biochemical techniques coupled with careful developmental studies demonstrated a common origin for most cells responsible for production of bioregulators.

Many of these cells, previously thought to be ectodermally and endodermally derived, possessed a property previously ascribed only to amine-secreting neurons. Cells with the ability to accumulate amino acid precursors and convert these precursors into biologically active amine neurotransmitters by removing their carboxyl acidic group were described as **APUD cells**: amine content and amine precursor uptake and decarboxylation cells. This property also was shared by melanin-producing skin cells that, similar to the amine-secreting neurons of sympathetic ganglia, were derived from special embryonic neural ectoderm cells called neural crest cells. During early development, neural crest cells develop as paired masses of cells at intervals along the embryonic nerve cord, migrate to other locations, and give rise to the sympathetic ganglia, melanin-producing skin cells, secretory cells of the adrenal medulla, and components of the skull and branchial skeletal elements. The discovery of this APUD property in many peptide-secreting endocrine and neuroendocrine cells prompted A.G.E. Pearse to propose that all cells with APUD characteristics have the same neural origins including parathyroid cells, calcitonin-secreting cells of the ultimobranchial body, gastrointestinal endocrine cells, and even some pituitary cells. Later, elegant experiments with bird embryos by N. LeDouarin and C. LeLievre verified that the calcitonin-secreting cells of the avian ultimobranchial glands were of neural crest origin although the matrix of the gland itself developed as an outpocketing of gut endoderm. They transplanted quail neural crest cells with a cytological marker into chicken embryos and observed them migrating to and finally residing in the ultimobranchial glands. Similar evidence was obtained for the parathyroid gland secretory cells in the frog *Rana temporaria*. Earlier efforts that showed a neural origin for the tropic hormone-secreting cells of the pituitary as well as the neurosecretory neurons of the hypothalamus apparently have been confirmed in studies by Sakae Kikuyama and his associates who transplanted pigmented neural ridge tissue into albino Japanese toads, *Bufo japonicus*, and were able to trace their migration into the neuroendocrine system. Thus, we now recognize that most endocrine and neuroendocrine cells are of neural origin with the exception of the steroid-secreting cells of the gonads and adrenal cortex (mesodermal), endocrine cells of the kidney (mesodermal), and possibly the thyroid follicular cells.

In addition to the recognition of APUD characteristics between neural cells and established endocrine cells, it was noted that neuroendocrine-like cells appeared not only diffusely distributed within the GI tract but also in gills of fishes, lungs of amphibians and mammals (so-called clear cells), and in skin. These neural-like cells were termed **paraneurons** by Tsuneo Fujita and were found to synthesize many of the same bioregulators found in the nervous system. Some paraneurons have APUD characteristics and some are even innervated. A few function as chemosensory receptors. Some paraneurons have been demonstrated to have paracrine–like actions locally, and this may be a general role for these paraneurons that are found in epithelia.

The portion of the adenohypophysis that makes contact with the pars nervosa of the neurohypophysis is defined as the pars intermedia. Indeed, differentiation of the pars intermedia occurs only if physical contact takes place between the developing adenohypophysis and the infundibulum that will become the pars nervosa.

The major portion of the adenohypophysis originally was designated as the **pars anterior**, and a variety of cellular types were identified there by selective staining procedures. In these animals lacking a true pars intermedia, the pars anterior was called the pars distalis. However, this latter term is now applied routinely as if it were synonymous with the pars anterior, especially since pars distalis was the appropriate term for adult humans and was so named in most textbooks. Because of extensive use of pars distalis in the literature for both anatomical designations, we use the term "pars distalis" exclusively in this textbook. Likewise, the term **"anterior lobe"** is applied loosely to mean either the pars distalis or the pars anterior plus the pars intermedia. **"Posterior lobe"** often is used in place of neurointermediate lobe, but at other times this term indicates only the pars nervosa in animals lacking a pars intermedia. Because of their variable meanings, the terms "anterior lobe" and "posterior lobe" are not used here.

1. Pars Tuberalis

The pars tuberalis is characteristic of all tetrapod vertebrates, but understanding of its physiological significance is limited. The presence of cells containing certain tropic hormones has led to the suggestion that the pars tuberalis is only an extension of the pars distalis related primarily to reproduction. However, recent studies have demonstrated that the pars tuberalis is an important endocrine link between the pineal gland and the prolactin-secreting cells of the pars distalis (see pineal gland discussion ahead).

Structurally the cells of the pars tuberalis are connected to the cerebrospinal fluid of the third ventricle in the brain through cellular processes originating in modified **ependymal cells** known as **tanycytes**. Ependymal cells are epithelial cells that line the ventricles of the brain and form a protective layer that surrounds the nervous system. It has been suggested that tanycytes may selectively remove molecules, including various types of regulators, from cerebrospinal fluid and transfer them to cells of the pars tuberalis, causing the latter to release their stored products. Although this is a highly speculative idea, such an interesting anatomical relationship demands some imaginative research to provide a better understanding of both tanycytes and the cells of the pars tuberalis.

2. Pars Intermedia

Only one glandular cell type appears in the mammalian pars intermedia, and it is responsible for secretion of the peptide hormone melanocyte-stimulating hormone or **melanotropin (α-MSH)**. An alternative name for α-MSH is melanophore-stimulating hormone, based on its effects in a unique pigment cell not found in mammals, the melanophore (see Chapter 5). In mammals, α-MSH stimulates skin cells, known as **melanocytes**, to synthesize a brown pigment, **melanin**, which causes increased deposition of pigment in the skin or hair. The term **neurointermediate lobe** designates both the pars intermedia and the pars nervosa as an anatomical unit although they are not functionally related. In some species, the pars intermedia is separated from the remainder of the adenohypophysis by a cavity or cleft. Some mammals, such as whales, manatees, elephants, armadillo, pangolin, beaver, and adult humans, lack a pars intermedia. Most of those mammals lacking a pars intermedia lack hair and/or have few if any melanocytes.

3. Pars Distalis

Five cellular types are present in the pars distalis and are responsible for secretion of six pituitary tropic hormones: **corticotropin**, or adrenocorticotropic hormone (**ACTH**); **thyrotropin**, or thyroid-stimulating hormone (**TSH**); **growth hormone**, or somatotropin (**GH**); **prolactin** (**PRL**); and two **gonadotropins**, or gonadotropic hormones (**GTHs**). The two GTHs are **follicle-stimulating hormone** or follitropin (**FSH**) and **luteinizing hormone** or lutropin (**LH**), both of which are named for their effects in female mammals but have equally important and similar roles in males. All of these hormones are polypeptides or proteins. In addition, α-MSH, a peptide secreted from the pars intermedia, often is included as a tropic hormone. A listing of the pituitary tropic hormones, alternative names for them, their targets, and their general physiological roles are summarized in Table 4-1. The names most commonly found in the modern literature on vertebrate endocrinology are emphasized in this textbook.

In addition, peptides known as **lipotropins (LPH)** and endorphins (e.g., **β-endorphin**) may be released from the adenohypophysis. Although not listed here as tropic hormones, they may perform endocrine functions. β-endorphin is one of several peptides known as **endogenous opioid peptides (EOPs)** that bind to the same receptors as the drug morphine, an exogenous opioid derived from the plant product opium. The term "endorphin" as a contraction of "endogenous morphine" was suggested for the natural internal substance that bound to what had been called **opioid receptors** in the CNS.

B. Cellular Types of the Adenohypophysis

Differentiation of pituitary cell types requires the interaction of a number of transcription factors (e.g., the **pituitary-specific transcription factor, Pit-1**) and differentiation or growth factors (e.g., **steroidogenic factor 1, SF1**) as outlined in Table 4-2. The cellular types in the pars distalis and the pars intermedia first were distinguished by utilizing special dyes in particular staining combinations. This differential uptake of dyes is due to the differential affinity of cytoplasmic granules for these dyes. Some cytoplasmic granules bound acidic dyes, and cells with these granules were termed acidophilic cells or **acidophils** (*philos*, love). Other granules bound basic dyes, and the cells containing these granules were termed **basophils**. A pituitary basophil was defined as a cell that was stained by the aniline blue dye of the Mallory trichrome staining method. However, since aniline blue is in reality an acidic dye, some investigators have preferred to use the term **cyanophil** (*cyanos*, blue) to designate these cells. Cells that do not contain stainable cytoplasmic granules are called **chromophobes** (*phobos*, fear of color). They are also known as **non-granulated cells**.

Various types of basophils or acidophils may be distinguished from one another in terms of their specific affinities for other dyes. A listing of dyes used to distinguish pituitary cellular types is found in Table 4-3, and a common nomenclature of the hormone-secreting cells of the adenohypophysis is provided in Table 4-4. Although a cell type now is identified routinely by immunocytochemistry for the hormone it secretes, knowledge of stainable features of secretory cells is helpful when interpreting the older mammalian literature and especially the comparative literature prior to the availability of specific antibodies for tropic hormones. This nomenclature appears even in recent publications, often without explanation of the terms.

The electron microscope also has been used to characterize cellular types of the pars distalis on the basis of general cellular morphology and the size and shape of electron-dense cytoplasmic storage granules containing tropic hormones (Table 4-5). A combination of ultrastructural, tinctorial (staining with dyes), and immunocytochemical techniques leaves little doubt as to the cellular origins of the tropic hormones. Ultrastructural features of some pars distalis cells can be seen in Figure 4-7.

Table 4-3. Some Regulatory Factors Involved in Pituitary Tropic Cell Development

Factor	Abbreviation	Cell type affected	Action
Pituitary-specific transcription factor	Pit-1	Thyrotrope, lactotrope, somatotrope	Necessary for their differentiation
Steroidogenic factor 1	SF-1	Gonadotrope	Makes cell responsive to GnRH
LIM/homeobox gene-3	Lhx3	All cells except corticotropes	Necessary for differentiation

Table 4-4. Some of the Dyes Used in Cytological Observation of Adenohypophysial Cells and Their Abbreviations

Dye or staining procedure	Abbreviation	Chemical specificity (if known)
1. Aldehyde fuchsin	AF	—
2. Alcian blue	AB	Disulfide bonds, mucopolysaccharides
3. Periodic acid–Schiff	PAS	Glycoproteins, mucopolysaccharides
4. Orange G	OG	—
5. Azocarmine	AZ	—
6. Lead hematoxylin	PbH	—
7. Iron hematoxylin	FeH	—

Table 4-5. Some Light and Electron Microscopic Features of Cellular Types in the Mammalian Pars Distalis

Cellular type	Tropic hormone secreted	Stainability[a] for light microscope	In situ granule size (nm)
Thyrotrope (β basophil)	TSH	PAS(+), AF(+)	150
Gonadotrope (δ basophil)	FSH, LH	PAS(+), AF(−)	200
Corticotrope	ACTH	Weakly PAS(+), AF(+); maybe PbH(+)	200
Lactotrope (ε acidophil)	PRL	Azocarmine(+)	600–900
Somatotrope (α acidophil)	GH	OG(+)	Variable to 350

[a] See Table 4-4 for dye abbreviations.

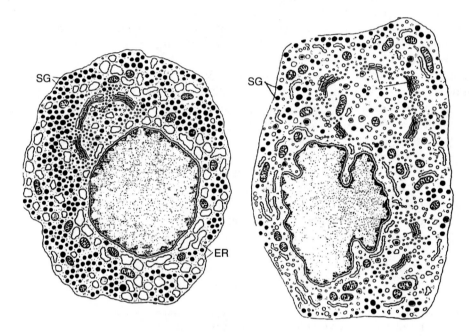

Figure 4-7. **Gonadotrope (left) and corticotrope (right) cell types.** Note the differences in abundance and size of electron-dense granules. Compare to the lactotrope and somatotrope in Figure 4-8. (From Norman, A. W., and Litwack, G. (1992). "Hormones." Academic Press, San Diego.)

1. Cytology of the Pars Distalis

Originally using differential staining combined with experimental manipulations, it was determined that there was one cellular type responsible for synthesis and release of each tropic hormone with one exception. These initial observations were later supported and refined by immunocytochemical studies using antibodies prepared against each pituitary hormone. There are two different stainable acidophils in the pars distalis, one responsible for secretion of GH and one for PRL. A weakly staining basophilic cell is responsible for synthesis of ACTH. However, only two strongly basophilic cells are found, and they are responsible for secretion of three glycoprotein tropic hormones: one secretes TSH and the other secretes LH and FSH. The two gonadotropins (GTHs) generally are produced in the same cell type based on immunochemistry, ultrastructure, and staining properties, although some of these cells may produce predominantly one gonadotropin (either LH or FSH). In the following descriptions, the traditional mammalian designation for each of these five cellular types is given. The cells responsible for secreting tropic hormones are designated with the suffix "**trope.**" Because tropic hormones were formerly called "trophic hormones," some authors still refer to the cell types with the suffix "**troph.**"

The **thyrotrope** is the least common of the secretory cell types in the pars distalis. Thyrotropes have long cytoplasmic processes and contain spherical secretory granules. They occur primarily in the anterior-medial portion of the pars distalis and show little variations with sex or age.

Despite the chemical similarity of GTHs and TSH (see ahead), the **gonadotrope** has been readily distinguishable from the thyrotrope by cytological and immunological techniques. Gonadotropes represent about 15–20% of the pars distalis cells and are distributed throughout the pars distalis. Two populations of spherical or slightly irregular secretory granules can be distinguished on the basis of size. At least three gonadotropic subtypes were identified by differences in immunoreactivity. One subtype contains only FSH, one contains only LH, and the third contains both LH and FSH.

Two acidophilic cell types in the pars distalis are considered to be sources for GH and PRL, respectively (Figure 4-8). The **somatotrope** is the most abundant cell type in the pars distalis, representing about 50% of the cells, and is found mostly along the lateral margins of the pars distalis. The second acidophil is called a **lactotrope** and secretes PRL. The lactotropes account for between 10–25% of the cells in the pars distalis, with the lower figure being common in men and nulliparous (never having borne children) women. There are relatively few PRL-secreting cells in children. Lactotropes are distributed throughout the pars distalis, often found associated with gonadotropes. At least two lactotropes have been identified using ultrastructural criteria. One is very common, a sparsely granular cell with smaller spherical, oval, or irregular granules. The second type is uncommon, is densely granular, and typically occurs adjacent to capillaries. A third acidophilic cell type has been described, the **mammosomatotrope**, which secretes both GH and PRL, especially during pregnancy.

Corticotropin-secreting cells or **corticotropes** were identified as being intermediate in stainability between chromophobes and basophils (i.e., weak basophils). Corticotropes are located in a central wedge within the

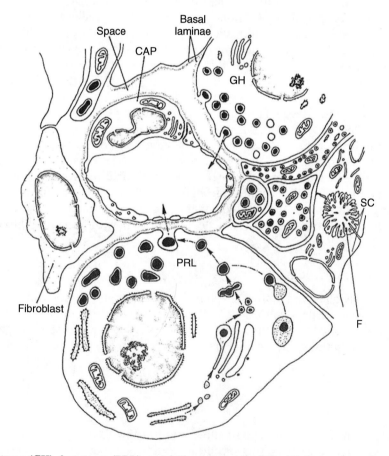

Figure 4-8. **Somatotrope (GH), lactotrope (PRL), and follicostellate cells (SC).** All three cell types are located near a capillary (CAP). The GH and PRL cells are distinguished by the different size and relative abundance of secretion granules whereas the SC are not granulated and show a tendency to form a follicular structure (F) where they contact one another.

pars distalis and represent 10–15% of the total cells. They contain a variety of granules that are somewhat larger than those of thyrotropes and are immunoreactive for ACTH, LPH, and β-endorphin.

Corticotropes also are immunoreactive for the protein **cytokeratin** that occurs in the perinuclear area and typically is not found in other tropic cells. The number of corticotropes does not vary with age or sex but may vary markedly in a number of pathological states (see Chapter 8).

Careful studies of hormone distribution, receptors present in pituitary tropic cells, and the presence of mRNA molecules have painted a much more dynamic picture of the pars distalis than previously thought. Not only do we have multiple populations of GTH-secreting cells and PRL-secreting cells, but we are finding some cells that are making a greater variety of tropic hormones than previously suspected. For example, not only do some gonadotropes produce GTHs but they may also produce GH. Furthermore, these GTH-GH cells possess receptors for both hypothalamic-releasing hormones suggesting that these cells are secreting both hormones. Corticotropes have been observed to vary with respect to the type of receptors they express for **corticotropin-releasing hormone (CRH)** and in their ability to also bind the neuropeptide vasopressin. Using cDNA probes, investigators have discovered the presence of mRNAs for more than one tropic hormone in pituitary tropic cells implying that, if the appropriate signals are received by these cells, they could begin secretion of alternative hormones. These new developments suggest a much more dynamic pituitary cytology than previously believed.

A sixth cellular type found in the mammalian pars distalis is the non-granulated cell or chromophobe that is not distinguished by selective staining techniques. Non-granulated cells may represent inactive, depleted, or undifferentiated cells, and some of the latter may differentiate into either basophils or acidophils, depending upon the stage of development, physiological conditions, or in response to experimental manipulations. One type of non-granulated cell is the **null cell** that has no special histologic, immunoreactive, or ultrastructural features other than presence of a few small cytoplasmic granules. Null cells are thought to be the source of certain pituitary adenomas. A special type of non-granulated cell, the **follicostellate cell**, has been observed in all vertebrates with the aid of the electron microscope. Follicostellate cells exhibit the **S-100 protein**, a characteristic of neuroglial cells in the brain, and the S-100 protein is not found in any other cells of the adenohypophysis. The cytoplasmic processes of these glial-related stellate (star-shaped) cells are very long and form a sort of network or reticulum between capillaries throughout the pars distalis. They are called "follicular" because of the way their stellate processes will sometimes surround or enclose tiny spaces. Each of these follicles consists of an extracellular space surrounded completely by processes of the follicostellate cells and are filled with fluid (Figure 4-8). Microvilli and sometimes cilia project into the follicular lumina of these follicles. The follicostellate cells may perform a supportive or nutritional function and are known to act as phagocytic scavenger cells. They are probably not the source of any tropic hormones, but they do produce paracrine secretions including interleukin (IL-6), basic **fibroblastic growth factor (bFGF)**, and **vascular endothelial cell growth factor (VEGF)**. Secretions from follicostellate cells in culture attenuate release of GH, PRL, and LH following administration of substances that normally evoke their release. Finally, recent evidence suggests that follicostellate cells have properties of stem cells and may differentiate into other cell types.

2. Cytology of the Pars Intermedia

The melanotrope is the only glandular epithelial cell in the mammalian pars intermedia. The pars intermedia also contains non-granulated stellate cells of unknown function that are interspersed among the α-MSH-secreting cells. In most mammals, the cleft that separates the pars intermedia from the pars distalis is lined by ependymal-like cells called **epithelial cleft cells**. The cleft cells often are ciliated, but their functional role has not been worked out.

3. Cytology of the Pars Tuberalis

Several cell types have been reported in the pars tuberalis of mammals. One cell type reacts specifically with antibody to pituitary LH, and a second type specifically binds antibody to TSH. Occasionally, one or two rare cells are observed in primates that bind antibody to ACTH and GH. Another special cell type has been discovered recently. This cell secretes a peptide that stimulates PRL secretion by lactotropes in the pars distalis (see ahead). The majority of pars tuberalis cells are chromophobic in most mammals, but all are stainable types in humans. The pars tuberalis may represent a "fragment" of the pars distalis, and it may function as an additional, but limited, source of tropic hormones.

C. Subdivisions of the Neurohypophysis

The mammalian neurohypophysis consists of two distinct neurohemal components, the median eminence and the pars nervosa. The median eminence is defined as the more anterior portion of the neurohypophysis that has a blood supply in common with the adenohypophysis; specifically, the portal system. (Note that in some terminologies the median eminence is considered to be a subdivision of the hypothalamus but is considered by Green as a neurohemal subdivision of the neurohyphophysis.) An abundant but separate blood supply characterizes the pars nervosa (Figures 4-3 and 4-6), which is that posterior portion of the neurohypophysis in contact with the pars intermedia. In species lacking a pars intermedia, the pars nervosa is defined on the basis of which neuropeptides are present (see ahead). Both the median eminence and the pars nervosa are composed of capillaries, pituicytes, and axonal tips of NS neurons originating in hypothalamic NS nuclei. Pituicytes probably are derived from ependymal or neuroglial cells, and they could play a role as supportive elements or may be involved actively in storage and release of neurohormones from the neurohypophysis, similar to the role of stellate cells of the adenohypophysis.

II. The Mammalian Hypothalamus

The NS nuclei of the hypothalamus and **preoptic area (POA**; Figure 4-9) produce neurohormones that are stored in the neurohypophysis. Axons from these nuclei travel either to the median eminence (Figure 4-10) or to the pars nervosa. The neurohormones associated with the median eminence and adenohypophysis are the hypothalamic-releasing hormones and can be identified as either **releasing hormones (RHs)**, or **release-inhibiting hormones (RIHs)**, depending on whether they stimulate or inhibit tropic hormone release from the adenohypophysis (Table 4-1). Initially, these neurohormones were named as "factors" until their specific chemical structures were known. Some researchers still refer to some or all of them as releasing factors or release-inhibiting factors rather than hormones. These regulating hormones are mostly small peptides composed of as few as three to as many as 44 amino acids. One is simply a catecholamine (dopamine) derived from a single amino acid. The neurohormones associated with the pars nervosa are all very similar in structure (Figure 4-11). Each is a peptide consisting of nine amino acid residues. The name "octapeptide" was used originally for these neurohormones because the two cysteine residues at positions 1 and 6 form a disulfide bridge to become cystine. Formation of this disulfide bond results in conversion of six amino acid residues into the characteristic five amino acid-ring structure with a side chain of three amino acids, hence the original name

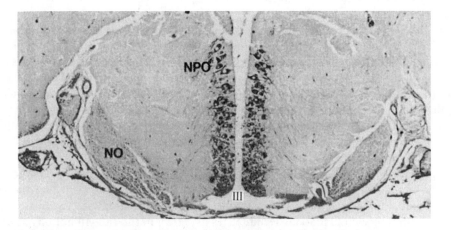

Figure 4-9.   **Neurosecretory neurons in the nucleus preopticus (NPO) of the eel.** NO, optic nerve; III, third ventricle. (From Matsumoto, A., and Ishii, S. (1992). "Atlas of Endocrine Organs." Springer-Verlag, Berlin.)

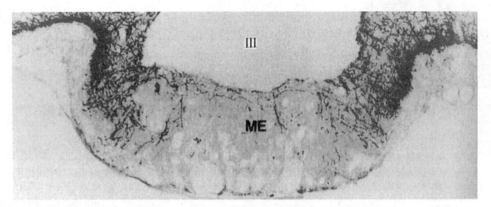

Figure 4-10. **The rat median eminence**. Immunoreactive gonadotropin-releasing hormone (GnRH) in nerve fibers stained in the lateral areas of the median eminence (ME). (From Matsumoto, A., and Ishii, S. (1992). "Atlas of Endocrine Ograns." Springer-Verlag, Berlin.)

Vasopressin-like peptides

Name	Amino acid sequence
Arginine vasopressin	C-Y-F-Q-N-C-P-R-G-NH$_2$
Lysine vasopressin	C-Y-F -Q-N-C-P-*K*-G-NH$_2$
Phenypressin	C-*F*- F-*R*-N-C-P-*K*-G-NH$_2$
Arginine vasotocin	C-Y- *I-R*- N-C-P-R-G-NH$_2$

Oxytocin-like peptides

Name	Amino acid sequence
Oxytocin	C-Y-I-Q-N-C-P-L G-NH$_2$
Mesotocin	C-Y-I-Q-N-C-P-*I* -G-NH$_2$

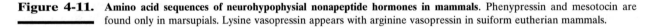

Figure 4-11. **Amino acid sequences of neurohypophysial nonapeptide hormones in mammals**. Phenypressin and mesotocin are found only in marsupials. Lysine vasopressin appears with arginine vasopressin in suiform eutherian mammals.

of octapeptide. However, because there are nine residues numbered 1 to 9, these peptides now are referred to as the **nonapeptide neurohormones** of the pars nervosa.

Five nonapeptides are stored in the adult mammalian pars nervosa and have been identified in the hypothalamus, although not all occur in the same species. These nonapeptides include the neutral nonapeptide **oxytocin (OXY)**, as well as the basic nonapeptides **arginine vasopressin (AVP), lysine vasopressin (LVP)** in suiform mammals, and **phenypressin (PVP)** in macropodid marsupials (kangaroos and wallabies). In addition, **mesotocin (MST)** that is charactertistic of non-mammalian tetrapods (see Chapter 5) is found in some species as well as OXY and in others instead of OXY.

The region of the mammalian brain that controls pars distalis function consists primarily of bilateral (paired) NS nuclei, including the **anterior hypothalamic nucleus (AHN), suprachiasmatic nucleus (SCN), ventromedial nucleus (VMN), dorsomedial nucleus (DMN), posterior hypothalamic nucleus (PHN), supraoptic nucleus (SON), paraventricular nucleus (PVN), periventricular nucleus (PERIVN)**, and **arcuate nucleus (ARC)** (Figure 4-12). Although technically the paired nuclei of the POA are not anatomically part of the hypothalamus, they usually are included in discussions of hypothalamic control because they function as part of the HPG axis. Collectively, these bilateral nuclei are responsible for producing the hypothalamic-releasing neurohormones that regulate release of tropic hormones from the hypophysis and for production of the nonapeptide neurohormones of the pars nervosa. In the HPG axis it was noted in both male and female rats that the releasing hormone contents of the VMN, DMN, and PVN on the right side were greater than on the left side of the brain. Other studies support a functional dominance of nuclei on the right side of the brain in control of gonad function as well as for thyroid and adrenal cortex (see readings at end of chapter). Although the possibilities of such functional asymmetries as shown in the rat will not be a focal point in future discussions, the student should never assume that paired structures—whether they occur in the brain or as paired structures elsewhere in the body—are always the same on both sides of the body.

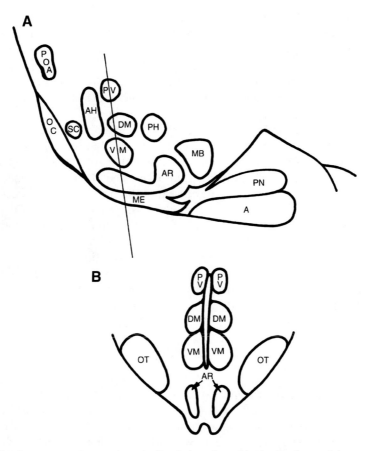

Figure 4-12. **Hypothalamic neurosecretory centers**. A. Saggital section of brain showing nuclei on one side. B. Cross-section of brain showing paired nature of nuclei. The nuclei depicted here are as follows: AH, anterior hypothalamic; AR, arcuate; DM, dorsomedial; PH, posterior hypothalamic; POA, preoptic area; paraventricular, PVN; suprachiasmatic (SC); ventromedial, VM. A, adenohypophysis; MB, mammillary body; ME, median eminence; OC, optic chiasm; OT, optic tract; PN, pars nervosa.

Much of our initial knowledge about the functional roles for these hypothalamic NS centers was accumulated from observing the effects on pituitary tropic hormone secretion of lesions or of localized electrical stimulation in the hypothalamus and POA as well as from studies involving implants of crystalline hormones into these regions. Some cautions for interpretation of data obtained from such studies are in order, however. The use of disruptive lesions, for example, requires careful bilateral placement of comparable lesions and leaves some uncertainty as to exactly what was destroyed by the lesions. Alterations in pituitary function following placement of lesions might involve destruction of the NS neurons that elaborate a given hypothalamic-releasing hormone or may only disrupt a NS tract. Furthermore, the lesion might have damaged non-NS neurons that would normally modulate the activity of certain NS neurons. Damage to vascular elements of the median eminence might also alter tropic hormone release patterns. Ideally, secretion of all tropic hormones should be monitored following placement of a particular lesion; yet, for practical reasons, this is rarely done. Usually only one (such as TSH) or, at most, two tropic hormone systems are examined, whereas others (e.g., PRL, LH, FSH, ACTH, and GH in this example) often are ignored. Lastly, it is difficult to establish suitable controls for some of these procedures. In spite of such drawbacks, the use of these approaches in combination with immunocytochemical techniques has helped to establish the location of NS centers responsible for secreting each hypothalamic neuropeptide.

A. Sexual Differences in the Hypothalamus

A variety of sexual dimorphisms have been described in the mammalian brain, especially in the hypothalamus. These dimorphisms are related to differing reproductive functions by the hypopthalamic centers of males and females, and they are important in puberty and in the regulation of reproductive cycles and reproductive behavior (see Chapter 10). Androgens secreted early in development are generally responsible for establishing these dimorphisms although estrogens may play a role in females. Extensive studies in rodents have established that conversion of androgens to estrogens by the enzyme P450 aromatase is involved in establishing the masculinization of the hypothalamus, but it is not clear this is the mechanism of the androgenic effect in other mammals including primates. In the medial preoptic area of the rat (mPOA), there is a striking difference in the density of neurons and size of the nucleus that is larger in males (2.5 to 5X that of females). This area is known as the **sexually dimorphic nucleus (SDN)**. Although similar differences have been observed in other mammals (e.g., guinea pigs, gerbils, ferrets, monkeys, and humans), mice do not exhibit this SDN. Studies have shown that male rats switched from a diet containing soy phytoestrogens (e.g., genistein) to a phytoestrogen-free diet exhibited a significantly reduced SDN suggesting that exogenous estrogen exposure might be responsible for this dimorphism. A marked sexual dimorphism (being better developed in males than in females) also has been described in the mammalian **vomeronasal organ (VNO)** and the associated accessory olfactory bulb, some regions of the bed nucleus of the stria terminalis, and the medial amygdala. These regions all exhibit steroid receptors and are especially responsive to pheromones in rodents.

The presence of sexual dimorphisms in humans and their associations with androgens are controversial. Anatomical studies that have demonstrated differences in the human brain are not always repeatable, and studies using brain imaging techniques of living brains are needed. No differences in the region referred to as the SDN in humans is present in children and there is no experimental evidence demonstrating that androgens affect sexual differentiation of this region.

B. Hypothalamic-Releasing Hormones

Numerous studies have confirmed that the hypothalamus exerts a direct influence over functioning of the adenohypophysis. Microscopic observations indicate the absence of neural connections between the mammalian hypothalamus and the adenohypophysis such as seen in teleost fishes. The discovery of the portal system led to the establishment of what is now termed the **neurovascular hypothesis**: that hypothalamic neurohormones released into the portal circulation are responsible for controlling tropic hormone release from the adenohypophysis. Severing the portal connections or transplanting the pituitary to some avascular site elsewhere in the body causes marked changes in the secretory pattern of the tropic hormones. These operations usually are followed by a marked reduction in circulating levels of TSH, FSH, LH, GH, and ACTH, whereas PRL and α-MSH levels increase. These observations led to the initial interpretation that release of TSH, GH, ACTH, and the gonadotropins is primarily under stimulatory control (via releasing hormones) and that release of α-MSH and PRL is normally under inhibitory control (via release-inhibiting hormones). This initial interpretation soon was modified as we learned more about the many factors that influence tropic hormone release (see ahead). If the severed blood vessels of the portal system are allowed to regenerate so that blood may again flow from the median eminence to the adenohypophysis, the normal secretory patterns for the tropic hormones resume. These latter observations support strongly the neurovascular hypothesis of hypothalamic control over tropic hormone release in mammals.

In recent years, many hypothalamic regulatory hormones have been proposed and their chemical identities established. Andrew Schally and Roger Guillemin shared a Nobel Prize for the initial isolation and characterization of **thyrotropin-releasing hormone, TRH**, and **gonadotropin-releasing hormone, GnRH**, respectively. Soon, with the advent of vastly improved biochemical techniques, other regulatory neurohormones were identified.

Each hypothalamic regulatory hormone is named for the tropic hormone it was first shown to influence and is designated according to whether it causes release (RH) or is release-inhibiting (RIH). The relative importance of RHs or RIHs for the various tropic hormones differs for each tropic hormone but is consistent for different mammalian species as well as for many non-mammalian vertebrates (see Chapter 5).

C. Control of Hypothalamic Hormone Release

Release of hypothalamic regulatory hormones is influenced primarily by neural activity and negative or positive feedback mechanisms of certain hormones. The following accounts represent a generalized pattern of control in mammals, but individual species may vary significantly from this pattern.

The predominant feedback loop involves production of blood-borne hormones or metabolites resulting from the actions of tropic hormones on specific peripheral target cells (Figure 4-1). This feedback may affect NS neurons in the hypothalamus directly. Feedback also may alter the sensitivity of pituitary cells to hypothalamic RHs and RIHs or affect other neurons that innervate the hypothalamic NS neurons. Feedback effects by tropic hormones and even by RHs and RIHs have been documented, but, for simplicity, we will focus our attention on the predominant feedback mechanism described above. You will recall from Chapter 1 that most feedback is of the negative type but that enhancement of responsiveness or even positive feedback may occur, such as the estrogen induction of the midcycle gonadotropin surge characteristic of female mammals (see Chapter 10).

1. Hypothalamic Hormones (Factors)

Regulation of tropic hormone release is accomplished directly by hypothalamic neurohormones as illustrated in Figure 4-13. In addition, neuronal input to these NS neurons can modulate their activity as can direct feedback from circulating hormones. Most of the RHs and RIHs are peptides as are some of the neuronal neurotransmitters that influence their release. In addition, a variety of non-peptide neurotransmitters (i.e., acetylcholine, dopamine, norepinephrine, serotonin, and GABA) affect tropic hormone release through their effects at the hypothalamic level. A specific neurotransmitter may stimulate release of one tropic hormone

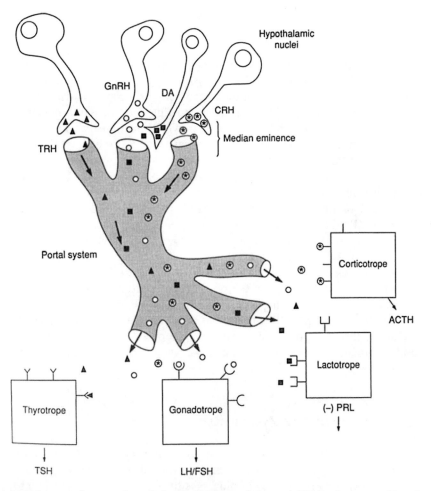

Figure 4-13. **Origin and targets for some hypothalamic-releasing and release-inhibiting hormones.** Note that each hypothalamic hormone travels through the portal system and binds to receptors on different pars distalis cell types, evoking tropic hormone release. TRH, thyrotropin-releasing hormone; GnRH, gonadotropin-releasing hormone; CRH, corticotropin-releasing hormone; DA, dopamine or prolactin release-inhibiting hormone; TSH, thyrotropin; LH, luteinizing hormone; FSH, follicle-stimulating hormone; PRL, prolactin; ACTH, corticotropin.

and inhibit release of another depending on the nature of their synaptic connections. Conversely, two or more different molecules might justifiably be termed an RH or RIH for a particular tropic hormone.

Many pharmacological studies of nervous regulation of hypothalamic/POA NS centers have been conducted, employing neurotransmitters or drugs that either mimic (agonists) or block (antagonists) the activity of various known neurotransmitters (see Chapter 2). Studies of this type have led to identification of neurons that regulate release of individual hypothalamic-releasing hormones. For example, application of dopamine to cultured pituitary cells with and without co-cultured hypothalamic/POA tissue has made it possible to distinguish between the indirect stimulatory activity of dopamine on LH release via a neurotransmitter role in the hypothalamus/POA and its direct inhibitory action as a neurohormone on PRL release. Utilization of catecholamines and related drugs *in vivo* and *in vitro* also has contributed much to our understanding of neuronal regulation of hormone release.

The response of NS neurons to specific neurotransmitters and neuromodulators of pituitary cells to neurohormones is determined by the presence of specific receptors for these substances on the cell membranes of the NS neurons. For example, the inhibitory action of dopamine on PRL release mentioned above is accomplished through the binding of dopamine to receptors in the plasmalemma of the PRL-secreting cells. The ergot alkaloids, such as **ergocornine** and **ergocryptine**, can mimic the action of dopamine by binding to another receptor on the PRL cell membrane termed an α-receptor. Stimulation of this α-receptor by a PRL-RH might ordinarily evoke PRL release, but the use of these α-receptor blocking drugs (α-blockers) can completely inhibit hormone release even in the absence of the PRL-RIH.

D. Paracrine Factors in the Adenohypophysis

The discovery of many known regulatory peptides in cells of the adenohypophysis first suggested possible paracrine roles for tropic cell secretions as well as possible paracrine secretions from some of the nongranulated cell types. Follicostellate cells, for example, have been proposed to form a chemical communication network throughout the adenohypophysis. Most of the supporting data for paracrine and sometimes autocrine functions for various peptides come from culture systems in which the density and physical relationship of cell types may be very different from conditions within the pituitary gland. For example, renin, renin substrate, and **angiotensin II (ANG-II)** have been reported from gonadotropes in the rat and from lactotropes in humans. Release of PRL is stimulated in cultures of both rat and human cells by ANG-II. However, the importance of these factors *in vivo* is still unclear.

An important paracrine regulator in the adenohypophysis is the polypeptide known as **pituitary adenylate cyclase activating peptide (PACAP)**. PACAP is a member of the secretin-glucagon family of peptides (see Table 3-4 and Figure 4-14). This peptide appears in two forms that are functionally indistinguishable (27 and 38 amino acids). PACAP enhances the release of all pars distalis tropic hormones since release by their releasing hormones is triggered in each case by increased intracellular levels of cAMP. It appears that PACAP is secreted by a variety of cell types in the pituitary in addition to the stellate cells.

One of the **natriuretic peptides** (see Chapter 8) known as **CNP** may be an important paracrine factor in the hypothalamus and the pituitary. CNP is related to **atrial natriuretic peptide (ANP)** that is important in the body's effort to combat chronic hypertension. Specific receptors for CNP are found on GnRH neurons in the ARC nucleus and on gonadotropes in the pars distalis. The exact role of CNP in gonadotropin release is not yet established, however.

III. Tropic Hormones of the Adenohypophysis

Numerous bioassays have been developed for quantitatively measuring tropic hormone activity, although current techniques for measuring gene action and immunological identification procedures generally have superceded the use of bioassays. A brief survey of bioassays for tropic hormones can be found in Appendix D.

The tropic hormones are separable into three distinct chemical categories (Table 4-6). The hormones within each category exhibit considerable overlap in chemical structures (that is, amino acid sequences) and in some cases overlap in biological activities as well, especially when administered in pharmacological doses. Category I includes the glycoprotein hormones: TSH, FSH, and LH. Each of these hormones is composed of two

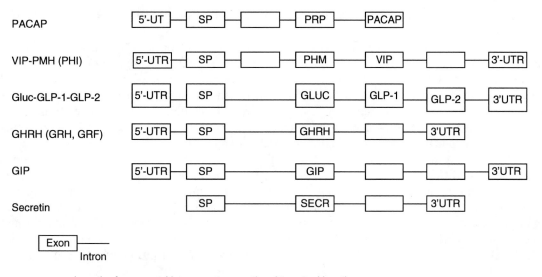

Figure 4-14. **Human genes for the secretin-glucagon family of peptides**. SP, signal peptide; see Appendix A or text for other abbreviations.

Table 4-6. Chemical Categories of Some Tropic and Placental Peptide/Protein Hormones

Category	Name	Site of synthesis
I	Thyrotropin (TSH)	Adenohypophysis: pars distalis
	Luteinizing hormone (LH)	Adenohypophysis: pars distalis
	Follicle-stimulating hormone (FSH)	Adenohypophysis: pars distalis
	Chorionic gonadotropin (CG)	Placenta
	Chorionic thyrotropin (CTSH)	Placenta
	Menopausal gonadotropin	Adenohypophysis: pars distalis
II	Growth hormone (GH)	Adenohypophysis: pars distalis; placenta
	Prolactin (PRL)	Adenohypophysis: pars distalis; placenta
	Chorionic sommatomammotropin (CS)	Placenta
III	Corticotropin (ACTH)	Adenohypophysis: pars distalis
	α-Melanotropin (α-MSH)	Adenohypophysis: pars intermedia
	β-Endorphin	Adenohypophysis: pars distalis and pars intermedia
	Chorionic corticotropin (CC)	Placenta

polypeptide subunits, each containing specific carbohydrate moieties. GH and PRL constitute the category II tropic hormones. Both PRL and GH are fairly large, folded polypeptide chains, and they exhibit considerable structural and some functional overlap. Category III includes smaller peptides: ACTH, α-MSH, LPH, and endorphins. All of these category III molecules have a common prohormone, have overlapping amino acid sequences, and exhibit some overlap in their biological actions.

In addition to pituitary tropic hormones, certain tropic hormones of similar chemical structure and biological activity are produced in the placental mammals. As many as five tropic-like hormones have been isolated from the chorionic (fetal) portion of the placenta (see Chapter 10), including **chorionic gonadotropin (CG)**, which is primarily LH-like in both structure and function, and **chorionic somatomammotropin (CS)**, which has some GH but mostly PRL-like activity. Both a **chorionic thyrotropin (CT)** and a **chorionic corticotropin (CC)** have been isolated from human placentas and may be secreted in other mammals. Pregnant mares produce large quantities of a placental gonadotropin that has both strong FSH-like and LH-like properties. This glycoprotein hormone is termed **pregnant mare serum gonadotropin (PMSG)**. The importance of these placental hormones in pregnancy is discussed in Chapter 10. A variant pituitary gonadotropin occurs in postmenopausal women and is called **menopausal gonadotropin (MG)**. Human MG is basically FSH-like and is produced by the postmenopausal adenohypophysis. Large amounts are secreted in response to failure of the ovaries to produce adequate levels of estrogens.

Much of our initial knowledge concerning the structure and function of tropic hormones initially came about as a result of the availability of pituitary glands and placentas from slaughtered domestic livestock. Huge quantities of starting tissue were needed in those days to yield one mg of pure hormone. Modern advances in biochemical techniques have reduced drastically the amount of tissue needed and has increased the efficiency of extraction and consequently the availability of purified tropic hormones from many animal sources. Techniques of genetic engineering have made it possible to develop culture systems to synthesize large quantities of a specific tropic hormone for research and clinical uses.

Since there are many structural variations in these polypeptides when isolated from different animals, and some corresponding differences in biological activity, it is important to designate the source of the hormone used in experimental studies. This is especially true when using mammalian hormones in non-mammals where a molecule that performs a particular function in mammals may provide different results in a non-mammal. Investigators who study mammalian tropic hormones usually designate the source of the hormone such as bovine (cattle), ovine (sheep), porcine (pig), cervine (deer), equine (horse), caprine (goat), and murine (rodent). An additional lower-case letter preceding the abbreviation of a tropic hormone usually designates

---

Box 4B.   Antibody Specificity and Measurement of Tropic Hormones

There are a number of drawbacks to widely employing RIAs for measurement of circulating peptide/protein hormone levels. Production of antibodies against hormones purified from pituitary glands may result in an antibody that reacts against some portion of a preprohormone or prohormone that is released from the cell rather than against the circulating biologically active form. Use of such antibodies that interact with differing proportions of active and inactive hormones might yield results that do not correlate with biological bioassay data since preprohormones and prohormones may react with the antibody but not bind to the receptors on target cells. Some peptide hormones may occur in different sizes (number of amino acids) or have some molecules altered through conjugation to another molecule (e.g., acetylation) resulting in different forms with different biological potencies with respect to receptor binding and activation but that all bind equally well to the antibody used in the RIA or ELISA. Furthermore, the close similarities in structure among the various tropic hormones of a given category (for example, PRL, GH, and CS) may result in cross-reactivities to the antibody produced against only one hormone because all in this category have gross structural similarities. The extremely similar structures of GHs and PRLs within and among species make measurements by RIAs for either PRL or GH difficult, and extreme caution should be used when interpreting RIA data, especially the use of antibodies to mammalian PRL to measure PRL levels in non-mammals. There is a common heptapeptide core (seven amino acids) in α-MSH, ACTH, and LPH, and this similarity in structure is reflected clearly by overlapping biological activity. Corticotropin has considerable α-MSH activity, and LPH has rather low ACTH activity but strong α-MSH action. Melanotropin has both weak ACTH and LPH activity. These overlaps in function affect interpretation of bioassayable data on α-MSH activity; i.e., which peptide is actually being measured by the bioassay? Similar questions should be raised with respect to the actual specificity of α-MSH or ACTH antibodies for RIAs or ELISAs.

The specificity of the antibody for the structure of the purified hormone antigen makes it difficult to use one antibody prepared against oFSH to estimate circulating levels of FSH in another species where differences in amino acid sequences of this species' tropic hormones might result in reduced cross-reactivity to the biologically active hormone or the cross-reactivity to another glycoprotein (LH or TSH). These problems of variability and structural similarities make it absolutely essential that any RIA be validated in several ways (including by bioassay) especially if the species used for the antibody preparation is not phylogenetically close to the species in which it is being used to measure hormone levels. The development of the immunoradiometric assays of recent years has improved the selectivity of identifying specific molecules in plasma samples with less interference from closely related molecules or fragments (see Chapter 3).

the species source. For example, bovine GH is designated bGH, GH prepared from human genes is hGH and bullfrog GH is bfGH. This method of designating the source may cause some confusion as purified hormones from a greater number of species become available, but it is a useful shorthand for indicating the source.

The activities of the various tropic hormones first were determined by bioassays (see Chapter 3). The classical bioassays for each tropic hormone can be found in Appendix D. These biological approaches still may be used in the biochemical isolation and characterization of tropic hormones, especially in non-mammals and in studies where purified hormones are not available. Once highly purified hormones became available, radioimmunoassays (RIA) and ELISAs (see Chapter 3) were developed for the mammalian tropic hormones and now are routinely employed to measure circulating levels.

A. Category I Tropic Hormones

All of the mammalian glycoprotein tropic hormones examined to date are composed of two peptide subunits (Figure 4-15) with an assortment of carbohydrate moieties attached. Molecular weights for these glycoproteins are about 32 kDa. The biological half-lives for TSH and LH in mammals are about 60 minutes whereas that of FSH is about 3X longer. The longer half-life for FSH is attributed at least in part to differences in its unique carbohydrate components.

Each glycoprotein tropic hormone consists of two subunits, an **α-subunit** and a **β-subunit**. The α-subunit is identical in all three adenohypophysial glycoproteins as well as in chorionic gonadotropin. The β-subunit is specific to each hormone and is responsible for its unique biological activity. Hence, RIA procedures that employ antibodies made against β-subunits are more accurate and show less cross-reactivity with other glycoprotein hormones.

Glycoprotein subunits are each synthesized as a separate prosubunit. Each prosubunit is coded by a different gene, modified post-translationally (including the addition of carbohydrates), and then the α- and β-subunits are coupled to form a heterodimer. Although the α-subunits of category 1 tropic hormones are nearly identical in amino acid composition, there is considerable variation among the β-subunits of LH, FSH, and TSH. The α- and β-subunit genes for hLH are located on different chromosomes (6 and 19, respectively). Both β-subunit genes for hLH and hCG occur on chromosome 19, suggesting that the βhCG gene arose by a relatively recent duplication of the βLH gene that occurred about the time mammals evolved from reptiles. Considerable overlap occurs between β-subunits of hLH and hCG, which have very similar biological activities.

The carbohydrate components represent 15–30% of the molecular weight of the glycoprotein subunits and the resulting heterodimer hormones. Glycoprotein hormones also show considerable specificity in their carbohydrate composition. For example, FSHs contain larger quantities of sialic acid than do the others, and the sialic acid is largely associated with the FSH β-subunit. Sialic acid protects FSH from rapid degradation by the liver. Treatment of FSH with the enzyme neuraminidase selectively removes sialic acid, reduces the biological activity of FSH, and allows it to be degraded more rapidly.

It is relatively easy with chemical procedures to dissociate these glycoprotein hormones into their respective subunits. These separated subunits have little if any biological activity when administered to animals. It is possible to recombine the dissociated subunits and restore full biological activity. Any α-subunit can be combined with any β-subunit resulting in a fully active hormone characteristic of the source of the β-subunit. Thus, when an α-subunit isolated from TSH is combined with a β-subunit from FSH, a glycoprotein with

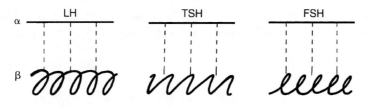

Figure 4-15. **Generalized structures of pituitary glycoprotein hormones.** The α-subunit is common to all three hormone, but the β-subunit coded for by a different gene is unique to each hormone and is responsible for the type of biological activity shown by the mature heterodimer.

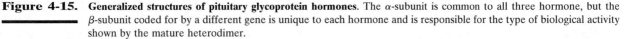

FSH activity results. Thyrotropes and gonadotropes produce excessive amounts of α-subunits indicating that regulation is directed at the unique β-subunit genes.

1. LH: Actions

Synthesis of androgens in both males and females is caused by LH action on the testes and ovaries. It also can be caused by chorionic gonadotropins. LH acts through a G-protein-based, cAMP second messenger system (see Chapter 3). Gamete release (sperm release in males and ovulation in females) also is under the control of LH. In females, LH causes formation of the corpus luteum from the ruptured ovarian follicles remaining after ovulation, and also may stimulate the corpus luteum of the ovary to secrete progesterone (see Chapter 10).

Since three pituitary tropic hormones were named for their actions in females (PRL, FSH, and LH), an effort was mounted some years ago to rename LH for its action on the androgen-producing cells that occur between the seminiferous tubules of the testis rather than for inducing corpus luteum formation (luteinization) in the female. Hence, it was suggested that LH be renamed the **interstitial cell-stimulating hormone (ICSH)** for its action on the steroidogenic interstitial cell of the testis (also called the Leydig cell) and the interstitial cell of the ovary (see Chapter 10). Although the use of ICSH occurs sporadically in the literature, LH has prevailed and is used today by most endocrinologists.

2. FSH: Actions

Like LH, FSH binds to a membrane receptor and stimulates cAMP production as a second messenger. Whereas the major actions for LH are stimulation of androgen synthesis and gamete release in both sexes, FSH is primarily involved with gamete preparation: that is, ovarian follicle development in females and spermatogenesis in males. In females and to a lesser extent in males, FSH also stimulates the conversion of androgens into estrogens through the induction of the enzyme P450 aromatase (see Chapter 3). This enzyme also is very important in converting androgens to estrogens in the male brain.

3. TSH: Actions

TSH operates via a cAMP-dependent mechanism to increase synthesis of thyroid hormones, cause release of stored thyroid hormones, and secondarily increase iodide uptake by cells of the thyroid. However, these measurements provide no consistent information concerning rates of thyroid hormone synthesis and release (see Chapter 6 for more details of TSH-stimulated thyroid events).

Humans may produce variant TSHs, one of which is associated with a pathological condition known as Graves' disease. Normal hTSH has a biological half-life of about 0.25 hours. The so-called **long-acting thyroid-stimulator (LATS)** in Graves' disease has a biological half-life of 7.5 hours. Furthermore in rats, TSH causes maximal radioiodide uptake in 4 hours whereas LATS continues to produce elevated uptake 12 hours after administration. LATS is not a product of the pituitary but is an aberrant immunoglobulin that is not influenced by negative feedback of elevated thyroid hormones (see Chapter 6 for more information on Graves' disease).

B. Category II Tropic Hormones

Two pituitary tropic hormones, GH and PRL, plus the placental tropic hormone, CS, comprise category II. Multiple copies of the genes for hGH and hCS are found in humans on chromosome 17 whereas multiple copies of the hPRL gene occur on chromosome 6. Hence, multiple forms may occur in the plasma of one individual. PRL and GH are large, single-polypeptide hormones of similar structure (Figure 4-16) and molecular weight (about 22 to 23 kDa). Human CS is similar to both hGH and hPRL although in other mammals CS may be structurally more like PRL than GH. There is an 85% homology between hGH and hCS as well as considerable overlap with hPRL; hence the name "somatomammotropin." CS also is known as **placental lactogen**, but this older name, though still in use, doesn't reflect its GH-like actions. It is estimated that duplication of the GH gene and evolution of the CS gene occurred between 85 and 100 MYBP. This is a

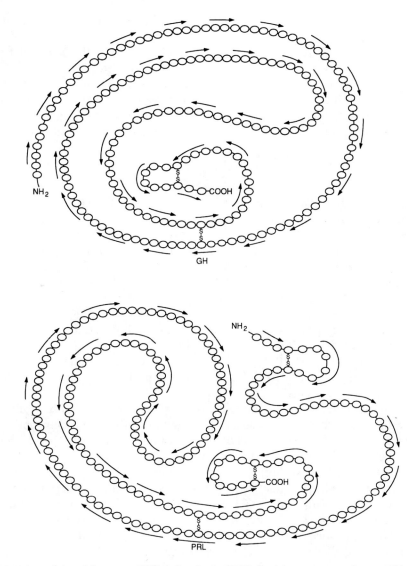

Figure 4-16. **Comparison of growth hormone (GH) and prolactin (PRL).** Both hormones are of comparable size, exhibit considerable overlap in amino acid sequence, and may have similar actions in some systems. GH typically has two disulfide bonds whereas PRL typically has three.

relatively recent event compared to the separation of the GH and PRL genes estimated to have occurred about 400 MYBP.

The human placenta also produces the pituitary forms of GH and PRL. Placental PRL accumulates in amniotic fluid. A smaller (16 kDa) variant of pituitary PRL also has been isolated from the rat placenta. A 20 kDa variant of pituitary hGH has been demonstrated during the second half of pregnancy. A similar molecule is produced in the pituitary by alternative processing of mRNA from the normal GH gene but does not appear in the circulation.

Both GH and PRL appear in the circulation as monomers as well as dimers (e.g., "big" GH) or oligomeres (e.g., "big-big" GH). These multiple forms are measureable by RIA but the monomers have greater biological activity. In addition, GH, at least in humans and rabbits, is known to interact with a plasma **GH-binding protein**, complicating further the picture of circulating levels. Because of the heterogeneity of category II hormones, all references to GH or PRL are to the normal monomeric forms unless indicated.

Both GH and PRL produce a number of common effects on osmoregulation (renal function, intestinal fluid absorption), selective tissue growth (prostate gland, sebaceous gland), lactation, and other processes. These common actions are related to their structural similarity. However, PRL and hCS, unlike GH, only have weak effects on body growth and metabolism.

Membrane receptors for GH and PRL are monomeric proteins that span the cell membrane only once, yet they lack enzymatic activity (see Chapter 3). Both PRL and GH receptors are similar to one another and neither receptor activates adenylyl cyclase. The GH receptor undergoes dimerization and then interacts with Janus kinase, an intracellular tyrosine kinase, that mediates the action of GH in target cells (see above). The extracellular domain of the hGH receptor is identical to the serum hGH-binding protein mentioned earlier, suggesting the plasma-binding protein may be a hydrolysis product from the membrane receptor.

1. GH: Actions

Growth hormone is often described as a protein anabolic hormone because it stimulates incorporation of amino acids into proteins and has a negative effect on nitrogen excretion. Growth hormone represents about one-half of the total hormone content of the human adenohypophysis, which emphasizes its importance in adults as well as during the years of maximal growth. It has been characterized chemically as a protein composed of 191 amino acids (MW = 21.5 kDa) having a biological half-life in blood of 20 to 40 minutes. hGH has been synthesized in the laboratory and is available for clinical purposes. hCS also consists of 191 amino acids, of which 161 are identical to those in hGH; yet, as mentioned earlier, hCS has rather low GH activity.

Crude GH preparations consist of a collection of protein isohormones. Each form is thought to have its own actions, and collectively they produce all the effects normally attributed to pituitary GH activity. The gene responsible for synthesis of the 21,500-Da form of GH has been cloned and inserted successfully into the genome of mice. Growth rates of mice with the inserted genes and growth rates of their offspring are about twice that of normal mice. This approach to GH therapy has important implications for future treatment of GH-based growth deficiencies in humans.

Growth hormone stimulates absorption of amino acids and protein synthesis, especially by skeletal muscle cells. It cooperates with insulin to channel utilization of amino acids, fatty acids, and carbohydrates into storage following a meal. Furthermore, GH becomes an important regulator of blood glucose and amino acid utilization in the absence of insulin during short-term and long-term starvation.

Circulating levels of hGH are highest during the period of maximal growth (ages 2 to 17 years). A daily secretory rhythm becomes established at about 4 years of age and continues throughout adult life. This pattern of GH secretion is both irregular and spontaneous, depending upon the physiological state of the individual, but episodes of GH release are frequently correlated with the onset of deep sleep.

Optimal growth-promoting actions of GH are obtained in hypophysectomized animals only when thyroid hormones are administered together with GH. This relationship between thyroid hormones and GH has been described as a synergism; that is, the growth response elicited by combined therapy with thyroid hormones and GH in hypophysectomized animals is greater than predicted by adding together the responses obtained with each hormone administered alone. Either thyroid hormones or GH will reinitiate some growth in hypophysectomized animals, but complete resumption of normal growth requires combined therapy. Furthermore, intact animals that exhibit thyroid deficiencies grow slowly and abnormally (see Chapter 6).

Thyroid hormones may influence synthesis of GH in intact rats, but their actions pertinent to hypophysectomized animals is a peripheral one. Thyroid hormones maintain a "responsive state" in target cells so that they are more sensitive to GH and other regulators (see Chapter 6 for more details of this "permissive" effect).

The effects of steroid hormones on growth are complex. Androgens and estrogens can increase the responsiveness of human tissues to hGH but to a lesser extent than do thyroid hormones. The mechanism of this steroid effect is not understood. Steroids, especially androgenic ones, have important effects on amino acid and carbohydrate metabolism unrelated to the roles of GH (see Chapter 12). Androgens are known to stimulate protein synthesis and hypertrophy of skeletal muscle, and estrogens selectively increase protein synthesis in the uterus. Conversely, the increase in androgens and estrogens associated with the onset of puberty causes cessation in proliferation of the epiphyseal plates at the ends of long bones of the appendicular skeleton and render these tissues unresponsive to GH. This results in a permanent cessation of growth in stature.

Direct metabolic actions of GH on protein synthesis, amino acid transport, and lipolysis have been reported in several tissues. However, these growth effects of GH are mediated indirectly by the GH-stimulated production of two peptide regulators in the liver or, in some cases, directly in target tissues. These peptides were first called **sulfation factors** because of effects on incorporation of sulfate into cartilage during GH-stimulated cartilage growth, a phenomenon that could not be invoked by direct application of GH to cartilage cells *in vitro*. Later, they became known as **somatomedins** since they mediated the actions of the somatotropic hormone GH. These peptide growth stimulators are structurally related to insulin and have some insulin-like activity, in addition to their growth-promoting actions, due to their ability to bind to the insulin receptor. Later, they acquired the names of **insulin-like growth factors (IGF-I, IGF-II)**. IGF-II is secreted primarily during fetal growth and IGF-I is secreted primarily in children and adults. The liver, then, can be considered a target endocrine gland for GH since it synthesizes and releases IGFs into the circulation, thus constituting the HPH axis. IGFs are transported in the blood while complexed to specific plasma **IGF-binding proteins**. In other target tissues, IGFs synthesized by GH target cells may be necessary for producing GH-linked effects in these targets (e.g., in cartilage and bone). Levels of both IGF-I and IGF-binding proteins are depressed in hypothyroid patients and elevated in hyperthyroid patients, indicating thyroid hormones can affect GH actions through their actions at the liver as well as at other GH target cells.

In adult mammals, IGF-I binds to a receptor that is very similar to the receptor for insulin and that can even bind insulin weakly. In contrast, IGF-II is primarily a fetal growth factor with a unique receptor, and it may be secreted under the influence of hCS in humans. IGF-II has only weak insulin-like activity and doesn't bind well to adult insulin or IGF receptors. However, both IGFs are powerful mitogens in their appropriate target cells (i.e., they stimulate cellular division or mitosis). Circulating levels of hIGF-I increase at about 6 to 8 years of age and peak during puberty. Lower, relatively constant levels of IGF-I are characteristic of adults.

2. Prolactin: Actions

Prolactin consists of a single chain of 199 amino acids (23 kDa) and, like GH, occurs as multiple isohormones. It produces a variety of distinctive actions in animals, including effects associated with reproduction, growth, osmoregulation, and the integument (Table 4-7). Furthermore, PRL may produce synergistic actions with ovarian, testicular, thyroid, and adrenal hormones. The best-known action for PRL is the lactogenic effect on the mammary gland of females for which the hormone was named. PRL stimulates DNA synthesis, cellular

Table 4-7. Prolactin Actions in Mammals

Actions related to reproduction	Actions related to water and electrolyte balance
Mammary development and lactation	Lactation
Preputial gland size and activity	Increased Na$^+$ retention at renal level
Synergism with androgen on male sex accessory glands	Corticotropic
Luteotropic in rodents	Actions on integumentary structures
Fertility in dwarf mice	Mammary development and lactation
Increased testis cholesterol	Sebaceous and preputial gland size and activity
Increased androgen binding in human prostate	Hair maturation
Stimulation of glucuronidase activity in rodent testis	Actions on steroid-dependent targets or synergisms
Parental behavior	with steroids
Decreased copulatory activity in male rabbits	Mammary growth (ovarian steroids)
Advanced puberty in rats	Milk secretion (corticosteroids)
Vaginal mucification in rats	Sebaceous and preputial gland secretion (gonadal and
Antiovulatory and antiluteinizing actions in rats	cortical steroids)
Relaxation of uterine cervix in rats	Growth and secretion of male sex accessory
Reduced catabolism of progesterone by rat uterus	glands (androgens)
Inhibition of myometrial contractions	Luteotropic action (estrogens?)
Increased estradiol binding by rat uterus	Renal Na$^+$ reabsorption (aldosterone?) and
Decreased GTH release	renotropic action (androgens)
Actions related to growth and development	Spermatogenesis (androgens)
Mammary development	Advanced puberty (gonadal steroids)
Sebaceous and preputial gland growth	Hair growth (androgens, corticosteroids)
Hair growth	Vaginal mucification in rats (estrogen and
Erythropoietic actions	progesterone)
Renotropic actions	
Spermatogenic actions	
Male sex accessory development	

proliferation, and the synthesis of milk proteins (casein and lactalbumin), free fatty acids, and lactose by the glandular epithelium of the mammary gland. hCS from the placenta produces a similar effect.

In some species (i.e., rats, sheep), PRL may influence the synthesis of progesterone by the corpus luteum of the postovulatory ovary. This action was responsible for the older name for prolactin, the **luteotropic hormone, LTH**. There also is evidence in male mammals for effects of PRL on certain sex accessory structures. These reproductive actions of PRL are discussed in Chapter 10 with respect to the overall regulation of reproduction in mammals.

Like the situation for GH, PRL actions on the mammary gland and possibly on other targets requires an interaction with additional hormones. Estrogens favor cell proliferation and growth of the mammary gland, making the mammary more responsive to PRL. Glucocorticoids also potentiate the actions of PRL in all species examined. Progesterone inhibits PRL actions on the mammary gland and can block lactogenesis. One hypothesis suggests progesterone competes for glucocorticoid binding and/or blocks gene activation by glucocorticoids. The stimulatory actions of insulin on the mammary gland may be related to its IGF-like activity that mimics an action of PRL.

C. Category III Tropic Hormones

This category comprises several hormones derived from the same precursor, a prohormone known as **pro-opiomelanocortin** or **POMC**, and includes ACTH, α-MSH, LPH, and the EOP, β-endorphin. POMC-related peptides are found in cells of the brain, the pars distalis, and the pars intermedia (when present). All of the category III molecules produced in the pituitary are a result of variations in post-translational processing of POMC and consequently exhibit considerable overlap in their biological activities due to possession of similar amino acid sequences (see Figure 4-17).

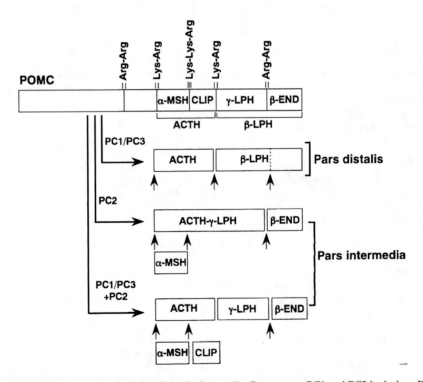

Figure 4-17. **Fates of proopiomelanocortin (POMC) in pituitary cells.** Convertases PC1 and PC3 hydrolyze POMC in corticotropes of the pars distalis to yield mainly ACTH and β-lipotropin (LPH). PC2 separates POMC into α-MSH (melanotropin) and β-endorphin (β-END). If PC1, PC2, and PC3 are all active in the melanotrope, the result is α-MSH, corticotropin-like peptide (CLIP), γ-LPH, and β-END. (Based on Mizuno, K., and Matsuo, H. (1994). Processing of peptide hormone precursors. *In* H. Imura, ed. "The Pituitary Gland," 2nd Ed. Raven Press Ltd., New York, pp. 153–178.)

In corticotropes of the pars distalis, POMC is cleaved to produce ACTH (39 amino acids), an N-terminal **16K fragment** (molecular weight = 16,000) with no known biological activity, and a large form (91 amino acids) of LPH known as β-lipotropin or **β-LPH**, representing the C-terminal portion of POMC. β-LPH may be cleaved again to form a 58-amino acid fragment called **γ-LPH** (consisting of residues 1–58 of β-LPH) and β-endorphin (residues 61–91 of β-LPH). In melanotropes of the pars intermedia, ACTH is cleaved further to yield α-MSH (residues 1–13 of ACTH) and a **corticotropin-like peptide** called **CLIP** (residues 18–39 of ACTH). In the brain, **proenkephalin** (enkephalin meaning "in the head") is the precursor for either the opioid pentapeptide **met-enkephalin** or the opioid pentapeptide **leu-enkephalin** which differ only at position 5. **Dynorphin** is a larger opioid peptide occurring in two forms (13 or 16 amino acids) derived from a POMC-like prohormone called **prodynorphin** (also known as proenkephalin B). There are two smaller, partly homologous peptide versions of the dynorphins called **α-and β-neoendorphins**. The enkephalins, dynorphins, and endorphins all have the same four or five N-terminal amino acids that are important for binding to opiate receptors.

The amide of α-MSH and β-endorphin may be acetylated by an interaction with N-acetyltransferase and acetyl coenzyme A. This reaction occurs post-translationally in the secretory granules of melanotropes. Thus, a high proportion of α-MSH and β-endorphin are acetylated prior to release.

1. Corticotropin (ACTH)

Corticotropin stimulates the adrenal cortex (see Chapter 8) to secrete glucocorticoids (cortisol and/or corticosterone), hormones that alter protein and carbohydrate metabolism (see Chapter 12). ACTH purified from several mammalian sources (e.g., bovine, porcine, ovine, human) consists of 39 amino acids in a single peptide chain with a molecular weight of about 4500. Amino acids 1–23 of ACTH have full biological activity, 1–19 have 80% of full activity, but the fragment 1–16 has very little ACTH biological activity. Amino acids 24–39 are obviously outside that region of the molecule responsible for its biological activity. All ACTH fragments containing residues 1–13 also have α-MSH activity (see ahead). Hence, although CLIP has considerable amino acid homology to part of the intact ACTH molecule, it has no ACTH-like or α-MSH-like biological activity because it lacks the essential first 13 amino acids. The presence of multiple-sized fragments of $ACTH_{39}$ in the circulation has implications for the efficacy of RIA procedures for both ACTH and α-MSH with antibodies that may or may not have overlapping affinities (see also Box 4B). The amino acid sequences of several mammalian ACTHs are compared in Table 4-8.

2. Melanotropin (α-MSH)

In mammals, the epidermal melanin-producing cell is the melanocyte that synthesizes melanin under the influence of α-MSH but extrudes it into the extracellular compartment where it is accumulated in **keratinocytes** (keratin-containing epithelial cells). Animals that change from a white "winter coat" to a brown "summer coat" employ the services of α-MSH to stimulate melanin production for the summer coat. Hypophysectomy of the short-tailed weasel during the winters causes the summer coat to be white like the winter coat. Treatment of hypophysectomized weasels with either α-MSH or ACTH (which has inherent α-MSH-like action) is sufficient to cause regrowth of the normal brown summer coat.

Table 4-8. Structural Variation of Active Portion of Mammalian ACTHs

Source of ACTH	1	....	25	26	27	28	29	30	31	32	33	....	39
Porcine	Ser	....	Asn	Gly	Ala	Glu	Asp	Glu	Leu-	Ala	Glu	....	Phe
Ovine	Ser	....	Asp	Gly	Ala	Glu	Asp	Glu	Ser	Ala	Gln	....	Phe
Bovine	Ser	....	Asn	Gly	Ala	Glu	Asp	Glu	Ser	Ala	Gln	....	Phe
Human	Ser	....	Asn	Gly	Ala	Glu	Asp	Glu	Ser	Ala	Glu	....	Phe

The adenohypophyses of all vertebrates tested by bioassay (see Appendix D) possess α-MSH activity, including some mammals and all birds that lack a pars intermedia. This activity may reside in ACTH or possibly in LPH that also contains some MSH-like sequences (see ahead). As mentioned above, α-MSH and CLIP are released following the hydrolysis of ACTH in melanotropes. α-MSH usually is acetylated prior to release, slowing its degradation and increasing its biological activity. It is not possible to distinguish MSH-like activity caused by α-MSH or by ACTH or ACTH fragments that also bind readily to α-MSH receptors and activate them. The physiological roles for α-MSH in pigmentation are not known in birds or in most mammals, but a role in feeding behavior has been described (see Chapter 12).

Two additional forms of MSH have been isolated from the mammalian pars intermedia. One of these forms, β-MSH, is found within the LPH sequence and if separated from the rest of the peptide will exhibit MSH activity. Similarly, a γ-MSH occurs as part of the LPH sequence of amino acids. It is not clear that either of these melanotropins is of any physiological relevance since under normal circumstances, they do not appear to be released as free peptides into the circulation. α-MSH probably is the true melanotropin and β-MSH and γ-MSH may simply be artifacts of extraction. Consequently, only α-MSH is discussed ahead, but the reader should be aware that the other peptide forms bind to the same receptors as α-MSH although with lower affinity.

3. Lipotropins (LPHs)

In addition to its role as a precursor for endorphins, LPHs have been proposed as hormones that stimulate lipolysis in adipose tissue (that is, hydrolysis of fats to free fatty acids and glycerol). Lipotropins, presumably of pituitary origin, have been identified in the systemic circulation, but levels of circulating LPHs have not been linked to observed changes in lipid metabolism, leaving open the question of any physiological role for LPHs. Other lipolytic hormones appear to be much more potent than the LPH peptides, further questioning their importance as lipolytic factors *in vivo* (see Chapter 12). LPHs may have some importance as sources for the production of endorphins (see below).

4. The Endorphins and Enkephalins

Morphine is an opiate analgesic (pain-killing) drug that binds to specific receptors in the central nervous system. Scientists postulated that there also would be endogenous compounds that produce analgesic opiate-like (morphine) effects on the central nervous system. A search for endogenous analgesics has resulted in identification and chemical characterization of two groups of EOPs. The larger EOPs include the dynorphins, β-endorphin, and some C-terminal hydrolysis products of β-endorphin that are acetylated at the N-terminal end. However, these additional alterations to β-endorphin markedly reduce its analgesic properties. The pentapeptide enkephalins also bind to opioid receptors. The distribution of endorphins in the pituitary and central nervous system parallels that observed for ACTH and LPHs indicating they are products of POMC hydrolysis. The enkephalins and dynorphins are produced from a different but related prohormone and are localized in other neurons. Painful stimuli elevate levels of endorphins and enkephalins in the CSF, and they appear to exhibit the features required for endogenous opiate-like agents. The endorphins function as neuromodulators or neurotransmitters within the central nervous system through their morphine-like actions. The action of morphine, a non-peptide, is blocked by closely related pharmaceuticals such as **naloxone** (Figure 4-18). The effects of endorphins also are blocked by naloxone implying closeness in mechanisms of action for morphine and the endorphins that bind to similar receptors. Three types of opioid receptors have been identified with differing affinities for the various opioids (see Table 4-9).

In addition to their involvement with pain perception, endorphins influence release of neurotransmitters affecting tropic hormone release and can inhibit oxytocin release (see Figure 4-19). The possible roles for endorphins and enkephalins as regulators of behavior, especially as related to painful stimuli, and their possible endocrine implications represent an exciting new area of neuroendocrinology.

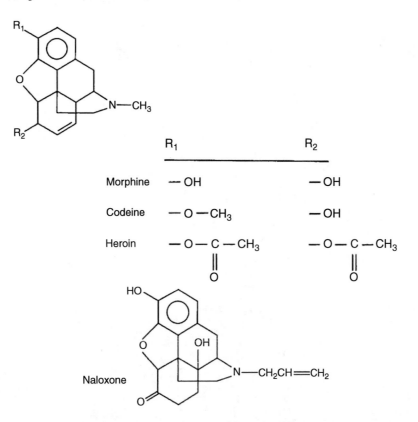

Figure 4-18. **Chemical structures of opiate and anti-opiate (naloxone) drugs.** Three common opiates (morphine, heroin, codeine) differ according to the groups attached to the carbon rings at R_1 and R_2.

Table 4-9. Affinity of Opioids for Major Opioid Receptor Types

	Receptor types		
Opioid	μ Receptor (mu)	δ Receptor (delta)	κ Receptor (kappa)
Morphine	High	Low	None
Naloxone (antagonist)	High	Low	None
β-Endorphin	High	Low	None
Enkephalins	Low	High	None
Dynorphin	None	Low	High

IV. Regulation of Tropic Hormone Secretion in Mammals

The nature and actions of the various RHs and RIHs involved, what the major feedback loops are, and how other neural factors may influence secretion of a tropic hormone are discussed below for each of the tropic hormones. In addition, an overall scheme that summarizes or models each tropic hormone regulatory system is provided (see Figure 4-20).

A. Regulation of Thyrotropin Secretion

Release of TSH is under stimulatory control as evidenced by the lack of TSH release following disruption of the portal vessels or explanting of the adenohypophysis. The major factor controlling release is a hypothalamic tripeptide known as **thyrotropin-releasing hormone (TRH)** or **thyroliberin.** The TRH prohormone may have from four to seven copies of the TRH peptide embedded within itself. There is no confirmed thyroid

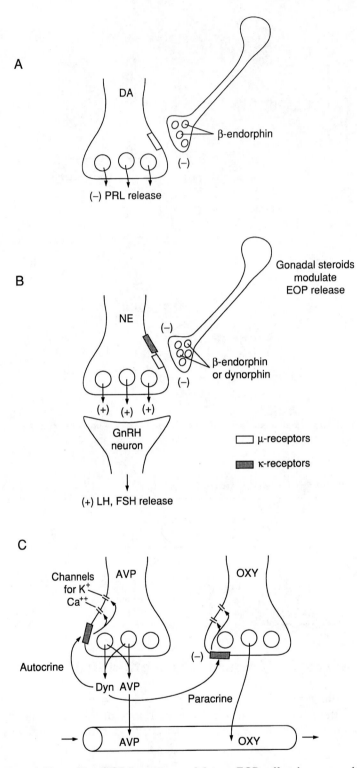

Figure 4-19. **Endogenous opioid peptides (EOPs) as neuromodulators.** EOPs affect hormone release in at least three ways as exemplified with specific examples here. They can (A) increase PRL release by blocking the release of dopamine (DA) which normally blocks PRL release; (B) inhibit norepinephrine (NE) stimulation of GnRH release; (C) prevent oxytocin (OXY) release when AVP is being released from the pars nervosa. Dyn = dynorphin.

1. Hypothalamus

POA	Preoptic area
ARC	Arcuate
PERIVN	Periventricular
PVN	Paraventricular
SO	Supraoptic
VMN	Ventromedial

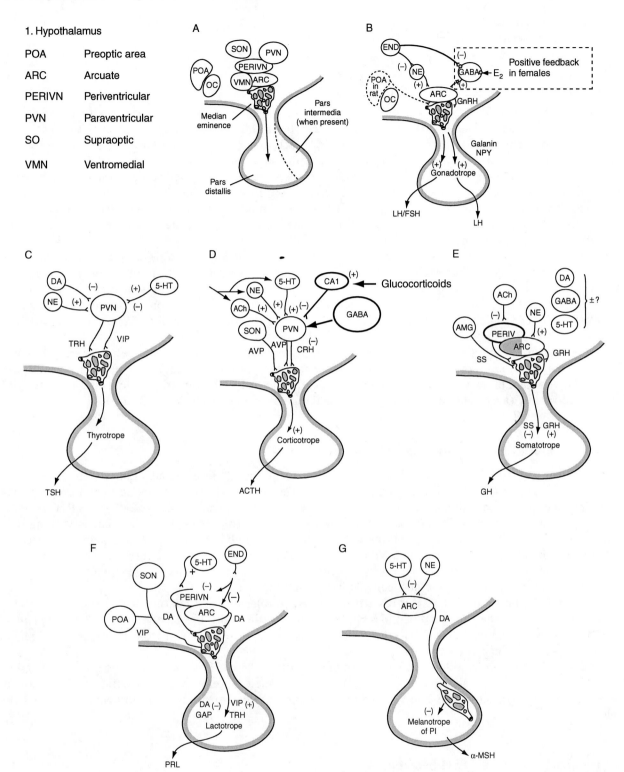

Figure 4-20. **Factor affecting tropic hormone release**. (A) Identification of principal sources for hypothalamic hormones. (B) Control of LH and FSH release. (C) Control of TSH release. (D) Control of ACTH release. (E) Control of GH release. (F) Control of PRL release. (G) Control of α-MSH release. See Appendix A or text for explanation of abbreviations.

release-inhibiting hormone, but a number of other hypothalamic factors may be involved in regulating TSH release. The factors controlling TSH release are summarized in Figure 4-20c.

1. Thyrotropin-Releasing Hormone (TRH)

The tripeptide TRH (Table 4-1) was one of the first hypothalamic regulatory hormones to be identified chemically. It is found in the NS neurons of many nuclei but in highest concentration in the PVN that sends TRH-immunoreactive fibers to the median emergence. TRH appears in the portal system blood following electrical stimulation of the appropriate regions of hypothalamus, and causes release of TSH *in vivo* and *in vitro* from the adenohypophysis. TRH binds to a G-protein coupled receptor that works through IP_3 to activate phosphokinase C (PKC; see Chapter 3). In turn, PKC phosphorylates transcriptions factors, such as Pit-1, that can activate transcription of the $TSH\beta$ gene. IP_3 also elevates intracellular Ca^{2+} and facilitates release of TSH from the thyrotrope. A second neurohormone, **vasoactive intestinal peptide (VIP)**, stimulates the cAMP second messenger system and also activates TSH secretion.

Extrahypothalamic TRH also is present in other brain regions, the spinal cord, the pineal gland, and the neurohypophysis as well as in some other tissues. The common occurrence of TRH outside the hypothalamus and its presence in extrahypothalamic regions of the nervous system of mammals, non-mammalian vertebrates, and even invertebrates have led to the suggestion that TRH may also function as a neuromodulator or neurotransmitter. Administration of synthetic TRH causes depression of firing in certain brain neurons, and pituitary-like TRH receptors have been demonstrated in many brain areas.

The biological half-life for TRH in peripheral blood is very short (2 minutes in mice) apparently because peptidases in the blood rapidly inactivate TRH. Were it not for post-translational modifications of both the C- and N-terminal amino acids that slow peptidase degradation of TRH, this tripeptide would be destroyed even more rapidly (a pyroglutamate on the N-terminal end and an amidated C-terminal end).

B. Other Neural Factors Affecting TSH Secretion

Both stimulatory and inhibitory neural control of TRH release occurs in mammals. Experimental studies in rodents have demonstrated that TRH neurons in the PVN are innervated by dopaminergic and norepinephrine-secreting neurons. Stimulation of norepinephrine-secreting neurons can evoke release of TRH whereas dopamine is an inhibitor of TRH release. The stimulatory role of norepinephrine in humans is supported but not confirmed. Serotoninergic fibers have been shown to inhibit TRH release although some studies indicate a stimulatory role for serotonin. Effects of serotonin in humans are based largely on use of pharmacological agents known to influence serotonergic neurons or serotonin receptors. These studies are somewhat controversial in interpretation, and no clear role has been established.

The peptide **leptin** stimulates TRH mRNA production and releases TRH but only from hypothalamic neurons of the PVN. It is suggested that peptides implicated in appetite control [e.g., leptin, α-MSH, **neuropeptide Y (NPY), galanin**] can influence TRH release in mammals and are related to thyroid hormone involvement in metabolism (see Chapters 6 and 12).

Somatostatin, another hypothalamic neurohormone associated with GH secretion (see below), can function as a TSH-RIH, but its physiological role has not been confirmed. Release of somatostatin can be inhibited by adrenergic α_2-agonists, which is in keeping with the known stimulatory action of norepinephrine on TSH release.

C. Feedback Effects on TSH Secretion

Feedback of thyroid hormones occurs primarily at the thyrotropic cells in the pars distalis and reduces their sensitivity to TRH. The plasma concentration of T_4 is considered to be the most important plasma cue, and pituitary thyrotropes contain a deiodinase that converts T_4 to T_3 prior to binding to nuclear thyroid receptors (TRs). Occupied TRs interfere with the activation of other transcription factors such as Pit-1 that normally would release TSH. Additional evidence suggests that inhibition of the hypothalamic dopaminergic and serotonergic neurons by thyroid hormones is also important in feedback regulation of the HPT axis.

Studies with other neurotransmitters (e.g., acetylcholine, histamine, GABA) and related pharmacological agents exhibit diverse effects but have provided little insight into the control of TSH release. They do suggest there can be many subtle influences on the HPT axis, and this may be important in clinical studies as well as in implications of environmental pharmaceuticals on possible endocrine disruption of the HPT axis.

D. Regulation of Gonadotropin (GTH) Secretion by GnRH

Release of the GTHs is largely under stimulatory control similar to that described for TSH. A **gonadotropin inhibitory hormone (GnIH)** has been isolated from avian brains (see Chapter 5), and these observations were extended to three rodent species in 2006. This recent discovery will undoubtedly change future discussions of GTH bioregulation in mammals, but the account here is limited to the role of GnRH. Release of both LH and FSH is caused by a decapeptide (10 amino acids; Table 4-1) called gonadotropin-releasing hormone (GnRH). Because earlier studies had focused on the actions of this peptide on release of LH, it was first named **luteinizing hormone-releasing hormone (LHRH)** and sometimes is called **luliberin**. However, its dual action causing release of both LH and FSH implies that GnRH is a more appropriate name and is used commonly today. Existence of a specific **FSH-RH** has long been speculated on physiological evidence, but the actual molecule responsible has remained elusive. Neural and neurohormonal factors affecting GTH secretion are summarized in Figure 4-20c.

Since mammalian GnRH was first synthesized, approximately 1400 synthetic analogues have been created, including analogues that are even more potent stimulatory agents than native GnRH as well as inhibitors that can block the action of endogenous GnRH. One super-releaser has approximately 150 times the potency of native GnRH. All of the releasing analogues liberate both FSH and LH under most conditions. Under certain circumstances, exogenous GnRH can inhibit gonadotropin secretion, too (see ahead).

It was soon discovered that a second form of GnRH is present in the mammalian midbrain but was not associated with the HPG axis. This second GnRH in mammals is identical to a form first found in the midbrain of chickens (called **chicken II**) as well as in all other vertebrates examined. Soon, other molecular forms of this decapeptide were isolated from various species and in different brain regions and each was named for the species source. An alternative nomenclature (used here) has been proposed for naming GnRH molecules according to where they are found within the brain (Figure 4-21; see also Chapter 5). The GnRH form in the hypothalamus that is responsible for GTH release in mammals first was designated as **mGnRH** and more recently has been termed **GnRH-1** regardless of the amino acid sequence of the molecule found in the hypothalamus (Figure 4-22) The midbrain form, that uniformly in mammals is the chicken II form, is now called **GnRH-2**. A third location for GnRH is restricted to the telencephalon and is called **GnRH-3**. Thus, in this nomenclature, salmon GnRH (sGnRH) would be sGnRH-1 when located in the hypothalamus but sGnRH-2 when found in the telencephalon. A further discussion of the various vertebrate GnRHs and their nomenclature is provided in Chapter 5.

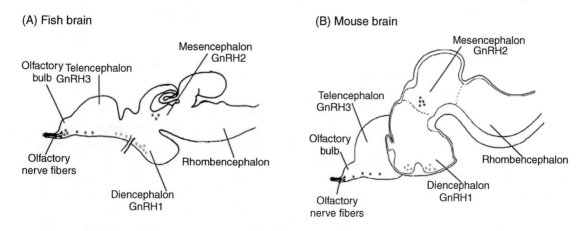

Figure 4-21. **Distribution of the forms of GnRH in the brain.** See text for explanation of abbreviations. [Reprinted with permission from Whitlock, K. E. (2005). Origin and development of GnRH neurons. *Trends Endocr. Metab.* **16**, 145–151. Elsevier Science Inc.] See color insert, plate 5.

GnRH1-Hypothalamic Form	GnRH2-Mesencephalic Form	GnRH3-Telencephalic Form
human GnRH1	human GnRH2	goldfish GnRH3
tree Shrew GnRH1	rhesus monkey GnRH2	zebrafish GnRH3
pig GnRH1	tree Shrew GnRH2	salmon GnRHA3
rat/mouse GnRH1	musk Shrew GnRH2	salmon GnRHB3
chicken GnRH1	goldfish GnRH2	midshipman GnRH3
Xenopus GnRH1	catfish GnRH2	cichlid GnRH3
catfish GnRH1	cichlid GnRH2	seabream GnRH3
cichlid GnRH1	seabream GnRH2	medaka GnRH3
seabream GnRH1	medaka GnRH2	seabass GnRH3
medaka GnRH1	seabass GnRH2	
seabass GnRH1	eel GnRH2	
eel GnRH1		

Figure 4-22. Comparison of schemes for naming GnRH molecules.

Endogenous GnRH-1 originates in NS neurons located from the POA to the medial basal hypothalamus, depending on the species. In rats and mice, most of the GnRH-1 immunoreactive cells sending fibers to the median eminence are located in the POA, anterior to the optic chiasm. In guinea pigs and humans, the medial basal hypothalamus (mainly the ARC nucleus) is the major residence for GnRH-1 neurons. GnRH-1 immunoreactive cells also have been identified in the olfactory region, and recent studies support the hypothesis that at least some of the hypothalamic GnRH-1 cells migrated from the olfactory region into the hypothalamic area (see below).

GnRH-1 cells also contain other regulatory molecules including the **delta sleep-inducing peptide (DSIP)** and the peptide galanin. Nothing is known about the importance of DSIP in GnRH-neurons with respect to reproduction, but galanin may be released along with GnRH and is itself a releaser of LH. Galanin has no effect on FSH release, however. Furthermore, galanin content varies in GnRH-neurons of females during the reproductive cycle. Synthesis of galanin peaks just prior to ovulation and may participate in the generation of the midcycle surge in LH that brings about ovulation and subsequent corpus luteum formation in the ovary (see Chapter 10).

Neurons that secrete GnRH-1 do not form a discrete, compact nucleus but develop an interconnected network that produces an endogenous, synchronized, pulsatile pattern of GnRH-1 release. This network is the **GnRH pulse generator**. Special GnRH neurons called **GT-1 neurons** (a special cell line derived from transgenic mice) exhibit an oscillatory pattern of GnRH release *in vitro* and, together with some related cell lines, have provided a model system for studying the GnRH pulse generator.

GT-1 neurons synthesize and exhibit pulsatile release of GnRH but do not carry any biochemical glial cell markers. The absence of glial markers supports the contention that these cultures consist only of neurons. The pulsatile nature of their secretion implies an endogenous oscillator controlling this behavior, and experiments suggest an autocrine role for GnRH-1 to control its own release. From these experiments, researchers have concluded that operation of the endogenous oscillator depends on Ca^{2+} influx through **voltage-sensitive calcium channels (VSCCs)** and an autocrine positive feedback of released GnRH which causes additional GnRH release.

The pulsatile nature of GnRH-1 secretion is essential to stimulate FSH and LH secretion from the pituitary. Hence administration of chronic, non-pulsatile doses of GnRH or GnRH analogues may prevent rather than stimulate gonadotropin release, possibly due to prolonged down-regulation of GnRH receptors.

Ultrashort negative feedback has been established for GnRH on normal GnRH-secreting neurons of the rat hypothalamus both *in vivo* and *in vitro*. The mechanism for this autofeedback is not clear, but it could occur through recurrent collateral fibers of GnRH neurons that synapse on their own cell body or dendrites. GT-1 neurons do have GnRH receptors and binding of GnRH to these receptors is associated with a rapid, dose-dependent increase in intracellular Ca^{2+}. This results in a two-phase response involving an initial phospholipase C-mediated, inositol trisphosphate (IP_3)-dependent mobilization of Ca^{2+} (see Chapter 2) and a sustained entrance of Ca^{2+} through VSCCs. The phospholipase C system activates other internal mechanisms involving phospholipase D and diacyl glycerol (DAG) that sustain activation of protein kinase C.

Initial binding of GnRH activates additional GnRH release (positive feedback) but soon is followed by inhibition and loss of spontaneous pulsatility (negative feedback). These dual autocrine actions of GnRH result in regular pulsatile episodes of GnRH release into the medium. Additional mechanisms for activating

GnRH release in GT-1 cells have been demonstrated and these may influence the *in vivo* responses of GnRH-secreting neurons. Among the agents that can affect Ca^{2+} mobilation in GnRH cells are the peptides called **endothelins** (Figure 4-23) and catecholamines (dopamine, norepinephrine, and epinephrine). Receptor channels for glutamate and GABA are also present on GnRH neurons and may be important modulators of the hypothesized endogenous oscillator controlling pulsatile GnRH release.

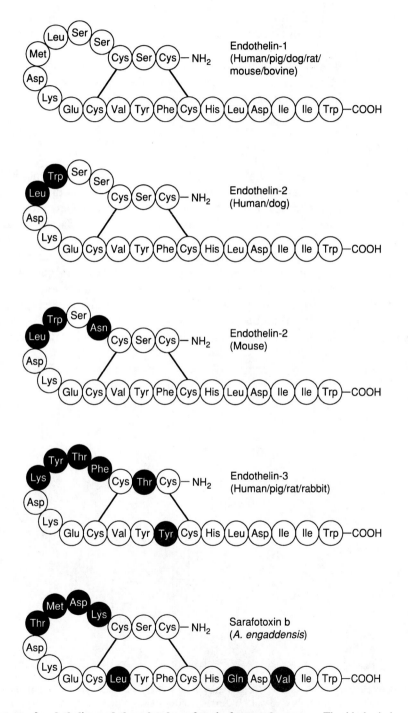

Figure 4-23. **Structure of endothelins and the related sarafotoxin from snake venom.** The black circles represent amino acids not present in the sequence of endothelin-1. (Modified from Masaki, T. Endothelins: homeostatic and compensatory actions in the circulatory and endocrine systems. *Endocrine Rev.* **14**, 256–268 (1993). © The Endocrine Society.)

1. GnRH-1: Action

GnRH-1 operating through a cAMP-dependent mechanism causes release of both FSH and LH from gonadotropes in the adenohypophysis, although a greater amount of LH release is always observed following administration of synthetic GnRH. Prolonged treatment with most GnRH agonistic analogues results in down-regulation of GnRH receptors, however, and chronic administration causes a reduction in gonadotropin release. Pulsatile administration of GnRH or GnRH analogues is necessary to stimulate natural patterns of GTH secretion.

The half-life of GnRH is very short, for it is rapidly degraded in peripheral plasma. The short-term success of several potent synthetic analogues of GnRH appears to be related to their relative resistance to degradation by blood peptidases.

GnRH-2 has been identified immunologically in extrahypothalamic nervous tissue and in the pineal gland of some species. Similarly, GnRH-2, like TRH, can cause depression of neural function in the central nervous system. Thus, GnRH-2 may play a physiological role as a neuromodulator or neurotransmitter.

2. Origin of GnRH-1 Cells

Studies of early amphibian development showed that the precursors of adenohypophysial cells as well as certain hypothalamic neurons have their origins in portions of the embryonic neural ridge. From these studies, we have learned in both amphibians and mammals that one of these neural ridge derivatives, the **nasal placode**, is the origin of GnRH-1 secreting neurons of the hypothalamus as well as olfactory neurons that eventually make up the olfactory, terminal, and vomeronasal nerves. Nasal placodes are bilateral structures responsible for development of both left and right olfactory tracts. The olfactory neurons migrate first from the nasal region and contact the forebrain, inducing formation of the olfactory bulbs (Figure 4-24). The NS neurons follow an extracellular matrix laid down by olfactory neurons along their migration route and are identifiable by their secretion of GnRH-1. The degree of migration of these NS cells in different species probably explains the variability in GnRH distribution. Ablation (surgical destruction or extirpation) of both nasal placodes in amphibians results in the absence of GnRH-1 cells in the hypothalamus. Unilateral ablation results in absence

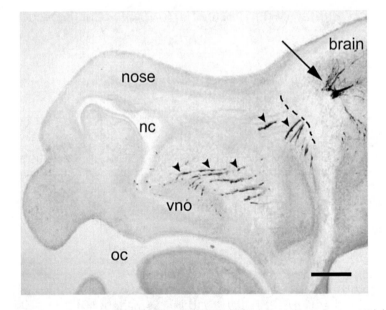

Figure 4-24. **Gonadotropin-releasing hormone (GnRH) migration in the mouse embryo**. Immunostaining of GnRH of a sagittal section of the head on embryo day 13.5. Arrow indicates GnRH neurons already located in the brain whereas the arrow heads designate migrating GnRH neurons still in the nasal compartment. nc, nasal cavity; oc, oral cavity; vno, vomeronasal organ. The dotted line designates the cribiform plate separating the nasal region from the brain. Courtesy of Dr. John Gill and Dr. Pei-San Tsai, University of Colorado.

of GnRH cells only on the side of the ablation. Similarly, a genetically based abnormality known as **Kallmann's syndrome** in humans results in a failure for nasal placode cells to migrate and produces patients with anosmia and hypogonadism.

3. Other Neural Factors Affecting Gonadotropin Secretion

Secretion of GnRH is under the stimulatory control of NE-secreting neurons in both rats and primates. Activity of these NE-secreting neurons as well as the GABA-secreting neurons can be depressed by neurons secreting β-endorphin. The only other neurotransmitter with distinct stimulatory actions on gonadotropin release is **glutamate**, an excitatory amino acid neurotransmitter. The actions of cholinergic, serotonergic, and dopaminergic factors on GnRH-1 and gonadotropin release are based largely on pharmacological studies and are considered controversial due to the variety of reported effects.

E. Feedback Effects on Gonadotropin Secretion

Gonadal steroids generally have negative feedback effects on gonadotropin release at the level of the gonadotropes, reducing their sensitivity to GnRH. Selective negative feedback on FSH secretion occurs at the gonadotrope, reducing FSH output but not LH output in response to GnRH-1. This feedback is accomplished through FSH-dependent production by the gonads of a peptide known as **inhibin**. The predominence of LH in the midcycle surge of gonadotropin at ovulation in females is due in part to this selective action of inhibin. Galanin released at this time from the hypothalamus enhances release of LH, thus contributing to the LH surge that precedes ovulation. Further discussion of inhibin and other peptides involved in ovulation can be found in Chapter 10.

Positive feedback also occurs in the gonadal axis of female mammals and is responsible for the midcycle surge of LH that stimulates ovulation. Explanation of the estrogen-induced, preovulatory GnRH-1 surge in females is complicated by the absence of estrogen receptors (ERs) on the GnRH-1 neurons. However, GABA-secreting neurons that innervate GnRH-1 neurons can stimulate GnRH-1 release. These GABA neurons also possess ERs and may be responsible for the GnRH-1 surge. Part of the inhibitory action of endorphins on GnRH-1 release is through inhibition of these GABA neurons. This scheme is summarized in Figure 4-20b. Rupture of the ovarian follicle at ovulation causes a reduction in estradiol synthesis and in the secretion of progesterone by the corpus luteum in the ovary and reinstates negative feedback on hypothalamic secretion of GnRH-1 (see Chapter 10).

F. Regulation of Growth Hormone Secretion

Although initial studies involving transection of the portal system or explant of the pituitary implied that release of GH was under stimulatory hypothalamic control, we now know it is under both inhibitory and stimulatory control by neurohormones. Secretion of GH is episodic; that is, it occurs in bursts separated by longer intervals of lowered release. For example, in rats, GH is secreted at intervals of about 3 hours. In humans, maximal episodes of GH release occur during sleep (Figure 4-25). The major neural and neurohormonal factors influencing GH secretion are summarized in Figure 4-20e.

1. GH Release-Inhibiting Hormone (Somatostatin)

Release of GH *in vivo* is controlled primarily by a GH release-inhibiting peptide (GHRIH), more commonly called **somatostatin (SST)**. However, even in the absence of SST, a releasing hormone known variously as somatocrinin, somatoliberin, or **growth hormone-releasing hormone (GHRH = GRH = GRF)** is necessary to stimulate GH release. The episodic bursts of GH release occur during periods of lowered SST levels and elevated GHRH.

The PERIV nucleus of the anterior hypothalamus and the amygdala of the limbic system are the sources for most of the SST-containing nerve terminals in the median eminence. This tetradecapeptide (14 AA; Table 4-1)

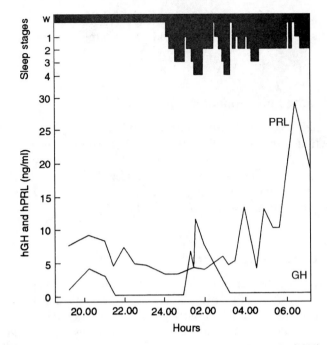

Figure 4-25. **Diurnal patterns of GH and PRL release**. (From Baulieu, E., and Kelly, P. (1990). "Hormones: From Molecules to Disease," p. 206. Chapman & Hall, London.)

is a strong inhibitor of GH release. SST_{14} appears to work through a GTP-dependent G_i-protein that prevents the elevation of cAMP necessary to provoke GH release (see Chapter 3).

SST also occurs in extrahypothalamic nervous tissue (both brain and spinal cord). Multiple SST-receptors have been identified and their differential distribution in the CNS and peripheral tissues described. A number of possible neuromodulator/neurotransmitter functions in the central nervous system have been suggested, similar to the case for the other major releasing hormones. It is also present in the mucosa of the stomach where it locally inhibits release of the gastric hormone, gastrin, and in the pancreatic islets where it inhibits both glucagon and insulin release (see Chapter 12). A larger form of SST (SST_{28}) was extracted first from the gut and pancreatic tissues and later was shown to exist in nerve endings of the median eminence along with the tetradecapeptide. Studies have since shown that SST_{28} is released in equal or greater amounts than SST_{14} into portal blood. Furthermore, pituitary receptors show stronger binding affinity for the larger peptide. Both forms of SST apparently are produced from the same prohormone.

2. Growth Hormone-Releasing Hormone (GHRH)

A potent peptide releaser of GH was first isolated and characterized from a human pancreatic tumor associated with an unusual case of excessive GH secretion resulting in clinical condition called acromegaly (see clinical discussion ahead). The same gene was later found to be active in the hypothalamus. In human, porcine, bovine, ovine, and caprine mammals, GHRH isolated from the ARC nucleus is composed of 44 amino acid residues and is related chemically to the secretin-glucagon family of peptides (see Chapter 3, Table 3-4). In the rat, GHRH consists of only 43 amino acids and differs considerably in amino acid composition from the other mammalian GHRHs. The significance of this deviation in rat GHRH structure is unknown.

GHRH-immunoreactive fibers extend from the ARC nucleus to the median eminence. Some neurons in the ARC nucleus contain dopamine and neurotensin as well as GHRH. Others exhibit GHRH colocalized with dopamine and galanin. A potent GHRH-releasing peptide was discovered and later identified as the peptide **ghrelin**, previously found in the gastrointestinal tract. Ghrelin, like GHRH, is found in neurons of the ARC nucleus and probably plays an important role in GHRH secretion and hence in GH release. It also has important effects on appetite (see Chapter 12).

3. Other Neural Factors Affecting GH Secretion

There is no shortage of investigations that have reported the effects of pharmacological and/or disruptive techniques on GH secretion. However, there are considerable conflicting data, and it is difficult to determine whether effects observed are direct or indirect. Furthermore, it is often difficult to ascertain whether an effect is mediated through control of SST or GHRH release. For example, an increase in GH secretion could represent either a decrease in SST release, an increase in GHRH release, or both.

Factors which have been shown to elicit GH release under certain conditions include neurotransmitters (norepinephrine, dopamine, serotonin, GABA, NPY), opiates, VIP, thyroid hormones, glucocorticoids, and estrogens. Inhibition of GH secretion has been reported following treatment with a variety of neural factors (GABA, serotonin, substance P, neurotensin), large quantities of glucocorticoids, and androgens. From this brief summary, it seems clear that catecholamines are stimulatory. Serotonin is usually stimulatory, probably acting through effects on norepinephrine-secreting neurons. The dichotomous actions of GABA could be due to its ability to inhibit release of SST and GHRH under different conditions. Substance P and neurotensin increase SST release, explaining their prevention of GH secretion.

Some of the confusion as to roles of various regulators on GH release stems from species differences. For example, stress, which is usually associated with elevated glucocorticoids, generally increases GH secretion in primates, inhibits GH secretion in rodents, and has no effect in domestic ungulates. Moderate exercise causes GH release in humans. Total food deprivation increases GH secretion in primates as well as in domestic ungulates.

G. Feedback Effects on GH Secretion

Many of the actions of GH on body growth are mediated by IGF-I and IGF-II produced in the liver and secreted into the general circulation under the direction of GH rather than by GH itself. Plasma IGF-I reduces release of GH through negative feedback.

GH produces metabolic effects including elevation of glucose and free fatty acid levels as well as decreases in plasma amino acids. These metabolic products can affect GH release, but it appears they play no major physiological role. Elevated glucose can decrease GH output and insulin-induced hypoglycemia elevates GH release. High levels of free fatty acids also depress GH levels, and, conversely, depressed fatty acid levels elevate GH release. Both glucose and free fatty acid feedback effects are consistent with the reduction in both following insulin injection.

GH release is especially sensitive to one amino acid, arginine. Infusion of arginine causes a marked increase in GH release. However, other amino acids are not very effective stimulators of GH release, and no elevation in circulating GH is observed following consumption of a high-protein meal. Hence, the physiological importance of amino acid feedback is unclear.

H. Regulation of Prolactin Secretion

Prolactin has the distinction of being the only pituitary tropic hormone for which there is evidence for two distinct RHs and RIHs although most authorities favor only one of each. The primary control over PRL release, as mentioned earlier, is inhibitory in mammals, and the pituitary releases PRL when freed either surgically or chemically from hypothalamic control. This is in marked contrast to the situation with GH where both the absence of SST and the presence of GHRH are necessary to elicit secretion. Consequently, ectopic or explanted pituitaries spontaneously release large quantities of PRL.

In lactating mammals, suckling or electrical stimulation of the teat sends neural input to the hypothalamus and evokes release of the nonapeptide oxytocin into the circulation, causing contraction of cells lining the ducts of the mammary glands and milk ejection. This **neuroendocrine reflex** also stimulates a delayed release of PRL which stimulates the mammary gland to replace lost milk. Major neural and neurohormonal factors affecting PRL release are summarized in Figure 4-20f.

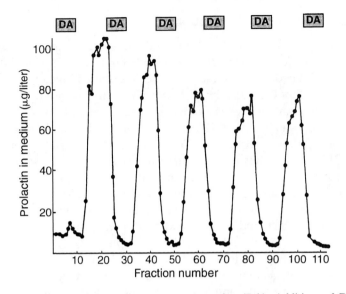

Figure 4-26. **Response of perifused rat pituitary lactotropes to dopamine (DA).** Additions of DA immediately depresses the spontaneous secretion of PRL normally seen *in vitro*. (From Martini, L., and Besser, G. M. (1977). "Clinical Neuroendocrinology." Academic Press, New York.)

1. Prolactin-Releasing (PRH) and Release-Inhibiting Hormones (PRIH)

The consensus is that mammalian **prolactin release-inhibiting hormone (PRIH)** is the catecholamine neurotransmitter, dopamine, which is a potent inhibitor of PRL release *in vivo* or *in vitro* (Figure 4-26). Dopamine is released from hypothalamic neurons in the ARC nucleus and periventricular hypothalamus as a neurohormone. It is elevated in the portal system under physiological conditions where PRL release is inhibited.

Two additional PRIH candidates have been proposed. The first is GABA which has been shown to block PRL release *in vivo* and *in vitro* by direct action on lactotropes. However, large amounts of GABA are required to inhibit PRL release and such levels are not found in either portal or peripheral blood samples, indicating that GABA probably is not a physiological PRIH.

There is also support for a peptide PRIH that can inhibit PRL release. This peptide PRIH is the 56-amino acid C-terminal fragment of the GnRH prohormone. Inhibition of PRL release often accompanies GTH secretion. However, it is not confirmed that this **GnRH-associated peptide (GAP)** is a physiological regulator.

Like the situation for GH, there is evidence for an endogenous factor or factors that stimulate PRL release. This **PRL-releasing hormone (PRH)** at first was thought to be the tripeptide already named TRH since administration of synthetic TRH stimulates PRL release as well as TSH release at least under some conditions. However, the neuropeptide VIP stimulates PRL release during suckling when TRH is ineffective. Administration of TRH to suckling mice causes elevated TSH release but no increase in PRL release such as caused by VIP. Furthermore, TSH release is not observed during normal suckling.

A peptide first isolated as an orphan receptor was thought to be a potent releaser of PRL both *in vitro* and *in vivo*. This **prolactin-releasing peptide (PrRP)** releases PRL when administered in low doses but is not as potent as TRH. It does not cause GH release. PrRP apparently is widely distributed in the brain and has been shown to modulate many unrelated physiological events including lactation, stress, body weight homeostasis, feeding behavior, and gastric motility. It also is a potent releaser of PRL in fishes. Much needs to be learned about this newest PRL releaser before we can determine its physiological roles with certainty, but numerous observations suggest it is not a PRH at physiological levels where it does affect appetite (see Chapter 12).

Recent studies have demonstrated a peptide, called **tuberalin**, that is produced in the pars tuberalis. Tuberalin can stimulate release of PRL from lactotropes and is believed to be an important regulator related to photoperiodic effects on PRL release (see pineal gland discussion ahead).

2. Other Neural Factors Affecting Prolactin Secretion

Several neuropeptides evoke PRL release under experimental conditions, including neurotensin, epidermal growth factor (EGF), and EOPs. The opioids apparently block the activity of dopamine-secreting neurons that normally prevent PRL release. SST also can inhibit PRL release. GABA, which can directly inhibit PRL release at the lactotrope, can also stimulate PRL release through actions on hypothalamic neurons. It is not clear whether these actions of SST and GABA have any physiological significance.

I. Feedback and Other Chemical Effects on Prolactin Secretion

The major feedback loop established in rats involves PRL feeding back directly on hypothalamic dopaminergic neurons. PRL also increases GABA synthesis and release into the portal circulation, supporting its inhibitory action on the lactotrope as part of the feedback mechanism rather than as a true PRIH.

Estrogens modulate PRL release in rats and to a lesser extent in sheep by enhancing the sensitivity of lactotropes to hypothalamic PRHs. This effect may involve an estrogen-induced reduction in their sensitivity to dopamine by altering receptor levels and/or intracellular second messenger systems. Estradiol is concentrated by certain GABA-secreting neurons, decreasing their activity and possibly releasing some PRH-secreting neurons from tonic GABA inhibition.

Gonadotropes release the octapeptide angiotensin-II (ANG-II) in response to GnRH-1. ANG-II then binds to specific receptors on nearby lactotropes. This potentially paracrine action on the lactotrope may have some importance for PRL release but confirmatory studies are needed.

J. Regulation of Corticotropin Secretion

Corticotropin secretion by corticotropes of the pars distalis is primarily under stimulatory regulation by the neuropeptide **corticotropin-releasing hormone (CRH)**. CRH is also called **corticoliberin** although this name is not in general use. Physiological evidence has been presented that suggests the existence of an inhibitory hypothalamic factor as well. Although ACTH and α-MSH are synthesized by hydrolysis of the same preprohormone in the melanotrope and the corticotrope (see ahead), there are many differences in the regulation of their release. Secretion of ACTH stimulates synthesis and release of cortisol (e.g., humans) or corticosterone (e.g., rats) or both (e.g., deer) from the adrenal cortex (see Chapter 8), and the circadian rhythm of ACTH secretion is reflected in a similar rhythm for corticosteroid release. In humans, there is a gradual decrease in ACTH plasma levels with the onset of sleep to a minimum at about midnight (see Chapter 2, Figure 2-3). Then, a series of bursts of ACTH release occurs, culminating in maximal plasma levels of ACTH and cortisol at about 6 a.m. Following these peaks, there is a gradual decline in both hormones during the daylight hours with occasional bursts of secretion. Release of ACTH may occur following a mid-day meal but not an evening meal. In nocturnally active rats, the pattern of corticosterone secretion is the reverse of that seen in diurnal humans. Major neural and neurohormonal factors affecting ACTH release are summarized in Figure 4-20d.

1. Corticotropin-Releasing Hormone (CRH) or Factor (CRF)

CRH consists of 41 amino acid residues and it releases ACTH from the corticotrope *in vivo* and *in vitro*. The highest hypothalamic levels of CRH in rats and humans are in the PVN and ARC nucleus. In rats and humans, AVP and CRH have been colocalized in the same hypothalamic neurons. CRH in rats occurs in the highest concentration within neuronal endings located in the median eminence where it exceeds concentrations in other brain regions by 10 to 100 times. CRH occurs in other forebrain nuclei (e.g., central nucleus of the amygdala) as well as in other regions of the brain (e.g., substantia nigra of the midbrain). In addition to its role in ACTH secretion from the pituitary, CRH probably functions as a neuromodulator in other brain regions including the olfactory bulb, cerebral cortex, cerebellum, hippocampus, and amygdala.

Human and rat CRHs are identical peptides but oCRH differs from these at seven residues. There is considerable homology of CRH (at 20 positions) to **sauvagine**, a 40-residue peptide isolated from skin of the

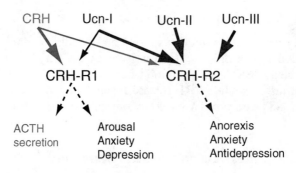

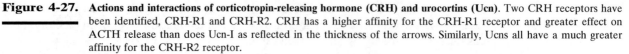

Figure 4-27. **Actions and interactions of corticotropin-releasing hormone (CRH) and urocortins (Ucn).** Two CRH receptors have been identified, CRH-R1 and CRH-R2. CRH has a higher affinity for the CRH-R1 receptor and greater effect on ACTH release than does Ucn-I as reflected in the thickness of the arrows. Similarly, Ucns all have a much greater affinity for the CRH-R2 receptor.

frog, *Phylomedusa sauvagii*, as well as overlap with the structure of a hypotensive agent, **urotensin I**, isolated from the spinal cord and urophysis of teleostean fishes (see Chapter 5).

Additional members of the CRH-like family of peptides (Table 4-9) in mammals are called **urocotrins**. Three urocortins have been identified: **urocortin I (Ucn-I), urocortin II (Ucn-II),** and **urocortin III (Ucn-III).** Ucn-I is present in neurons of the midbrain as well as in cells of the GI tract, testes, cardiac muscle, thymus, spleen, and skin, suggesting diverse actions (Figure 4-27). Ucn-II and III are found primarily in the hypothalamus. Two receptors that bind CRH and the urocortins also have been described and usually are called **CRF-R1** and **CRF-R2**. CRH and Ucn-I both bind to CRF-R1 that is the more prevalent receptor type in the brain and pituitary. All three urocortins bind to CRF-R2 that has been demonstrated in the hypothalamus as well as in peripheral sites including the digestive tract, arteries, lung, and skeletal muscle. CRH binds strongly to CRF-R1 but binds much less strongly to CRF-R2 than do the urocortins. Urocortins as well as injected CRH inhibit gastric secretion, decrease blood pressure, and reduce inflammation. These actions of CRH treatment are probably pharmacological, and the urocortins are probably the physiological mediators of these effects. A unique form of CRF-R2 (βCRF-R2) with affinity for Ucn-II and Ucn-III occurs in heart muscle and is involved with regulation of cardiac output.

ACTH release also is stimulated by the nonapeptide **arginine vasopressin (AVP)**, and there is good evidence to support a physiological role for AVP in enhancing the responsiveness of corticotropes to CRH. AVP may be colocalized with CRH in the same hypothalamic neurons. During stress (see Chapter 8), the ratio of secreted AVP to CRH increases from 2:1 to as high as 9:1. Apparently, AVP released from the median eminence acts directly upon corticotropes to markedly increase their sensitivity to CRH and prevents shutdown of ACTH secretion via corticosteroid feedback on CRH release (see ahead). CRH-like bioactivity in the supraoptic nucleus is due primarily to the presence of AVP and not CRH whereas the major CRH-like bioactivity in the PVN is due to CRH.

Although the Battleboro strain of rats lacks the ability to synthesize AVP, these rats still show a stress response. However, extracts from Battleboro hypothalami exhibit only 20% of the CRH activity demonstrated in normal rats. Addition of AVP restores ACTH-releasing activity to 100% in these rats.

CRH is also a potential bioregulator of LH and GH release at the level of the hypothalamus. These effects do not involve opioid neurons, but the exact mechanism is unknown. CRH can stimulate GHRH release and inhibit SST release and might explain its effect on GH. The reduction in LH release when CRH is elevated may provide a mechanism whereby stress shuts down the reproductive axis.

2. Other Neural Factors Affecting ACTH Secretion

In addition to CRH and AVP, release of ACTH occurs following administration of several classical neurotransmitters (norepinpehrine, epinephrine, serotonin, acetylcholine) and a variety of neuropeptides (OXY, VIP, PHI, ANG-II). Although all of these compounds have been reported within nerve fibers of the median eminence, none of them appears to be of major importance in influencing ACTH release. GABA, however, has direct inhibitory actions on paraventricular CRH neurons as well as on corticotropes in rats, although data concerning the action of GABA on ACTH secretion in humans are conflicting.

K. Feedback Effects on ACTH Secretion

Negative feedback occurs through the actions of glucocorticoids both on CRH neurons in the hypothalamus and corticotropes in the pars distalis. Glucocorticoids are known to feed back via mineralocorticoid receptors (MR = GR-1; see Chapter 3) on CA1 neurons in the hippocampus that in turn innervate CRH neurons in the hypothalamus, but bind to glucocorticoid receptors (GR = GR-2) in the corticotropes. During chronic stress as mentioned previously, the output of AVP, which is not subject to glucocorticoid feedback, increases. As a result, the sensitivity of corticotropes to CRH is enhanced. This action probably helps to sustain prolonged elevation of glucocorticoids in the face of negative feedback on CRH release during chronic stress.

L. Regulation of Melanotropin (α-MSH) Secretion

Melanotropin is released in large amounts when the pituitary is transplanted to an ectopic site or placed *in vitro*, indicating chronic inhibition of α-MSH release is the normal condition. Although evidence exists for stimulatory factors regulating α-MSH release, it seems that removal of inhibitory controls is most important for eliciting α-MSH release. A summary of major neural and neurohormonal factors affecting α-MSH release is provided in Figure 4-20g.

The predominant form of circulating α-MSH is acetylated α-MSH. αMSH is produced by hydrolysis of ACTH within the melanotrope. Three separate MSH molecules have been identified in extracts of mammalian pituitaries, but only α-MSH appears to be released from POMC *in vivo* and occurs in the circulation. Hydrolysis of the 16-K fragment can yield γ-MSH (18 amino acids) and β-MSH (22 amino acids) as hydrolysis products of LPH.

1. Melanotropin-Releasing (MRH) and Release-Inhibiting Hormones (MRIH)

It is not always clear whether α-MSH release is controlled by a neurohormone or by direct innervation from hypothalamic neurons. Dopamine appears to be the physiological **melanotropin release-inhibiting hormone (MRIH)** in numerous species. Several peptides possess intrinsic MRIH-like activity, but they may not be physiologically relevant. Extrahypothalamic MRIH activity has been demonstrated, and at least one of the synthetic releasers of α-MSH is an antidepressant when administered to humans.

2. Feedback Effects on α-MSH Secretion

There does not appear to be any direct feedback mechanism operating on α-MSH release. Stimulation of melanocytes by α-MSH does not release anything into the circulation that would be a feedback candidate. Perhaps the strong negative control of α-MSH release precludes the requirement for negative feedback.

V. The Nonapeptide Hormones

The hypothalamic nonapeptide neurohormones are synthesized in the SON and the PVN. Most of these neurons project their axons to the pars nervosa although some neurons connect to the median eminence. Nonapeptides stored in the pars nervosa can be released from neurosecretory neuronal endings directly into the general circulation in response to neural stimulation. The targets for these hormones are located at considerable distances from the pars nervosa (for example, kidney, mammary gland, uterus).

Two neurohypophysial nonapeptide hormones (usually AVP and OXY) are present in the pars nervosa of most adult mammals. **Lysine vasopressin (LVP)**, a variant of AVP, is produced by members of the mammalian order Suina, which includes peccaries, domestic pigs, and the hippopotamus. Most of the species in this group

Table 4-10. Distribution of Basic and Neutral Nonapeptides in Mammals

Mammals		Basic	Neutral
Prototheria	Echidna, platypus	AVP	OXY
Metatheria	Common opossum, four-eyed possum	LVP	OXY
	American opossum, bandicoot	LVP	MST
	Dasyuroids	AVP	MST
	Macropodids ('roos, wallabies)	LVP, PVP	OXY, MST
Eutheria	Suiformes (hippo, wild pigs)	LVP, AVP	OXY
	Suiformes (domestic pig)	LVP	OXY
	All others	AVP	OXY

secrete both AVP and LVP in addition to OXY, but the domestic pig secretes only LVP. **Phenypressin (PVP)**, a unique vasopressin-like molecule, replaces vasopressin in the pars nervosa of marsupials (Table 4-10).

Fetal mammals secrete a molecule that at first appears to be a hybrid of AVP and OXY, being composed of the side chain of AVP with the ring structure of OXY. This nonapeptide is known as **arginine vasotocin (AVT)** and is characteristic of adult non-mammalian vertebrates (Figure 4-11). The pineal gland of at least some adult mammals also contains AVT.

The vasopressins (AVP, LVP) and PVP function as antidiuretic agents, increasing the ability of the kidneys to reabsorb water from the glomerular filtrate, reducing urine volume (antidiuresis). At higher doses, vasopressins cause vasoconstriction and can elevate blood pressure (pressor effect). This action may increase glomerular filtration and water excretion (diuresis). AVT produces similar actions in non-mammals and may play an osmoregulatory role in fetal mammals.

As mentioned earlier, OXY stimulates contraction of myoepithelial cells lining the ducts of the mammary glands and causes ejection of milk. The stimulatory action of OXY on the smooth muscle of the uterus is related to the induction of labor and the birth process. OXY also stimulates contractions in oviducts as well as in the vas deferens (sperm duct) of males.

Nonapeptide hormones, of course, are synthesized as part of larger propeptides. Early studies established the presence of additional peptides in the pars nervosa extracts that lacked biological activity in the nonapeptide bioassays. These peptides first were thought to play some carrier function to bring the nonapeptides to the secretory granules and were named **neurophysins**. The first stains specific for staining the secretions of the pars nervosa that allowed us to trace the neurosecretory neurons to their source in the hypothalamus were actually staining these neurophysins. We now recognize two distinct propeptides, **prooxyphysin** (also called prooxytocin) and **propressophysin** (provasopressin), as the prohormones for OXY and the vasopressins, respectively (Figure 4-28). When prooxyophysin is hydrolyzed, it yields OXY plus **neurophysin I**, a peptide of 92 amino acids. Hydrolysis of propressophysin yields vasopressin, **neurophysin II** (93 amino acids), and a short, unnamed glycopeptide (39 amino acids).

A. The Biological Actions of Vasopressins

As we have already discussed, the main physiological role for vasopressins appears to be an antidiuretic action on the kidney with a secondary role in elevating blood pressure through effects on vascular smooth muscle. OXY causes contraction of reproductive tract smooth muscles in both males and females and contraction of myoepithelial cells lining the ducts of the mammary gland in females.

A brief examination of the amino acid composition of the nonapeptides reveals the bases for their biological activities. Antidiuretic and pressor activites apparently require a basic amino acid at position 8, and these actions are enhanced by phenylalanine at position 3. Peptides with neutral amino acids at position 8 exhibit predominately OXY-like actions, and the appearance of isoleucine at position 3 enhances that effect (see Figure 4-11).

As already mentioned, vasopressins and OXY may act as neurotransmitters or neuromodulators in the central nervous system and AVP enhances release of ACTH from the pituitary. Furthermore, a number of metabolic actions for both neurohormones have been reported, but it is not clear how important these putative roles are in relation to the dominant metabolic hormones such as GH, glucocorticoids, and insulin (see Chapter 12).

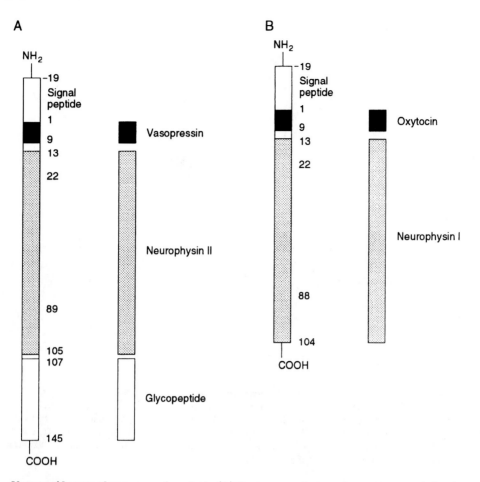

Figure 4-28. **Nonapeptide preprohormones and products.** (A) Prepropressophysin undergoes post-translational processing to yield three peptides: vasopressin, neurophysin II, and a glycopeptide. (B) Preprooxyphysin gives rise to two peptides: oxytocin and neurophysin I. (From Baulieu, E., and Kelly, P. (1990). "Hormones: From Molecules to Disease," p. 206. Chapman & Hall, London.)

1. Antidiuresis and Blood Vascular Effects: Vasopressins

In the kidney, blood pressure determines the **glomerular filtration rate** at which water and solutes are filtered through capillary tufts known as glomeruli and enter the nephrons as the **glomerular filtrate**. Normally, the filtrate lacks plasma proteins and the cellular components of the blood plasma, and, initially, the concentrations of solutes such as Na^+ and glucose in the filtrate are identical to blood plasma. Numerous mechanisms operate to return solutes and most of the water back to the blood vascular system. If something interferes with the reabsorption process, a larger than normal volume of urine will be produced; i.e., diuresis. Should more reabsorption occur than normal, more fluid is reabsorbed and antidiuresis results. Regulation of water reabsorption is critical to maintaining normal blood volume and blood pressure. Likewise, any marked changes in blood volume and concomitant changes in blood pressure will have effects on glomerular filtration rate and may lead to antidiuresis or diuresis.

Vasopressins act on the cells lining the collecting ducts by binding to V_2 receptors on the serosal surface of the cells of the collecting duct in the kidney. This G-protein coupled V_2 receptor activates cAMP-based intracellular mechanisms that produce two effects. Phosphorylation of special cytoplasmic proteins called **aquaporins** causes them to interact with the luminal cell surface and allow water to enter the collecting duct cell. In addition, genes are activated to synthesize more aquaporin molecules. Water pumped into the cell then leaves passively through additional aquaporin molecules on the serosal surface (see Figure 4-29). From here, water moves osmotically into the blood resulting in an increase in both total blood volume and blood

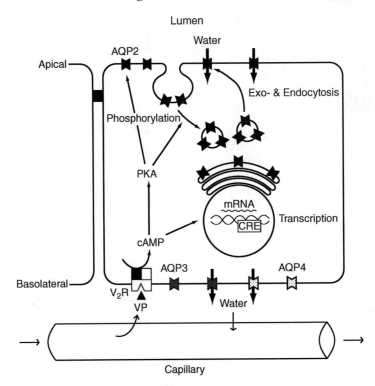

Figure 4-29. **Vasopressin actions on aquaporins and water transport.** Vasopressin binds to the V_2-receptor and via a cAMP second messenger system stimulates synthesis of aquaporins. cAMP also activates protein kinase A that through phosphorylation directs the movements of newly synthesized aquaporin molecules to the cell surface where they can participate in water transport. [Reprinted with permission from Sasaki, S., Ishibashi, K., and Marumo, F. (1998). AQUAPORIN-2 AND -3: Representatives of Two Subgroups of the Aquaporin Family Colocalized in the Kidney Collecting Duct. *Ann. Rev. Physiol. 60,* 199–200.]

pressure. This reuptake of water from the glomerular filtrate reduces the volume of urine formed and elevates its solute concentration.

An increase in blood osmotic concentration and/or a decrease in blood pressure triggers release of vasopressin which causes increased water reabsorption, antidiuresis, and a homeostatic decrease in blood osmotic concentration and/or elevation of blood pressure. Similarly, an increase in blood pressure and/or a decrease in blood osmotic concentration represses vasopressin secretion and causes diuresis with a corresponding drop in blood volume and pressure. Thus, vasopressins are important in the minute-to-minute regulation of blood volume and pressure as water uptake occurs in the intestine. A secondary action of vasopressins occurs in the brain where it stimulates thirst. Consumption of water will also add fluid to the blood vascular system and will increase blood pressure.

High doses of vasopressins cause contraction of arteriole smooth muscle and elevate blood pressure. This in turn increases the glomerular filtration rate sufficiently to override the normal antidiuretic action of the hormone and produces a net diuresis. Secretion of sufficient vasopressin to bring about arteriole constriction and attendant diuresis probably occurs following severe drops in blood pressure such as following hemorrhage. Neural regulation as well as other endocrine regulators of blood pressure, such as the angiotensins (see Chapter 8), may be more important regulators than vasopressins, however.

2. Natriuretic Peptides (NPs)

Chronic high blood pressure can cause the release of **atrial natriuretic peptide (ANP)** from the heart into the general circulation (Figure 4-30). Initially named for its discovery in the artrium, ANP also is synthesized in the ventricles and is produced in the brain as well. The brain produces a second but less potent NP called **BNP** that is also produced by the heart. Studies show that the major circulating forms of NPs are from the heart and not from the brain. A third NP, **CNP**, also has been described. NPs primarily produce their effects at the level of the kidney and at the adrenal cortex but also have effects in the central nervous system, accelerating

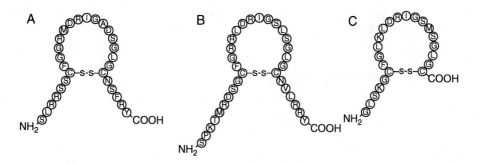

Figure 4-30. **Natriuretic peptides.** (Reprinted by permission of the publisher from Samson, W. K. Natriuretic peptides. A family of hormones. *Trends in Endocr. Metab.* **3**, 86–90. Copyright 1992 Elsevier Science Inc.)

sodium loss and hence promoting diuresis and lowering blood pressure. In addition, ANP inhibits release of vasopressin and further accelerates diuresis in an attempt to compensate homeostatically for the high blood pressure. NPs are released under conditions of chronic hypertension and have been shown to block secretion of aldosterone and AVP (see Chapter 8).

3. Other Factors Affecting Vasopressin Secretion

Ethyl alcohol has an inhibitory effect on release of vasopressins. Hence, consumption of alcoholic beverages produces a diuresis by increasing blood volume, blood pressure, and glomerular filtration rate as well as through reduction in the efficiency of the reabsorption of water in the kidney. This inhibition of vasopressin release by alcohol may be prolonged even after blood pressure returns to normal so that excessive dehydration occurs, contributing to production of the severe headaches often associated with hangovers.

4. AVP and Corticotropin Release

The hypothalamus also is the source of AVP that potentiates ACTH release from the adenohypophysis, but, in this case, it is released directly into the portal system and does not come from the pars nervosa. This effect on ACTH release apparently is very important in prolonging the stress response (see Chapter 8).

B. Uterotonic and Milk Ejection Activities: Oxytocin

The contraction of the uterine smooth muscle caused by OXY was almost immediately recognized as a methodology for artificially inducing labor in women, and it has been employed extensively for this purpose as well as to stimulate clamping down of the uterine muscles after birth to reduce postpartum bleeding. It was many years, however, before it was proven that OXY actually participates in the natural induction of labor in humans and other mammals.

OXY not only produces rhythmic contractions in the female reproductive tract, but it is responsible for contraction of the vas deferens and epididymis during ejaculation by males. The pleasurable sensation of orgasm involves rhythmic contractions of reproductive smooth muscle in both men and women and is induced by OXY as well.

In women, cows, and other female mammals, release of milk from the mammary glands is also induced by OXY. Exposure of mammary glands to estrogens stimulates development of the glands and the myoepithelial cells that line the ducts. Prolactin causes the epithelial cells of the mammary glands to synthesize milk, and OXY causes contraction of the myoepithelial cells lining the ducts to cause milk ejection.

Release of OXY is brought about through a neuroendocrine reflex. Suckling of the newborn on the nipple sends neural impulses to the brain that reach the hypothalamus and direct the release of OXY from the pars nervosa into the general circulation. Sufficient OXY in the circulation also can stimulate rhythmic oviduct contractions leading, in the mother, to a pleasurable sensation during suckling.

Like AVP, administration of OXY has been shown to have effects on tropic hormone release. However, no distinct endogenous role for OXY as a releasing hormone has been verified.

C. Nonapeptide Neurohormones and Behavior

Parental behavior in mammals is affected by nonapeptides. Among a group of rodents known as voles, some species such as the prairie vole, *Microtus ochrogaster*, are monogamous whereas other species such as the meadow vole, *Microtus pennsylvanicus*, are non-monogamous. Both males and females of the monogamous prairie voles spend considerable time tending to pups in their nest (60–70% of their time) whereas male meadow voles spend only about 15% of their time tending the nest and even females spend only 35%. The distribution of OXY neurons differs in the brains of these two species, and corticosterone and AVP levels are high in prairie voles during periods of parental behavior. Maternal behavior in mice is regulated by nine genes of which one gene produces the prohormone for OXY. AVP not only induces parental behavior in males but it also increases aggression toward strange males. In rats, OXY induces lordosis posture in females, a position of submission and acceptance to mounting and copulation by an amorous male. OXY also stimulates female sheep (ewes) to nurture their young.

Peptides related to OXY and vasopressins have been localized in neurons of a number of invertebrates (see Chapter 5, Table 5-15) and have been shown to have behavioral roles. One of these peptides, **conopressin**, has been shown to regulate ejaculatory behavior in male snails and regulates egg laying and female reproductive behavior. **Annetocin** in earthworms is expressed in the subesophageal ganglion and regulates egg laying and other reproductive movements.

Experiments in which OXY was administered in a nasal spray have shown an increase in the sense of trust between people when compared to others receiving a placebo nasal spray. Researchers suggest that this "trust" role for OXY may be important in the formation of bonds between offspring and their mother. The possibility that there may be roles for neural nonapeptides in human behavior may have important implications for parental social behavior.

VI. The Pineal Gland

The human pineal gland was described by Galen during the second century as a structural (supportive) element within the brain. Much later, in 1646, Rene Descartes reasoned that the pineal was the location of the soul because it was an unpaired structure within an otherwise bilateral brain. It was, however, not until three centuries later that scientists determined what the soul was doing through the pineal gland. McCord and Allen in the early 1900s observed that pineal extracts caused blanching (lightening of the skin) of amphibian larvae by causing a concentration of melanin within the melanophores. Later, the pineal was discovered to play an important role in the control of seasonal reproduction.

The epithalamus represents the roof of the diencephalic portion of the brain that has differentiated into a variety of secretory structures in vertebrates as well as into photoreceptors (Figure 4-31). The **pineal gland** or **epiphysis** and the nearby **parapineal** are known as the **epiphysial complex**. Two additional prominent dorsal evaginations of the brain occur in the epithalamus: the **paraphysis** and the **dorsal sac**.

The pineal complex is connected to an adjacent ependymal structure, the **subcommissural organ of Dendy (SCO)**. The ependymal cells of the SCO produce a secretion rich in disulfide bonds and cysteine. This secretion is similar to that observed in the pineal ependyma. The major secretory product of the SCO is a non-cellular fiber that in some species extends into the central canal of the spinal cord for its entire length. This structure is known as **Reissner's fiber**. Its significance is not clear. The SCO and its Reissner's fiber have been described in vertebrates from cyclostomes to mammals. Once it was supposed that Reissner's fiber was involved in regulating posture through tension produced in it by flexion of the body. This tension presumably operated through influences of Reissner's fiber on pressure-sensitive neurons. A more plausible suggestion is the possibility that Reissner's fiber contributes to formation of cerebrospinal fluid. Formation and dissolution of the fiber into the cerebrospinal fluid (CSF) have been documented as a temperature-dependent process in the frog *Rana esculenta*. Reissner's fiber also binds biogenic amines (epinephrine, norepinephrine) present in the CSF in both *R. esculenta* and in mammals (cows, cats). Studies with mammals and reptiles suggest a functional relationship among the pineal complex, the SCO, and the adrenal

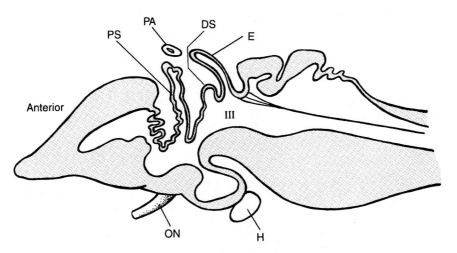

Figure 4-31. **Epithalamic structures.** Among the evaginations that develop from the roof of the epithalamus are the epiphysis cerebri or pineal (E), the parietal or parapineal organ (PA), the dorsal sac (DS), and the paraphysis (PS). ON, optic nerve; H, hypophysis or pituitary.

cortex, but the nature of that relationship remains somewhat obscure. Cytological activation of the SCO in the lizard *Lacerta s. sicula* has been correlated positively with seasonal activities of adrenal cortical cells and of testicular steroidogenic cells. The actual role or roles for the SCO and its secretory products must await further research, but preliminary data would suggest it is somehow related to activity of the pineal complex.

A. The Pineal Gland and Melatonin

Many years after the observation that pineal extracts caused the skin of frogs to lighten, Lerner and his coworkers succeeded in isolating and characterizing the active skin-lightening agent, 5-methoxyl-N-acetyltryptamine, or **melatonin**. Subsequently, a number of biologically active indoleamines and related compounds have been isolated from pineal tissue including melatonin and **serotonin (5-HT)**. Both melatonin and serotonin are secreted by the pineal into the blood and each has its unique actions. The initial substrate for synthesis of the indoleamines is the amino acid tryptophan that is converted to serotonin and then to melatonin (see Chapter 3, Figure 3-5).

B. Functions of the Pineal Gland in Mammals

A central action for the pineal gland is the regulation of endogenous rhythms, a role probably related to the primitive role of the epiphysial complex as a photoreceptive organ. The mammalian pineal gland also has been implicated as an inhibitor of reproductive and thyroid activity. Recently, the pineal has come under scrutiny as a potential regulator of aging and of the immune system. Some confirmed actions of melatonin are summarized in Table 4-11.

1. The Pineal and Endogenous Rhythms

Melatonin in the blood exhibits a distinct diurnal rhythm. Levels are greater at night than during the day in almost every species examined, and the circadian rhythm usually persists under constant dark conditions. Plasma melatonin rhythm is a consequence of a circadian rhythm in activity of the rate-limiting enzyme ***N*-acetyltransferase (NAT)** (Figure 4-32). This enzymatic rhythm is controlled by neural signals from the SCN of the hypothalamus that probably controls a number of circadian rhythms in mammals. Information on photoperiod detected by the retina is responsible for entraining the SCN to light/dark cycles. Blood levels of melatonin are greatest during the dark or the **scotophase** of the day-night cycle and lowest during

Table 4-11. Summary of Nonreproductive Actions of Melatonin and the Pineal in Mammals

Target	Description of action
Melanophores (melanocytes)	Melatonin implants in weasels, *Mustela erminea*, cause them to grow white coats (typical of winter) in the spring instead of brown coats
Hair	Melatonin inhibits hair growth of intact or pinealectomized mice
Connective tissue	Pinealectomy reduces permeability of subcutaneous connective tissue
Adrenal cortex	Pineal substance, adrenoglomerulotropin, claimed to stimulate aldosterone release
	Pineal may alter release of ACTH from adenohypophysis
Parathyroid	Pinealectomy of rat caused hypertrophy of parathyroids, which was reduced by administration of pineal extract or melatonin
Cardiovascular system	Vasopressor activity reported for pineal extracts, probably due to presence of AVT
Immune response	Chronic administration of pineal extracts caused leukocytosis, lymph node hypertrophy, and an increase in mitotic activity in the spleen. Probably it was a simple immunological response to antigens in the extract
Thyroid	Melatonin or pineal extracts inhibit thyroid function, possibly through regulation of TSH release from the adenohypophysis

Figure 4-32. **Serotonin and melatonin levels related to photoperiod and activity.** Both the quantity of melatonin and activity of the rate-limiting enzyme *N*-acetyl transferase (NAT) in the pineal gland of chickens increases during the photophase. Similar observations have been made in mammals. (From Binkley, S. A. (1990). "The Clockwork Sparrow: Time, Clocks, and Calendars in Biological Organisms." Prentice-Hall, Englewood Cliffs, NJ.)

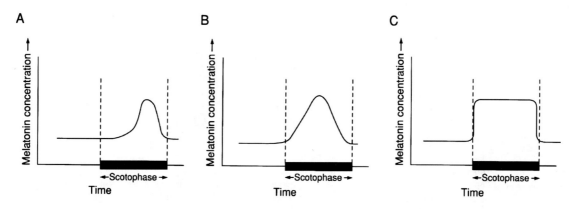

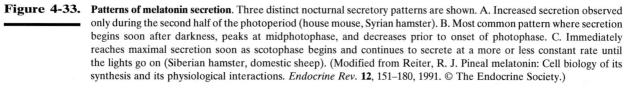

Figure 4-33. **Patterns of melatonin secretion.** Three distinct nocturnal secretory patterns are shown. A. Increased secretion observed only during the second half of the photoperiod (house mouse, Syrian hamster). B. Most common pattern where secretion begins soon after darkness, peaks at midphotophase, and decreases prior to onset of photophase. C. Immediately reaches maximal secretion soon as scotophase begins and continues to secrete at a more or less constant rate until the lights go on (Siberian hamster, domestic sheep). (Modified from Reiter, R. J. Pineal melatonin: Cell biology of its synthesis and its physiological interactions. *Endocrine Rev.* **12**, 151–180, 1991. © The Endocrine Society.)

the **photophase** (daylight portion). Nighttime melatonin secretion occurs in three basic patterns showing differences in latency of the response after light disappears or in the temporal relationship to when light returns (Figure 4-33).

Most studies of pineal activity and light have been done in rodent species that show greater sensitivity to light than do large mammals such as humans and sheep. Nevertheless, similar mechanisms appear to be operating in most species. Light stimulates the retina of the eye that generates neural impulses via two pathways to alter pineal secretion (Figure 4-34). The **retinohypothalamic pathway** innervates the SCN that in turn operates through the brain stem and spinal cord to reduce the activity of sympathetic fibers traveling from the **superior cervical ganglion (SCG)** to the pinealocytes of the pineal gland. Normally, these postganglionic fibers release NE that increases cAMP in the pinealocytes causing secretion of melatonin. These NE-secreting neurons also release the peptide NPY that modulates the responsiveness of pineal cells to NE (Figure 4-35). Elevated cAMP is associated with increased activity of NAT and subsequent melatonin synthesis. Light shining on the retina reduces NE input to the pineal, reducing cAMP levels, NAT activity, and melatonin synthesis via this pathway. Lesions in the retinohypothalamic pathway or the SCN do not necessarily abolish pineal secretory rhythms and led to the discovery of a second pathway between the retina and the brain stem that travels via the inferior accessory optic tract (Figure 4-34).

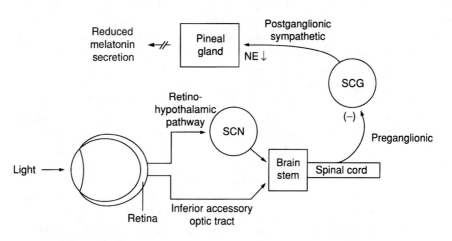

Figure 4-34. **Regulation of pineal secretion by light.** Light received by the retina inhibits pineal secretion via two central mechanisms. See text for details as well as Figure 4-35.

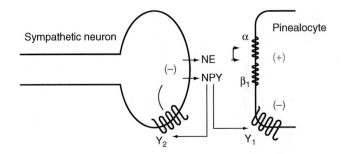

Figure 4-35. **Neuropeptide Y (NPY) and its interactions with norepinephrine (NE).** Activation of the release of melatonin is accomplished by NE secreted by sympathetic postgangionic neurons from the superior cervical ganglion. NPY acts as a local inhibitor to shut off the response to NE and also prevent additional NE release. Adrenergic receptors: α, β_1. NPY receptors: Y_1, Y_2.

2. The Pineal Gland and Development

During pregnancy, the fetus must rely on the mother not only for nutrients and removal of metabolic wastes but also for information about the environment. Evidence supports a role for melatonin from the mother in providing the fetus with information on the day-night cycle. Thus, melatonin acts like a pheromone to the fetus to appraise it of environmental conditions. Even after birth, melatonin passes from the mother to the newborn through milk until the offspring's pineal begins its own rhythmic secretion.

3. Pineal Secretions and Reproduction

Major effects of the pineal gland in mammals are related to reproduction and are most pronounced in species that breed only during spring or fall. In 1941, Fiske reported that keeping rats under conditions of constant light increased the frequency of estrus (a time of enhanced female receptivity to the male; see Chapter 10). Several years later, Wurtman discovered that pinealectomy also increased the frequency of estrus in rats maintained under normal photoperiods, and a surge of investigation was launched into possible roles of photoperiod, the pineal gland, and melatonin in controlling sexual maturity and reproductive cycles in mammals. Animals whose annual reproductive cycles are controlled by photoperiod (length of photophase and/or scotophase) are termed photoperiodic. A mass of data soon appeared to suggest that melatonin released from the pineal gland acted through either the blood or cerebrospinal fluid on the hypothalamus or directly on the pituitary to lower circulating LH levels in photoperiodic animals. As mentioned above, light inhibits sympathetic input to the pineal, resulting in decreased melatonin synthesis followed by increased levels of LH leading to estrus.

Considerable evidence has accumulated from clinical studies that implicate the pineal gland in controlling the onset of puberty in humans, although little experimental work on humans is available. Circulating melatonin decreases by 75% between the ages of 7 to 12 years when LH levels are observed to rise. Furthermore, many cases of precocial puberty, especially in males, are associated with non-secreting pineal tumors that reduce melatonin output and allow for an early release of LH and consequent gonadal stimulation (for additional information on puberty and reproduction, see Chapter 10).

Many studies of the relationship between pineal and gonadal function have been conducted with the golden hamster, *Mesocricetus auratus*. This animal exhibits marked gonadal collapse when subjected to short photoperiods (less than 12 hours of light per day) when the daily period of elevated plasma melatonin is longest. Pinealectomized golden hamsters do not exhibit gonadal collapse when subjected to short photoperiods, and subdermal melatonin implants (administered in silastic capsules) cause testicular atrophy in hamsters maintained on long photoperiods.

Some studies have provided a different explanation for the effects of light on estrus. Pinealectomy or injection of massive doses of melatonin never produces marked effects on rat reproduction, and some workers have not found any effect of melatonin on rat reproduction. One study, in fact, reported stimulation of rat gonads by melatonin treatments. If rats are made anosmic (olfaction blocked either mechanically or surgically) and are blinded, more marked gonadal atrophy occurs than was seen following pinealectomy alone.

For many mammals, longer photoperiods stimulate gonadal development only at certain times and at other times the animal does not respond; that is, it is **photorefractory**. Many photoperiodic animals exhibit photorefractoriness after breeding and cannot be induced to reenter the breeding condition. Support for a stimulatory gonadal role by melatonin has been reported by Thorpe and Herbert for the ferret, in which melatonin may be responsible for bringing the animal out of photorefractoriness. Here, melatonin treatment restores the gonadal growth response to long photoperiod in photorefractory (postbreeding) ferrets maintained on artificially long photoperiods. In Djungarian hamsters, photorefractoriness appears in a different form. Short photoperiods cause gonadal collapse due to inhibitory effects of elevated melatonin secretion on the reproductive endocrine axis. However, after a period of continued short-day exposure, the animals develop photorefractoriness to the short photoperiod, and the gonads undergo **recrudescence** (= regrowth).

Ependymal cells of fetal human and rat pineals synthesize AVT. If AVT is administered to neonatal mice during the period when the brain is undergoing sexual differentiation, increased growth of reproductive organs upon entering adulthood is observed. In contrast, if AVT is administered after the brain has undergone sexual differentiation, the growth of accessory organs and in some cases growth of the gonads themselves are inhibited.

The hypertrophy of the remaining ovary after unilateral ovariectomy of mice is a response to increased GTH levels caused by an effective reduction in circulating estrogens (a feedback effect). AVT administered intraperitoneally or directly into the third ventricle of the brain prevents this **compensatory ovarian hypertrophy (COH)**. Much less AVT is required if it is administered through the third ventricle than if it is given intraperitoneally. Several related basic nonapeptides, including AVP and LVP, also inhibit COH, but OXY is ineffective. All of the nonapeptides active at inhibiting COH have an identical ring structure and a basic amino acid at position 8. Treatment of these active molecules with mercaptoethanol disrupts the disulfide bridges necessary for maintenance of the ring structure. Such reduced nonapeptides no longer prevent COH; in fact, they enhance it.

The presence of several hypothalamic peptides including AVT, OXY, AVP, TRH, and SST has been demonstrated in human pineals. In addition to sympathetic innervation coming indirectly from the SCN through the SCG, numerous peptidergic fibers are found in the pineal gland that originate in other brain regions (e.g., the PVN and habenular nucleus). Immunoreactive VIP, NPY, AVP, and OXY have been demonstrated in pineal nerve endings. This peptidergic innervation probably modulates or fine-tunes pineal function. For example, receptors for VIP are present on pinealocytes, and binding of VIP to these receptors activates a cAMP-mediated increase in NAT function. This mechanism enhances the stimulation of cAMP and NAT by NE.

C. The Pineal Gland and Other Tropic Hormones

In addition to the inhibition of GTH secretion, melatonin may have important influences on secretion of other tropic hormones as well (Figure 4-36). Thyroid function in at least some mammals is strongly affected by photoperiod that appears to be acting through the control of melatonin secretion. Melatonin treatment reduces thyroid function presumably by limiting hypothalamic secretion of TRH and not by a direct action at the thyrotropic cells of the pars distalis.

The rise in PRL release observed in rats at the onset of the photophase has been linked to a reduction in melatonin release. Long photoperiods are correlated with increased PRL secretion in ruminant ungulates (sheep, cattle, goats), and melatonin treatment decreases PRL secretions in both sheep and goats, although not in cattle. Pinealectomy or denervation of the pineal sometimes produces increased PRL secretion in goats and sheep but has no effect in cattle. Similarly, pineal activity is associated with seasonal breeding in sheep and goats but is not associated with reproduction in cattle. This difference among ungulates may be due to artificial selection as a result of selective breeding of cattle over many centuries.

The explanation for this pineal effect apparently lies with the pars tuberalis. Cells in the pars tuberalis that produce tuberalin possess melatonin receptors, and their secretion is inhibited by melatonin. Thus, pinealectomy removes melatonin inhibition and can result in secretion of PRL.

Evidence for an effect of melatonin on ACTH release relies mainly on a few observations. Exogenous corticosteroids stimulate melatonin release that in turn might be involved in reducing ACTH release as part of a negative feedback loop. Furthermore, whereas the HPA axis reduces immune functions, melatonin, possibly acting at the hypothalamus and reducing ACTH release, can enhance certain immune functions. Melatonin also may enhance directly the functioning of the immune response system, and it has been proposed that it

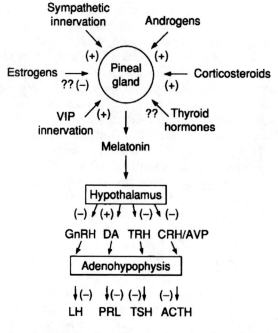

Figure 4-36. **Melatonin regulates hypothalamic functions.** The pineal receives input from hormones as well as sympathetic neural innervation that affects melatonin secretion. Melatonin in turn can block secretion of hypothalamic-releasing hormones (GnRH, TRH, CRH/AVP) as well as stimulate DA release, the PRL release-inhibiting hormone. Gonadal, thyroid, and adrenal hormones may provide negative feedback input through the pineal.

may increase immune surveillance and decrease the incidence of cancer. Clinical studies have not substantiated such claims, however.

D. The Pineal Gland and Aging

Biological aging is a complex phenomenon that is complicated often by attendant pathologies. There are many theories as to the causes and progression of aging, and no single explanation seems adequate. One popular theory of aging involves the formation and accumulation of **free radicals**, compounds that can interact with and damage particular proteins, phospholipids, nucleic acids, and sugars. One of the most dangerous free radicals is produced during the breakdown of hydrogen peroxide. The presence of melatonin in certain *in-vitro* systems reduces free radicals whereas 5-HT, the predominant pineal secretion during daylight hours, elevates free radicals. In a number of pathological disorders (including Parkinson's disease, atherosclerosis, muscular dystrophy, multiple sclerosis, and rheumatoid arthritis), free radicals are known to be responsible for cell damage related to protein aggregations. As a mammal ages, the SCN of the hypothalamus, which can send important regulatory messages to the pineal as well as to cells controlling pituitary function, becomes dysfunctional and the pineal gland reduces production of melatonin and elevates production of 5-HT.

Another influence of the pineal on aging may be related to effects of melatonin on the immune response system. In contrast, 5-HT of pineal origin may impair immune functions. Since decreased immune functions in general are associated with aging, melatonin may have a dual retarding effect on the aging process (e.g., by reducing free radicals and enhancing immune surveillance). Clinical studies do not support the use of melatonin as an anti-aging drug, however, and because of the many potential effects of melatonin on other systems, the Endocrine Society recommends extreme caution in its use for any purpose.

E. Other Factors Affecting the Pineal

In addition to the well-known actions of light on the pineal gland, hypophysectomy, stress, and gonadal steroids all influence pineal function. Some of these effects suggest that the pineal may participate in feedback mechanisms of steroid hormones on tropic hormone secretion (Figure 4-36). For example, androgens (e.g., testosterone, dihydrotestosterone) inhibit MAO activity in the pineal, which in turn allows for increased melatonin synthesis. Increased melatonin can reduce LH release and in turn decrease androgen levels. In contrast, estrogens can increase MAO activity and decrease pineal secretion of melatonin, bringing about enhancement of GTH release. Hypophysectomy or administration of histamine also reduces melatonin synthesis by reducing activity of HIOMT. Acute stress stimulates pineal activity, presumably through enhanced sympathetic stimulation. Chronic stress (for example, starvation) is associated with elevated corticosteroids that reduce pineal MAO activity and allow for increased melatonin production. Thus, stress working through these two pathways may depress reproductive function by reducing activity of the pineal gland.

F. Extrapineal Sources of Melatonin

The **harderian gland**, or Harder's lacrimal gland, was described by Harder in 1694 in the red deer. It is located directly behind and around the eye in all vertebrates that possess nictitating membranes (reptiles, birds, and most mammals). In humans, the harderian gland is poorly developed (rudimentary). Reddish porphyrin pigments present in the harderian gland undergo fluctuations correlated with lighting conditions. Prior to 12 days of age, the rat harderian gland contains little porphyrin pigment. Blinded 12-day-old rats exhibit an increase in pineal 5-HT as well as HIOMT activity during the scotophase, but this rhythm is abolished if the harderian glands also are removed. Melatonin synthesis has been demonstrated in the rat harderian gland, and continuous illumination causes enlargement of the rat harderian gland and an increase in HIOMT activity. Harderian HIOMT differs somewhat from the HIOMT found in the pineal gland and from that found in the retina of the eye. In contrast, continuous illumination decreases pineal weight and pineal HIOMT activity. The importance of these observations to overall involvement of pineal indoles or harderian indoles to observations on reproduction or other pineal-influenced processes remains to be determined.

The retina of the eye may be another viable source for melatonin, but the nocturnal increase in circulating melatonin is clearly of pineal origin. Retinal melatonin appears to regulate melanin distribution within the retina. Pinealectomy does not eliminate melatonin from the circulation but typically reduces it to daytime levels. Circulating melatonin during the photophase appears to be due to retinal and/or harderian gland production.

VII. Clinical Aspects of the Neuroendocrine System

Only disorders associated with the pars nervosa nonapeptides, growth hormone secretion, and general pituitary dysfunction are considered here. Discussions of clinical problems that involve the HPT, HPG, and HPA axes are delayed until after specific discussions of these axes in later chapters (see Chapters 6, 8, 10, 12, and 14).

A. Disorders of the Hypothalamus

A rare clinical disorder of the hypothalamus is **diabetes insipidus**. The patient produces an abnormally large volume (3 to 30 liters/day) of dilute urine. This diuresis is most commonly due to the absence of AVP that normally controls water reabsorption in the kidney. Forty to 50% of such patients are **idiopathic** (i.e., denoting a disease of unknown cause) and exhibit no other evidence of neuroendocrine dysfunction. Some of these patients have been identified at autopsy as having degeneration of the SON and the PVN. About 15% of the cases are related to the presence of tumors within the brain, producing pressure on the SON and PVN and indirectly reducing secretion of AVP. Physical damage (such as a brain lesion) or certain infections (e.g., encephalitis) account for the remainder. **Nephrogenic diabetes insipidus** is the result of a failure of the kidney tubules to respond to normal or above-normal levels of AVP.

The **syndrome of inappropriate antidiuresis (SIAD)** is caused by excessive AVP release. High levels of AVP result in excessive water retention, elevated blood pressure, and reduced urine production. Drugs such as demeclocycline block the action of AVP on the kidney and are used to treat this condition. However, long-term use of such drugs induces nephrogenic diabetes insipidus. Medications that control AVP release from the pars nervosa often are not uniformly effective and can influence other hypothalamic functions.

B. Disorders Associated with the Pineal Gland

Tumors within the central nervous system are responsible for a number of other disorders. One of the more dramatic consequences is **sexual precocity** (accelerated sexual maturation; see Chapter 10 for a technical description of precocity). Precocity is much more common in males. About one-fourth of precocity cases are correlated with the presence of a pineal tumor, and 95% of these occur in males. A number of other cases of sexual precocity are associated with hypothalamic tumors, most of which also are found in males. One type of tumor, associated with precocity, the **harmatoma**, occurs in the posterior hypothalamus. It consists of masses of partially disoriented glial and ganglion cells or of normal cells located in abnormal sites. Harmatomas may secrete GnRH that could explain their effects on early sexual maturation. Other causes for precocity are discussed in Chapter 10.

Melatonin also is thought to play a role in **circadian dysrhythmia**: the disruption of normal body rhythms due to air travel. Crossing one or more time zones in a 24-hr period results in a significant change in the photoperiod relationship and causes biological rhythms to get out of phase with the day-night cycle; hence, dysrhythmia. Crossing numerous time zones within 24 hr magnifies this disruptive effect. People often feel out-of-sorts when these rhythms are disrupted. Oral administration of melatonin is claimed to help reset the pineal and restore normal rhythms so that the traveler feels in tune with her environment. Similarly, melatonin has been claimed to have sleep-promoting effects that would help one adjust to new time zones. Many elderly people claim that self-administered melatonin helps them sleep as well although clinical studies are still controversial on this point.

Melatonin has been implicated in a variety of psychiatric disorders. Alterations in melatonin production are known to be associated with **seasonal affective disorder (SAD)**, bipolar disorder, unipolar depression, bulemia, anorexia, schizophrenia, panic disorder, and obsessive compulsive disorder. The manic high in bipolar disorder is associated with elevated melatonin secretion whereas the depression phase is accompanied by reduced melatonin secretion. High and low melatonin are correlated also with low and high glucocorticoid levels, respectively, in bipolar disorder. It is not clear whether the pineal is involved in the onset of these disorders or is a consequence of other causative disturbances.

C. Disorders of the Adenohypophysis

Pituitary chromophobe adenomas are the most common source of pituitary-related problems. An adenoma is a benign or noncarcinogenic glandular tumor. They rarely secrete any hormones (occasionally GH and rarely PRL, TSH, or ACTH), and their effects usually are due to pressure on the brain or optic chiasm caused by growth of the tumor. Most patients experience severe headaches and visual disturbances (even blindness can result). Sometimes the production of one or more pituitary hormones may be reduced. Other adenomas may secrete excessive amounts of PRL (prolactinomas). Rarely, TSH, ACTH, or GTHs may be products of pituitary adenomas, and their clinical impacts are discussed in Chapters 6, 8, and 10, respectively. Surgical removal of the adenoma is the most common treatment and is highly successful.

Acromegaly is a spectacular, although rather rare, disorder of GH regulation that has been publicized heavily. It affects from 3 to 40 individuals per million people in the United States each year. When it occurs in children, it can lead to **gigantism**. It is a well-known disorder because acromegaly was the first disorder of the pituitary gland to be recognized and because it can produce giants. Acromegaly is caused by overproduction of GH due either to the absence of adequate SST to suppress GH release or by the absence of negative feedback to suppress release. Growth hormone-secreting tumors are unaffected by normal control mechanisms and release GH autonomously. Approximately half of acromegalic patients are deficient in one or more additional pituitary hormones, usually the GTHs, due to the growth of the GH tumor that compresses other cell types. Not only do such patients exhibit excessive growth, but body proportions become distorted. When acromegaly develops in adults, only the body proportions become distorted since growth in stature has ceased and cannot be reinitiated with any quantity of GH. In adults, cartilage in joints proliferates under the influence of GH-dependent IGFs resulting in abnormally proportioned hands and elongate jaws. The nose and ears, whose supporting tissue is cartilage, enlarge markedly causing distortion in appearance. There also are marked effects on other systems; for example, excessive sweating and secretion of sebum by the skin, enlargement of the heart, and hypertension may develop. Life expectancy is shortened considerably for these victims. Use of excessive amounts of GH by people to augment muscle growth in order to improve physical performance can produce similar effects to those of acromegaly. Excessive use of exogenous GH also has been associated with increased incidence of liver cancer.

Removal of the pituitary GH tumor has been the classical method for treating acromegaly although this can also produce deficiencies of other pituitary hormones. Use of a synthetic GH-receptor antagonist that blocks formation of IGFs can bring growth into normal limits although it doesn't address the initial cause of the disorder.

In contrast, lack of sufficient GH during early life can cause short stature. However, other explanations for subnormal growth are known. Furthermore, it is important to distinguish between **short stature** with normal body proportions and **dwarfism** where the individual exhibits distorted features. **Laron-type dwarfism** occurs in humans with normal GH levels but very low IGF blood levels. Due to possession of a mutant allele, the liver of these patients lacks GH receptors and does not secrete IGFs. GH-binding proteins are absent from the blood as well. In contrast, African pygmies lack the binding proteins for GH but show the normal pattern for growth proportions but exhibit short stature. The inability to maintain normal circulating levels of GH causes total growth to be reduced.

Partial or total **hypopituitarism** refers to selective or total absence of pituitary hormones. These defects may reside in the adenohypophysis itself (primary disorder) or be due to hypothalamic dysfunction (secondary disorder).

There has been considerable interest in the role(s) of EOPs on mental disturbances such as depression and schizophrenia. Clinical studies, however, have yielded mixed results, and it is not clear whether mental illness is associated with EOPs. CRH and TRH deficiencies or excesses also have been correlated with certain psychological disturbances.

VIII. Summary

The adenohypophysis produces tropic hormones and consists of a pars distalis, a pars intermedia, and a pars tuberalis. The embryonic origin of the adenohypophysis appears to be neural in origin similar to the neurohypophysis and hypothalamus. The pars distalis produces GH, PRL, GTHs, (FSH, LH), ACTH, TSH, and endorphins (EOPs). Four of the tropic hormones and their endocrine target glands constitute the major hypothalamus-pituitary (HP) axes of the neuroendocrine system: HPG (gonad), HPT (thyroid), HPA (adrenal), HPH (hepatic or liver). The posterior portion of the adenohypophysis is the pars intermedia, which is responsible for synthesis of α-MSH and endorphins. A number of mammals lack a pars intermedia. The pars tuberalis contains some stainable cell types and secretes tuberalin that stimulates PRL release.

The neurohypophysis forms from the infundibulum and consists of an anterior neurohemal area, the median eminence, and a more posterior neurohemal structure, the pars nervosa. The median eminence stores the hypothalamic-releasing hormones (RHs and RIHs) produced in hypothalamic nuclei that regulate tropic hormone release from the adenohypophysis. The portal system connects the median eminence to the adenohypophysis and brings RHs and RIHs to the tropic hormone-producing cells. The pars nervosa has no common blood supply with the adenohypophysis. It is responsible for storage of nonapeptide neurohormones (usually AVP and OXY) produced in the hypothalamus until they are released into the general circulation.

There are three categories of tropic hormones based on chemical structure. Category I includes the glycoproteins, LH, FSH, and TSH. Category II includes the large peptides, GH and PRL. Category III includes the very similar smaller peptides, ACTH, α-MSH, and LPH. Structural similarities suggest that LPH may be related to the endorphins, which are linked to opiate actions on the mammalian central nervous system. Placentas of mammals produce up to four tropic-like hormones, including CG (LH-like), CS (PRL-like and GH-like to some degree), CT (TSH-like), and CC (ACTH-like) as well as PRL and GH. Pregnant mare serum gonadotropin is a chorionic-type GTH with both FSH- and LH-like properties. Menopausal gonadotropin is FSH-like and is produced by the pituitary of postmenopausal women.

The NS nuclei controlling tropic hormone release are generally located in the preoptic area or the ventral region of the hypothalmus. Aminergic and peptidergic neurons terminate in the median eminence where they regulate release of RHs and RIHs into the portal circulation. These NS neurons are innervated by regular neurons (e.g., aminergic, cholinergic, serotonergic, and/or peptidergic) which influence their release. These regulating neurons may be responsive to hormones or other factors as well.

TSH release is stimulated by TRH secreted primarily by neurons in the paraventricular nucleus. TRH release can be increased by VIP, NE, and E and inhibited by 5-HT and DA. SST also blocks TSH release. Thyroid hormones feedback primarily on the thyrotropes with only minor effects in the hypothalamus.

GTH release (LH and FSH) is induced by pulsatile secretion of GnRH-1 from the ARC that in turn is stimulated by NE but inhibited by opioid-secreting neurons. Negative feedback occurs generally through actions of gonadal steroids at the hypothalamus neurons or on gonadotropes. Inhibin secreted by the gonads feeds back specifically to limit FSH release from the gonadotrope whereas galanin from the hypothalamus enhances LH release. Positive feedback by estrogens appears to operate through GABA neurons that innervate GnRH-1 neurons.

GH release is under strong inhibitory control by hypothalamic SST, but GHRH is necessary to evoke release in the absence of SST. SST comes primarily from the PERIV nucleus and the amygdala of the limbic system. GHRH is produced in the ARC nucleus. Many neural and NS factors (e.g., ghrelin) can affect GH release, but the pathway and physiological importance of most observations are unclear. Catecholamines are always stimulatory. Many actions of GH are mediated by IGFs and the latter form the primary negative feedback on GH release. Metabolites (glucose, free fatty acids, arginine) can affect GH release, but their physiological role is uncertain.

PRL release, like GH, is under strong inhibitory control by dopamine acting as a neurohormone from the ARC and PERIV nuclei. It also can be inhibited by GAP although a physiological role for GAP is not clear. Unlike the situation for GH, no PRH seems necessary to get PRL release in the absence of DA inhibition. During suckling, however, hypothalamic VIP is an important stimulant. Estrogens enhance the sensitivity of lactotropes to VIP. Tuberalin from the pars tuberalis stimulates PRL release. Although TRH has been shown to induce PRL release, it may not be a physiological releaser. Negative feedback may occur through direct actions of PRL on hypothalamic neurons.

ACTH secretion is stimulated by CRH, and AVP enhances the sensitivity of corticotropes to CRH. Corticotropes also produce β-LPH from which they release β-endorphin. β-LPH and ACTH are produced from the same preprohormone, POMC. CRH is produced primarily in the PVN and ARC nucleus, and greatest levels are observed in the median eminence. AVP in the median eminence comes primarily from the PVN. Glucocorticoids provide negative feedback directly on corticotropes via GRs and indirectly on hypothalamic CRH neurons via MR on CA1 hippocampal neurons. GABA neurons play an important inhibitory role over CRH release. In chronic stress, glucocorticoid feedback is in part overcome by elevated AVP.

Release of melanotropin (α-MSH), like PRL, is inhibited by dopamine, probably acting as a neurohormone (MRIH), and no MRH is necessary. Melanotropes first produce ACTH from a POMC and then hydrolyze it further to α-MSH and CLIP prior to release. Like corticotropes, they also release β-endorphin into the general circulation. There is little evidence for negative feedback on α-MSH release.

NS neurons in the SON and PVN produce the nonapeptides AVP and OXY which are stored in the pars nervosa. A few mammals make LVP as well as AVP, and marsupials produce PVP instead of AVP, and some marsupials secrete MST. Fetal mammals produce AVT instead of AVP and OXY.

The major secretory product of the pineal gland or epiphysis is melatonin although peptides such as AVT are secreted as well. The pineal receives innervation from several sources. In mammals, the most important pathway is the sympathetic innervation of pinealocytes that is controlled by two retinal pathways both passing through the superior cervical ganglion. One of these pathways involves the hypothalamic SCN, a major determiner of biological rhythms in mammals. Pineal secretion of melatonin is inhibited by light, and the pineal gland plays a major role in mediating seasonal and daily endocrine activity primarily through effects on the hypothalamus. Melatonin generally acts as an anti-gonadal, anti-adrenal, or anti-thyroid factor. It is also an anti-PRL factor through its inhibition of tuberalin secretion. The pineal may have a role in delaying aging and enhancing immune surveillance.

Suggested Reading

Books

Brown, R. E. (1994). "An Introduction to Neuroendocrinology." Cambridge Univ. Press, New York.
Colmers, W. F., and Wahlestedt, C. (1993). "The Biology of Neuropeptide Y and Related Peptides." Humana Press, Totowa, NJ.

Imura, H. (1994). "The Pituitary Gland," 2nd Ed., Comprehensive Endocrinology Revised Series. Raven, New York.

Melmed, S. (1995). "The Pituitary." Blackwell, Cambridge, MA.

Motta, M. (1991). "Brain Endocrinology," 2nd Ed., Comprehensive Endocrinology Revised Series. Raven, New York.

Muller, E. E., and Nistico, G. (1989). "Brain Messengers and the Pituitary." Academic Press, San Diego.

Nemeroff, C. B. (1992). "Neuroendocrinology." CRC Press, Boca Raton, FL.

North, W. G. (1993). "The Neurohypophysis: A Window on Brain Function," Vol. 689. N.Y. Acad. Sci., New York.

Parhar, I. S., and Sakuma, Y. (1997). GnRH Neurons: Gene to Behavior. Brain Shuppan, Tokyo.

Pierpaoli, W., Regelson, W., and Fabris, N. (1994). The aging clock: The pineal gland and other pacemakers in the progression of aging and carcinogenesis. N.Y. Acad. Sci., New York.

Reiter, R. J. (1994). "The Pineal Gland and Melatonin." CRC Press, Boca Raton, FL.

Saito, T., Kurokawa, K., and Yoshida, S. (1995). "Neurohypophysis: Recent Progress of Vasopressin and Oxytocin." Elsevier, Amsterdam.

Articles

General/Miscellaneous

Armstrong, D. L., and White, R. E. (1994). Natriuretic peptides and receptors. *Sci. Am. Sci. Med.* **Mar/Apr**, 34–43.

Baker, B. I. (1994). Melanin-concentrating hormone updated. *Trends Endocr. Metab.* **5**, 120–126.

Beck-Peccoz, P., Persani L., and Faglia, G. (1992). Glycoprotein hormone α-subunit in pituitary adenoma. *Trends Endocr. Metab.* **3**, 41–45.

Besedovsky, H. O., and Del Ray, A. (1996). Immune-neuro-endocrine interactions: Facts and hypotheses. *Endocr. Rev.* **17**, 64–102.

Brann, D. W., and Mahesh, V. B. (1992). Excitatory amino acid neurotransmission: Evidence for a role in neuroendocrine regulation. *Trends Endocr. Metab.* **3**, 122–126.

Crowley, W. R., and Armstrong, W. E. (1992). Neurochemical regulation of oxytocin secretion in lactation. *Endocr. Rev.* **13**, 33–65.

Deschepper, C. F. (1991). The renin-angiotensin system in the pituitary gland. *Trends Endocr. Metab.* 104–107.

Dubois, P. M., and El Amraouci, A. (1995). Embryology of the pituitary. *Trends Endocri. Metab.* **6**, 1–7.

Evans. J. J. (2002). The anterior pituitary gland is mysterious, alluring and useful. *Archives Physiol. Biochem.* **110**, 3–8.

Fannon, S. A., Vidaver, R. M., and Marts, S. A. (2002). Sex, cells and signals in the developing brain. *Trends Neurosci.* **25**, 334–335.

Fauquier, T., Lacampagne, A., Travo, P., Bauer, K., and Mollard, P. (2002). Hidden face of the anterior pituitary. *Trends Endocr. Metab.* **13**, 304–309.

Gershon, M. D. (1993). Development of the neural crest. *J. Neurobiol.* **24**, 141–145.

Green, J. D. (1951). The comparative anatomy of the hypophysis with special reference to its blood supply at innervation. *Am. J. Anat.* **88**, 225–311.

Guillemin, R. (2005). Hypothalamic hormones a.k.a. hypothalamic releasing factors. *J. Endocr.* **184**, 11–28.

Hammer, G. D., and Ingraham, H. A. (1999). Steroidogenic factor-1: Its role in endocrine organ development and differentiation. *Frontiers in Neuroendocr.* **20**, 199–223.

Houben, H., and Denef, C. (1990). Regulatory peptides produced in the anterior pituitary. *Trends Endocri. Metab.* **1**, 398–403.

Inoue, K., Mogi, C., Ogawa, S., Tomida, M., and Miyai, S. (2002). Are folliculo-stellate cells in the anterior pituitary gland supportive cells or organ-specific stem cells? *Archives Physiol. Biochem.* **110**, 50–53.

Kobayashi, H., Yamaguichi, Y., and Uemura, H. (1999). The median eminence. A mediator in the regulation of the pituitary by the brain. *In* Prasada Rao and Peter (Eds.,). "Neural Regulation in the Vertebrate Endocrine System." Kluwer Academic/Plenum Publishers, New York, pp. 1–22.

Pearse, A. G. E., and Takor Takor, T. (1976). Neuroendocrine embryology and the APUD concept. *Clin. Endocrinol.* **5**, Suppl. 229s–244s.

Pissios, P., and Maratos-Flier, E. (2003). Melanin-concentrating hormone: from fish skin to skinny mammals. *Trends Endocr. Metab.* **14**, 243–248.

Rawlings, S. R., and Hezareh, M. (1996). Pituitary adenylate cyclase-activating polypeptide (PACAP) and PACAP/vasoactive intestinal polypeptide receptors: Actions on the anterior pituitary gland. *Endocr. Rev.* **1**, 4–29.

Reiter, R. J. (1991). Pineal gland: Interface between the photoperiodic environment and the endocrine system. *Trends Endocr. Metab.* **2**, 13–19.

Reiter, R. J. (1991). Pineal melatonin: Cell biology of its synthesis and its physiological interactions. *Endocr. Rev.* **12**, 151–180.

Saarela, S., and Reiter, R. J. (1994). Function of melatonin in thermoregulatory processes. *Life Sci.* **54**, 295–311.

Said, S. I. (1991). Vasoactive intestinal peptide: Biologic role in health and disease. *Trends Endocr. Metab.* **2**, 107–112.

Samson, W. K. (1992). Natriuretic peptides: A family of hormones. *Trends Endocr. Metab.* **3**, 86–90.

Schwartz, J., and Cherny, R. (1992). Intercellular communication within the anterior pituitary influencing the secretion of hypophysial hormones. *Endocr. Rev.* **13**, 453–475.

Spangelo, B. L., and MacLeod, R. M. (1990). The role of immunopeptides in the regulation of anterior pituitary hormone release. *Trends Endocr. Metab.* **1**, 408–412.

Steele, M. K. (1992). The role of brain angiotensin II in the regulation of luteinizing hormone and prolactin secretion. *Trends Endocr. Metab.* **3**, 295–301.

Stojilkovic, S. S. (2001). A novel view of the function of pituitary folliculo-stellate cell network. *Trends Endocr. Metab.* **12**, 378–380.

Swabb, D. F., Hofman, M. A., Lucassen, P. J., Purba, J. S., Raadsheer, F. C., and Van de Nes, J. A. P. (1993). Functional neuroanatomy and neuropathology of the human hypothalamus. *Anat. Embroyl.* **187**, 317–330.

Gonadotropins and Releasing Hormones

Bakker, J., and Balm, M. J. (2000). Neuroendocrine regulation of GnRH release in induced ovulators. *Frontiers in Neuroendocr.* **21**, 220–262.

Barbieri, R. L. (1992). Clinical applications of GnRH and its analogues. *Trends Endocrinol. Metab.* **3**, 30–34.

Beitins, I. Z., and Padmanabhan, V. (1991). Bioactive follicle-stimulating hormone. *Trends Endocr. Metab.* **2**, 145–151.

Bentley, G. E., Kreigsfeld, L. J., Osugi, T., Ukena, K., O'Brien, S., Perfito, N., Moore, I. T., Tsutsui, K., and Wingfield, J. C. (2006). Interactions of gonadotropin-releasing hormone (GnRH) and gonadotropin-inhibitory hormone (GnIH) in birds and mammals. *Journal of Experimental Zoology* **305A**, 807–814.

Dode, C., and Hardelin, J.-P. (2004). Kallmann syndrome: Fibroblast growth factor signaling insufficiency? *J. Molec. Med.* **82**, 725–734.

Gharib, S. D., Wierman, M. E., Shupnik, M. A., and Chin, W. W. (1990). Molecular biology of the pituitary gonadotropins. *Endocr. Rev.* **11**, 177–198.

Knobil, E. (1992). Remembrance: The discovery of the hypothalamic gonadotropin-releasing hormone pulse generator and of its physiological significance. *Endocr.* **131**, 1005–1006.

Kriegsfeld, L. J., Mei, D. F., Bentley, G. E., Ubuka, T., Mason, A. O., Inoue, K., Ukena, K., Tsutsui, K., and Silver, R. (2006). Identification of a gonadotropin-inhibitory system in the brains of mammals. *Proc. NSA USA* **103**, 2410–2415.

Krsmanovic, L. Z., Stojilkovic, S. S., and Catt, K. J. (1996). Pulsatile gonadotropin-releasing hormone release. *Trends Endocr. Metab.* **7**, 56–59.

Neill, J. D. (2002). Minireview: GnRH and GnRH receptor genes in the human genome. *Endocr.* **143**, 737–743.

Petit, C. (1993). Molecular basis of the X-chromosome-linked Kallmann's syndrome. *Trends Endocr. Metab.* **4**, 8–13.

Rissman, E. F. (1996). Behavioral regulation of gonadotropin-releasing hormone. *Biol. Reprod.* **54**, 413–419.

Schwanzel-Fukuda, M., Jorgenson, K. L., Bergen, H. T., Weesner, G. D., and Pfaff, D. W. (1992). Biology of normal luteinizing hormone-releasing hormone neurons during and after their migration from olfactory placode. *Endocr. Rev.* **13**, 623–634.

Stojilkovic, S. S., Krsmanovic, L. Z., Spergel, D. J., and Catt, K. J. (1994). Gonadotropin-releasing hormone neurons: Intrinsic pulsatility and receptor-mediated regulation. *Trends Endocr. Metab.* **5**, 201–209.

Tobet, S. A., Bless, E. P., and Schwarting, G. A. (2001). Developmental aspect of the gonadotropin-releasing hormone system. *Molec. Cell. Endocr.* **185**, 173–184.

Tsai, P.-S., and Weiner, R. I. (1996). Regulation of gonadotropin-releasing hormone neurons by basic fibroblast growth factor. *Trends Endocr. Metab.* **7**, 65–68.

Wierman, M. E., Pawlowski, J. E., Allen, M. P., Xu, M., Linseman, D. A., and Nielson-Preiss, S. (2004). Molecular mechanisms of gonadotropin-releasing hormone neuronal migration. *Trends Endocr. Metab.* **15**, 96–102.

TSH and Releasing Hormones

Magner, J. A. (1990). Thyroid-stimulating hormone: Biosynthesis, cell biology, and bioactivity. *Endocr. Rev.* **11**, 354–385.

Tixier-Vidal, A., and Faivre-Baumann, A. (1992). Ontogeny of thyrotropin-releasing hormone biosynthesis and release of hypothalamic neurons. *Trends Endocr. Metab.* **3**, 59–64.

GH, PRL, and Releasing Hormones

Amselem, S., Duquesnoy, P., and Goosens, M. (1991). Molecular basis of Laron dwarfism. *Trends Endocr. Metab.* **2**, 35–40.

Barkum, A. L. (1992). Acromegaly. *Trends Endocr. Metab.* **3**, 205–210.

Baumann, G. (1991). Growth hormone heterogeneity: Isohormones, variants, and binding proteins. *Endocr. Rev.* **12**, 424–449.

Baxter, R. C. (1993). Circulating binding proteins for the insulinlike growth factors. *Trends Endocr. Metab.* **4**, 91–96.

Ben-Johnathan, N., and Lie, J.-W. (1992). Pituitary lactotrophs: Endocrine, paracrine, juxtacrine, and autocrine interactions. *Trends Endocr. Metab.* **3**, 254–258.

Corpas, E., Harman, S. M., and Blackman, M. R. (1993). Human GH and human aging. *Endocr. Rev.* **14**, 20–39.

Devsa, J., Lima, L., and Tresguerres, J. A. F. (1992). Neuroendocrine control of growth hormone secretion in humans. *Trends Endocrinol. Metab.* **3**, 175–182.

Dieguez, C., and Casanueva, F. F. (1995). Influence of metabolic substrates and obesity on growth hormone secretion. *Trends Endocr. Metab.* **6**, 55–59.

Frawley, L. S. (1994). Role of the hypophyseal neurointermediate lobe in the dynamic release of prolactin. *Trends Endocr. Metab.* **5**, 107–112.

Goffin, V., Binart, N., Touraine, P., Keey, P. A. (2002). Prolactin: The new biology of an old hormone. *Ann. Rev. Physiol.* **64**, 47–67.

Herrington, A. C. (1994). New frontiers in the molecular mechanisms of growth hormone action. *Mol. Cell. Endocr.* **100**, 39–44.

Korbonits, M., and Grossman, A. B. (1995). Growth hormone releasing peptide and its analogues: Novel stimuli to growth hormone release. *Trends Endocr. Metab.* **6**, 43–49.

LeRoith, D., Adamo, M., Werner, H., and Roberts, C. T., Jr. (1991). Insulinlike growth factors and their receptors as growth regulators in normal physiology and pathologic states. *Trends Endocr. Metab.* **2**, 134–139.

Lewis, U. J. (1992). Growth hormone: What is it and what does it do? *Trends Endocr. Metab.* **3**, 117–121.

Sinha, Y. N. (1992). Prolactin variants. *Trends Endocr. Metab.* **3**, 100–106.

Sun, B., Fujiwara, K., Adachi, S., and Inoue, K. (2005). Physiological roles of prolactin-releasing peptide., *Regulatory Peptides* **126**, 27–33.

POMC Derivatives

Lightman, S. L., Windle, R. J., Ma, X.-A., Harbuz, M. S., Shanks, N. M., Julian, M. D., Wood, S. A., Kershaw, Y. M., and Ingram, C. D. (2002). Hypothalamic-pituitary-adrenal function. *Archives Physiol. Biochem.* **110**, 90–93.

Margioris, A. N. (1993). Opioids in neural and nonneural tissues. *Trends Endocr. Metab.* **4**, 163–168.

Moore, H.-P. H., Andersen, J. M., Eaton, B. A., Grabe, M., Haugwitz, M., Wu, M. M., and Machen, T. E. (2002). Biosynthesis and secretion of pituitary hormones: Dynamics and Regulation. *Archives Physiol. Biochem.* **110**, 16–25.

Orth, D. N. (1992). Corticotropin-releasing hormone in humans. *Endocr. Rev.* **13**, 164–191.

Plotsky, P. M., Cunningham, E. T., and Widmaier, E. P. (1989). Catecholaminergic modulation of corticotropin-releasing factor and adrenocorticotropin secretion. *Endocr. Rev.* **10**, 437–458.

Solomon, S. (1993). Corticostatins. *Trends Endocr. Metab.* **4**, 260–264.

Endothelins

Battistini, B., D'Orleans-Juste, P., and Sirois, P. (1993). Endothelins: Circulating plasma levels and presence other biologic fluids. *Lab. Invest.* **68**, 600–628.

Macrae, A. D., and Bloom, S. R. (1992). Endothelin: An endocrine role. *Trends Endocr. Metab.* **3**, 153–157.

Masaki, T. (1993). Endothelins: Homeostatic and compensatory actions in the circulatory and endocrine system *Endocr. Rev.* **14**, 256–268.

Stojilkovic, S. S., and Catt, K. J. (1992). Neuroendocrine actions of endothelins. *Trends Pharmacol. Sci.* 385–391.

Pineal and Melatonin

Arendt, J. (1998). Melatonin and the pineal gland: influence on mammalian seasonal and circadian physiology. *Rev. Reproduction* **3**, 13–22.

5

The Hypothalamus-Pituitary System in Non-Mammalian Vertebrates

The following chapter describes the major features of the hypothalamus-pituitary (HP) axes of non-mammalian vertebrates as contrasted with those previously given for mammals in Chapter 4. Hormones and anatomical features described in Chapter 4 that also appear in non-mammals are not redefined, although their names appear with abbreviations the first time they are used. If the reader is not familiar with non-mammalian vertebrates, a brief discussion of the evolutionary relationships and importance of various vertebrate taxonomic groups listed here can be found in Chapter 1.

The HP system is unique to the vertebrate chordates, and no invertebrate chordate—or for that matter any other invertebrate phylum—exhibits an endocrine gland so closely integrated with the brain as the vertebrate pituitary. However, there is evidence of a homologous system in the primitive cephalochordate known as amphioxus (*Branchiostoma*) that was elucidated by the efforts of Aubrey Gorbman and his collaborators. A shallow epithelial groove located in the oral cavity of *Branchiostoma* appears in close proximity to the simple dorsal nervous system of this animal (Figure 5-1). It is known as **Hatschek's pit** and has been found to react positively to antibodies against substance P, met-enkephalin, cholecystokinin (CCK), mammalian luteinizing hormone (LH), and the enzyme aromatase ($P450_{aro}$) that coverts certain androgens into estrogens (see Chapter 3). Hatschek's pit also expresses **Pit-1**, a transcription factor unique to the developing vertebrate pituitary. In another group of invertebrate chordates, the ascidians or tunicates, we find the neural gland complex consisting of a cerebral ganglion and the dorsal strand (Figure 5-2) that also is associated with the oral cavity. A number of neuropeptides of endocrine significance have been isolated from tunicates including corticotropin (ACTH), prolactin (PRL), gonadotropin-releasing hormone (GnRH), and nonapeptides. In addition, cells containing ACTH as well as corticotropin-like peptide (CLIP) also contain the proopiomelanocortin (POMC) processing enzymes, PC1 and PC2. The embryological association of all three structures (pituitary, Hatschek's pit, neural gland complex) with the nasal placodes together with the presence of similar bioregulators and enzymes is strongly suggestive of homology.

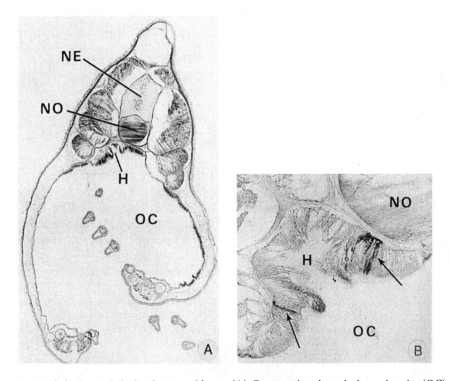

Figure 5-1. **Hatschek's pit in the cephalochordate, amphioxus.** (A) Cross-section through the oral cavity (OC) of an adult animal showing two basic chordate features: the dorsal nerve cord (NE) and the notochord (NO). Hatschek's pit (H) appears on the dorsal pharyngeal surface similar to the location of Rathke's pouch in vertebrate embryos. (B) Enlargement of Hatscheck's pit showing immunoreactive metenkephalin-like material (arrows). [From Nozaki, M., and Gorbman, A. (1992). The question of functional homology of Hatschek's pit of amphioxus (*Branchiostoma belcheri*) and the vertebrate adenohypophysis. *Zool. Sci.* **9**, 387–395.]

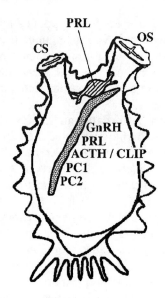

Figure 5-2. **The neural complex of a tunicate.** Ganglion, striped; Dorsal strand, dotted. [From Kawamura, K., Kouki, T., Kawahara, G., and Kikuyama, S. (2002). Hypophyseal development in vertebrates from amphibians to mammals. *Gen. Comp. Endocr.* **126**, 130–135.]

With few exceptions, the brain structures responsible for secretion of neuropeptides in vertebrates are paired areas although contributions of right and left nuclei may not always be equal as discussed in Chapter 4. However, in discussing the presence of these secretory areas or nuclei and their related neuropeptides, it is often cumbersome to refer always to their paired nature. In the following accounts, the reader should assume all nuclei are paired or bilateral even though they may be referred to in the singular (see Figure 4-12).

A major developmental difference in formation of the brains of fishes and tetrapods has made it more difficult to identify homologous brain centers. In development of the teleost brain, for example, the neural tube turns itself outwardly whereas in the tetrapod brain, the growth occurs inwardly. Thus the mammalian hippocampus, for example, is located deep within the brain whereas in teleosts the putative hippocampus occurs on the lateral dorsal surface of the brain.

I. The Fishes

The piscine HP system is separable into the same major divisions as that of mammals: hypothalamus, neurohypophysis, and adenohypophysis (Figure 5-3). Much of the following account is based on pioneering anatomical studies of the HP axis in primitive fishes done by Michael Lagios. These and other studies are summarized in "The Pituitary Gland: A Comparative Account" by Holmes and Ball (see "Suggested Reading" at end of chapter). Some marked differences from mammals occur in fishes. There is no pars tuberalis in fishes, although a possibly homologous structure, the pars ventralis, occurs in elasmobranchs (chondrichthyeans). The neurohypophysis of lampreys, sharks, and non-teleost bony fish groups is separable into a median eminence

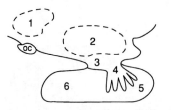

Figure 5-3. **Generalized hypothalamo-hypophysial axis in fishes.** 1, Preoptic area; 2, hypothalamus; 3, median eminence (when present); 4, pars nervosa; 5, pars intermedia; 6, pars distalis. 4 and 5 together constitute the neurointermediate lobe. OC = optic chiasm.

and a pars nervosa. The median eminence is connected to the adenohypophysis by a portal system. However, there is no median eminence and no portal system in hagfishes and teleosts.

In most fishes, the pars distalis of the fish adenohypophysis is differentiated into two subregions or zones, each with its special cell types. Two different terminologies have been proposed for the subregions of the piscine adenohypophysis. The nomenclature proposed by Green is used here in favor of the alternative system proposed by Pickford and Atz because the Green system is similar to mammalian terminologies (Figure 5-4) and is used most commonly in the literature. During this discussion, each term is defined initially, followed by the italicized terms proposed by Pickford and Atz, in parentheses. There are three distinct zones recognized in the adenohypophysis by both schemes. The most anterior and rostral (dorsal) portion of the piscine adenohypophysis often consists of follicles of cells and is termed the **rostral pars distalis** (*proadenohypophysis*). The remainder of the pars distalis comprises the **proximal pars distalis** (*mesoadenohypophysis*). The third region is the **pars intermedia** (*meta-adenohypophysis*). Each of these regions of the adenohypophysis is readily distinguished cytologically and generally each contains different cell types that produce different tropic hormones. The cell types found in each region and the hormones they are thought to produce are summarized in Table 5-1. Distribution of cell types is illustrated in Figure 5-5. Although alternative schemes have been proposed, the classification scheme for pituitary cell types used here is the same one described for mammals in Chapter 4.

The fish pars intermedia is intimately interdigitated with the pars nervosa of the neurohypophysis to form a **neurointermediate lobe**. Posterior to the neurointermediate lobe in cartilaginous fishes and most bony fishes is a unique structure formed from the floor of the diencephalon called the **saccus vasculosus**. This structure is probably derived from ependymal cells. It is especially prominent in some groups, but its function is unknown. The saccus vasculosus is a prominent feature with possible endocrine function that evolved among early jawed fishes (see ahead).

For our discussions of hypothalamic control of hypophysial functions, we shall focus on two regions in which the majority of neurosecretory (NS) neurons reside (Figure 5-2). The first area is located just anterior and dorsal to the optic chiasm and is called the **preoptic area (POA)**. This subregion marks the telencephalic and diencephalic boundary and usually is considered part of the telencephalon. Endocrinologists often include it when they are discussing the hypothalamic control of pituitary function as though it were part of the hypothalamus, a habit continued here. The second subregion includes the hypothalamus proper. With the exception of the preoptic nucleus of hagfishes (see ahead), the NS nuclei of the HP system are all paired structures. Other telencephalic and mesencephalic structures may produce similar peptides or may be targets

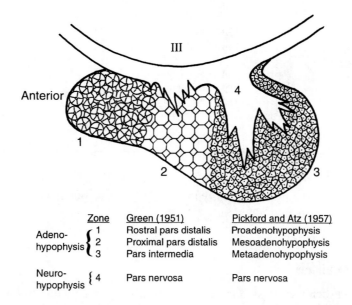

	Zone	Green (1951)	Pickford and Atz (1957)
Adeno-hypophysis	1	Rostral pars distalis	Proadenohypophysis
	2	Proximal pars distalis	Mesoadenohypophysis
	3	Pars intermedia	Metaadenohypophysis
Neuro-hypophysis	4	Pars nervosa	Pars nervosa

Figure 5-4. **Regions of the fish adenohypophysis.** The terminologies of Green (1951) and Pickford and Atz (1957) are compared for the three histologically distinct regions (1, 2, and 3). Only the Green nomenclature is used in the text.

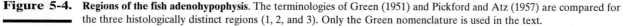

Table 5-1. Comparative Cytology of the Pars Distalis from Representatives of Different Vertebrate Groups

Hormone	Vertebrate group	Cellular type	Alternate names	Ultrastructural determination of cytoplasmic granule size (nm)
TSH	Chondrichthyes: Selachians	Type 1 basophil	Type I	90–120
	Osteichthyes			
	Holosteans	Type 1 basophil (amphophil)		—
	Teleosts	Type 1 basophil	δ-Basophil	400
	Amphibia: Anurans	Type 1 basophil		150–400
	Reptiles	Type 1 basophil		300–400 × 200–250
	Birds	Type 1 basophil	δ-Basophil	50, 100, 200
	Mammals	Type 1 basophil	β-Basophil	150
GTH	Chondrichthyes: Selachians	Type 2 basophil	Type V, VI	100–700
	Osteichthyes			
	Holosteans	Type 2 basophil		
	Teleosts	Type 2 basophil	β- and γ-Basophils	60–160; 80–240
	Amphibia: Anurans	Type 2 basophil		Polymorphous to 900
	Reptiles	Type 2 basophil		150–270; 600–800
	Birds	Type 2 basophil	β-Basophil; γ-basophil	120–200 120–400
	Mammals	Type 2 basophil	δ-Basophil	200
ACTH	Chondrichthyes: Selachians	Type 3 basophil	Type II	140
	Osteichthyes			
	Holosteans		Acidophil	
	Teleosts	Type 3 basophil	ε-Cell	110–250
	Amphibia: Anurans	Type 3 basophil		100–200
	Reptiles	Type 3 basophil (amphophil)		—
	Birds	Type 3 basophil	ε-Cell	150–300
	Mammals	Type 3 basophil		200
PRL	Chondrichthyes: Selachians	Type 1 acidophil	Type IV	263
	Osteichthyes			
	Holosteans	Type 1 acidophil		—
	Teleosts	Type 1 acidophil	η-Cell	Polymorphic; 170–350
	Amphibia: Anurans	Type 1 acidophil		180–500
	Reptiles	Type 1 acidophil		—
	Birds	Type 1 acidophil	η-Cell	Polymorphic; 250–300
	Mammals	Type 1 acidophil	ε-Acidophil	Polymorphic; 600–900
GH	Chondrichthyes: Selachians	Type 2 acidophil	Type III	200
	Osteichthyes			
	Holosteans	Type 2 acidophil		—
	Teleosts	Type 2 acidophil	α-Cell	—
	Amphibia: Anurans	Type 2 acidophil		180–250
	Reptiles	Type 2 acidophil		310
	Birds	Type 2 acidophil	α-Acidophil	250–300
	Mammals	Type 2 acidophil	α-Acidophil	350

for fibers secreting peptides usually associated with the HP system, but they are not thought to be central players in the regulation of endocrine function.

A. Agnathan (Jawless) Fishes

Our knowledge of the neuroendocrine system of agnathan fishes is largely due to the early studies by Aubrey Gorbman that have been continued largely through the efforts of Stacia Sower and her colleagues at the University of New Hampshire as well as by Japanese scientists, most notably Hiroshi Kawauchi.

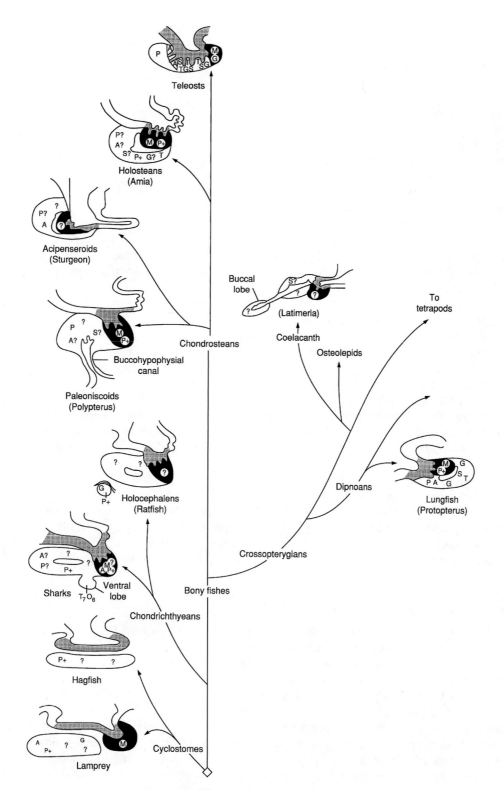

Figure 5-5. **Comparative anatomy of the fish pituitary**. The neurohypophysis in indicated by oblique lines and the pars intermedia is shown in black. Approximate distributions of cell types secreting tropic hormones are indicated by letters. A, corticotropin; G, gonadotropins; M, melanotropin; P, prolactin; P+, somatolactin; S, growth hormone or somatotropin; T, thyrotropin, ?, unidentified. [Modified from Schreibman, M. P. (1986). Pituitary Gland. *In* "Vertebrate Endocrinology: Fundamentals and Biomedical Implications. Volume 1, Morphological Considerations" (P. K. T. Pang and M. P. Schreibman, Eds.), pp. 11–56. Academic Press, Orlando, FL.]

B. The Myxinoids (Hagfishes)

The Atlantic and Pacific hagfishes possess the most primitive HP system among the chordates (Figure 5-5). The hagfish system lacks many of the features that characterize other piscine and tetrapod groups. Furthermore, hagfishes are much more primitive in many respects than even their closest living agnathan relatives, the lampreys (Petromyzontidae).

The hagfish brain has several NS regions. Anterior and dorsal to the optic chiasm is the **preoptic nucleus (PON)** that appears to produce NS products that are stored in the neurohypophysis, a neurohemal area comparable to the mammalian pars nervosa. There is, however, no anterior neurohemal region in the Atlantic hagfish comparable to the median eminence, although a very primitive anterior neurohemal area has been described for the Pacific hagfish and has been termed a median eminence. The presence of gonadotropin-releasing hormone (GnRH) has been demonstrated in the Atlantic hagfish, *Myxine glutinosa*, and shown to vary seasonally with reproductive state.

The origin of the adenohypophysis of hagfishes appears to be from endoderm rather than from ectoderm, presenting an additional puzzle with respect to the origin of the pituitary. Furthermore, it raises the question of possible homology of the hagfish adenohypophysis to that of other vertebrates and supports the viewpoint that hagfishes are abberant vertebrates, are not on the mainline evolutionary pathway, and cannot readily be compared to vertebrates.

The hagfish adenohypophysis is not differentiated into subregions; that is, there is no discernable pars distalis or pars intermedia. The adenohypophysis is composed primarily of non-stainable cells with rare PAS(+) basophils or an occasional acidophil. Electron micrographs of the hagfish adenohypophysis show rare granular cells with cytoplasmic granules of 100–200-nm diameter. These granular cells are believed to represent the two rare stainable cell types identifiable with the light microscope. When hagfish adenohypophysial tissue is cultured *in vitro*, no observable changes take place in either granular or nongranular cells.

Certain cells of the myxinoid adenohypophysis exhibit cytological modifications where they make contact with the neurohypophysis. These altered cells collectively are termed **modified adenohypophysial tissue**, and it has been proposed that this apparent induction by neurohypophysial tissue represents phylogenetically the origin of the pars intermedia. In other vertebrates, the pars intermedia develops following contact of the presumptive adenohypophysis with the neurohypophysis.

Bioassays of hagfish pituitaries for PRL activity have proven negative, and anti-ovine PRL antibody does not bind to hagfish adenohypophysial cells. Hypophysectomy of Pacific hagfish produces no convincing alterations in either thyroid or gonadal tissue. Bioassayable ACTH-like and thyrotropin (TSH)-like activities have been demonstrated in pituitary extracts of a Pacific hagfish, *Eptatretus stouti*, and gonadotropin (GTH) activity has been demonstrated in the pituitary of *Eptatretus burgeri*, a shallow-water, seasonally breeding hagfish. Obviously, the hagfishes demonstrate a very primitive stage of HP interaction.

C. Lampreys (Petromyzontids)

In the lampreys (Figure 5-6), the more anterior rostral pars distalis is composed of basophils and non-stainable cells as well as carminophils. Immunocytochemical staining has identified corticotropes mainly in the rostral pars distalis. A carminophilic cell containing growth hormone (GH)/PRL-like immunoreactive occupies the dorsal portion of the proximal pars distalis. The ventral portion of the proximal pars distalis consists of what appears to be an LH-like basophil although distinct GTHs have not been isolated to date from lampreys. Finally, a melanotrope has been identified in the pars intermedia.

The distinct pars nervosa and the pars intermedia form a well-developed neurointermediate lobe. Peptidergic neurons terminate in the pars nervosa where the single nonapeptide neurohormone arginine vasotocin (AVT) is stored. A second anterior neurohemal region is associated with the pars distalis and has been referred to as a median eminence. However, this structure is devoid of portal blood vessels so it is unlikely that it functions as a median eminence. Studies do show that materials can diffuse readily from the brain into the adenohypophysis via this putative median eminence.

There are more NS nuclei identifiable in the lamprey brain than have been demonstrated in their relatives, the hagfishes. Two major NS centers occur in the lamprey brain anterior and dorsal to the optic chiasm: the **medial** and **lateral anterior preoptic areas** as well as the preoptic nucleus. Both GnRH and PRL have been identified in neurons of the preoptic area using immunocytochemistry. GnRH occurs in olfactory regions, too.

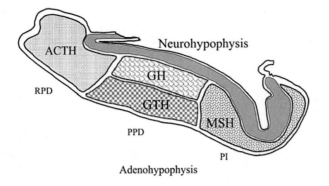

Figure 5-6. **Pituitary of the sea lamprey.** Regions known to be responsible for secretion of tropic hormones are identified. [From Kawauchi, H., and Sower, S. A. (2006). The dawn and evolution of hormones in the adenohypophysis. *Gen. and Comp. Endocri.* **148**, 3–19.]

Two additional NS areas are found in the hypothalamus: the **anterior hypothalamic area** and the **dorsal** and **ventral periventricular arcuate nuclei** (see Figure 5-7).

D. Chondrichthyean Fishes

The chondrichthyean fishes represent a side road off the main line of vertebrate evolution. Once a dominant marine group, they are represented today by elasmobranchs or selachians (the sharks, rays, and skates) and a small group of fishes known as the holocephalans (chimaeras or ratfishes). However, they do retain numerous features of the HP system that probably evolved in ancient fishes that gave rise to this group as well as to the bony fishes.

1. Sharks, Rays, and Skates (Elasmobranchs)

The elasmobranch HP system possesses two anatomical features not found in agnathan fishes. The **pars ventralis** represents a fourth subdivision of the adenohypophysis unique to elasmobranchs. It is located ventral to the proximal pars distalis to which it is connected by a stalk (Figure 5-5). Localization of GTH and TSH activity in the pars ventralis has prompted some investigators to suggest that the pars ventralis is homologous to the pars tuberalis of the tetrapod adenohypophysis, but this seems unlikely (see Chapter 4). The terms "rostral" and "proximal" may be somewhat misleading when applied to the elasmobranch pars distalis because of the presence of the ventral lobe which is probably homologous to part of the proximal pars distalis of teleost fishes. These regions are sometimes designated as the rostral, median, and ventral lobes of the pars distalis. The distribution of cell types in the elasmobranch pituitary is summarized in Table 5-1.

The second feature appearing for the first time in elasmobranchs is the saccus vasculosus derived from the hypothalamic ependyma and located immediately posterior to the neurointermediate lobe. It is not as well-developed as its homologue in bony fishes, but it does possess the unique **coronet** cell type characteristic of the saccus vasculosus of bony fishes (see Figure 5-8). Immunoreactive melanin-concentrating hormone (MCH) has been colocalized with melanotropin (α-MSH) in the saccus vasculosus of the shark, *Scyliorhinus*.

The neurointermediate lobe shows extensive interdigitation of neural and endocrine cells. The pars nervosa stores some unique nonapeptides in addition to AVT. These hormones are presumably produced in the preoptic nucleus. The pars intermedia contains only one cell type associated with α-MSH activity.

There is a well-developed median eminence with a portal system connecting it to the pars distalis. The median eminence consists of anterior and posterior neurohemal areas. The posterior region receives both peptidergic and aminergic NS axons and appears to be linked by portal vessels to the proximal pars distalis but not to the ventral lobe. There is considerably less NS material in the anterior neurohemal area that appears to be connected by capillaries to the rostral pars distalis. It is tempting to suggest that the median eminence has differentiated in these fishes to increase the efficiency of delivering hypothalamic neurohormones to specific adenohypophysial cells.

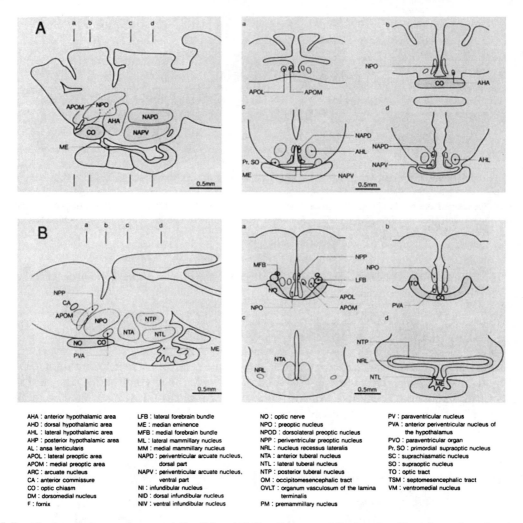

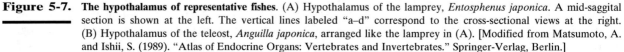

AHA : anterior hypothalamic area	LFB : lateral forebrain bundle	NO : optic nerve	PV : paraventricular nucleus
AHD : dorsal hypothalamic area	ME : median eminence	NPO : preoptic nucleus	PVA : anterior periventricular nucleus of
AHL : lateral hypothalamic area	MFB : medial forebrain bundle	NPOD : dorsolateral preoptic nucleus	the hypothalamus
AHP : posterior hypothalamic area	ML : lateral mammillary nucleus	NPP : periventricular preoptic nucleus	PVO : paraventricular organ
AL : ansa lenticularis	MM : medial mammillary nucleus	NRL : nucleus recessus lateralis	Pr. SO : primordial supraoptic nucleus
APOL : lateral preoptic area	NAPD : periventricular arcuate nucleus,	NTA : anterior tuberal nucleus	SC : suprachiasmatic nucleus
APOM : medial preoptic area	dorsal part	NTL : lateral tuberal nucleus	SO : supraoptic nucleus
ARC : arcuate nucleus	NAPV : periventricular arcuate nucleus,	NTP : posterior tuberal nucleus	TO : optic tract
CA : anterior commissure	ventral part	OM : occipitomesencephalic tract	TSM : septomesencephalic tract
CO : optic chiasm	NI : infundibular nucleus	OVLT : organum vasculosum of the lamina	VM : ventromedial nucleus
DM : dorsomedial nucleus	NID : dorsal infundibular nucleus	terminalis	
F : fornix	NIV : ventral infundibular nucleus	PM : premammillary nucleus	

Figure 5-7. **The hypothalamus of representative fishes.** (A) Hypothalamus of the lamprey, *Entosphenus japonica*. A mid-saggital section is shown at the left. The vertical lines labeled "a–d" correspond to the cross-sectional views at the right. (B) Hypothalamus of the teleost, *Anguilla japonica*, arranged like the lamprey in (A). [Modified from Matsumoto, A. and Ishii, S. (1989). "Atlas of Endocrine Organs: Vertebrates and Invertebrates." Springer-Verlag, Berlin.]

2. Ratfishes (Holocephalans)

The pituitary of ratfishes is readily subdivided cytologically into rostral pars distalis, proximal pars distalis, and pars intermedia. Although several cell types have been demonstrated with selective staining procedures, no experimental studies have verified which cells produce which tropic hormones.

Like elasmobranchs, holocephalans possess a unique region associated with the adenohypophysis, called the **pharyngeal lobe**. This structure is located in the roof of the mouth outside the cranium and is not connected to the adenohypophysis proper. The pharyngeal lobe consists of follicles and may be homologous to the follicular rostral pars distalis of bony fishes. On the other hand, it may be homologous to the ventral lobe of the elasmobranch and the buccal lobe of the coelacanth pituitary (see ahead).

The ratfish neurohypophysis includes a prominent median eminence connected to the rostral pars distalis and the proximal pars distalis by a portal system.

Somatostatin (SST), thyrotropin-releasing hormone (TRH), and GnRH immunoreactivities are present in the ratfish hypothalamus. The pars nervosa is mingled with the pars intermedia of the adenohypophysis to form a typical neurointermediate lobe. AVT and oxytocin (OXY) are present in the ratfish pars nervosa and represent a unique occurrence of OXY among fishes. A well-developed saccus vasculosus is also present.

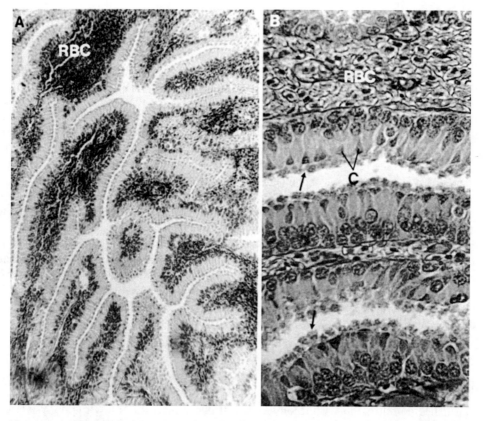

Figure 5-8. **The saccus vasculosus of rainbow trout, *Oncorhynchus mykiss*.** (A) Coronet cells (arrow) and ependymal secretory cells. (B) Higher magnification showing mucoid secretory products (arrows) of saccus vasculosus cells.

E. Bony Ray-Finned Fishes (Actinopterygians)

Four taxonomically distinct groups of ray-finned fishes are recognized traditionally by most authorities, and those names are used here (see Chapter 1). Three of these (polypterans, chondrosteans, and holosteans) are considered to represent more primitive fish groups whereas the fourth group (teleosts) is recognized as the most evolutionary advanced of these fishes. The embryonic origin of the fish adenohypophysis should be reexamined in the light of recent understandings of the neural origin of the tetrapod pituitary (see Chapter 4).

1. Polypteran Fishes (*Polypterus* and *Calamoichthyes*)

The ancient African polypterid fishes possess all the typical piscine pituitary features including rostral and proximal divisions of the pars distalis, a neurointermediate lobe, and a saccus vasculosus. As adults, they retain a connection between the hypophysis and the mouth cavity called the **buccohypophysial canal** (*bucco*, mouth). This canal is believed to be a remnant originally connecting the pituitary to the oral cavity (Figure 5-5). The buccohypophysial canal or duct is lined with a weakly staining cell type that does not appear to be associated with production of any tropic hormones.

The polypteran pars nervosa contains AVT and an OXY-like nonapeptide known as **isotocin (IST)** secreted by the preoptic nucleus. These two neurohormones are characteristic of all ray-finned fishes. A portal system with a defined median eminence is well-developed. Peptidergic fiber tracts travel from the PON via the median eminence to terminate in the pars nervosa. Aminergic neurons that terminate in the median eminence probably originate in the preoptic region, too.

2. Chondrostean Fishes (Sturgeons, Paddlefishes)

There is less information concerning the HP system of chondrostean fishes than for any other ray-finned bony fishes. However, chondrostean fishes are very large, long-lived species with very limited distributions and hence are difficult to study. There is no buccohypophysial canal in chondrosteans, but a hypophysial cavity is present. This cavity separates the pars distalis and pars intermedia and may be homologous to the buccohypophysial canal and/or the hypophysial cleft described in some mammals. The pars distalis consists of a rostral zone and a proximal zone (rostral and proximal pars distalis). Numerous follicles occur throughout the pars distalis, and their lumina, which are filled with a basophilic colloidal material, are considered by some to be remnants of the hypophysial cavity. The entire pars distalis may be homologous to the proximal pars distalis of teleost fishes, and the terms "rostral pars distalis" and "proximal pars distalis" may not be applicable to the two apparent zones of the chondrostean pars distalis.

The pars intermedia of sturgeons is large and closely associated with the pars nervosa, forming a typical neurointermediate lobe. The pars nervosa is basically hollow and is similar in appearance to the saccus vasculosus. Both peptidergic and aminergic fibers have been reported in the pars nervosa.

The hypothalamus contains a well-developed PON that provides peptidergic fibers to the pars nervosa. The **nucleus lateralis tuberis (NLT)** is a new nucleus in bony fishes and consists of peptidergic and aminergic neurons. There is a well-developed median eminence consisting of aminergic axonal endings from the NLT. The median eminence is separated from the pars distalis by a connective tissue sheath so that no neurons penetrate the pars distalis. A portal system is present and probably conducts neurohormones from the median eminence to the pars distalis. Immunoreactive corticotropin-releasing hormone (CRH) has been demonstrated in the POA, the NLT, and the median eminence of sturgeon.

3. Holostean Fishes (Gars and Bowfin)

Adult holostean fishes do not exhibit a buccohypophysial duct nor is there any hypophysial cleft although a transient hypophysial cleft does appear during development of the pituitary. The adenohypophysis consists of a follicular rostral pars distalis, a proximal pars distalis, and a pars intermedia that interdigitates with the pars nervosa to form a neurointermediate lobe.

The PON has separated into two distinct portions, the dorsal **pars magnocellularis** made up of larger NS neurons and the ventral **pars parvocellularis** of smaller cells. Peptidergic fibers from the PON pass to the pars nervosa where nonapeptide hormones (AVT and IST) are stored. Aminergic fibers also appear in the pars nervosa and are believed to come at least in part from the NLT.

The median eminence is connected to the pars distalis by a well-developed portal system. In addition, there are a limited number of peptidergic and aminergic axons that penetrate the pars distalis. However, only aminergic fibers are associated with the median eminence of the bowfin, *Amia calva*. Here, in these near-relatives of the teleost fishes, is the modest beginning of a shift from neurovascular control to neuroglandular control of the adenohypophysis directly by neurons of the hypothalamus as is seen among the teleosts.

4. Teleost Fishes

The HP systems of numerous teleost species have been studied in detail. Excellent neuroanatomical atlases are available for a number of species including goldfish, zebrafish, and numerous salmonids. In view of the vast adaptive radiation that teleosts have undergone, it is not surprising to find considerable variability in this system. Although only a relatively few species have been examined, they have been examined in greater detail than for other piscine groups, and the various cell types have been identified and their secretions characterized chemically. There is a strong tendency for localization of cell types in particular regions of the adenohypophysis (Figures 5-9 and 5-10). This anatomical arrangement has aided scientists in determining what hormone each cell type produces. Unlike the situation with mammals, two kinds of GTH-secreting cells have been demonstrated in the teleost proximal pars distalis. Although early studies indicated there was only one LH-like GTH in teleosts, two GTHs have been described because it was initially thought they were distinct from those of tetrapods. These teleost GTHs were named **GTH-I** and **GTH-II**. GTH-I is like follicle-stimulating hormone (FSH-like) and controls androgen and estrogen synthesis as well as spermatogenesis and

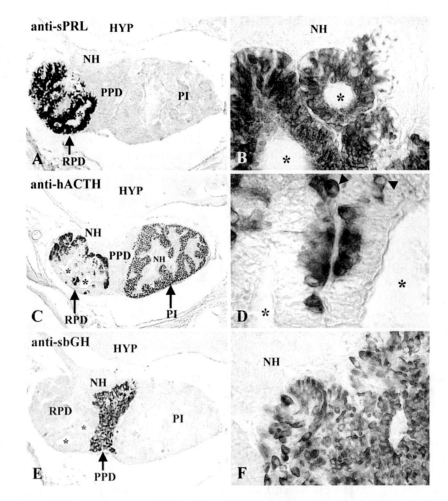

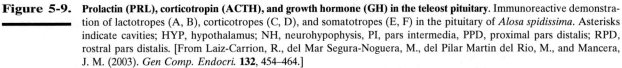

Figure 5-9. **Prolactin (PRL), corticotropin (ACTH), and growth hormone (GH) in the teleost pituitary.** Immunoreactive demonstration of lactotropes (A, B), corticotropes (C, D), and somatotropes (E, F) in the pituitary of *Alosa spidissima*. Asterisks indicate cavities; HYP, hypothalamus; NH, neurohypophysis, PI, pars intermedia, PPD, proximal pars distalis; RPD, rostral pars distalis. [From Laiz-Carrion, R., del Mar Segura-Noguera, M., del Pilar Martin del Rio, M., and Mancera, J. M. (2003). *Gen Comp. Endocri.* **132**, 454–464.]

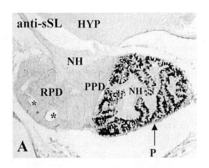

Figure 5-10. **Somatolactin (SL) cells in teleost pars intermedia.** Immunoreactive SL cells in the teleost, *Alosa sapidissima*. See Figure 5-9 for explanation of abbreviations. [From Laiz-Carrion, R., del Mar Segura-Noguera, M., del Pilar Martin del Rio, M., and Mancera, J. M. (2003). *Gen. Comp. Endocri.* **132**, 454–464.]

oogenesis. GTH-II is LH-like and responsible for production of a progesterone-like hormone, final gamete maturation, and ovulation or sperm release.

Teleosts exhibit extensive innervation of the pars distalis by preoptic and hypothalamic neurons. There is no distinct portal system and hence no true median eminence in most species examined, and the control of tropic hormone release is **neuroglandular** by direct peptidergic or aminergic innervation rather than **neurovascular** as found in many ancient fishes and in the tetrapods (see Table 5-2). Some neurons make direct synaptic connections to the pituitary cells whereas the axons of others end on the pituitary basement membrane, and their secretions must diffuse through the basement membrane to reach receptors on the pituitary cells.

The pars intermedia is intimately associated with the pars nervosa of the neurohypophysis to form a neurointermediate lobe as described for the elasmobranchs and more ancient bony fishes. Direct innervation from the pars nervosa is responsible for controlling α-MSH release from the pars intermedia. In addition to α-MSH-secreting cells, a PAS(+)-cell type, the **PIPAS cell**, is present in the pars intermedia of teleosts with the exception of the salmonids. This cell secretes a unique hormone named somatolactin (see ahead). A similarly staining cell also occurs in the pars intermedia of some more ancient bony fishes (i.e., *A. calva* and *Polypterus*).

The diversity of teleosts makes generalizations about the hypothalamic distribution of neuropeptides very difficult. Furthermore, development and extensive application of immunohistochemistry to the teleost brain have resulted as they did for mammals in the discovery that neuropeptides may appear in many neurons that are not associated directly with the activity of the HP system. For example, in addition to the hypothalamus, immunoreactive GnRH neurons may be found in the anteriormost olfactory regions of the brain as well as in the midbrain. Similarly, the amount of TRH present in the telencephalon typically is much greater than in the hypothalamus. The anatomy of the brain of the Japanese eel, *Anguilla japonica*, serves as a representative but not necessarily typical teleost (Figure 5-6).

There are numerous neurosecretory centers in the teleost brain, and considerable variation in the names applied to them. Hence, only general descriptions are provided here, and the interested reader should consult the references at the end of this chapter for specific sources. Axons of neurosecretory neurons follow well-defined tracts to the pars distalis or the neurointermediate lobe of the pituitary whereas others may connect with a variety of other brain structures. The preoptic area located anterior to the optic chiasm sports several specialized areas in the eel. In addition to the PON, there are also medial and lateral POAs as well as the anterior periventricular nucleus of the anterior hypothalamus that is a major source of dopaminergic axons ending in the pars distalis. Magnocellular and parvocellular NS neurons of the PON have been reported to contain either growth hormone-releasing hormone (GHRH), GnRH, SST, CRH, or AVT as well as neuropeptide Y (NPY), vasoactive intestinal peptide (VIP), and others. The suprachiasmatic nucleus (SCN) also sends axons to the pituitary.

The basal and caudal hypothalamus contains several neurosecretory centers. The NLT is separated into anterior, posterior, and lateral parts that are principally responsible for secretion of thyrotropin-releasing hormone (TRH) and MCH as well as GHRH, SST, NPY, GnRH, CRH, urotensin-I, AVT, and others.

Table 5-2. Presence of Neuropeptides in Neurons Contacting Secretory Cells of the Adenohypophysis of the Sea Bass, *Dicentrarchus labrax*[a,b]

Region	Secretory cell type	Peptides present
Rostral pars distalis	ACTH cells	SS, GHRH, CRH, AVT, IST, SP, NT, GAL
	PRL cells	GAL
Proximal pars distalis	GH cells	SS, GHRH, AVT, IST, CCK, SP, NPY, GAL
	GTH cells	GnRH, IST, GHRH, AVT
	TSH cells	GHRH, CRH, AVT, IST, SP, GAL
Pars intermedia	MSH cells	GHRH, CRH, MCH, AVT, IST, SP
	PAS(+)cells	GHRH, CRH, MCH, AVT, IST, SP

[a] See text or Appendix A for explanation of peptide abbreviations.

[b] After Moons, L., Cambré, M., Ollevier, F., and Vandesande, F. (1989). Immunocytochemical demonstration of close relationships between neuropeptidergic nerve fibers and hormone-producing cell types in the adenohypophysis of the sea bass (*Dicentrarchus labrax*). *Gen. Comp. Endocri.* **73**, 270.

Immunoreactive α-MSH also has been demonstrated in the NLT of carp and rainbow trout. Dopaminergic, serotinergic, and noradrenergic fibers also travel from the paraventricular organ, the nucleus recessus lateralis, and the nucleus recessus posterioris to the pituitary in many species. These neurons play important roles in the regulation of reproduction (see Chapter 11).

Two types of CRH and CRH-secreting cells have been described in the common sucker, *Catostomus commersoni*. CRH-containing cells in the PON react best to antisera for mCRH and often contain the nonapeptide AVT. In contrast, the axonal processes of CRH cells in the NLT react to antibodies for sauvagine and urotensin-I and do not contain AVT. Experimental studies suggest that the preoptic CRH colocalized with AVT is responsible for controlling release of ACTH whereas CRH in the NLT controls synthesis. These observations also suggest an ACTH-releasing role for AVT that is similar to the role for arginine vasopressin (AVP) in mammals. A similar pattern for CRH distribution has been reported for several species of eel (*Anguilla* spp.). In goldfish, synthesis and release of ACTH appear to be under control of CRH from the NLT. The complexity of connections in this system is exemplified by the observations that in the sea bass, *Dicentrarchus labrax*, the corticotropic cells of the pars distalis apparently are contacted by a variety of neurons containing AVT, CRH, neurotensin, GHRH, or SST.

Preoptic GnRH-1 neurons are larger in brains of males of naturally sex-changing teleosts (e.g., wrasses) with respect to number and/or size. A similar sexual dimorphism in the size of POA GnRH neurons is reported for goldfish, a species that does not change sex naturally. No sexual dimorphism was evident in AVT neurons in goldfish. However, males of the marine goby, *Trimma okinawae*, one of four teleost species that are known to naturally change sex more than once, exhibit smaller AVT neurons in the POA. Change of the male to a female is accompanied by an increase in the size of these AVT neurons that again become smaller when that female later changes back to a male. GnRH-2 neurons are associated with the teleost midbrain. The role of GnRH-3 neurons in the telencephalon is not known. The GnRH-4 neurons that have their origin in the diencephalon appear to regulate pituitary GTH release like the GnRH-1 neurons that migrated from the olfactory placode (see Chapter 4 as well as discussion ahead).

F. Bony Fishes: The Lobe-Finned Fishes (Sarcopterygians)

Although they once thrived in the ancient oceans and radiated in many directions, only two lobe-finned groups have living representatives. The dipnoans or lungfishes are represented by three genera comprising seven species. The two species of living crossopterygians are thought to be very close to the long-extinct crossopterygian fishes that gave rise to amphibians. The HP system of *Neoceratodus* is similar to that of primitive bony fishes including possession of a neurointermediate lobe. There is a follicular rostral pars distalis containing cells that secrete ACTH and PRL. In contrast, the pituitary systems of the African and South American lungfishes structurally are more similar to those of tetrapods, especially amphibians. For example, there is less regionalization of cell types in the adenohypophysis and no neurointermediate lobe. However, this similarity with amphibians could be the result of parallel or convergent evolution. In general, hypothalamic regulation in lungfishes appears to be neurovascular as in primitive actinopterygians rather than neuroglandular as in teleosts. The pars tuberalis, a landmark tetrapod feature, is, however, missing in all living lungfishes as well as in the coelacanths.

The HP system of the coelacanths is much more piscine-like (Figure 5-5) than it is tetrapod-like. The anatomy of the adenohypophysis is much like that of the elasmobranchs. There is a **buccal lobe** in the pars distalis which, based on the cell types present there, may be homologous to the ventral lobe of elasmobranchs. The pars distalis may be subdivided into rostral and proximal portions with stainable cell types appearing that are distributed similarly to those of teleosts. The pars intermedia forms a typical neurointermediate lobe with the pars nervosa as in other bony fishes. Unlike teleosts, there is a distinct median eminence connected to the adenohypophysis by a well-developed portal system, particularly in the proximal region. However, some NS axons appear to penetrate the proximal pars distalis similar to the situation described for the holostean fish, *A. calva*.

Although the sarcopterygian fishes represent descendents of fishes ancestral to the tetrapods, extant members of this group provide no transitional stages with respect to anatomical features of the HP system. However, the distribution and structure of α-MSH and the structure of PRL isolated from the Australian lungfish are more like tetrapods than like other bony fishes.

II. The Tetrapod Vertebrates: Anatomical Considerations

The neuroendocrine systems of tetrapods exhibit most of the characteristics described for mammals but lack the major features that characterize the fishes. The median eminence and pars nervosa are well-developed, distinct neurohemal structures. There is no remnant or suggestion of a saccus vasculosus in tetrapods. The amphibian pars distalis shows a tendency for cell regionalization, and the pars distalis of reptiles and birds consists of two somewhat distinct zones. However, these zones are not anatomically separated as are the rostral and proximal zones in fishes although the distribution of cell types is similar from anterior to posterior. The pars tuberalis is a consistent tetrapod feature and appears to have secretory cells. A putative role for the pars tuberalis in controlling PRL release from the pars distalis has been proposed for mammals (see Chapter 4), but no role has been established for any non-mammals.

The tetrapod hypothalamus becomes progressively differentiated into more distinct nuclei from amphibians to reptiles and then to birds and mammals although they are never as distinct as they appear in drawings (Figure 5-11). Although some direct neural control of the pars intermedia is present in amphibians, there is a predominance of neurovascular control rather than direct neural control of adenohypophysial function in all tetrapods.

A. Amphibians

The amphibian HP axis has most of the features characteristic of the tetrapod system (Figure 5-12), including the presence of a pars tuberalis (Figure 5-13). The prominent preoptic area (Figure 5-11) contains several NS centers including the lateral and medial POAs and the PON we saw in the fishes. GnRH-1, GnRH-associated peptide (GAP), GHRH, SST, AVT, TRH, CRH, and another OXY-like nonapeptide mesotocin (MST) have been reported in the preoptic region. In addition, there is a distinct SCN and a **ventromedial nucleus (VMN)**. AVT has been reported in the SCN of bullfrogs. The **infundibular nucleus (IFN)** located in the basal hypothalamus supplies both aminergic and peptidergic axons to the median eminence. This IFN is separable into **dorsal (NID)** and **ventral (NIV)** components and is homologous to at least part of the major hypophysiotropic region of the mammalian hypothalamus. The exact relationship between the IFN of amphibians and the NLT of fishes is uncertain. Immunoreactive-like TRH, SST, NPY, and atrial natriuretic peptide (ANP) have been identified in the NID whereas TRH, α-MSH, and NPY occur in the NIV. Pituitary adenylyl cyclase-activating peptide (PACAP) has been demonstrated in the POA as well as in the NID and NIV, and PACAP-immunoreactive axons appear in the median eminence suggesting a role in controlling pituitary function. The similarity of amino acid sequences in PACAP and the secretin-glucagon family of peptides (see Table 3-4 or 4-14) suggests one should be cautious when interpreting immunoreactive data since antisera to PACAP may cross-react with other members of the family including VIP and glucose-dependent insulinotropic peptide (GIP). Experimental studies have demonstrated that purified mammalian PACAP stimulates cAMP production and calcium mobilization in anuran pars distalis cells.

Sexual dimorphism has been described in the amphibian brain. The number of neurons in the anterior POA of leopard frogs (*Rana pipiens*) is dependent on androgens whereas the number of neurons in the posterior tuberculum (TP) is estrogen-dependent. Furthermore, the distribution of AVT also is sexually dimorphic in the brain.

The pars nervosa of the amphibian neurohypophysis receives peptidergic fibers originating in the magnocellular neurons of the PON and is the storage site for at least two nonapeptide hormones (AVT and MST). TRH is colocalized in neurons containing MST in the pars nervosa. A tract of ANP-reactive axons travels from the dorsal hypothalamus through the median eminence to enter the pars nervosa. AVT-secreting cell bodies in the POA and axonal endings in the pars nervosa also contain GHRH. Neurons containing immunoreactive MCH project from the anuran PON to the pars nervosa. These neurons also contain α-MSH although α-MSH neurons originating in the NIV do not contain MCH. There is no tendency for development of a neurointermediate lobe in amphibians.

The amphibian adenohypophysis consists of pars tuberalis, pars intermedia, and pars distalis. Based upon ultrastructural comparison of cytoplasmic granules and other features, there appear to be two separate granular cell types in the anuran pars tuberalis similar to those described in mammals. There also appears to be a neural pathway extending from the ependymal lining of the third ventricle to the pars tuberalis, but no functional correlation has been reported.

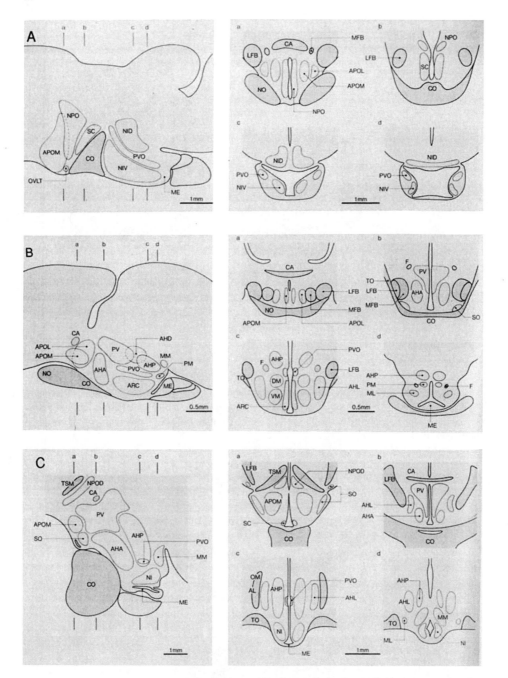

Figure 5-11. **The hypothalamus of representative nonmammlian tetrapods.** (A) Hypothalamus of the bullfrog *Rana catesbeiana*. (B) Hypothalamus of the snake, *Elaphe conscpicillata*. (C) Hypothalamus of the Japanese quail, *Coturnix coturnix japonicus*. See Figure 5-7 for explanation of symbols. [Modified from Matsumoto, A., and Ishii, S. (1989). "Atlas of Endocrine Organs: Vertebrates and Invertebrates." Springer-Verlag, Berlin.]

The amphibian pars intermedia has a poor vascular supply, but it is directly innervated by aminergic neurons thought to originate in the caudal aminergic nuclei of the hypothalamus. Release of α-MSH appears to be under direct neural control of aminergic neurons but is also affected by peptidergic fibers. NPY- and ANP-immunoreactive neurons enter the pars intermedia of anurans, and NPY inhibits release of α-MSH whereas ANP is stimulatory. MST also causes α-MSH release although it may not be a true α-MSH-releasing hormone.

The pars distalis is not separable into discrete regions although there is a tendency for some regionalization of cell types (Figure 5-14). Caudate amphibians exhibit greater regionalization than do anuran species. Careful

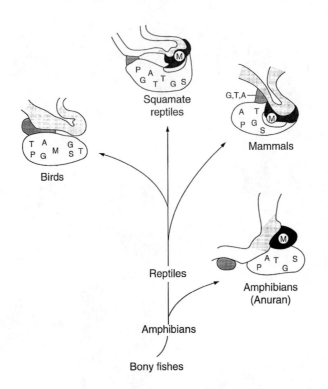

Figure 5-12. **Comparative anatomy of the tetrapod pituitary.** See Figure 5-5 for explanation of symbols. [Modified from Schreibman, M. P. (1986). Pituitary gland. *In* "Vertebrate Endocrinology: Fundamentals and Biomedical Implications. Volume 1, Morphological Considerations" (P. K. T. Pang and M. P. Schreibman, Eds.), pp. 11–56. Academic Press, Orlando, FL.]

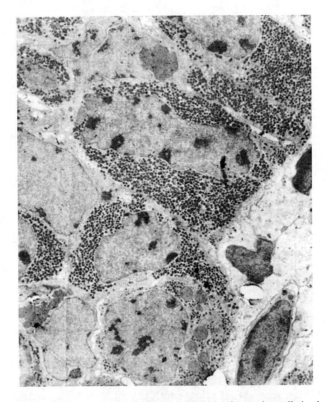

Figure 5-13. **Amphibian pars tuberalis.** Transmission electron micrograph of granular cells in the pars tuberalis of the frog, *Rana pipiens*. Two cell types can be identified on the basis of granule size. (Photograph courtesy of Dr. Kevin T. Fitzgerald.)

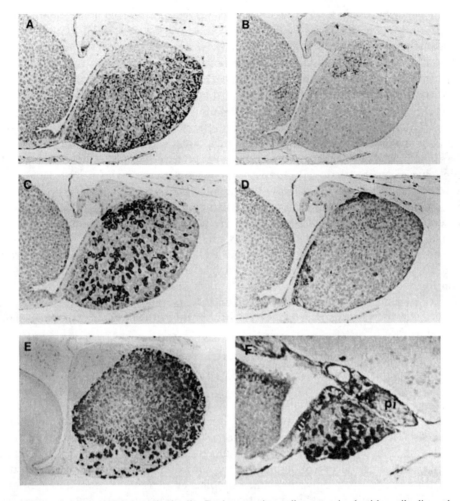

Figure 5-14. **Cytology of the amphibian pars distalis.** Dark-appearing cells are stained with antibodies selective for different pituitary hormones. (A) Immunoreactive prolactin-secreting cells. (B) Immunoreactive growth hormone-secreting cells. (C) Immunoreactive FSH-secreting cells. (D) Immunoreactive LH-secreting cells. (E) Immunoreactive corticotropin-secreting cells. (F) Immunoreactive thyrotropin-secreting cells. (A–D) Japanese newt, *Cynops pyrrhogaster*; (E), adult bullfrog, *Rana catesbeiana*; (F) postmetamorphic toad, *Bufo calamita*. [(A–D) are courtesy of Shigeyasu Tanaka and Sakae Kikuyama, Waseda University, Tokyo. (E) is reprinted with permission from Tanaka, S., Park, M. K., Hayashi, H., Hanaoka, Y., Wakabayashi, K., and Kurosomi, K. (1990). Immunocytochemical mlocalization of the subunits of glycoprotein hormones (LH, FSH, and TSH) in the bullfrog pituitary gland using monoclonal antibodies and polyclonal antiserum. *Gen. Comp. Endocri.* **77**, 88–97. Academic Press, San Diego. (F) is reprinted with permission from Garcia-Navarro, S., Malagon, M. M., and Garcia-Navarro, F. (1988). Immunohistochemical localization of thyrotropic cells during amphibian metamorphosis: A sterological study. *Gen. Comp. Endocri.* **71**, 116–123, Academic Press, San Diego.]

cytological studies have been performed on many amphibian species, often coupled with experimental manipulations, bioassays or correlation with specific life history events. Unfortunately, there has been considerable disagreement among researchers in this area with respect to establishment of specific sources for the various tropic hormones. The cytology of the pituitary of *Rana temporaria* can serve as an example of the basic amphibian condition (Table 5-1).

B. Reptiles

The reptilian hypothalamus is depicted in Figure 5-11. In reptiles, there is no longer a PON, but the medial and lateral POAs are present. Replacing the PON are the separate **supraoptic nucleus (SON)** and the

paraventricular nucleus (PVN) that are characteristic of amniote vertebrates. These nuclei consist of peptidergic NS neurons that terminate in the pars nervosa and produce the octapeptide neurohormones AVT and MST. CRH has been colocalized with AVT in some neurons of the PVN. The hypothalamus is separated into **anterior, dorsal**, and **posterior hypothalamic areas, paraventricular organs, periventricular nucleus (PERIV)**, and both **ventral** and **dorsal medial nuclei**. The IFN, also called the **arcuate (ARC) nucleus**, is considered to be homologous to the NIV of the amphibian IFN and the ARC nucleus (= IFN) of birds as well as to the major hypophysiotropic area of the mammalian hypothalamus. Aminergic and peptidergic NS fibers (including neurons containing GnRH-1) originate in this nucleus and terminate in the median eminence. Immunoreactive-MCH is present in neurons of the PERIV and lateral hypothalamic nuclei of a turtle, a lizard, and two snake species, but these fibers project to other brain regions and probably do not influence the pituitary.

The adenohypophysis is well-developed in most reptiles, and it consists of a pars distalis, a pars tuberalis, and a pars intermedia (Figure 5-12). The Rhynchocephalia (*Sphenodon punctatus*), Chelonia (turtles), and Crocodilia are thought to represent the primitive reptilian condition. The pars distalis appears as two distinct regions reminiscent of the condition in bony fishes. There is a rostral or **cephalic lobe** and a **caudal lobe** in the pars distalis, and the distribution of cell types in these lobes is similar to that described for fishes (Table 5-1). The pars tuberalis is well-developed in the Rhynchocephalia, Chelonia, and Crocodilia, but it is greatly reduced and sometimes absent in lizards. In adult snakes, the pars tuberalis is completely absent. There is no explanation for this apparent disappearance of the pars tuberalis in squamates.

Although the intermediate lobes of many lizards and burrowing snakes are markedly reduced or absent, some reptiles have well-developed intermediate lobes. It is especially elaborate in certain chelonians, crocodilians, snakes, and anoline lizards.

C. Birds

The avian HP system differs from that of other tetrapods (and fishes) in that the pars intermedia is absent in adults of all species, a condition seen in many reptiles as well. A well-developed pars tuberalis is present, and the pars distalis consists of cephalic and caudal lobes homologous to those described for reptiles (Figure 5-12).

Unlike mammals, the primary capillaries of the portal system in birds lie superficially or in grooves on the surface rather than penetrating the pars tuberalis to form the complex vascular bed seen in mammals.

The hypophysiotropic region of the hypothalamus supplies aminergic and peptidergic fibers to the median eminence. The region anterior and dorsal to the optic chiasm is occupied by the medial anterior POA, a dorsal PON, SCN, PVN, and SON (Figure 5-11). As in reptiles and mammals, the SON and the PVN are primarily responsible for secretion of the nonapeptide neurohormones. Immunoreactive oCRH also has been localized in the PVN. The hypothalamus itself includes the anterior and lateral hypothalamic areas, paraventricular organ, and an IFN (= ARC).

Two sexually dimorphic brain regions are known for birds. In quail, the males exhibit a larger medial preoptic nucleus (mPON) with greater levels of aromatase activity. This nucleus is innervated by both AVT and catecholaminergic neurons and controls male copulatory behavior. Testosterone blood levels are responsible for activating this center, but the testosterone must be converted to estradiol to have any effect. Administration of either steroid, then, can induce male copulatory behavior. Any reduction in circulating testosterone levels such as would occur following castration or placement of the birds on a non-stimulatory photoperiod (short days) results in regression of the mPON. The second sexually dimorphic region is the song control region of passerine (song) birds which is larger in males that do the majority of singing. In wrens that sing duets, there is no marked difference in this region whereas there is a marked difference in one species of wren in which only the male sings. Although clearly a sex-related phenomenon, it is not clear that this dimorphism has a hormonal basis.

In some birds (i.e., the pigeon, the Japanese quail, and the white-crowned sparrow), the median eminence is separable into an anterior neurohemal area and a more posterior neurohemal area similar to that described for elasmobranchs. Each of these areas has its own portal connection to the pars distalis, which consists of a cephalic and a caudal lobe. It is not certain how widespread this phenomenon of two media eminentia is among other avian species. However, such potential regionalization of both the median eminence and the pars distalis could represent a mechanism to increase the efficiency of delivery of hypothalamic neurohormones to cell types regionalized in various parts of the pars distalis (Table 5-1). This neurovascular specialization is analogous to the system of direct innervation of pars distalis cells that was observed in teleosts.

III. Tropic Hormones of Non-Mammalian Vertebrates

The same categories of tropic hormones are found in non-mammals as were discussed for mammals in Chapter 4. Each category represents a gene family. Category I includes the glycoprotein hormones LH, FSH, and TSH. Growth hormone (GH) and PRL as well as **somatolactin (SL)** in teleosts constitute hormones of Category II, and the derivatives of **proopiomelanocortin (POMC)** represent Category III (ACTH, α-MSH, CLIP, endorphins).

A. Category I: Gonadotropins (GTHs) and Thyrotropin (TSH)

Purified GTHs isolated from non-mammalian species are similar to those of mammals. Mammalian GTHs have been examined extensively for activity in lower vertebrates (see reading list at end of this chapter). Generally, the hormonal control of reproduction involves two GTHs with LH-like and FSH-like activities. The apparent failure to find two GTHs in squamate reptiles may be due to derived secondary reliance on only one GTH with synthesis of the other repressed. Specific activity for both mammalian FSH and LH in non-mammals may be related to biological half-life differences between the two hormones when they are examined *in vivo* and emphasizes the need for good *in-vitro* bioassays in a variety of vertebrates comparing mammalian and non-mammalian GTHs.

It was proposed a number of years ago that the most primitive glycoprotein hormone was an LH-like molecule. Later, the LH gene duplicated and became modified to produce a TSH-like hormone. FSH presumably diverged even later from TSH. Support for this hypothesis was based in part on observations of inherent thyroid-stimulating activity of mammalian LHs tested in more primitive vertebrates. However, Category I tropic hormones have now been isolated from an array of jawed fish groups and all of the tetrapod groups, and the β-subunits have been examined for homologies. TSHβ, LHβ, and FSHβ subunits cluster regardless of the species from which they are derived (Figure 5-15). Furthermore, LHβ and FSHβ appear to be more closely related with TSHβ subunits forming a separate cluster. This relationship is in keeping with the hypothesis that the ancestral LHβ gene underwent duplication and one form diverged into a TSHβ gene. Following a second genome duplication, another copy of the LHβ gene mutated into the FSHβ. This later creation of the FSHβ gene would have had less time to diverge from the LHβ gene than the TSHβ gene has had. Within each glycoprotein type, then, the species separate according to their phylogenetic history. The single exception seems to be the LHβ isolated from tilapia (teleost) that is more like the TSHβ subunits of other vertebrate groups than it is like other LHβ subunits.

1. Gonadotropins (GTHs) in Agnathan Fishes

Physiological and immunocytochemical evidence indicates GTHs are present in the proximal pars distalis of the lamprey, but only recently have Hiroshi Kawauchi and Stacia Sower using cDNA cloning techniques identified a putative GTHβ subunit whose expression is stimulated by lamprey GnRH. No data are available for hagfishes.

2. Gonadotropins (GTHs) in Chondrichthyean Fishes

Gonadotropin activity is present in both the proximal pars distalis and the ventral lobe of elasmobranchs. Antibody to mammalian GTHs binds to cells of the ventral lobe. Bioassay of the elasmobranch proximal pars distalis reveals the presence of an LH-like GTH that will stimulate oocyte maturation in the clawed frog *Xenopus laevis*. Both LHβ and FSHβ subunits have been sequenced from a shark (*Scyliorhinus canicula*) and shown to be unique from those of all other gnathostomes.

3. Gonadotropins (GTHs) in Bony Fishes

Early studies of teleost GTHs suggested a single LH-like GTH in teleosts was present. Mammalian FSH appeared to be inactive in teleosts and mammalian LH was able to support the entire reproductive process.

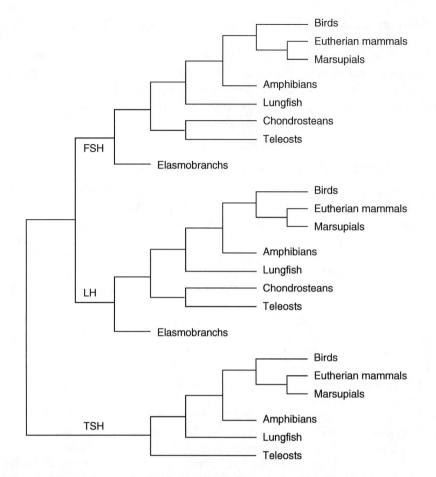

Figure 5-15. **Phylogeny of β-subunit genes for the glycoprotein tropic hormones**. Note that the genes for each tropic hormone form a distinct cluster for all species examined. [Based on studies by Oba, Y., Hirai, T., Yoshiura, Y., Kobayashi, T., and Nagahama, Y. (2001). Fish gonadotropin and thyrotropin receptors: The evolution of glycoprotein hormone receptors in vertebrates. *Comp. Biochem. Physiol. B* **129**, 441–448; Querat, B., Arai, Y., Henry, A., Akama, Y., Longhurst, T. J., and Joss, J. M. P. (2004). Pituitary glycoprotein hormone β subunits in the Australian lungfish and estimation of the relative evolution rate of these subunits within vertebrates. *Biol. Reprod.* **70**, 356–363.]

Furthermore, antibody directed against mammalian LH bound to salmon gonadotropic basophils, but antibody against mammalian FSH did not. GTHs purified from salmon, carp, and rainbow trout were attributed high LH-like activity when tested with the frog spermiation bioassay, as did pituitary extracts prepared from lungfishes. This spermiation reaction, however, subsequently has been shown to respond to highly purified FSH as well as LH and should not have been interpreted as evidence for the exclusive LH nature of teleost gonadotropin. Furthermore, removal of sialic acid, a carbohydrate in higher concentration in mammalian FSH than in LH reduced the activity of salmon GTH prior to its assay in the lizard testicular bioassay (see Appendix D), suggesting salmon GTH has FSH-like properties, too.

More recent analyses of teleost GTH preparations confirmed the presence of two glycoprotein molecules that originally were termed GTH-I and GTH-II. These teleost GTHs consist of α and β subunits like the GTHs of tetrapods. The pituitary content of GTH-I is much greater than GTH-II (e.g., 100X greater in juvenile coho salmon) and is also present in greater amounts in the blood of salmon undergoing vitellogenesis or spermatogenesis. Although both hormones show similar potencies in stimulating steroidogenesis and gamete release *in vitro*, GTH-II apparently is released primarily during the final step of gonadal maturation when it stimulates synthesis of the steroid **17,20β-dihydroxy-4-pregnen-3-one (DHP)**. Initially, DHP was named the **oocyte maturational steroid hormone** but later it was shown to cause spermiation in males, too. Immunocytochemical studies have demonstrated that GTH-I and GTH-II are produced in separate pituitary cell types, and physiological studies show that they functionally resemble mammalian FSH and LH, respectively. Consequently, the terms FSH and LH were adopted at the 6th International Symposium on the Reproductive Physiology of Fishes in 1999 to replace the names GTH-I and GTH-II, respectively. A comparison of GTH receptors also shows that fish FSH receptors are more closely aligned with tetrapod FSH receptors and that fish LH receptors are more like tetrapod LH receptors. These observations further support the validity of using the names "LH" and "FSH" for teleost GTHs.

A non-glycoprotein GTH preparation that stimulated uptake from the blood of protein precursors utilized in yolk synthesis by growing oocytes (i.e., vitellogenesis) has been prepared from pituitaries of a few teleost species. This "GTH" does not consist of subunits like other GTHs, appears to be limited in its distribution among the teleosts, and is of uncertain significance.

4. Gonadotropins (GTHs) in Amphibians

Two distinct GTHs have been isolated and purified from several urodeles and anurans. Purified bullfrog LH and FSH both stimulated spermatogenesis and spermiation in bullfrogs, but only bullfrog LH elevated plasma androgen levels. Some species specificity is associated with these GTHs. For example, salamander (*Ambystoma*) LH was not as effective as bullfrog LH in raising plasma androgen levels in bullfrogs. Conversely, *Ambystoma* LH was more effective than bullfrog LH in *Ambystoma*, although the latter was considerably more effective than *Ambystoma* FSH.

Bullfrog LH is more effective than ovine LH in stimulating progesterone synthesis in amphibians. Bullfrog LH also stimulates reptilian and avian thyroids, emphasizing the structural closeness of LH and TSH molecules and their actions.

These studies reveal that non-mammalian GTHs can be expected to differ markedly in structure and function both when compared to their mammalian counterparts and among more closely related species. Caution must be applied before assuming an LH of species-X will be more LH-like in its action when tested in species-Y or that a molecule labeled as an LH can even be called that when applied to another species where it might induce FSH-like effects. This diversity in action may be due in part to variability in receptor structures that might recognize different regions of these molecules or respond to subtle changes in shape of the same region due to variations in amino acid sequences.

5. Gonadotropins (GTHs) in Reptiles

Studies employing injections of mammalian hormones into squamate reptiles have emphasized a role for FSH-like GTHs but suggest no role for LH-like hormones. Earlier data might be interpreted as a consequence of a very short biological half-life for injected mammalian LH or that mammalian FSH might be similar enough to both a squamate FSH and LH to possess both activities. Purification of gonadotropic activity from squamate reptiles, however, has verified that only one FSH-like molecule is present, although both FSH-like and LH-like GTHs have been isolated from chelonians and crocodilians. Presence of only one molecular species of GTH in squamates does not rule out the possibility that this molecule has intrinsic FSH-like and LH-like activities. Since both FSH- and LH-like GTHs are found in other reptiles, the squamate condition is probably secondarily derived and does not represent a primitive condition.

There is great variability in the responses of reptilian tissues to GTHs purified from different vertebrate groups. Testicular weight maintenance in hypophysectomized *Anolis carolinensis* is readily maintained by FSH-like hormones purified from mammals, birds, reptiles or amphibians, but this testicular parameter is very insensitive to LH-like gonadotropins from any source. Nevertheless, plasma androgen levels in hypophysectomized *A. carolinensis* may be elevated by either FSH-like or LH-like GTHs from almost any source. Similar effects on plasma levels of androgens or on androgen synthesis by minced testes *in vitro* have been observed for crocodilians. The situation in chelonians is not clear as testes of some species do not respond to LH-like hormones *in vitro*, whereas at least one species (*Chrysemys picta*) does respond to *in-vivo* injections of mammalian LH but not as well as it responds to mammalian FSH. The reptilian ovary, like the testis, exhibits broad sensitivity to mammalian and other FSHs and LHs. FSHs are generally the most effective GTHs in reptiles, although there are some conflicting reports regarding this point.

6. Gonadotropins (GTHs) in Birds

Birds conform to the typical mammalian pattern of two GTHs, LH, and FSH, although avian species are rather insensitive to mammalian FSH and LH preparations. Two separate GTHs have been extracted and partially purified from domestic galliform birds. However, studies of the duck support existence of only one GTH.

Chicken LH stimulates interstitial cells in the testis of chickens or Japanese quail, and the seminiferous tubules are stimulated by chicken FSH. Mammalian LH and avian LH are reported to be more effective than FSHs in stimulating androgen production by chicken interstitial cells *in vitro*. Some conflicting reports suggest that avian FSH and LH are more nearly equal in their actions on minced pigeon or chicken testes, however. Reptilian LH is more effective than reptilian FSH in stimulating androgen production by the avian testis. Purified amphibian GTHs (both LH-like and FSH-like) are equally effective, although their overall activity in birds is low.

7. Thyrotropin (TSH) in Vertebrates

Mammalian TSHs have been shown to stimulate thyroid function in representatives of all vertebrate groups although it is ineffective in hagfishes. Similarly, pituitary extracts from most non-mammals exhibit TSH-like activity when tested in mammals. The specific actions of TSH on non-mammalian thyroid glands and the functions of thyroid hormones in non-mammals are similar to those for mammals (see Chapters 4 and 7). Although non-mammalian TSHs have not been studied to the extent that non-mammalian GTHs have, it is apparent that β-subunits of teleosts, amphibians, and birds cluster with mammalian TSH β-subunits and are distinctly separate from vertebrate GTH β-subunits (Figure 5-15). Interestingly, the TSH β-subunit from sturgeon is more like those of tetrapods than like several species of teleosts. Furthermore, TSH receptors isolated from amago salmon cluster with tetrapod TSH receptors and not fish or tetrapod GTH receptors. Purified bullfrog TSH is thyrotropic in both anurans and caudate amphibians but is ineffective on thyroids of reptiles and birds.

B. Category II Tropic Hormones: Prolactin (PRL) and Growth Hormone (GH)

As discussed in Chapter 4, PRL and GH are chemically very similar molecules. This similarity in structure has resulted in considerable confusion about the actions of these hormones in non-mammals, especially when based on the observations of treating non-mammals with mammalian PRL and GH.

PRL has more than 300 different actions in vertebrates and it is almost impossible to characterize this hormone (see "Suggested Reading" at the end of chapter). Many of the reported actions of PRL (Table 5-3) may be grouped into six general categories: (1) water and electrolyte balance; (2) growth and development; (3) metabolism; (4) behavior; (5) reproduction; and (6) immunoprotection.

The most primitive role for PRL is the regulation of osmotic-ionic balance, with the other actions being acquired later among vertebrates during evolution. Certainly, the major role for PRL in teleosts is related to osmotic regulation in fresh water. Even in humans, PRL has osmoregulatory actions in development, and release of PRL can be induced following alterations in blood osmotic pressure. Regardless of the multiplicity of roles or even the establishment that it may be primarily an osmoregulatory hormone, the name "prolactin" for this hormone is here to stay.

PRL provides an excellent example for demonstrating the evolution of endocrine systems. There have been evolutionary changes in the structure of the PRL molecule as evidenced by the failure of fish PRLs to work in avian and mammalian bioassays, although mammalian PRLs retain piscine activity (see Appendix D). The antigenic portion of piscine PRLs is similar to mammals as evidenced by the binding of mammalian PRL antibodies to the lactotropes of the piscine rostral pars distalis. Furthermore, new PRL target tissues have evolved (for example, the crop sac of birds and the mammary glands of mammals) that possess receptors specific for the "newer" portions of the molecules. This is evidenced by the failure of the piscine PRLs to activate responses in avian and mammalian tissues. It is unfortunate that there are no bioassays employing reptilian tissues and that purified reptilian PRLs are not available to fill in this part of the evolutionary changes that appear to be supported by studies with the bioassays of the other major groups.

Mammalian GHs are effective in most non-mammals, and most non-mammalian preparations exhibit GH activity in mammals. The differences among vertebrate GHs are exemplified by their varied effectiveness when

Table 5-3. Prolactin Actions in Non-Mammalian Vertebrates

Actions related to reproduction
  Teleosts
    Skin mucous secretion (e.g., discus "milk")
    Reduction of toxic effects of estrogen
    Growth and secretion of seminal vesicles
    Parental behavior (nest building, fin fanning, buccal incubation of eggs)
    Maintenance of brood pouch in male seahorse
    Gonadotropic
  Amphibians
    Water drive (prior to reproduction)
    Secretion of oviductal jelly
    Spermatogenic and/or antispermatogenic
    Ovulation
    Stimulation of cloacal gland development
  Reptiles
    Antigonadotropic
  Birds
    Production of crop "milk"
    Formation of brood patch
    Antigonadal
    Premigratory restlessness
    Parental behavior
    Synergism with steroids on female reproductive tract
    Suppression of sexual phase of reproductive cycle
Actions related to growth and development
  Teleosts
    Proliferation of melanocytes
    Growth of seminal vesicles
    Renal glomerular growth, tubule stimulation and proliferation
  Amphibians
    Tail and gill growth
    Limb regeneration
    Proliferation of melanophores
    Structural changes accompanying water drive
    Brain growth in tadpoles
    Cloacal gland development
    Ultimobranchial stimulation
  Reptiles
    Tail regeneration
    Skin sloughing
  Birds
    Proliferation of pigeon crop sac mucosa
    Epidermal hyperplasia in brood patch
    Feather growth
    Development of female reproductive tract
Actions related to water and electrolyte balance
  Cyclostomes
    Electrolyte metabolism in hagfish
  Teleosts
    Survival of hypophysectomized euryhaline freshwater species
    Restoration of water turnover in hypophysectomized *Fundulus kansae*
    Restoration of plasma Na^+ and Ca^{2+} in hypophysectomized eels when given with cortisol
    Skin, buccal, and gill mucus secretion
    Reduced gill Na^+ efflux (reduced permeability)
    Reduced gill permeability to water
    Inhibition of gill Na^+/K^+-ATPase
    Renotropic action (increased glomerular size)
    Increased urinary water elimination and decreased salt excretion
    Stimulation of renal Na^+/K^+-ATPase
    Decreased water absorption and increased Na^+ absorption in flounder bladder
    Decreased salt and water absorption from eel gut

continues

Table 5-3.—*Continued*

Actions related to water and electrolyte balance (cont.)
  Amphibians
    Skin and electrolyte changes associated with water drive, metamorphosis
    Sodium and water transport across toad bladder
    Restoration of plasma Na^+ in hypophysectomized newts
    Possible hypercalcemia in toads
  Reptiles
    Restoration of plasma Na^+ levels in hypophysectomized lizard
  Birds
    Stimulation of nasal (orbital) salt gland secretion
Actions on integumentary structures
  Teleosts
    Reduced gill Na^+ efflux
    Reduced gill permeability to water
    Inhibition of gill Na^+/K^+-ATPase
    Restoration of water turnover in hypophysectomized *Fundulus kansae*
    Skin, buccal, and gill mucus secretion
    Melanogenesis and proliferation of melanocytes (synergism with MSH)
    Dispersal of yellow pigment in cutaneous xanthophores (?)
    Maintenance of brood pouch in male seahorse
  Amphibians
    Skin changes associated with water drive
    Proliferation of melanophores
    Effects on toad bladder
    Skin yellowing in frogs
  Reptiles
    Epidermal sloughing
  Birds
    Production of crop "milk"
    Formation of brood patch
    Stimulation of feather growth
    Stimulation of nasal gland secretion
Actions on steroid-dependent targets or synergisms with steroids on targets
  Cyclostomes
    Electrolyte metabolism in hagfish
  Teleosts
    Na^+ retention by gills (corticosteroids)
    Na^+ retention by kidney (corticosteroids)
    Salt and water movement in gut (corticosteroids)
    Synergism with androgens on catfish seminal vesicles
    Dispersal of yellow pigment in xanthophores (corticosteroids) (?)
    Maintenance of brood pouch in male seahorse (corticosteroids)
  Amphibians
    Stimulation of oviductal jelly secretion (estrogens and progestogens)
    Na^+ transport across anuran bladder (aldosterone)
    Water-driven structural changes (sex steroids)
    Spermatogenesis (androgens)
    Cloacal gland development (androgens)
  Reptiles
    Restoration of plasma Na^+ levels in hypophysectomized lizard (corticosteroids)
    Antigonadotropic actions (sex steroids?)
  Birds
    Formation of brood patch (synergism with ovarian or testicular steroids)
    Parental behavior (possible progesterone synergism)
    Synergism with estrogens and progestogens on female reproductive tract
    Stimulation of nasal (orbital) gland secretion (corticosteroids)
    Stimulation of feather growth (sex steroids in some species)
    Antigonadotropic actions (sex steroids?)

tested in a single system such as the rat tibia bioassay (see Appendix D). Comparative functional studies are hampered further by the structural similarity of GH and PRL. For example, PRL has clear growth-promoting actions in larval amphibians.

Structural analyses of GHs from fishes and tetrapods suggest a molecular phylogeny that recognizes a distinct dichotomy with most teleosts diverging from other bony fishes and from the tetrapods (Figure 5-16). Interestingly, lungfish GH and amphibian GH form a separate cluster. GH has been characterized from adult sea lampreys and shown to stimulate insulin-like growth factor (IGF) mRNA production in the lamprey liver as it does in mammals (see Chapter 4). The confirmation of a GH gene in lampreys together with the absence of assayable PRL suggests that GH is the most primitive member of Category II tropic hormones and that PRL appeared subsequent to a gene duplication. IGF genes have been cloned from a hagfish, the cephalochordate amphioxus, and a tunicate although GH has been identified only in the hagfish. The crocodilians and birds form a subcluster distinct from other tetrapods. Primate GHs are distinctly mammalian and do not appear to be closely related structurally to non-mammalian hormones.

1. Category II Hormones (PRL & GH) in Agnathans and Chondrichthyeans

Antibodies to mammalian PRLs don't work very well in hagfishes or lampreys, and only negative bioassays for PRL have been obtained from hagfish pituitaries. However, lamprey pituitaries do contain bioassayable PRL, based on responses observed in the xanthophore-expanding *Gillichthyes* bioassay (see Appendix D). Similarly, testing of pituitary extracts from elasmobranchs in the *Gillichthyes* bioassay indicates PRL activity in the rostral pars distalis. No bioassays of holocephalan pituitaries have been reported.

The presence of a GH gene has been identified in the sea lamprey where it also has been shown to stimulate IGF production in lamprey liver. GH also has been isolated and characterized from sharks and is structurally unique from lungfish GH and the GHs of several teleosts. IGF activity also has been demonstrated for two sharks, *Squalus acanthias* and *Mustelus canis*, although no definite link to GH has been established.

2. Category II Hormones (PRL, GH, and SL) in Bony Fishes

As mentioned previously, PRL plays an important role in osmotic regulation in freshwater teleosts (Table 5-3). PRL has been shown to alter ion and water movements in gill, kidney, intestine, urinary bladder, and skin. It also stimulates mucus secretion by gill, intestine, and skin. Mucus secretion and aspects of parental care by both male and female blue discus fish, *Symphysodon aequifasciata*, is stimulated by PRL, and this mucus is used by their offspring as a food source. Additionally, PRL has been implicated in male parental behavior by bluegill sunfish, *Lepomis machrochirus*, and three-spined sticklebacks, *Gasterosteus aculeatus*.

Several teleost PRLs and lungfish PRL have been purified. Teleost PRLs have little biological activity in amniote bioassays, but they work well in amphibians and teleost biooassays (see Appendix D). Purified PRLs prepared from teleosts are all missing the N-terminal disulfide bond that characterizes PRLs from sturgeon, lungfishes, and all tetrapods (Figure 4-16). Hence, teleost GHs structurally resemble mammalian GH more closely than mammalian PRL (see fish hormone in Figure 5-17 and compare to hormones in Figure 4-16). Furthermore, two PRL genes and hence two separate forms of PRL are present in teleosts, no doubt another reflection of the second genome duplication believed to have occurred early in teleost evolution.

Mammalian GHs are very active in promoting growth of fishes, and polypterid, chondrostean, holostean, and teleost pituitaries exhibit GH activity in the mammalian tibia bioassay (see Appendix D). Additionally, there is a marked influence of thyroid hormones on growth in teleosts. Thyroid hormones accelerate growth in fishes, and thyroid hormone treatment restores growth rates to normal in radiothyroidectomized rainbow trout (see Chapter 7). Although it has not been demonstrated conclusively, it is reasonable to assume a synergistic relationship between thyroid hormones and GHs similar to that reported for mammals. Androgens also produce a positive effect on growth of salmonid fishes, suggesting a protein anabolic action for these steroids that is probably independent of the action of GH.

GH secretion correlates directly with induction of IGF-I mRNA in livers of growing coho salmon, and similar relationships between GH and IGF-I levels have been reported for rainbow trout, long-jawed mudsucker (*Gillichthyes*), and Japanese eels (*Anguilla*). Transfer of juvenile coho salmon prematurely into seawater decreases IGF-I levels and growth although GH levels increase. In coho salmon, GH appears to be important

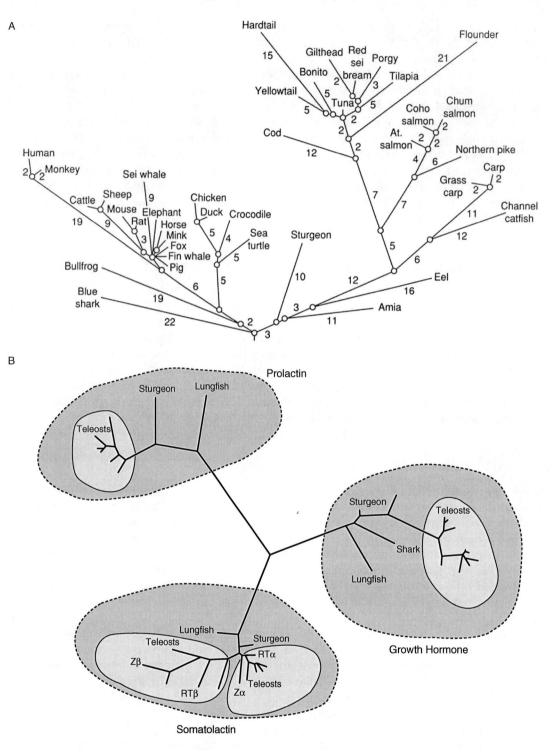

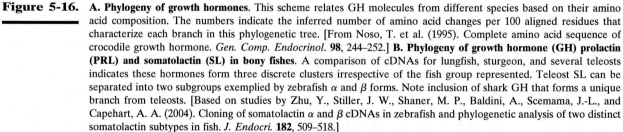

Figure 5-16. **A. Phylogeny of growth hormones.** This scheme relates GH molecules from different species based on their amino acid composition. The numbers indicate the inferred number of amino acid changes per 100 aligned residues that characterize each branch in this phylogenetic tree. [From Noso, T. et al. (1995). Complete amino acid sequence of crocodile growth hormone. *Gen. Comp. Endocrinol.* **98**, 244–252.] **B. Phylogeny of growth hormone (GH) prolactin (PRL) and somatolactin (SL) in bony fishes.** A comparison of cDNAs for lungfish, sturgeon, and several teleosts indicates these hormones form three discrete clusters irrespective of the fish group represented. Teleost SL can be separated into two subgroups exemplified by zebrafish α and β forms. Note inclusion of shark GH that forms a unique branch from teleosts. [Based on studies by Zhu, Y., Stiller, J. W., Shaner, M. P., Baldini, A., Scemama, J.-L., and Capehart, A. A. (2004). Cloning of somatolactin α and β cDNAs in zebrafish and phylogenetic analysis of two distinct somatolactin subtypes in fish. *J. Endocri.* **182**, 509–518.]

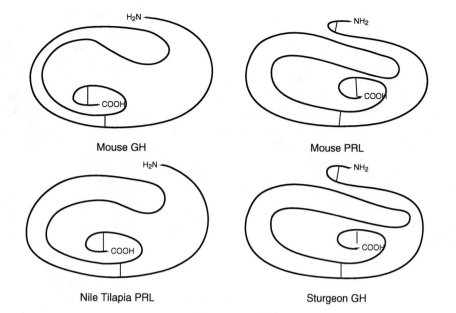

Figure 5-17. Comparison of teleost prolactin (PRL) and growth hormone (GH) to mammalian forms.

for seawater adaptation although it does not seem to be important in adaptation to seawater by young tilapia. IGF-binding proteins are described for several species, and GH-binding proteins have been characterized from rainbow trout. These observations suggest that involvement of GH and IGF-I in growth of teleosts is similar to mammals.

Madeleine Olivereau in France correlated the cytological appearance of PIPAS cells in the pars intermedia of teleosts with low-calcium environments and named them **calcium-sensitive cells.** In the early 1990s, a new teleost hormone was reported by M. Ono and associates from the pars intermedia of Japanese flounder (*Paralichthys olivaeus*) and by Marilyn Rand-Weaver and coworkers from the Atlantic cod, *Gadus morhua*. The new hormone was named **somatolactin (SL)** because it was similar in structure to both GH and PRL. SL was shown by immunocytochemistry in several teleosts to reside in the PIPAS cells. In salmonids, such as the rainbow trout (*Oncorhynchus mykiss*), which lack cells with PIPAS features, there are non-PIPAS cells in the pars intermedia that bind antibodies to SL. These SL-immunoreactive cells are stimulated cytologically by placing rainbow trout in low-calcium environments and are cytologically repressed when the fish are in high-calcium environments.

SL has been shown to produce effects on pigment cells, calcium balance, reproduction, and metabolism of phosphate and lipid. Rising plasma levels of SL also have been correlated with smolting of seaward-migrating salmonids as well as with gonadal maturation. Plasma SL peaks at spawning in Pacific salmon (*Oncorhynchus keta, O. kisutch, O. nerka*) and in *Mugil cephalus* although it is not known if these correlations are related to metabolism or to reproductive functions. Furthermore, SL stimulates steroidogenesis in ovarian or testicular fragments isolated from coho salmon, although SL is less potent in this regard than is FSH. This possible steroidogenic role for SL is similar to effects reported for exogenous GH and PRL in several teleosts and suggests the action of these latter hormones may be a reflection of their chemical similarity to SL.

Isolation and characterization of SLs from diverse teleost species have identified two subfamilies of SL. Some species exhibit only one type whereas others have both an SLα and an SLβ. The discovery of these dissimilar SL genes may explain in part the diversity of functions so far ascribed to SLs. Genes similar to SLα have been cloned from sturgeon (chondrostean) and the African lungfish, and there is evidence for SL in a shark as well.

3. Category II Hormones (PRL & GH) in the Amphibians

PRLs from most amphibians cross-react with antibody to rat GH, and amphibian PRL is thought by some to be the larval GH of amphibians. Tiger salamanders were the only animals tested whose PRL did not cross-react with rat GH antibody. In addition to possible influences on larval growth, PRL is anti-metamorphic in both anurans and caudate amphibians; that is, it blocks metamorphosis from the aquatic larva to the semi-terrestrial or terrestrial juvenile form. Nevertheless, some PRL also is essential for normal metamorphosis (see Chapter 7). PRL induces water-driven behavior in newts and salamanders (see ahead) and influences secondary sexual characters associated with breeding. Integumentary effects of PRL related to water balance have been observed on the skin of newts and salamanders indicating that PRL affects water balance in anurans and caudate amphibians as it does in fishes. Japanese workers have isolated amphibian PRLs and developed specific radioimmunoassays for studying possible functions of PRL in activities such as breeding migrations.

The assessment of GHs in amphibians is complicated by the observation that PRL may be a larval growth hormone, whereas GH *per se* may operate only in transformed or metamorphosed individuals. Both GH and PRL have been isolated from frogs, *R. catesbeiana* and *R. pipiens*. The large number of similarities in the physical properties of amphibian and mammalian GHs and the similarities in amino acid composition suggest that there has been considerable conservatism expressed in the evolution of tetrapod GHs. Purified frog GHs are not as effective as bovine GH in the rat tibia bioassay, however (see Appendix D).

IGF activity has been demonstrated in *Bufo woodhousei* and *Xenopus laevis*, but no link to either PRL or GH has been established. This is an important area that demands more attention in all non-mammalian groups.

4. Category II Hormones (PRL & GH) in the Reptiles

The reptiles are the only major vertebrate group in which a PRL bioassay has not been developed, and little work has been done with PRL in reptiles. Mammalian PRL stimulates growth in juvenile snapping turtles, *Chelyldra serpentina*, and lizards, *Lacerta s. sicula*. Appetite is also stimulated in *Lacerta* by PRL. A possible effect on water balance has been reported in turtles in which PRL influenced glomerular filtration. Purified reptilian PRLs give positive responses in other vertebrate bioassays (Appendix D), and this PRL activity appears to be confined to the cephalic (rostral) lobe of the pars distalis.

Mammalian GH, like PRL, stimulates growth in juvenile snapping turtles and in the lizard *Lacerta* although the sites of action for GH and PRL in the lizard appear to be different. Growth hormone stimulates appetite in *Lacerta*, as reported for PRL, and also produces a marked increase in growth of the digestive tract (**splanchnomegaly**), an action reported for PRL in other vertebrate groups.

Purified GH has been prepared from the caudal lobe of adult snapping turtle pituitaries and sea turtles. Many characteristics of these GHs are similar to those of other tetrapods. Turtle GHs are very effective in the rat tibia bioassay. Crocodilian GH is structurally closer to GH isolated from birds than to other reptiles (Figure 5-16).

5. Category II Hormones (PRL & GH) in Birds

PRL and GH have been isolated from domesticated birds (e.g., chicken, duck, turkey, Japanese quail). The amino acid composition and electrophoretic properties of chicken PRL are similar to mammalian PRLs. Chicken PRL is structurally and functionally distinct from chicken GH.

GH activity has been demonstrated in pituitaries of chickens and turkeys by means of the mouse tibia bioassay. However, antibovine GH antibody apparently does not cross-react with chicken pituitary extracts nor does purified GH from duck pituitaries cross-react with rat GH antibody. These observations suggest unique differences in bird GHs that are probably more similar to crocodilian GH than to mammalian GHs.

PRL plays several essential roles in avian reproduction. The first established role for PRL in birds was the stimulation of a nutritious, cytogenous secretion by the pigeon crop sac called **crop milk** that was coughed up and fed to young birds. This led C. S. "Karl" Nicoll to develop the first non-mammalian bioassay for PRL, the **crop sac bioassay** (Appendix D). A second reproductive role for PRL in some birds is the development of a **brood patch**, a ventral portion of the body that becomes defeathered and highly vascularized during breeding. This region is is used for transferring warmth during incubation of the eggs. Richard E. Jones showed that estrogens synergize with PRL in formation of the brood patch. Elevated PRL is associated with males in a number of bird species where these males exhibit considerable parental care. A third role for PRL is to stimulate premigratory fattening and induction of migratory restlessness in birds. This restless behavior or

Zugunruhe appears just prior to the actual migration of many north temperate bird species. PRL secretion has also been implicated in the induction of photorefractoriness in migratory birds (see Chapter 11).

C. Category III Tropic Hormones: The POMC Group

As in mammals, ACTH-, α-MSH-, CLIP-, and endorphin-like peptides are all derived from the same precursor, POMC, as discussed in Chapter 4. In corticotropes of non-mammals, POMC, is hydroylzed to yield ACTH and β-endorphin whereas in the melanotrope the end products are α-MSH, CLIP, and β-endorphin. Furthermore, the occurrence of *N*-acetylation of α-MSH and β-endorphin is similar to mammals. The presence of additional peptide sequences with melanotropin activity (i.e., β-MSH and γ-MSH) has proven useful in examining phylogenetic relationships although, as discussed in Chapter 4, only α-MSH probably has a bioregulatory role.

Although there is considerable variation in the composition of POMC within each major group of gnathostome vertebrates (Figure 5-18), the ancestral gnathostome gene form is found in at least some members of each group. The POMC complex of tetrapods has not been so closely examined as in the fishes with respect to evolution of POMC. Robert Dores, Hiroshi Kawauchi, Stacia Sower, and others have focused on the evolution of this complex group of bioregulatory peptides in fishes. Analysis of POMC sequences identifies three major groupings among the fishes: the chondrichthyeans, the lungfishes, and the ray-finned bony fishes (Figure 5-19). In this latter grouping, chondrostean (sturgeons, paddlefishes) POMC separates from holostean (gar) POMC that is in turn distinct from teleost POMC. Teleosts differ from other vertebrates in the absence of the γ-MSH sequence. Elasmobranchs are unique in the possession of yet another MSH-like sequence named δ-MSH. Curiously, the lamprey has been found to have two separate POMC-like genes that result in production of ACTH-like and MSH-like biological activities (see ahead).

1. ACTH Actions in the Fishes

Little is known about ACTH actions in the more primitive fish groups and not much more is known about teleosts. Treatment of lampreys with mammalian ACTH causes cytological changes in the interrenal cells (homologous to the adrenocortical cells of mammals; see Chapter 9) that are suggestive of stimulation. ACTH

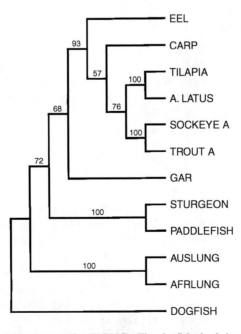

Figure 5-18. **Phylogeny of fish proopiomelanocortins (POMC).** The dogfish shark is used as the outgroup for this comparison. [From Alrubaian, J. (2003). *Gen. Comp. Endocri.* **132**, 384–390.]

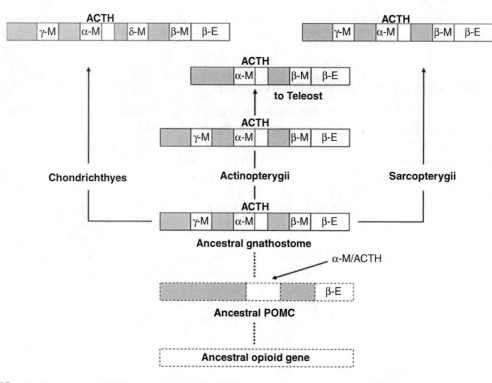

Figure 5-19. Corticotropin (ACTH) and melanotropin (MSHs) evolution. Four forms of MSH (α-M, β-M, γ-M, δ-M) are depicted in this scheme. The sarcopterygian branch would be similar to the tetrapod condition. [From Dores, R. M., and Lecaude, S. (2005). *Gen. Comp. Endocri.* **142**, 81–93.] See color insert, plate 6.

has been purified from lamprey and shark pituitaries, but its effects on interrenal tissue have not been studied. ACTH in teleosts stimulates secretion of cortisol.

2. ACTH Actions in Non-Mammalian Tetrapods

Activity of the steroidogenic enzyme $\Delta^5,3\beta$-hydroxysteroid dehydrogenase (3β-HSD) is enhanced in the bullfrog interrenal following treatment with ACTH. Blood levels of corticosterone are elevated by ACTH treatment and lowered by hypophysectomy in several anuran species. Similar responses of adrenal tissue to ACTH and hypophysectomy are reported for lizards, turtles, and birds. In addition, bird adrenals also respond to PRL and GH as well as to ACTH. In all tetrapods examined, ACTH seems to work through a cAMP-dependent mechanism as it does in mammals.

3. α-MSH Actions in Non-Mammals

Many vertebrates show changes in pigmentation or pigmentary patterns that are correlated with environmental factors or particular events in their life histories. Rapid pigmentary responses are under direct neural control, and the slower responses are generally the result of endocrine control or a combination of neural and endocrine control.

Vertebrates possess a variety of specialized, pigmented cells referred to as **chromatophores** (see Table 5-4). Chromatophores singly or in special combinations are the bases for color patterns associated with the integument. **Physiological color changes** involving displacement of pigment granules within a pigment cell are characteristic of many fishes, amphibians, and some reptiles. However, a physiological role in pigment changes has not been established for α-MSH in fishes where most of their pigment changes apparently are under direct, dual sympathetic-parasympathetic innervation, allowing for very rapid responses. In amphibians and some

Table 5-4. Vertebrate Chromatophores

Chromatophore	Organelle	Pigment	Color
Melanophore	Melanosomes	Melanins	Brown, black (yellow, red)
Iridophore (guanophore, leukophore)	Reflecting platelets	Guanine, adenine, hypoxanthine, uric acid	—
Xanthophore	Pterinosomes	Pteridines	Yellow, orange
	Carotenoid vesicles	Carotenoids	Yellow, orange, red
Erythrophore	Pterinosomes	Pteridines	Red, orange
	Carotenoid vesicles	Carotenoids	Yellow, orange, red

reptiles, α-MSH as well as melatonin influence physiological color changes. All vertebrates exhibit increases in the number of chromatophores and/or increases in the amount of pigment contained within or in the vicinity of the chromatophores in response to α-MSH. This type of color change is termed **morphological color change**.

One of the most important chromatophores of amphibians and some fishes are the dermal **melanophores** which contain melanin granules concentrated in special organelles called **melanosomes** (Figure 5-20). Melanophores differ from **melanocytes** that deposit their melanin products extracellularly (Figure 5-21). When melanosomes are concentrated around the nucleus of the melanophore, the skin appears lighter than when they are dispersed throughout the cytoplasm. The degree of concentration of melanosomes is inversely related to the darkness of the skin (see Appendix D). Coloration patterns in some vertebrates may be determined by the distribution of different types of chromatophores and by the relationship of dermal melanophores to other chromatophores. For example, the dark spots on the skin of the frog *Rana pipiens* are due to concentrations of melanocytes and extracellular deposition of melanin, whereas adjacent regions of the skin that may vary

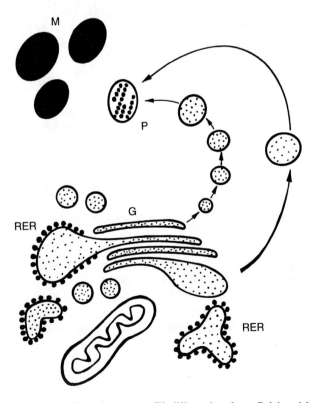

Figure 5-20. **Production of melanosomes.** Premelanosomes (P) differentiate from Golgi vesicles. They exhibit tyrosinase activity and synthesize melanin by polymerizing tyrosine. Once melanization of these organelles is complete, they are called melanosomes (M). RER, rough endoplasmic reticulum.

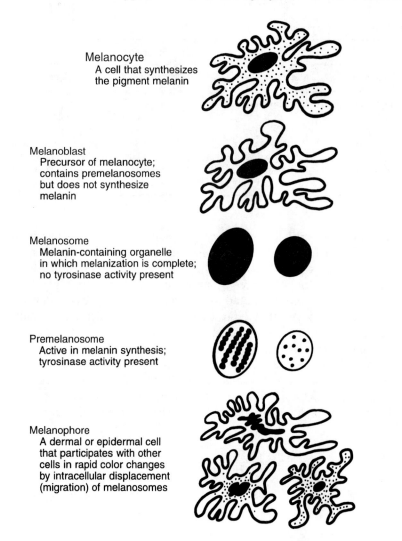

Melanocyte
A cell that synthesizes
the pigment melanin

Melanoblast
Precursor of melanocyte;
contains premelanosomes
but does not synthesize
melanin

Melanosome
Melanin-containing organelle
in which melanization is complete;
no tyrosinase activity present

Premelanosome
Active in melanin synthesis;
tyrosinase activity present

Melanophore
A dermal or epidermal cell
that participates with other
cells in rapid color changes
by intracellular displacement
(migration) of melanosomes

Figure 5-21. **Melanophores and melanocytes.** This terminology is based on the Sixth International Pigment Cell Conference held in 1966. Melanophores can disperse their melanosomes uniformly in the cytoplasm or concentrate them to varying degrees around the nucleus.

from light green to black are occupied exclusively by dermal melanophores and other chromatophores. The green color is produced by interactions of other chromatophores overlying the melanophores that are masked when the melanosomes are dispersed throughout the cytoplasm of the melanophore.

The dermal melanophore is the major target for α-MSH, and, in a few cases, other chromatophores may be affected. The actual mechanism of how melanosomes migrate in and out of the stellate processes of the melanophore is not completely understood. It appears that microtubules are essential for aggregation of the melanosomes, and these may be activated by α-MSH through the second messenger cAMP. Any experimental treatment known to interfere with microtubule formation, such as application of the drug **colchicine**, blocks melanosome aggregation. Ultrastructural observations, however, in some amphibian melanophores do not support the presence of microtubules oriented properly to cause melanosomes to disperse, and the role of microtubules needs further clarification.

4. MSH-like Activity in Agnathan Fishes

Hagfishes (*Myxinoidea*) show no ability to adapt to different backgrounds, suggesting no role for MSH-like peptides with respect to background adaptation. Early studies show that hypophysectomy of lampreys

(*Petromyzontidae*) produces permanent paling, presumably due to loss of MSH-like activity. In contrast, exogenous α-MSH causes melanosome dispersion in lampreys. Lamprey POMC contains two MSH-like sequences that do not correspond to any of the other vertebrate peptides with MSH-like activity: MSH A and MSH B. Curiously, MSH and ACTH in lampreys are coded by separate genes, a condition seemingly unique among the vertebrates. The prohormone for MSH is designated as POM and gives rise to MSH A and B as well as β-endorphin. The gene *POC* codes for ACTH, a different endorphin molecule, and a unique peptide called **nasohypophysial factor (NHF)**. This latter peptide consists of 121 amino acids, does not resemble any other pituitary peptide, and has no known function at this time. It is first expressed in the olfactory region during development but is confined to the pituitary in adults.

5. α-MSH in Chondrichthyean Fishes

Sharks adapt to background changes very slowly, requiring up to 100 hours to achieve maximal adaptation. Hypophysectomy abolishes this ability to "background adapt," whereas ectopic transplants of the neurointermediate lobe cause permanent darkening regardless of the background upon which the shark is placed. Melanophore responses to MSHs are paralleled by similar responses in xanthophores. In addition to α-MSH, the elasmobranch POMC contains β-MSH and γ-MSH as well as a unique sequence with melanotropic activity named δ-MSH.

6. α-MSH in Bony Fishes: Teleosts

The pigmentary responses of most fishes are under control of direct aminergic innervation of melanophores and other chromatophores (Tables 5-5 and 5-6), and α-MSH does not play a major role in physiological color changes. The melanophores of most species do not respond to either hypophysectomy or exogenous α-MSH, whereas others show only a limited response to α-MSH following denervation of the melanophores. Dispersion of pigments in melanophores of the goldfish *Carassius auratus* and erythrophores of the European minnow *Phoxinus phoxinus* occurs following treatment with α-MSH. In contrast, melanophore dispersion can be induced only in denervated melanophores of the killfish *Fundulus heteroclitus* because of the presence of overriding neural stimuli in intact fish.

α-MSH may play some role in morphological color changes in teleosts. Treatment of xanthic goldfish (goldfish normally lacking any melanophores) with α-MSH stimulates melanophore differentiation

Table 5-5. Drugs Causing Melanosome Dispersion When Injected Subcutaneously in the Opercular Area of the Fish *Scopthalmus aquosus*[a]

Drug	MED[b] (μg)
Serotonin blockers	
LSD-25	0.8
Dibenamine	0.2
Adrenergic blockers	
Dihydroxyergotamine	0.6
Propranolol	6.0
Depressants	
Pentobarbital sodium	80.0
Phenothiazine ataractics	
Chlorpromazine	0.8
Cholinergic substances	
Acetylcholine	No effect up to 500 μg

[a] Modified from Scott, G. T. (1972). The action of psychoactive drugs on pigment cells of lower vertebrates. *In* "Pigmentation: Its Genesis and Biologic Control" (V. Riley, Ed.), pp. 327–342. Appleton-Century-Crofts, New York.

[b] Minimum effective dose (three or four fish responding out of five fish tested).

Table 5-6. Drugs Causing Melanosome Aggregation When Injected Subcutaneously in the Opercular Area of the Fish *Scopthalmus aquosus*[a]

Drug	MED[b] (μg)	After pyrogallol[c] treatment (μg)
Epinephrine	0.04	0.00010
Isoproterenol	0.08	0.00002
Dopamine	0.02	0.02
Dopa	Inactive	Inactive
Phenylephrine	0.0002	0.0004
Melatonin	0.06	0.06
5-HT	0.1	2.0

[a] Modified from Scott, G. T. (1972). The action of psychoactive drugs on pigment cells of lower vertebrates. *In* "Pigmentation: Its Genesis and Biologic Control" (V. Riley, Ed.), pp. 327–342. Appleton-Century-Crofts, New York.

[b] MED, minimum effective dose (three or four fish responding out of five fish tested).

[c] Pyrogallol is an inhibitor of the enzyme catechol *O*-methyltransferase, which inactivates epinephrine and norepinephrine.

and melanogenesis. Hypophysectomy of *F. heteroclitus* causes a reduction in the number of melanophores, and treatment with α-MSH results in an increase in the number of melanophores.

MCH was isolated first from teleost pituitaries before it was demonstrated in mammals. It is a potent cyclic heptadecapeptide (17 amino acids) that causes concentration of teleost melanosomes but, in fact, produces weak melanosome dispersion in amphibian and reptilian melanophores. MCH also blocks ACTH and α-MSH release from teleost pituitaries.

7. α-MSH in Amphibians

Direct control of amphibian melanophores is under endocrine regulation, and there is no evidence for direct innervation of amphibian melanophores with the possible exception of limited neural control in *Rana pipiens*. However, release of α-MSH from the pars intermedia is under neural control in most amphibians.

Pigment organelles of another pigment cell, the **xanthophore**, are normally in an expanded state in most amphibians. In the tree frog *Hyla arenicolor*, however, the xanthophores are normally in an aggregated condition, and they may be dispersed by the application of α-MSH. An endogenous role for α-MSH on xanthophore pigment organelles has not been confirmed nor is it clear how widespread this phenomenon might be.

The aggregation of reflecting platelets in the **iridophore**, another special chromatophore, is stimulated by either cAMP or α-MSH. These iridophores possess α- and β-adrenergic receptors, and stimulation of the α-receptors produces dispersion of the reflecting platelets of the iridophore. These data suggest a possible role for catecholamines in iridophore regulation.

As mentioned earlier, MCH is present in the anuran brain, but no melanin-concentrating action has been demonstrated. In fact, MCH caused melanohore expansion in several studies. Additional work is needed to elucidate the physiological importance of MCH in amphibians.

8. α-MSH in Reptiles

Reptiles exhibit a variety of mechanisms for regulating dermal pigment cells, including neural and endocrine mechanisms. Unlike the well-established pattern of adrenergic innervation in most amphibians, no innervation of the pars intermedia has been observed at either the light or electron microscopic level in several lizard species. The primitive tuatara of New Zealand, *Sphenodon punctatus*, also exhibits no innervation of the pars intermedia, implying this may be a basic pattern that was established in the earliest of reptiles. Innervation of pigment cells does occur in some reptiles, and pigmentary control of dermal melanophores may be neural, endocrine, or both.

Color changes in the true chameleon *Chameleo pumilis* are under direct neural control, and α-MSH has no effect on the skin chromatophores. Melanophores of the closely related species *Chameleo jacksoni*, however, respond to both α-MSH and ACTH. The opposite extreme is found in the American chameleon, *Anolis carolinensis*, in which there is no general neural control over melanophore responses, and melanosome dispersion can be readily induced *in vitro* by application of α-MSH or cAMP to isolated pieces of *Anolis* skin. However, there is a patch of skin near the eye that darkens in response to catecholamines. Pretreatment with α-adrenergic-blocking agents obliterates the response of *Anolis* melanophores to α-MSH. Horned lizards, in the genus *Phrysonoma*, exhibit both neural and hormonal regulation of melanophores.

Neither xanthophores nor iridophores of *A. carolinensis* show any response to α-MSH. It is not known whether any non-melanin-containing chromatophores of other reptiles show any regulatory control.

9. α-MSH in Birds

Feather pigments (including melanin) are under the control of gonadal, thyroidal, and gonadotropic hormones and seem to be related to the loss of the pars intermedia and α-MSH in birds. The only reported action for α-MSH in birds possibly is related to a developmental action. Embryonic implants of chicken pituitaries cause formation of black feathers where normally only white feathers would develop. This effect can be mimicked by treatment with either α-MSH or ACTH.

D. Endorphins in Non-Mammals

β-endorphin and related molecules are produced by hydrolysis of POMC in the pituitaries of all vertebrates (or from POC or POM in lampreys). Endorphins are usually N-acetylated except in the cartilaginous dogfishes although it is N-acetylated in the ratfish. No physiological role has been established for the pituitary endorphins of non-mammals but it is assumed to have an analgesic action.

IV. Comparative Aspects of Hypothalamic Control of Pituitary Function in Non-Mammals

Numerous studies have documented the distribution of mammalian-like neuropeptides in the brains of non-mammals, but relatively little is known about the functional roles for most of these neuropeptides in non-mammals. In general, there is more plasticity in non-mammals with respect to the actions of neuropeptides that bear specific names related to their roles in mammals. When making comparisons, it is important to bear in mind that hypothalamic control in teleosts is primarily neuroglandular rather than neurovascular as in other fish groups and in tetrapods.

A. Category I: The Glycoprotein Hormones

The focus in studies of glycoprotein hormone regulation has been on the GTHs rather than on thyrotropin. In fact, it has been and continues to be a problem to determine what neuropeptide(s) is(are) the endogenous releaser for TSH in many cases. Consequently, the picture is more complete for GTH release where decapeptides similar or identical to mGnRH-1 are active releasers of GTHs.

1. Control of GTH Release

The embryonic origin of GnRH-secreting cells in non-mammals is similar to that described for mammals in Chapter 4. A considerable body of research has accumulated on the characterization of GnRHs in non-mammals and on their evolutionary relationships. In addition, a physiologically relevant **gonadotropin release-inhibiting hormone (GnIH)** has been discovered recently in birds by Kazoyoshi Tsutsui, George Bentley, and their associates. Chemically, GnIH is an RF-amide dodecapeptide (C-terminal end of the peptide is capped by arginine and phenylalanine, hence RF). This discovery may prove to have a considerable impact on our understandings of reproductive bioregulation in all vertebrates.

Table 5-7. GnRH Amino Acid Sequences

Source	Amino Acid sequence									
	1	2	3	4	5	6	7	8	9	10
Mammal	pE	H	W	S	Y	G	L	R	P	G-NH$_2$
Guinea pig	pE	Y	W	S	Y	G	V	R	P	G-NH$_2$
Chicken I	pE	H	W	S	Y	G	L	Q	P	G-NH$_2$
Frog	pE	H	W	S	Y	G	L	W	P	G-NH$_2$
Seabream[1]	pE	H	W	S	Y	G	L	S	P	G-NH$_2$
Salmon[1]	pE	H	W	S	Y	G	W	L	P	G-NH$_2$
Medaka[1]	pE	H	W	S	F	G	L	S	P	G-NH$_2$
Catfish[1]	pE	H	W	S	H	G	L	N	P	G-NH$_2$
Herring[1]	pE	H	W	S	H	G	L	S	P	G-NH$_2$
Dogfish Shark	pE	H	W	S	H	G	W	L	P	G-NH$_2$
Chicken II	pE	H	W	S	H	G	W	Y	P	G-NH$_2$
Lamprey III	pE	H	W	S	H	N	W	K	P	G-NH$_2$
Lamprey I	pE	H	Y	S	L	E	W	K	P	G-NH$_2$
Chelyosoma[2] I	pE	H	W	S	N	Y	F	L	P	G-NH$_2$
Chelyosoma[2] II	pE	H	W	S	L	C	H	A	P	G-NH$_2$
Ciona[2] I	pE	H	W	S	Y	A	L	S	P	G-NH$_2$
Ciona II	pE	H	W	S	L	A	L	S	P	G-NH$_2$
Ciona III	pE	H	W	S	N	Q	L	T	P	G-NH$_2$
Ciona IV	pE	H	W	S	Y	E	F	M	P	G-NH$_2$
Ciona V	pE	H	W	S	Y	E	Y	M	P	G-NH$_2$
Ciona VI	pE	H	W	S	K	G	Y	S	P	G-NH$_2$
Ciona VII	pE	H	W	S	N	K	L	A	P	G-NH$_2$

[1] teleost
[2] tunicate
[Based on Millar, R. P. (2005). Animal Reproduction. *Sci.* **88**, 5–28 (Elsevier).]

Numerous molecular variants of GnRH have been described in non-mammals including several forms in tunicates (Table 5-7). There are two ways to describe these diverse molecules that have GTH-releasing activity in vertebrates. One system involves simply naming them for the first species in which that molecular variant was discovered (see Table 5-7). The second method is based on the origins of the GnRHs and the pattern of migration they exhibit to their final resting place in the brain (Figure 4-21). In this scheme, GnRH-1 refers to GnRH-secreting cells that migrate from the olfactory epithelium to the preoptic-hypothalamus area and extend their axons to the median eminence. GnRH-2 refers to GnRH cells derived from the midbrain. GnRH-3 cells migrate from the olfactory placode but cease their movement and remain in the telencephalon. A final type, GnRH-4, is unique to advanced teleosts in having a diencephalic origin and limited migration only within that region. GnRH-4 appears to be involved in sexual differentiation but probably not in adult reproduction. The confusing part of this nomenclature scheme is that the same GnRH molecular form may be classified differently in diverse species depending on its distribution. A comparison of the two schemes is illustrated in Figure 4-22. A combination of both schemes is used here (e.g., salmon GnRH regulating pituitary function would be designated as sGnRH-1).

Mammalian GnRH (mGnRH-1) has been isolated from sheep, pigs, rats, mice, and humans as well as from amphibians. Two GnRH variants were found in chickens and were named **chicken-I (cGnRH-I)** and **chicken-II (cGnRH-II)**. These two forms are found in both birds and reptiles with chicken-I being a GnRH-1 and chicken-II being a GnRH-2 in all vertebrates. Teleosts have yielded several different molecular forms of GnRH-1. Salmon proved to have a unique decapeptide (**sGnRH**) that is found in several other teleost species as well. Unique GnRH-1 types were found in catfish (**cfGnRH**) and dogfish shark (**dfGnRH**). Lampreys were found to possess two new variants that were named **lamprey-I** and **lamprey-III (lGnRH-I and III)**. (A third peptide was named lamprey-II but it latter proved not to have GnRH activity.) Two additional teleost forms found in seabream (sb-GnRH) and medaka (md-GnRH) are GnRH-4 molecules. Frequently, more than one GnRH may perform as a GTH releaser when applied exogenously (Table 5-8), but only one is distributed appropriately to release GTHs (i.e., acts as a GnRH-1).

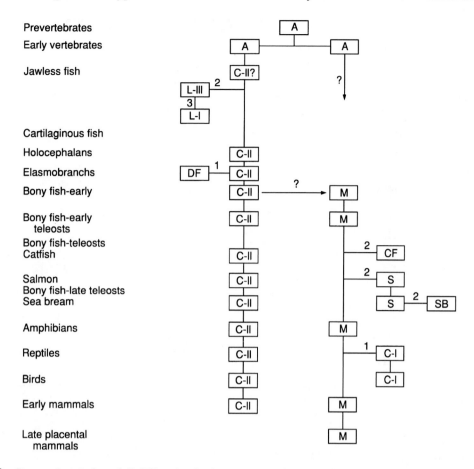

Figure 5-22. **Proposed evolution of GnRH molecules in vertebrates.** This hypothetical scheme focuses on the existence of an ancestral GnRH (A) that was present in the earliest vertebrates that may have undergone an earlier duplication resulting in the chicken-II form (C-II) and a mammalian GnRH (M) or the latter may have arisen from C-II in the early bony fishes. Names for vertebrate GnRHs: C-I, chicken-I; CF, catfish; DF, dogfish shark; L-I, L-III, lamprey forms; S, salmon; SB, sea bream. [From Sherwood, N. M., Parker, D. B., McRory, J. E., and Lescheid, D. W. (1994). Molecular evolution of growth hormone-releasing hormone and gonadotropin-releasing hormone. *In* "Fish Physiology" (N. M. Sherwood and C. L. Hew, Eds.), Vol. 13, pp. 3–66. Academic Press, San Diego.]

The work of Judy King, Robert Millar, and Nancy Sherwood led to a proposal for the evolution of vertebrate GnRH forms involving an early gene duplication and subsequent variation of one gene and relative conservatism of the other (Figure 5-22). This scheme is based in part on the observation that cGnRH-II is found in the midbrain of all gnathostome vertebrates and in part on the structures of the various decapeptides that are found with cGnRH-II and hence is hypothesized to be closest to the ancestral form. Later, following a gene duplication, one form of cGnRH-II gave rise to a second GnRH that became associated with release of pituitary GTHs. This second gene further mutated among teleosts into several forms and later gave rise to the form found in living reptiles and birds. Lampreys and hagfishes may have diverged from the ancestral pattern as evidenced by the presence of unique GnRHs and their unique forms of GnRH should not be considered ancestral forms. Caution must be applied whenever phylogenetic schemes are based upon only a fragment of a gene product, and such analyses should include the analysis of the entire GnRH gene.

The discovery of GnRH-like peptides among a variety of invertebrate species and their association with reproduction certainly has important implications for understanding the evolution of these peptides. Nine GnRH-like molecules have been isolated from tunicates (see Table 5-7), and both chicken and mammalian GnRH-1 stimulated gamete release in the tunicate, *Ciona intestinalis*. GnRH immunoreactive neurons have been identified in mollusks such as *Aplysia* and in a possible chordate ancestor, the hemichordate, *Saccoglossus bromophenolosus*. Exposure of a chitin (*Mopalia*) to either lamprey GnRH-I or tunicate tGnRH-2 dissolved in sea water stimulated gamete release. A GnRH-like molecule has been isolated from *Octopus*,

Table 5-8. Effects of Neural and Endocrine Factors on Gonadotropin Release in Non-Mammalian Vertebrates

Factor[a]	Effect	Teleosts	Amphibians	Reptiles	Birds
Mammalian GnRH	(+) Plasma androgens	×		×	×
Salmon GnRH	(+) GTH release		×	×	
Lamprey GnRH	(+) GTH release	×	○	○	
Dogfish GnRH	(+) GTH release	×			
Chicken GnRH-I	(+) GTH release	×	×	×/○	×
Chicken GnRH-II	(+) GTH release	×		×	
AVT	(+) GTH slightly			×	
DA, DA agonists	(−) Inhibit GTH release	×	×		
Arachidonic acid	(+) GTH release	×			
E_2	(+) Plasma androgens	×			
E_2	(−) GTH release			×	
T	(+) GTH release				×
T	(−) GTH release			×	
P_4, E_2	Enhanced GnRH stimulation of GTH release				×
VIP	(+) GTH release			○	×
TRH	(+) GTH release			○	
Ovine CRH	(+) GTH release			○	
GHRH	(+) GTH release			○	
Morphine	(+) GTH release				○
NPY	(+) GTH release	×			
Serotonin	(+) GTH release	×			

[a] E_2, estradiol; T, testosterone; P_4, progesterone. See text for other abbreviations.
[b] ×, effect; ○, no effect; blank, not tested.

but it is a slightly larger peptide than the traditional decapeptide of GnRH molecules, and its homology is uncertain.

Whereas the number of GnRH molecules present is fewer as we progress from tunicates to mammals, the same reduction seems to be true of GnRH receptors. Receptors for GnRH (GnRH-Rs) are found in several brain regions as well as in the pituitary gland. At least three types (and as many as five in some species) of GnRH-R have been described in teleosts although their distribution and relationship to the different forms of GnRH are not clear. Amphibians have as many as three genes coding for GnRH receptors. Mammals have two GnRH-Rs, but a number of mammals either have lost one of the genes or it has been inactivated (e.g., human, chimpanzees, sheep, cattle, and some rodents).

While searching for RF-amide types of neuropeptides in the avian brain, K. Tsutsui and associates discovered a novel neuropeptide that functions as a GnIH and inhibits GTH release. The first RF-amide peptide discovered was the cardioexcitatory FMRF-amide (Phe-Met-Arg-Phe-NH$_2$) neuropeptide isolated from the ganglia of a mollusk. A longer RF-amide was isolated from quail brain (SIKPSAYLPLRF-amide) that decreased GTH secretion in a dose-dependent manner. GnIH was found to reside principally in the PVN and GnIH-immunoreactive (ir) axons extended to the median eminence. This ir-GnIH peptide also is present in the PVN of seven song bird species. The gene has been cloned that produces a prohormone of 173 amino acids that includes the sequence of GnIH plus two similar related peptide sequences (GnIH-RP1 and GnIH-RP2). This gene also has been characterized in the white-crowned sparrow where the deduced sequence of GnIH is similar to the quail neuropeptide (SIKPFSNLPLRF-amide). Administration of purified GnIH to white crown sparrows decreases GnTH levels in a dose-dependent manner. Additionally, pinealectomy reduces the activity of the GnIH gene and decreases GnIH content of the PVN and the median eminence whereas melatonin restores GnIH levels in pinealectomized birds in a dose-dependent manner.

Numerous neuropeptides, amine neurotransmitters, and steroids have been shown to alter GTH release in vertebrates (see Table 5-8). These amines may operate at the level of the GnRH or GnIH neurons in the brain or at the pituitary. For example, dopamine directly inhibits release of GTHs from the teleost pituitary.

Feedback regulation of GTH release has been demonstrated in non-mammals and resembles that described for mammals. In teleosts, there is evidence for both positive feedback effects and negative feedback effects on GTH secretion depending on the stage of the reproductive cycle. Furthermore, exposure at very low levels (e.g., 0.1 to 1 ng/L) to exogenous natural and synthetic estrogenic compounds, including estradiol and the pharmaceutical **ethynylestradiol** (**EE$_2$**) commonly found in wastewater treatment plant effluents, can inhibit reproductive development in adult teleosts in both laboratory and field experiments, presumably by blocking GTH secretion. Similar observations of steroids on the inhibition of GTH secretion are known for other tetrapods as well.

2. Control of TSH Release

Although mTRH is an effective releaser of TSH in mammals and is present in the brain of all non-mammalian vertebrates examined so far, it is ineffective on TSH release in fishes and larval amphibians. Release of TSH in amphibians, reptiles, and birds is more responsive to mCRH than TRH, and several studies suggest CRH is the "TRH" of larval amphibians, too. Analysis of CRH receptors in a bullfrog and a chicken reveal that thyrotropes possess a different form of CRH receptor (CRH-R2) than are found on corticotropes (CRH-R1). In mammals, CRH has highest affinity for CRH-R1 and CRH-like peptides (e.g., urotensins and urocortins) show higher affinities for CRH-R2. Thus, the molecule we call "TRH" in mammals is probably not the "TRH" of non-mammals.

Experimental evidence suggests that the control of TSH release is less specific in non-mammals. Thyrotropes of non-mammalian tetrapods may release TSH not only in response to TRH and CRH but also to exogenous mGnRH, mGHRH, VIP, and the CRH-like peptides, sauvagine, and urotensin I (see Table 5-9). In chickens, TRH can stimulate TSH as well as GH release and the effect of TRH on both tropic hormones is inhibited by SST.

Teleosts represent an even greater anomaly in the control of TSH release. Not only are they unique among the vertebrates in having neuroglandular control rather than neurovascular control over TSH release, but TSH release is under inhibitory control. The possible significance of this condition is discussed in Chapter 7.

B. Category II: Growth Hormone (GH) and Prolactin (PRL)

Release of both category II tropic hormones are very similar to what has been observed in mammals. Notable exceptions are the neural control of PRL release exhibited in teleosts and the fact that PRL release in birds is entirely under stimulatory control.

Table 5-9. Effects of Neural and Endocrine Factors on Thyrotropin Release in Non-Mammalian Vertebrates

Factor[a]	Effect	Non-mammalian vertebrate group[b]					
				Amphibians			
		Chondrichthyes	Teleosts	Urodeles	Anurans	Reptiles	Birds
TRH	Increases plasma T$_4$			O/×[c]	×[c]	×	
TRH	Stimulates TSH release				×[c]/O	×	×
Ovine CRH	Stimulates TSH release			×	×	×	×
GnRH	Stimulates TSH release	×			×	O	
Mammalian GHRH	Stimulates TSH release				O	×	
DA	Stimulates TSH release					O	
NE	Stimulates TSH release					O	
VIP	Stimulates TSH release					×	×
Sauvagine	Stimulates TSH release					×	
Urotensin I	Stimulates TSH release					×	
SST	Inhibits TSH release		×				

[a] See text for abbreviations.
[b] ×, effect; O, no effect; blank, not tested.
[c] Observed only in metamorphosed adults.

1. Control of GH Release

Release of GH is altered predictably by mammalian hypothalamic neuropeptides (Table 5-10). Treatment of teleosts, amphibians, reptiles, and birds with mGHRH causes release of GH. Similarly, SST inhibits GH release in teleosts, amphibians, reptiles, and birds. Treatment with several other neuropeptides causes GH release including TRH (in amphibians, reptiles, birds), GnRH and NPY (teleosts), and ghrelin (amphibians and birds). The actions of catecholamines on GH release do not show any consistent pattern, and the response varies greatly among the vertebrates. The response to TRH and GHRH in birds can be blocked by IGF treatment, suggesting a negative feedback effect of IGFs may act on avian GH cells.

Soon after GH release was demonstrated in the goldfish following intraperitoneal injections of synthetic hGHRH, immunologically and chromatographically similar molecules were isolated from fishes. Apparently, the prohormone that yields GHRH in fishes also produces a peptide very much like the pituitary adenylate cyclase activating polypeptide (PACAP) described for mammals (see Chapter 4). However, in mammals, PACAP is a product of a separate gene. The mammalian PACAP precursor consists of PACAP and a GHRH-like peptide suggesting it is homologous to the fish GHRH gene. Immunoreactive hGHRH-like material also is present in amphibians, reptiles, and birds, and hGHRH stimulates GH release in frogs, turtles, and chickens. GHRH occurs in the NIV of the frog hypothalamus as well as in numerous areas unrelated to pituitary function. Furthermore, a PACAP-like peptide has been isolated from the frog *Rana esculenta*. The peptide ghrelin also has been shown to stimulate GH release in frogs. The relationship of GHRH-like and PACAP-like molecules in these vertebrate groups will be of special interest as we try to unravel the evolution of these genes.

SST is a GH release inhibitor in non-mammals as it is for mammals. In addition, it plays a paracrine inhibitory role in many peripheral tissues including the endocrine pancreas and the gastrointestinal tract (see Chapter 12). As many as three forms of SST have been isolated from the brains of fishes, and each can inhibit GH release. Furthermore, DA inhibits GH release in fishes under some conditions.

Two forms of SST have been isolated from frogs, and both inhibit hGHRH-stimulated GH release. One form is identical to mammalian SST_{14} (also called SS1) and the other is $[Pro^2, Met^{13}]SST_{14}(= SS2)$. Curiously, SST receptors are distributed throughout the pars distalis whereas somatotropes are limited to the dorsal portion. This suggests other sites of action for SST in the frog pituitary. SST_{14} has been isolated from both the tortoise, *Gophorus agassizii*, and the American alligator and both are identical to mSST.

In birds, both GHRH and TRH stimulate GH release whereas only SST is inhibitory. The release of GH and TSH, which is stimulated by TRH in the chicken, is inhibited by SST. Furthermore, TRH is a better releaser of GH than either GHRH or ghrelin.

Table 5-10. Effects of Neural and Endocrine Factors on Growth Hormone Release in Non-Mammalian Vertebrates

Factor[a]	Effect on growth hormone release	Non-mammalian vertebrate group[b]			
		Teleosts	Amphibians	Reptiles	Birds
Mammalian GHRH	Stimulates GH release	×	×	×	×
TRH	Stimulates GH release		×	×	×
Dogfish shark GnRH	Stimulates GH release	×			
Salmon GnRH	Stimulates GH release	×			
VIP	Stimulates GH release			×	
DA	Stimulates GH release	×		○	
DA	Inhibits GH release	×			
NPY	Stimulates GH release	×			
NE	Stimulates GH release			○/×	
NE	Inhibits GH release	×			
IGF	Suppresses response to TRH and GHRH				×
SST	Inhibits GH release	×	×	×	×
Morphine	Inhibits GH release				×
Serotonin	Inhibits GH release	×			
Ghrelin	Stimulates GH release				×

[a] See text for abbreviations.
[b] ×, effect; ○, no effect; blank, not tested.

2. Control of PRL Release

Observations on the effects of neural factors on PRL release in non-mammals is summarized in Table 5-11. The major control over PRL release seems to be inhibitory except in birds. Dopamine inhibits PRL release in teleosts and amphibians as well as do VIP and hGAP. This latter peptide is also a PRL release inhibitor in mammals. The inhibitory action of VIP in teleosts is somewhat unexpected in light of its stimulatory role in birds and mammals. **Peptide histidine isoleucine (PHI)** is a VIP-like peptide that also inhibits PRL release in teleosts. However, PHI can stimulate TSH release in amphibians. VIP and PHI are chemically related to PACAP and GHRH.

Stimulation of PRL release by TRH occurs in non-mammals as reported for mammals although the major control of PRL release in birds is stimulatory and appears to be under direct control by VIP. If this proves to be a common role for TRH in non-mammals, the abundance of TRH in the brains of non-mammals may be explained, at least in part. The peptide PrRH postulated in mammalian studies as a physiological PRH is present in fishes, and it has been shown to stimulate PRL release from the pituitary gland.

C. Category III: The POMC Group

Although the several peptides of the POMC group have a common precursor, the regulation of ACTH and α-MSH release is entirely different as it was for mammals (Chapter 4). Little is known about the control of endorphin release.

1. Control of ACTH Release

Synthetic oCRH is an effective releaser of ACTH in teleosts, amphibians, and birds (Table 5-12). The distribution of CRH immunoreactivity in reptiles is supportive of a similar role. In teleosts, the CRH-like peptides sauvagine and urotensin-I also can evoke ACTH release, but these CRH-like peptides so far have proven ineffective in amphibians. As in mammals, AVT or AVP also can stimulate ACTH release, but the details of this action have not been substantiated. The appearance of immunoreactive AVT-like material in the pars nervosa, together with CRH in the median eminence of bullfrog larvae at metamorphosis, supports an attendant releasing role. CRH levels in the POA are correlated with stress as well as foraging behavior in juvenile frogs. The CRH molecule also is a potent releaser of TSH in amphibians as mentioned earlier.

2. Control of α-MSH Release

Dopamine has proven to be the most potent hypothalamic inhibitor of α-MSH release, and several investigators have proposed that dopamine is the hypothalamic α-MSH release-inhibiting hormone (MRIH) in all

Table 5-11. Effects of Neural and Endocrine Factors on Prolactin Release in Non-Mammalian Vertebrates

Factor[a]	Effect on prolactin release	Non-mammalian vertebrate group[b]			
		Teleosts	Amphibians	Reptiles	Birds
Dopamine	Inhibits PRL release	×	×		
Apomorphine (DA agonist)	Inhibits PRL release	×			
Somatostatin	Inhibits PRL release	×			
VIP	Inhibits PRL release	×	×		
PHI	Inhibits PRL release	×			
PHI	Stimulates PRL release		×		
GAP	Inhibits PRL release	×	×		
TRH	Stimulates PRL release	×	×	×	×
pVIP	Stimulates PRL release				×

[a] See text for abbreviations.
[b] ×, effect; blank, not tested.

Table 5-12. Effects of Neural and Endocrine Factors on Corticotropin Release in Non-Mammalian Vertebrates

		Non-mammalian vertebrate group[b]			
Factor[a]	Effect	Teleosts	Amphibians	Reptiles	Birds
Ovine CRH	Elevates plasma corticoids	×	×		×
Sauvagine	Elevates plasma corticoids	×	○		
Urotensin-I	Elevates plasma corticoids	×	○		
AVT/AVP	Elevates plasma corticoids		×		×
DA antagonists	Elevates plasma corticoids				×
Morphine	Elevates plasma corticoids	×			
ANP	ACTH levels			○	
	Inhibits ACTH release	×			
NPY	Elevates ACTH			×	
ANG-I	Elevates plasma corticoids	○			

[a] See text for abbreviations.
[b] ×, effect; ○, no effect; blank, not tested.

non-mammals as well as in mammals (see Chapter 4). Both aminergic and peptidergic fibers penetrate into the dogfish pars intermedia. It has been hypothesized that the peptidergic fibers control synthesis of α-MSH and that aminergic fibers are responsible for controlling α-MSH release.

There have been reports of dual "innervation" of the pars intermedia in amphibians of a different type than reported for the cartilaginous fishes. Adrenergic fibers have been shown to penetrate the pars intermedia of *Rana temporaria* and *Bufo arenarum*, and two types of adrenergic fibers synapse with pars intermedia cells of *R. pipiens*. No innervation of the pars intermedia is observed in the African clawed frog *Xenopus laevis*, however. Dual control of α-MSH release as suggested for some anurans may operate through the presence of α- and β-adrenergic receptors in the plasmalemma of the pars intermedia cells. The catecholamines, dopamine, norepinephrine, and epinephrine, as well as α-receptor agonists such as phenylephrine all inhibit α-MSH release from the pars intermedia. Isoproterenol, a catecholamine agonist, stimulates α-MSH release by activating β-adrenergic receptors. This effect is blocked by antagonists of β-adrenergic receptors (e.g., propranolol). Known antagonists of α-receptors (for example, dibenamine and dihydroergotamine) block the inhibitory actions of the catecholamines.

Certain cautions must be employed when one is attempting to interpret the actions of various drugs on α-MSH release from the pars intermedia. Epinephrine, for example, inhibits MSH release when applied at higher doses (10^{-5} M) but stimulates α-MSH release when applied at lower doses (10^{-6} or 10^{-7} M). At higher dose, epinephrine saturates both α- and β-adrenergic receptors, but the α effect predominates. At lower doses, epinephrine is more readily bound to the β-adrenergic receptors so that the β effect predominates, and α-MSH is released. The observation that a certain compound stimulates release of MSH does not necessarily imply a normal *in-vivo* role for that substance or for the type of innervation it might suggest.

Studies of α-MSH release by hypothalamic factors in non-mammals are almost confined to teleosts and amphibians (see Table 5-13). In fishes, α-MSH release is caused by treatment with TRH or CRH as well as by sauvagine and urotensin-I. Both MCH and DA block α-MSH release in teleosts. Treatment with TRH causes α-MSH release in amphibians and sometimes in reptiles, but CRH-like peptides are ineffective.

V. Neurohormones of the Non-Mammalian Pars Nervosa

With the exception of the agnathan fishes, non-mammals typically produce two nonapeptides as described for mammals: one basic nonapeptide and a neutral one. In virtually every case, the basic peptide is AVT, and this nonapeptide is the only one found in the agnathans. There is considerable variation among the neutral nonapeptides of fishes. All of the vertebrate nonapeptides and their structures are provided in Table 5-14 as well as a comparison with some invertebrate peptides. The phylogeny of the vertebrate nonapeptide prohormones is provided in Figure 5-23. The biological activities of some of these neuropeptides are shown for five different bioassays in Appendix D.

Table 5-13. Effects of Neural and Endocrine Factors on Melanotropin Release in Non-Mammalian Vertebrates

Factor[a]	Effect on melanotropin release	Non-mammalian vertebrate group[b]		
		Teleosts	Amphibians	Reptiles
TRH	(+) MSH release	×	×	×/○
Ovine CRH	(+) MSH release	×	○	
Sauvagine	(+) MSH release	×	○	
Urotensin I	(+) MSH release	×	○	
MST/AVT	(+) MSH release		○	
MCH	(−) MSH release	×		
NPY	(−) TRH-induced MSH release		×	
DA	(−) MSH release	×	×	
Naloxone	(+) DA, which (−) MSH		×	

[a] See text for abbreviations.
[b] ×, effect; ○, no effect; blank, not tested.

Table 5-14. Nonapeptide Hormones in Animals

Vasopressin-like peptides

Name	Amino acid sequence	Animal group
Arginine vasopressin	**C-Y-F-Q-N-C-P-R-G-NH$_2$**	Mammals
Lysine vasopressin	**C-Y-F-Q-N-C-P-K-G-NH$_2$**	Suiformes
Phenypressin	**C-F-F-R-N-C-P-K-G-NH$_2$**	Marsupials
Arginine vasotocin	**C-Y- I-R- N-C-P-R-G-NH$_2$**	Non-mammals
Lysine conopressin	**C-F- I-R- N-C-P-K-G-NH$_2$**	Gastropod mollusks, leeches
Insect diuretic hormone	**C-L- I-T- N-C-P-K-G-NH$_2$**	Locust

Oxytocin-like peptides

Name	Amino acid sequence	Animal group
Oxytocin	**C-Y-I-Q-N-C-P-L G-NH$_2$**	Mammals
Mesotocin	**C-Y-I-Q-N-C-P-I-G-NH$_2$**	Lungfishes, amphibians, birds, reptiles, some marsupials
Isotocin	**C-Y-I- S-N-C-P-LG-NH$_2$**	Bony fishes
Aspargtocin	**C-Y-I-N-N-C-P-L G-NH$_2$**	Elasmobranchs
Asvatocin	**C-Y-I-N-N-C-P-VG-NH$_2$**	Elasmobranchs
Glumitocin	**C-Y-I-S-N-C-P-L G-NH$_2$**	Elasmobranchs
Phasvatocin	**C-Y-F-N-N-C-P-VG-NH$_2$**	Elasmobranchs
Valitocin	**C-Y-I-Q-N-C-P-VG-NH$_2$**	Elasmobranchs
Annectocin	**C-F-V-Q-N-C-P-TG-NH$_2$**	Earthworm (annelid)
Cephalotocin	**C-Y-F-Q-N-C-P-I-G-NH$_2$**	Octopus (mollusk)

Numerous attempts to develop meaningful phylogenetic trees based on the distribution of the nonapeptides have met with limited success. One reason lies in the early attempts to construct phylogeny based on only a small fraction of the parent molecule that is the direct gene product (prohormone). Consequently, much of the genetic information has been overlooked in these earlier schemes.

A second problem is the relatively small number of species in which the neurohypophysial nonapeptides have been identified with absolute certainty. The proliferation of forms in the chondrichthyean fishes suggests that we may eventually find a greater variety of these nonapeptide molecules in much larger taxa such as the teleost fishes or even in the reptiles than have been identified to date. Recent phylogenies based on genetic analysis and comparison of prohormones support the general pattern described for the nonapeptides. Hence, certain generalizations based only on the nonapeptide amino acid sequences are still valid, and it is very likely that AVT represents the most primitive (and possibly ancestral) form of nonapeptide in vertebrates from which the others evolved following one or two duplications of the AVT gene. The discovery of genes among invertebrates that produce similar peptides suggests that these peptides are ancient bioregulators that have acquired new roles in vertebrates.

Agnathan fishes produce only one nonapeptide, AVT, whereas other non-mammalian vertebrates produce two: one member of a variety of neutral nonapeptides plus the same basic peptide, AVT. In most bony fishes,

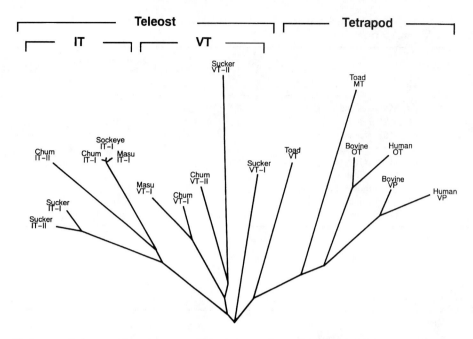

Figure 5-23. **Phylogeny of nonapeptide prohormones.** This phylogenetic tree is based on 119 amino acid residues. IT, isotocin (IST); VT, arginine vasotocin (AVT). The presence of two forms of IST and AVT in teleosts is consistent with the evidence for an additional genome duplication that occurred in their evolution. [From Urano, A., Kubokawa, K., and Hiraoka, S. (1994). Expression of vasotocin and isotocin gene family in the fish. *In* "Fish Physiology" (N. M. Sherwood and C. L. Hew, Eds.), pp. 101–132. Academic Press, San Diego.]

the neutral nonapeptide is isotocin (IST) whereas in amphibians, reptiles, and birds, the neutral nonapeptide is mesotocin (MST). Elasmobranchs produce one or two unique neutral nonapeptides (see Table 5-14). The spotted dogfish shark produces **phasvatocin (PhaT)** and **asvatocin (AsvT)** whereas the spiny dogfish produces a different pair of neutral nonapeptides, **aspargtocin (AspT)** and **valitocin (ValT)**. Rays and skates, however, produce only one, **glumitocin (GLT)**. In contrast, the holocephalan ratfish actually produces OXY, seemingly a unique appearance for this nonapeptide outside of mammals.

In general, studies of nonapeptide functions in non-mammals have focused on reproductive roles rather than osmoregulatory roles. In part, this was a consequence of early bioassays of AVT showing that it has considerable OXY-like activity on reproductive smooth muscle (see Appendix D). AVT was soon discovered to stimulate spawning reflexes in fishes as well as sperm release and/or egg laying in amphibians, reptiles, and birds. Furthermore, the sensitivity of oviducts to AVT is dependent on previous exposure to steroid hormones. Meanwhile, the neutral nonapeptides have largely been ignored, and we know little of the biological roles for MST in lungfishes and tetrapods (including the marsupials), IST in bony fishes, or the variety of neutral nonapeptides found in chondrichthyeans. AVT seems to be the more potent nonapeptide in non-mammals at stimulating reproductive smooth muscle, but physiological studies demonstrating a role for endogenous neutral secretions are lacking in non-mammals.

As discussed in Chapter 4, AVT has been replaced by AVP in adult mammals. OXY is found in almost all mammals with an exception of four of eight marsupials that produce MST. Two marsupials have been found to produce both OXY and MST. In addition, five marsupials (kangaroos and wallabies) produce phenypressin (PYP) instead of AVP and secrete both MST and OXY (see Table 4-10).

A limited number of studies have investigated the roles of nonapeptides in non-mammalian behaviors; studies of fishes by Andrew Bass and Matt Grober and their colleagues and in frogs by Sunny Boyd. For example, AVT is known to influence calling behavior in frogs as well as in some birds. AVT is linked to control of other reproductive behaviors in amphibians as demonstrated by Frank Moore and associates for the rough skinned newt, *Taricha granulosa*. They have linked corticosteroids and AVT to reproductive mating behavior. The molecular counterparts of vertebrate nonapeptides, **conopressin** in mollusks and **annectocin** in annelids, also have been linked to reproductive behaviors suggesting an ancient behavioral role for these peptides.

VI. The Epiphysial Complex

Almost all vertebrates exhibit one or two epithalamic structures that constitute the epiphysial complex (Figure 5-24). The components of this complex are the pineal organ and a more anterior projection, the parapineal organ. In fishes, amphibians, and some reptiles (lizards), these organs are basically sac-like diverticula that are more or less open to the third ventricle of the brain. They consist of a basal portion composed of sensory and ependymal (supportive) cells and may have an attached stalk with a distal end vesicle that contacts the dorsal brain case. These structures probably arose in primitive fishes as a pair of diverticula that for some reason later changed positions relative to one another. A well-developed parapineal organ has been retained only in cyclostomes and lizards, whereas the pineal organ is found in all vertebrate groups with the exception of crocodilians. In anamniotes, as well as in lizards, the pineal organ has retained both its sensory and endocrine functions. However, in other reptiles as well as birds and mammals, the pineal appears to be only an endocrine structure and often is termed simply the pineal gland.

The pineal gland secretes the amines melatonin and serotonin and possibly some small peptides, including AVT into the blood and possibly into the cerebrospinal fluid. Numerous studies have documented antigonadal actions of pineal extracts or melatonin in fishes, amphibians, reptiles, birds, and mammals. In addition, effects on thyroid function have been noted in some of these groups. Melatonin enhances certain aspects of the immune response system in mammals, but this role has not been confirmed for non-mammals. It is possible that these pineal actions are mediated via effects on the hypothalamus, or the specific sites of action may be at the target endocrine glands themselves.

The anteriormost evagination of the epiphysial complex that develops from the telencephalon is known as the **paraphysis**. The paraphysis is best seen in amphibians as a highly vascularized, sac-like diverticulum (Figure 5-24); it may function similarly to the choroid plexus in producing cerebrospinal fluid. The dorsal sac arises in most vertebrates as an epithalamic evagination just posterior to the paraphysis but anterior to the epiphysial complex. It is especially prominent in the ganoid fishes (chondrosteans, holosteans) and becomes

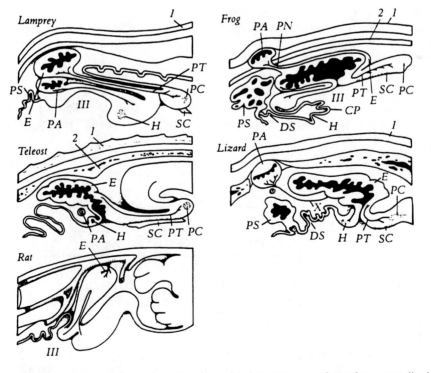

Figure 5-24. **The epiphysial complex.** The pineal gland and associated structures are shown for a generalized teleost, frog, lizard, and the rat. 1, skin; 2, skull; III, third ventricle; CP, choroids plexus; DS, dorsal sac; E, epiphysis (pineal); H, habenular commissure; PA, parietal (parapineal) organ; PC, posterior commissure; PN, pineal nerve; PS, paraphysis; PT, pineal tract; SC, subcommissural organ; X, parietal nerve.

less conspicuous in teleost fishes. In most vertebrates the dorsal sac contributes to formation of the choroid plexus, and these structures may be indistinguishable in the adult.

The pineal complex is connected to an adjacent ependymal structure, the **subcommissural organ** of Dendy (SCO). The ependymal cells of the SCO produce an aldehyde fuchsin-positive secretion rich in disulfide bonds and cysteine. This secretion is similar to that observed in the pineal ependyma. The major secretory product of the SCO is a noncellular fiber that in some species extends into the central canal of the spinal cord for its entire length. This structure is known as **Reissner's fiber**. Its significance is not clear (see Chapter 4). Cytological activation of the SCO in the lizard *Lacerta s. sicula* has been correlated positively with seasonal activities of adrenal cortical cells and of testicular steroidogenic cells. The actual role or roles for the SCO and its secretory products must await further research, but preliminary data would suggest it is somehow related to activity of the pineal complex.

Pineal function has been studied extensively in fishes and non-mammalian tetrapods, especially with respect to photoperiodic stimuli and daily and seasonal biological rhythms. After examining the experimental studies of melatonin on seasonal reproduction, Mayer et al. (see "Suggested Reading" at the end of this chapter) conclude that a role for melatonin in the photoperiodic control of reproduction in non-mammals is unwarranted. However, other reproductive roles have been demonstrated in non-mammals (see below). There is a progressive decrease in the correlation of the pineal as a photoreceptor and an increasing dependence upon the lateral eyes and the SCN-pineal pathway to control photoperiodically linked events such as seasonal reproduction and the secretion of melatonin. A summary of some of melatonin's actions in vertebrates is provided in Table 5-15.

A. Agnathan Fishes: Cyclostomes

The epiphysial complex of cyclostomes consists of a pineal organ and a parapineal organ, although the latter may be lacking in some species. Both organs possess variably shaped end vesicles that project dorsally against the roof of the brain case. The end vesicles contain sensory and ependymal cells structurally organized to suggest that they are photoreceptors. Efferent neural fibers from the pineal organ end at the posterior commissure, whereas those from the parapineal terminate at the habenular commissure. These organs probably relay photoperiodic information to other regions of the brain.

Nocturnal blanching has been observed in the ammocetes larvae of some lampreys, and epiphysial levels of HIOMT are correlated with nocturnal lightening of the skin in *Geotria australis*. Removal of the epiphysial complex causes persistent expansion of melanophores in *Lampetra planeri* and *G. australis* but not in *Mordax mordacia*, which lacks a parapineal organ and does not exhibit nocturnal lightening. Thus, melanophore expansion may be mediated via the parapineal. Hypophysectomy of cyclostomes also results in blanching due to the absence of α-MSH that normally stimulates melanophore expansion. The role of the parapineal may be to inhibit release of α-MSH, but melatonin could be the factor responsible for the observed melanophore contraction.

Table 5-15. Effects of Melatonin Treatment in Vertebrates

Effect	Vertebrate group					
	Agnatha	Osteichthyes	Amphibia	Reptilia	Aves	Mammalia
Concentration of melanosomes or inhibition of melanin synthesis	Yes	Yes	Yes	Yes		Yes
Preferred temperature		Increase	Decrease	Decrease		
Thermogenic effect on body temperature				Decrease	Decrease	Increase
Gonad function						
Adult		Stimulate/inhibit	Inhibit	Inhibit	Inhibit	Stimulate/inhibit
Juvenile					Stimulate	
Thyroid function	Stimulate?		Inhibit			Inhibit

There is evidence for a possible thyroid effect of the pineal organ of lampreys. Pinealectomy inhibits metamorphosis of the ammoecete to the adult body that normally is prevented by elevated thyroid hormones. However, additional data are needed to establish the site of action for pineal secretions.

B. Chondrichthyean Fishes

The shark pineal organ contains photosensory and supportive cells. No experimental data, however, have been reported, and the functional importance of the pineal is not known for these fishes. A parapineal organ has not been described for any species in this group. This vertebrate taxon demands further investigation.

C. Bony Fishes: Teleosts

The epiphysial complex of teleosts consists of a pineal organ (Figure 5-24) that is extremely variable in both size and degree of development. There is usually a prominent lumen, which in some cases is open to the third ventricle. Photosensory cells and ependymal cells are present in the pineals of several species. A reduced parapineal has been described in some teleosts.

Pigmentation, responses to light, and thyroid changes are influenced by the pineal organ in teleosts. Melanophore changes have been reported in several species of teleost, including rainbow trout, following injection of pharmacological amounts of melatonin. Some of these species also respond in a similar manner to epinephrine treatment. Other species respond only to epinephrine with no reaction to melatonin. Circulatory melatonin levels exhibit no correlations to adaptation by rainbow trout to different backgrounds, indicating that melatonin may not be a factor influencing normal pigmentary responses in this species. Furthermore, levels of HIOMT in rainbow trout pineals are not altered by either continuous light or darkness.

Control of pineal secretion appears to be determined by the presence or absence of light in teleosts and not by some endogenous mechanism or rhythm. Rainbow trout pineal glands *in vitro* were shown by William Gern to exhibit no endogenous secretory rhythm in melatonin secretion and to release melatonin only when in darkness. Similar observations have been reported by Japanese workers for goldfish pineals. Consequently, it appears that the pineal gland of teleosts may simply respond directly to light and may not be controlled through the lateral eyes and the SCN pathway as shown for mammals (see Chapter 4).

The white sucker, *Catostomus commersoni*, has been shown to respond to light intensity and/or thermal gradients. This sensitivity is mediated through the pineal. Shielding the pineal from light causes the fish to choose the warmer portion of horizontal temperature gradients or the better-illuminated portions of chambers maintained at a constant temperature. When the shield is removed, the fish returns to its original preference. The pineal may provide information on light intensity for use in mediating thermal behavior.

Structural correlations have been described between the pineal organ and phototactic responses by fishes. Species with a translucent covering over the pineal organ (a definitive pineal spot) exhibit predominantly positive phototaxis, whereas species with a pigmented, opaque skeletal covering do not show phototaxis. Species that have pigment cells located so that dispersal and concentration of pigment granules could regulate the intensity of light reaching the pineal organ exhibit responses varying from positive phototaxis to no response. The pineal organ might be involved in some other functions for the species showing no phototaxis. The presence of a pineal spot is more common in deep-sea fishes than in freshwater or shallow-water marine species and may relate to the influence of light on vertical migrations performed by deep-sea fishes.

Pinealectomy of *Poecilia reticulata* (guppy) causes pituitary enlargement and hyperplasia of the thyroid. This effect also occurs in *Fundulus heteroclitus* if pinealectomy is performed during the winter months (December through March). Pinealectomy between February and June produces no effect on the thyroid, however. The pituitary and thyroid of the characin, *Astyanax mexicanus*, are not affected by pinealectomy, but both stimulation and inhibition of the goldfish thyroid have been described. A possible influence of the pineal on gonadal development has been reported for *F. heteroclitus* and *F. similis*, but no relationship was found in goldfish or in the characin. Additional studies performed on a seasonal basis involving a large number of species and paying close attention to photoperiodic regimens are needed before any definitive statements can be made with respect to the pineal on thyroid or reproductive functions.

Melatonin has been measured in the retina of rainbow trout, and HIOMT is present in the retinas of several teleost species. Levels of melatonin in the trout retina exceed levels reported for the pineal. Melatonin may cause concentration of pigment in retinal melanophores to increase sensitivity of retinal cells in dim light.

D. The Pineal in Amphibians

The epiphysial complex of amphibians consists of a pineal organ, dorsal sac, choroid plexus, SCO, paraphysis, and often a parapineal organ (Figure 5-24). The proximal (basal) portion of the amphibian epiphysial complex contains HIOMT activity and melatonin. The retina of the eye has the same features. Pinealectomy reduces circulating melatonin to daytime levels, suggesting that the retina may be responsible for basal levels of melatonin in the blood.

As mentioned earlier, the role of melatonin on melanophores in larval amphibians was first suggested by the observations of McCord and Allen. Since that time, it has been shown that melatonin is the pineal agent responsible for the blanching of tadpoles or larval salamanders when held in the dark. As little as 0.1-ng/ml medium causes aggregation of melanin granules in melanophores of *Xenopus laevis* tadpoles. Plasma melatonin exhibits a distinct daily rhythm determined by photoperiod that is unaffected by temperature, suggesting the pineal could provide a cue to regulate seasonal events as well.

Attempts to relate pineal function or melatonin with thyroid function have been equivocal in amphibians. Pinealectomy of tadpoles of the midwife toad *Alytes obstetricans* accelerates metamorphosis, but a similar operation in larvae of the newt *Taricha torosa* is without effect. Earlier observations in *Bufo americanus*, however, indicate that feeding mammalian pineal to tadpoles accelerated metamorphosis. Pinealectomized larval tiger salamanders, *Ambystoma tigrinum*, exhibit decreased thyroidal uptake of injected radioiodide, but neither purified melatonin nor commercial bovine pineal powder influences iodide uptake of intact larvae. Numerous studies of anuran metamorphosis by Mary Wright and her collaborators have implicated the pineal gland in this process.

Reproduction may be under inhibitory influence of the pineal organ, at least in anurans. Accelerated gonadal development follows pinealectomy of *A. obstetricans* and *Hyla cinerea*. Gonadotropin-induced ovulation from *Rana pipiens* ovaries *in vitro* is inhibited by addition of melatonin to the culture medium. Bovine pineal extract similarly inhibited human chorionic gonadotropin-induced spermiation in male *R. esculenta*, but purified melatonin had no effect. This dichotomy of melatonin's influence in male and female anurans warrants further investigation. The possible influence of pineal principles on reproduction in urodeles has not been studied.

Unlike the other jawed vertebrates, some anurans have retained a well-developed parapineal end vesicle known also as the frontal organ or *stirnorgan* (Figure 5-24). Because of the presence of photosensory cells, the parapineal is often referred to as the parietal eye in these species. Photic information collected by the parietal eye is conducted directly to the pineal.

E. The Pineal in Reptiles

Reptiles can be separated into several groups on the basis of the anatomy of the epiphysial complex. Melatonin has been localized in the blood, pineal gland, and retinas of snakes, lizards, and turtles. Modern crocodilians have no pineal, parapineal, or parietal structures. Although a pineal is absent in alligators, melatonin (presumably of retinal origin) is present in the blood. Lizards possess an elaborate sac-like, pigmented pineal organ containing both photosensory and ependymal cells (Figure 5-24). The lumen of the lizard pineal lies close to the third ventricle but does not join with it. A parapineal organ penetrates the skull, forming a parietal spot on the surface. As in amphibians, the parapineal is often termed the parietal eye. Turtles and snakes have retained only the basal (glandular) portion of the pineal organ and have lost the end vesicle and stalk of the pineal organ as well as the complete parapineal organ. Nevertheless, the turtle pineal organ is the largest and the best-developed epiphysial structure among reptiles.

The parietal eye of lizards has been examined with respect to thyroid function, thermoregulation, and reproduction. The lizard parietal eye contains HIOMT activity suggesting that it also synthesizes melatonin, and removal of the parietal eye stimulates thyroid hyperplasia and oxygen consumption. These data suggest that melatonin or some other principle influences pituitary function although direct effects on the thyroid are not ruled out. Perhaps, the reptilian parietal eye is a photo/thermal radiation dosimeter that monitors solar radiation and, in turn, regulates daily activity patterns of lizards. Indeed, excision of the pineal or parietal eye alters thermal responses of numerous lizard species, and it may well be the major functional role for the epiphysial complex in lizards.

Definitive effects of the epiphysial complex on reproduction also have been reported in lizards. For example, excision of the parietal eye of the lizard *Anolis carolinensis* stimulates ovarian development in reproductively quiescent animals. This effect is blocked by administration of melatonin. In this lizard, long photoperiod and warm temperatures induce the onset of gonadal recrudescence. The parietal eye thus appears to be the transducer through which photoperiod influences reproduction in lizards. Treatment of male red-sided garter snakes with melatonin inhibits courtship behavior in males recently emerged from winter dens, suggesting that long photoperiod (short scotophase) is a permissive factor allowing for expression of breeding behavior.

F. The Pineal in Birds

The pineal organ of birds has been reduced to the glandular basal portion, the pineal gland. No parapineal or remnant thereof is present, and distinct photoreceptors are absent in the pineal. Structurally, the avian pineal exhibits considerable diversity, and it is composed of several cell types. The avian pineal is innervated by sympathetic fibers as reported for mammals.

Avian pineals are biochemically like their mammalian counterpart. Variations have been reported in HIOMT and NAT activities with respect to lighting conditions, but the most dramatic effects involve NAT. Activity of this enzyme exhibits a marked increase with onset of the scotophase, a peak about the middle of the scotophase, and a decrease rapidly following the onset of the photophase. Brief exposure to light at the peak of NAT activity causes a rapid reduction to photophase levels. Melatonin rhythms that correlate with rhythms in pineal NAT activity have been reported for brain, pineal, retina, and serum of birds. The brain and especially the hypothalamus in birds may be the primary site of action for melatonin and may explain effects of melatonin on gonadal function, thermoregulation, and locomotor activity.

Unlike mammals and the situation postulated for other vertebrates, the role of the pineal in the reproductive biology of birds may be progonadal. Pinealectomy inhibits androgen synthesis, whereas administration of melatonin stimulates androgen synthesis, presumably by altering gonadotropin release from the adenohypophysis. Pinealectomy of quail delays ovarian development, an observation that also supports a progonadal role. However, melatonin injections can decrease gonadal weight, suggesting that the progonadal agent might be a peptide that normally overpowers effects of endogenous melatonin on reproduction. Marked species differences may occur, however. For example, no effects of melatonin treatment on parameters of gonadal development and their relationship to photoperiod could be demonstrated in either white-throated sparrows or border canaries.

Neural control of melatonin secretion in birds also differs markedly in contrast to mammals where NE stimulates pineal secretion. In birds, increased activity of sympathetic fibers from the superior cervical ganglion decreases melatonin secretion in birds, and NE turnover is greatest during the photophase. This inhibitory action of NE appears to involve G_i-proteins in pinealocytes and subsequent reduction in cAMP formation, NAT activity, and melatonin synthesis and release. Pinealectomy abolishes endogenous body-temperature rhythms as well as free-running locomotor activity rhythms in house sparrows, *Passer domesticus*. Effects on locomotor activity appear to involve two pathways, one of which can bypass the pineal organ. Pinealectomized birds that have lost free-running locomotor activity in the dark still exhibit entrainment to light–dark cycles, supporting the presence of a bypass system. Both systems can be entrained by light, but the pineal has control only over the bypass system.

G. Evolution of Melatonin's Functions

An intriguing hypothesis, proposed by William Gern, for the original function of melatonin and the evolution of other functions is based on the presence of melatonin synthesizing systems in retinas, parietal eyes, and pineals and on the observations that pineals of more primitive vertebrate groups also are photoreceptive. Evidence suggests that both retinal and pineal melatonin exhibit nighttime (scotophasic) peaks of synthesis. This hypothesis proposes that melatonin was initially a local hormone for regulating the distribution of melanosomes in the retina. During the day, melanosomes are dispersed in retinal pigment cells that protect the photoreceptors from intense light. At night, elevated melatonin causes concentration of melanosomes and allows dim light to maximally stimulate the photoreceptors. This sensitivity of melanosomes to melatonin is retained in the melanophores of skin and brain ependyma of both modern fishes and amphibians.

Similar mechanisms presumably would operate in the photoreceptive outer portion of the pineal, in the parietal eye, and in the amphibian frontal organ. The increase in melatonin synthesis during the scotophase causes a greater proportion of melatonin to appear in the blood. Consequently, the scotophasic elevation in melatonin is a reliable internal cue for obtaining information about seasonal photoperiods. Information concerning length of the scotophase is reflected in circulating melatonin levels. Thus, according to Gern's hypothesis, the diurnal rhythm in melatonin has been co-opted as the blood-borne signal entraining a number of other internal events during the evolution of vertebrates.

VII. Summary

There is a progressive evolution of hypothalamic centers in vertebrates evident from examination of different vertebrates. The pattern of regulation has branched within the fishes with the most recent fishes (teleosts) exhibiting predominantly neuroglandular control of tropic hormone release. Primitive fishes, including the chondrichthyeans, and tetrapods have specialized in neurovascular control with the development of a distinct median eminence and a hypophysial portal blood system. The distinct regionalization of tropic cell types in the fish adenohypophysis is less marked in tetrapods. The adenohypophysis of fishes is usually separable into a rostral pars distalis, a proximal pars distalis, and a pars intermedia. The pars tuberalis of tetrapods is absent in fishes but a unique ependymal structure is evident, the saccus vasculosus. Lungfishes lack both a pars tuberalis and the saccus vasculosus.

All of the mammalian tropic hormones have a molecular counterpart among the non-mammals. Many non-mammalian functions can be stimulated by mammalian tropic hormones. The established occurrence of at least one hormone from each category in all gnathostomes (jawed vertebrates) suggests that early in vertebrate evolution three cell types differentiated [basophil, acidophil, and possibly PbH(+) cells], and each began elaboration of one of three types of molecules: glycoproteins (TSH, LH, FSH), large peptides (GH, PRL), and the POMC-related peptides (ACTH, MSH, endorphins), respectively. These three primitive molecular types attained functional significance as tropic hormones and gave rise via amino acid substitutions, modified cleavage of prohormones, or both, to the additional hormones that characterize each category.

Non-mammals produce the same tropic hormones as do mammals and there is considerable homology among them. Nevertheless, there is clear evidence of changes in the functions of these molecules related both to structural changes in the tropic hormones themselves and to alterations in receptors such that new functions have evolved in some cases. A new hormone, somatolactin, has been isolated from the pars intermedia of teleosts which may be involved in calcium regulation and/or reproduction.

Regulation of the release of tropic hormones in non-mammals follows the mammalian pattern for the most part. Many of the same neuropeptides are present in the brains of non-mammals as described for mammals but they show greater variations in their effects, often causing release of different tropic hormones than implied by their mammalian names.

Examinations on the actions of tropic hormones in non-mammals have resulted in development of numerous bioassays that have proven useful for quantifying levels during purification of tropic hormones. Furthermore, these bioassays are critical for measuring biological activity for a particular tropic hormone when purified sources from either mammalian or non-mammalian animals are not available. Because of structural similarities within tropic hormone categories, caution must be exercised when comparing the actions molecules from one species in different species, especially when making comparisons across larger taxa.

The most primitive nonapeptide is AVT that unlike other basic peptides has rather good uterotonic activity related to the oxytocin-like ring structure. Jawless fishes (agnathans) have only AVT, but all other vertebrates studied exhibit at least one basic (AVT in non-mammals) and one neutral nonapeptide (IST in most bony fishes; MST in amphibians, reptiles, birds, and marsupial mammals; oxytocin in placental mammals).

The major secretory product of the pineal gland is melatonin although peptides such as AVT may play important roles as well. Pineal secretion is inhibited by light, and the pineal gland plays a major role in mediating seasonal and daily endocrine activity primarily through effects on the hypothalamus. Melatonin generally acts as an antigonadal (except in birds), antithyroid, and anti-prolactin releasing factor. There also is evidence for a role of melatonin in thermoregulation of teleosts and reptiles.

Suggested Reading

Books

Bagnara, J. T., and Hadley, M. E. (1973). "Chromatophores and Color Change: The Comparative Physiology of Animal Pigmentation." Prentice-Hall, Englewood Cliffs, NJ.
Binkley, S. A. (1990). "The Clockwork Sparrow: Time, Clocks, and Calendars in Biological Organisms." Prentice Hall, Englewood Cliffs, NJ.
Chester-Jones, I., Ingleton, P. M., and Phillips, J. G. (1987). "Fundamentals of Comparative Vertebrate Endocrinology." Plenum, New York.
Holmes, R. L., and Ball, J. N. (1974). "The Pituitary Gland, a Comparative Account." Cambridge Univ. Press, Cambridge.

Articles

Acher, R. (1995). Evolution of neurohypophysial control of water homeostasis: Integrative biology of molecular, cellular and organismal aspects. In "Neurohypophysis: Recent Progress of Vasopressin and Oxytocin" (T. Saito, K. Kurokawa, and S. Yoshida, Eds.), pp. 39–54. Elsevier, Amsterdam.
Acher, R., Chauvet, J., and Rouille, Y. (1997). Adaptive evolution of water homeostasis regulation in amphibians: vasotocin and hydrins. Biol. Cell 89, 283–291.
Andersen, A. C., Tonon, M.-C., Pelletier, G., Conlon, J. M., Fasolo, A., and Vaudry, H. (1992). Neuropeptides in the amphibian brain. Intl. Rev. Cytol. 138, 89–210.
Ball, J. N. (1981). Hypothalamic control of the pars distalis in fishes, amphibians, and reptiles. Gen. Comp. Endocr. 44, 135–390.
Balment, R. J., Song, W., and Ashton, N. (2005). Urotensin II. Ancient hormone with new functions in vertebrate body fluid regulation. Ann. NY Acad. Sci. 1040, 66–73.
Bentley, G. E., Jensen, J. P., Kaur, G. J., Wacker, D. W., Tsutsui, K., and Wingfield, J. C. (2006). Rapid inhibition of female sexual behavior by gonadotropin-inhibitory hormone (GnIH). Hormones and Behavior, 49, 550–555.
Bern, H. A. (1983). Functional evolution of prolactin and growth hormone in lower vertebrates. Am. Zool. 23, 663–671.
Cooke, B., Hegstrom, C. D., Villeneuve, L. S., and Breedlove, S. M. (1998). Sexual differentiation of the vertebrate brain: Principles and mechanisms. Frontiers in Neuroendocr. 19, 323–362.
De Groef, B., Van der Geyten, S., Darras, V. M., and Kühn, E. R. (2006). Role of corticotropin-releasing hormone as a thyrotropin-releasing factor in non-mammalian vertebrates. Gen. Comp. Endocr. 146, 62–68.
Dufour, S., Weltzien, F. A., Seibert, M. E., Le Belle, N., Vidal, B., Vernier, P., and Pasqualini, C. (2005). Dopaminergic inhibition of reproduction in teleost fishes. Ecophysiological and evolutionary implications. Ann. NY Acad. Sci. 1040, 9–21.
Fernald, R. D., and White, R. B. (1999). Gonadotropin-releasing hormone genes: phylogeny, structure, and functions. Frontiers in Neuroendocr. 20, 224–240.
Fontaine, M., and Oliverau, M. (1975). Aspects of the organization and evolution of the vertebrate pituitary. Am. Zool. 15 (Suppl. 1), 61–81.
Gern, W. A., Nervina, J. M., and Greenhouse, S. S. (1987). Pineal involvement in seasonality of reproduction. In "Hormones and Reproduction in Fishes, Amphibians, and Reptiles" (D. O. Norris and R. E. Jones, Eds.), pp. 433–460. Plenum, New York.
Gonzalez, G. C., Belenky, M. A., Polenov, A. L., and Lederis, K. (1992). Comparative localization of corticotropin and corticotropin releasing factor-like peptides in the brain and hypophysis of a primitive vertebrate, the sturgeon Acipenser ruthenus L. J. Neurocytol. 21, 885–896.
Gorbman, A., and Sower, S. A. (2003). Evolution of the role of GnRH in animal (metazoan) biology. Gen. Comp. Endocr. 134, 207–213.
Green, J. D. (1951). The comparative anatomy of the hypophysis with special reference to its blood supply and innervation Am. J. Anat. 88, 225–311.
Han. Y.-S., Liao, I.-C., Tzeng, W.-N., and Yu, J. Y.-L. (2004). Cloning of the DNA for thyroid stimulating hormone β subunit and changes in activity of the pituitary-thyroid axis during silvering of the Japanese eel, Anguilla japonica. J. Mol. Endocr. 32, 179–194.
Hansen, G. N. (1983). Cell types in the adenohypophysis of the primitive actinopterygians, with special reference to immunocytochemical identification of pituitary hormone producing cells in the distal lobe. Acta Zool. Suppl. 1983, 1–87.
Hoyle, C. H. V. (1998). Neuropeptide families: Evolutionary perspectives. Regulatory Peptides. 73, 1–33.
Insel, T. R., and Young, L. J. (2000). Neuropeptides and the evolution of social behavior. Current Opinion in Neurobiol 10, 784–789.
Kawamura, K., and Kikuyama, S. (1992). Evidence that hypophysis and hypothalamus constitute a single entity from the primary stage of histogenesis. Development 115, 1–9.
Kawamura, K., and Kikuyama, S. (1995). Induction from posterior hypothalamus is essential for the development of the pituitary proopiomelanocortin (POMC) cells of the toad (Bufo japonicus). Cell and Tissue Res. 279, 233–239.
Kawamura, K., and Kouki, T., Kawahara, G. Kikuyama, S. (2002). Hypophyseal development in vertebrates from amphibians to mammals. Gen. Comp. Endocr. 126, 130–135.
Kawauchi, H., and Sower, S. A. (2006). The dawn and evolution of hormones in the adenohypophysis. Gen. Comp. Endocr., 148, 3–19.

Kikuyama, S., Inaco, H., Jenks, B. G., and Kawamura, K. (1993). Development of the ectopically transplanted primordium of epithelial hypophysis (anterior neural ridge) in *Bufo japonicus* embryos. *J. Exp. Zool.* **266**, 216–220.

Kloas, W. (1994). Localization of binding sites for atrial natriuretic peptide and angiotensin II in gill and kidney of various fish species. *In* "Fish Ecotoxicology and Ecophysiology" (T. Braunbeck, W. Hanke, and H. Segner, Eds.), pp. 367–384. VCH, Weinheim.

Klovens, J., and Schiöth, H. B. (2005). Agouti-related proteins (AGRPs) and Agouti-signaling peptide (ASIP) in fish and chicken. *Ann. NY Acad. Sci.* **1040**, 363–367.

Lederis, K., Fryer, J. N., Okawara, Y., Schronrock, C., and Richter, D. (1994). Corticotropin-releasing factors acting on the fish pituitary: Experimental and molecular analysis. *In* "Fish Physiology, Molecular Endocrinology" (N. M. Sherwood and C. L. Hew, Eds.), pp. 67–100. Academic Press, San Diego.

Lovejoy, D. A., Fischer, W. H., Ngamvongchon, S., Craig, A. G., Nahorniak, C. S., Peter, R. E., Rivier, J. E., and Sherwood, N. M. (1992). Distinct sequence of gonadotropin-releasing hormone (GnRH) in dogfish brain provides insight into GnRH evolution. *Proc. Natl. Acad. Sci. U.S.A.* **89**, 6373–6377.

Lovejoy, D. A., and Balment, R. J. (1999). Evolution and physiology of the corticotropin-releasing factor (CRF) family of neuropeptides in vertebrates. *Gen. Comp. Endocr.* **115**, 1–22.

Manzon, L. A. (2002). The role of prolactin in fish osmoregulation: A review. *Gen. Comp. Endocr.* **125**, 291–310.

Millar, R. P. (2005). GnRHs and GnRH receptors. *Animal Reprod. Sci.* **88**, 5–28.

Northcutt, R. G. and Muske, L. E. (1994). Multiple embryonic origins of gonadotropin-releasing hormone (GnRH) immunoreactive neurons. *Develop. Brain Res.* **78**, 279–290.

Nozaki, M., and Gorbman, A. (1992). The question of functional homology of Hatschek's pit of amphioxus (*Branchiostoma belcheri*) and the vertebrate adenohypophysis. *Zool. Sci.* **9**, 387–395.

Oba, Y., Hirai, T., Yoshiura, Y., Kobayashi, T., and Nagahama, Y. (2001). Fish gonadotropin and thyrotropin receptors: The evolution of glycoprotein hormone receptors in vertebrates. *Comp. Biochem. Phys. B* **129**, 441–448.

Ozaki, M., Ominato, K., Takahashi, A., Kawauchi, H., and Sower, S. A. (2001). Adenohypophysial cell types in the lamprey pituitary: Current state of the art. *Comp. Biochem. Phys. B* **129**, 303–309.

Pawson, A. J., Morgan, K., Maudsley, S. R., and Millar, R. P. (2003). Type II gonadotropin-releasing hormone (GnRH-II) in reproductive biology. *Reprod.* **126**, 271–278.

Peter, R. E. (1986). Vertebrate neurohormonal systems. *In* "Vertebrate Endocrinology: Fundamentals and Biomedical Implications. Volume 1, Morphological Considerations" (P. K. T. Pang and M. Schreibman, Eds.), pp. 57–104. Academic Press, San Diego.

Pickford, G. E., and Atz, J. W. (1957). "The Physiology of the Pituitary Gland of Fishes." New York Zoological Society, New York.

Querat, B., Arai, Y., Henry, A., Akama, Y., Longhurst, T. J., and Joss, J. M. P. (2004). Pituitary glycoprotein hormone β subunits in the Australian lungfish and estimation of the relative evolution rate of these subunits within vertebrates. *Biol. Reprod.* **70**, 356–363.

Reinecke, M., Betzler, D., Aoki, A., and Forssmann, W.-G. (1993). Atrial natriuretic peptides (ANP) in fish heart. *In* "Fish Ecotoxicology and Ecophysiology" (T. Braunbeck, W. Hanke, and H. Segner, Eds.), pp. 385–404. VCH, Weinheim.

Reiner, A. J. (1992). Neuropeptides in the nervous system. *In* "Biology of the Reptilia" (C. Gans and P. S. Ulinski, Eds.), Vol. 17, pp. 588–739. Univ. of Chicago Press, Chicago.

Sawyer, C. H. (1978). History of the neurovascular concept of hypothalamo–hypophysial control. *Biol. Reprod.* **18**, 325–328.

Schradin, C., and Anzenberger, G. (1999). Prolactin, the hormone of paternity. *News in Physiol. Sci.* **14**, 223–231.

Schreibman, M. P. (1986). Pituitary gland. *In* "Vertebrate Endocrinology: Fundamentals and Biomedical Implications. Volume 1, Morphological Considerations" (P. K. T. Pang and M. Schreibman, eds.), pp. 11–56. Academic Press, Orlando, FL.

Somoza, G. M., Miranda, L. A., Strobl-Mazzulla, P., Guilgur, L. G. (2002). Gonadotropin-releasing hormone (GnRH): From fish to mammalian brains. *Cell. Mol. Neurobiol.* **22**, 589–609.

Sower, S. A., and Kawauchi, H. (2001). Update: Brain and pituitary hormones of lampreys. *Comp. Biochem. Phys. B* **129**, 291–302.

Takahashi, A., and Kawauchi, H. (2006). Evolution of melanocortin systems in fish. *Gen. Comp. Endocr.* **148**, 85–94.

Takahashi, A., Nakata, O., Moriyama, S., Nozaki, M., Joss, J. M. P., Sower, S. A., Kawauchi, H. (2006). Occurrence of two functionally distinct proopiomelanocortin genes in all modern lampreys. *Gen. Comp. Endocr.* **148**, 72–78.

Urano, A., Kubokawa, K., and Hiraoka, S. (1994). Expression of the vasotocin and isotocin gene family in fish. *In* "Fish Physiology, Vol. XIII, Molecular Endocrinology of Fish" (N. M. Sherwood and C. L. Hew, Eds.), pp. 101–132. Academic Press, San Diego.

Watkins, W. B., and Choy, V. J. (1988). Identification of neurophyophysial peptides in the ovaries of several mammalian and nonmammalian species. *Peptide* **9**, 927–932.

Whitlock, K. E. (2005). Origin and development of GnRH neurons. *Trends Endocr. Metab.* **16**, 145–151.

Yaron, Z., Gur, G., Matemed, P., Rosenfeld, H., Elizur, A., and Levavi-Sivan, B. (2003). Regulation of fish gonadotropin. *Int. Rev. Cytol.* **225**, 131–185.

Zhu, Y., Stiller, J. W., Shaner, M. P., Baldini, A., Scemama, J.-L., and Capehart, A. A. (2004). Cloning of somatolactin α and β cDNAs in zebrafish and phylogenetic analysis of two distinct somatolactin subtypes in fish. *J. Endocr.* **182**, 509–518.

6

The Hypothalamus-Pituitary-Thyroid (HPT) Axis of Mammals

The thyroid gland (Figure 6-1) is unique among vertebrate endocrine glands in that it stores its secretory products (thyroid hormones) extracellularly. It is possibly the most highly vascularized endocrine gland in mammals and appears to be one of the oldest vertebrate endocrine glands phylogenetically (see Chapter 7). Thyroid function is regulated by the **hypothalamus-pituitary-thyroid (HPT)** axis (see Chapter 4). **Thyrotropin (TSH)** from the pituitary stimulates the synthesis of **tetraiodothyronine** or **thyroxine** (T_4). First, the amino acid tyrosine incorporated into a glycoprotein called **thyroglobulin (Tgb)** is iodinated and then two iodinated tyrosines are linked together to form T_4. Some T_4 is partially deiodinated to form the more active thyroid hormone **triiodothyronine** (T_3) prior to release from the thyroid gland. The structure of these compounds are provided in Chapter 3 (Figure 3-39).

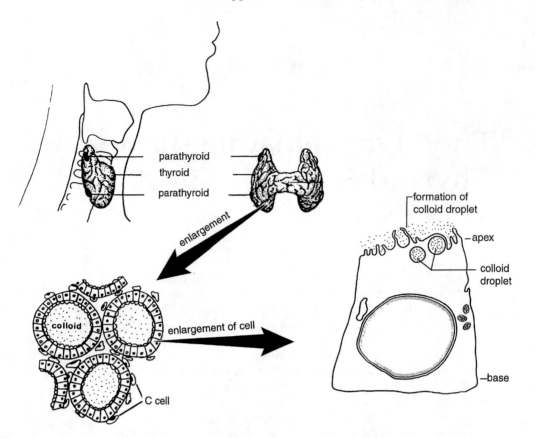

Figure 6-1. **The mammalian thyroid.** The thyroid gland is located in the neck region. It consists of many hollow follicles, each of which is filled with a proteinaceous fluid called colloid secreted by the follicle cells. Thyroxine synthesized by the follicle cells is stored in the colloid. The C-cells or parafollicular cells are of ultimobranchial origin and secrete the calcium-regulating hormone, calcitonin (see Chapter 14). Modified from McNabb, F. M. A. (1993). "Thyroid Hormones," Prentice Hall, Englewood Cliffs, NJ; Bolander, F. F. (1989). "Molecular Endocrinology," Academic Press, San Diego.

Thyroid hormones influence many aspects of reproduction, growth, differentiation, and metabolism. Many of these actions occur cooperatively with other hormones, and the thyroid hormones enhance their effectiveness. This cooperative role for thyroid hormones is referred to as a **permissive action** whereby thyroid hormones produce changes in target tissues that "allow" these tissues to be more responsive to another hormone, to neural stimulation, or possibly to certain environmental stimuli such as light. Thyroid hormones may maintain maximal sensitivity to other regulating agents in many types of tissues. The importance of thyroid hormones is reflected in the observation that the incidence of thyroid disease in humans is exceeded only by the incidence of diabetes mellitus (see Chapter 12).

Although rarely lethal, thyroid disorders have widespread effects in humans due to their many actions with other hormones. Of the more than 13 million thyroid disorders diagnosed in the USA, 11 million occur in women. This difference in incidence between males and females is not understood, although many cases are linked to pregnancy. Thyroid deficiencies that occur during pregnancy can have devastating effects on the development of the nervous system of the fetus, leading to extensive mental deficiencies. Thyroid deficiencies often develop so gradually that many thyroid disorders are not recognized by physicians.

I. Some Historical Aspects of Thyroid Physiology

Either deficient or excessive production of thyroid hormones may lead to serious pathological states with overt symptoms (Table 6-1). The first description of thyroid disease was of abnormal enlargement of the thyroid recognized by Chinese physicians about 3000 B.C. As a remedy, they recommended ingestion of seaweed and burned sponge or desiccated deer thyroids. The first two substances contained therapeutic quantities of

Table 6-1. Symptoms of Thyroid Deficiency and Hyperactivity in Humans

Type of symptom	Hypothyroid	Hyperthyroid
Appearance	Myxedema; deficient growth	Exophthalmus
Behavior	Mental retardation; mentally and physically sluggish; somnolent; sensitive to cold	Often quick mentally; restless, irritable, anxious, hyperkinetic; wakeful; sensitive to heat
Metabolism	Hypophagia; low basal metabolic rate; reduced QO_2^a of liver, kidney, and muscle *in vitro*; decrease in oxidative enzymes; constipation	Hyperphagia; high basal metabolic rate; increased QO_2 of liver, kidney, and muscle *in vitro*; increased oxidative enzymes; diarrhea
Muscle function	Weakness; hypotonia	Weakness; fibrillary twitchings, tremors

^{a} QO_2, respiratory quotient.

iodide, and the last contained sufficient thyroid hormones to alleviate the pathological symptoms in most cases. Hypothyroid deficiencies of this sort were not recognized in Western culture as clinical disorders until many centuries later. The **cretinism** syndrome was described clinically in Europe in 1526. Cretinism is manifested very early in life as a consequence of severe thyroid deficiency. This syndrome is characterized by dwarfism and a number of other physical abnormalities in addition to severe mental retardation, slow mental and physical activity, bradycardia (slowing of heart beat), and hypothermia. In 1880–1890, another clinical disorder in adults, **myxedema**, was linked to hypothyroid function. Myxedematous symptoms in adults are related to abnormal accumulation of water and protein throughout the body as well as to other disturbances in general metabolism. Accumulations of protein and fluid in the skin alter facial features, causing the patient to appear expressionless. In later stages of the disorder, the sufferer becomes less interested in both self and environment, and if untreated would eventually enter a coma and die. **Juvenile myxedema** is similar to cretinism except that early growth and development are normal but become severely retarded in later childhood. All of these clinical syndromes have the same basic cause: hypofunctioning of the thyroid gland.

Bauman discovered in 1896 that an organic iodine-containing compound could be extracted from thyroid glands. Subsequently, it was demonstrated that this "thyroidin" substance could reverse the adverse effects of iodide deficiency. In the early 1900s, the thyroid gland and its hormones were implicated in elevating basal metabolic rate, primarily through effects on certain tissues; for example, liver, kidney, and muscle. This observation has strongly influenced the direction of thyroid research in mammals as well as in many non-mammalian vertebrates. The action of thyroid hormones on metabolism is reflected in clinical thyroid states (Table 6-1).

The iodine-containing hormone T_4 was isolated, crystallized, and reported by Edward C. Kendall in 1915. This event marked a significant milestone, not only in thyroid research but in endocrinology as a whole, for T_4 was the first hormone to be isolated in pure form. It was not until 1952, however, that the second thyroid hormone, T_3, was identified by J. Gross and R. Pitt-Rivers. This second thyroid hormone was soon found to be more potent than T_4 as a thyroid hormone and is considered by many to be the active form of thyroid hormone (see below).

It was the discovery of **anti-thyroid drugs** in the early 1940s as well as the ready availability of radioactive isotopes of iodide (**radioiodide**) following developments in nuclear physics that provided essential tools for investigating thyroid gland functions. These discoveries provided diagnostic tools for assessing thyroid function (radioiodide) and chemicals (anti-thyroid drugs) suitable for blocking thyroid function. Radioiodide not only proved useful for clinical and laboratory work but also provided a label for thyroid molecules that made it possible to elucidate the details of thyroid hormone synthesis, metabolism, and mechanisms of action.

II. Development and Organization of the Mammalian Thyroid Gland

The mammalian thyroid gland consists of many epithelial follicles encapsulated by a connective tissue sheath. The gland is highly vascularized with a dense capillary network surrounding each follicle. The thyroid vasculature receives cholinergic innervation, and the follicle cells receive adrenergic (norepinephrine and dopamine) and peptidergic (e.g., neuropeptide Y, NPY; vasoactive inhibitory peptide, VIP) innervation.

Development of the thyroid gland begins by formation of a ventral bud in the floor of the embryonic pharynx (endoderm) between the first and second pharyngeal pouches. The gland initially differentiates as cellular cords that later separate into clusters of cells destined to become thyroid follicles. The cells of a cluster secrete a protein-rich fluid termed **colloid** that accumulates extracellularly in the center of the cluster. This secretory activity eventually leads to formation of a colloid-filled space, the **lumen** of the follicle, surrounded by a single layer of epithelial cells, the **thyroid epithelium** (Figure 6-1). The portion of the follicular cell that borders on the lumen of the follicle is known as the apex or **apical portion**. The nucleus is generally found in the **basal portion** of the cell that is farthest from the lumen and closest to the capillaries that surround each follicle.

In addition to capillaries and follicles, **parafollicular** or **C cells** occur in the regions between or adjacent to the follicles. Parafollicular cells may occur within the follicular epithelium or may even form separate follicular structures in some species. These cells are derived from another pharyngeal derivative, the **ultimobranchial body**, and secrete a hormone, **calcitonin**, that influences calcium metabolism (see Chapter 14). A comparison of parafollicular cells and follicular cells (Table 6-2) emphasizes their different structural and functional features. In some mammals the parathyroid glands also may be embedded within the mass of the thyroid (Figure 6-2). The parathyroids, like the parafollicular cells, have their origin nearby from the embryonic pharynx and in some species become embedded in the mass of thyroid follicles during development. The parathyroid glands are also discussed in Chapter 14. Unlike the thyroid follicular cells that appear to be of endodermal origin, the parafollicular cells and secretory cells of the parathyroid glands actually are of neural origin and migrate into the embryonic glands (see Chapter 4, Box 4A).

Table 6-2. Comparison of Characteristics of Thyroid Follicular and Parafollicular Cells

Thyroid follicular cell	Thyroid parafollicular cell
Absence of secretion granules	Large number of eosinophilic granules, 0.2-μm diameter; stain with silver nitrate
Endoplasmic reticulum cisternae of larger diameter, containing flocculent precipitate like that found in albumin-secreting cells	Many mitochondria and high level of the mitochondrial enzyme α-glycerophosphate dehydrogenase
Carbohydrate added at Golgi apparatus, which is rather inconspicuous in these cells	No lumenal surface present
	Nucleus more irregular in outline than those of follicular cells
Enlargement of Golgi apparatus from TSH treatment	Golgi apparatus prominent
Binds antibody to thyroglobulin but not to calcitonin	Binds antibody to calcitonin
Cytology not altered by high blood calcium level	Degranulation due to high blood calcium level
Readily accumulates iodide	

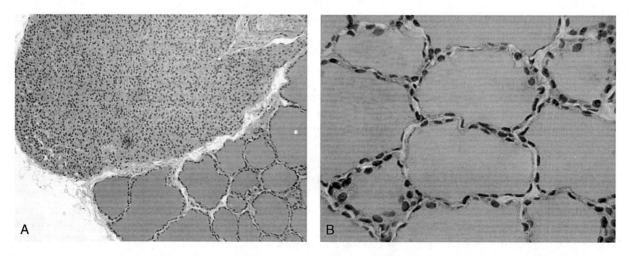

Figure 6-2. **Thyroid and parathyroid glands.** (A) Low magnification of compact parathyroid gland (above) embedded in the thyroid gland consisting of colloid-filled follicles (below). (B) High magnification of thyroid follicles with squamous epithelium surrounding colloid. See color insert, plate 7.

III. Synthesis, Secretion, Action, and Metabolism of Thyroid Hormones

The events related to the ability of thyroid follicles to synthesize and release thyroid hormones are discussed separately for simplicity, but it is important to keep in mind that many of these events may be occurring simultaneously (see Figure 6-3). The processes discussed in this section include:

1. Accumulation of inorganic iodide by follicular cells
2. Synthesis of Tgb, a glycoprotein that contains numerous tyrosine residues for hormone synthesis
3. Binding of inorganic iodide to tyrosine residues in Tgb
4. Synthesis of T from iodinated tyrosines
5. Storage of Tgb containing T_4 in the lumen of the follicle

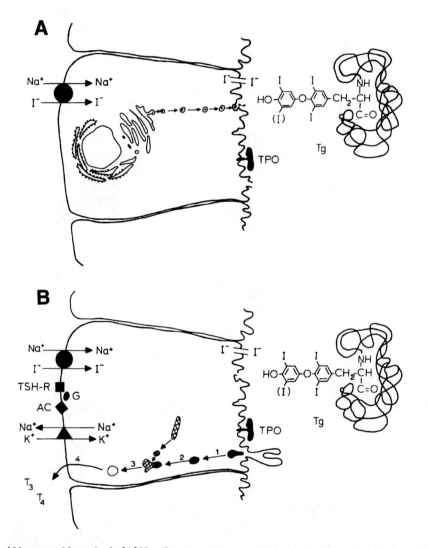

Figure 6-3. **Thyroid hormone biosynthesis.** [A] Na_+/I^- cotransport occurs at the basal surface of a follicular cell. The enzyme thyroid peroxidase (TPO) located at the apical surface is responsible for activating I^-, for iodinating thyroglobulin (Tgb), and for coupling iodinated tyrosines to form T_4. [B] Release of thyroid hormones requires engulfing colloid (endocytosis) to form intracellular endosomes that merge with lysosomes. This causes degradation of Tgb and liberation of T_4 from the basal surface of the cell into the blood. Some T_4 is deiodinated to T_3 or rT_3. DIT is deiodinated to MIT and then to tyrosine and iodide. The latter two products are recycled within the follicular cell. [Reprinted from Carrasco, N. Iodide transport in the thyroid gland. *Biochim. Biophys. Acta* **1154**, 65–82. © with permission of Elsevier Science4-NL, Sara Burgerhartstraat 5, 1055 KV Amsterdam, The Netherlands.]

6. Engulfing of colloid by follicular cells and hydrolysis of Tgb to release T_4 and subsequent conversion of some T_4 to T_3
7. Entry of T_3 and T_4 into the general circulation and their transport to targets

A. Dietary Iodide and Iodide Uptake

The principal source for inorganic iodide is dietary. In certain portions of the world, environmental iodide is in short supply in the environment; for example, the Great Lakes and Rocky Mountain regions of the US, northeastern Europe, and regions of Australia, Africa, and Asia (Figure 6-4). Consequently, in these regions human diets are low in naturally occurring iodide, and hypothyroid states commonly are encountered unless an iodide supplement is used. Iodide deficiency prevents normal synthesis of thyroid hormones, and feedback mechanisms cause excessive stimulation of thyroid glands by TSH. At one time, hypothyroid **goiters** or enlarged thyroids were common in people who inhabited these low-iodide regions or "goiter belts," but the addition of iodized salt to the diet restores thyroid hormone synthesis to normal and has almost eliminated this condition in developed countries. (The term "goiter" or "goitre" originally meant any tumor or abnormal glandular enlargement in the neck but has come to mean an enlarged thyroid.) Unfortunately, hypothyroidism due to low iodide still is rampant in developing countries where it has devastating effects on the well-being of millions of people.

Inorganic iodide is readily absorbed from the intestine into the blood and is selectively accumulated by thyroid follicular cells. There are energy-dependent, active transport mechanisms in both the follicular basal and apical cell membranes that are specific for iodide. Iodide is co-transported with Na^+ (**Na-I symporter, NIS**) at the basal membrane and transported across the apical membrane into the colloid by an apical porter called **pendrin**. Increased amounts of Tgb in the follicular lumen increases production of pendrin. Thus, uptake of iodide from the blood is enhanced by translocation of inorganic iodide at the apical surface and its conversion to organically bound forms (that is, iodinated tyrosines). The resulting concentration of iodide in the thyroid gland normally exceeds plasma levels by 20 to 40X and under some conditions may be even greater. Thyroidal iodide accumulation is not affected by other halide anions including Cl^-, Br^-, and Fl^-, but the iodide pump can be inhibited by excessive amounts of iodide. Patients with **Pendrin Syndrome** have a defective pendrin gene and are unable to retain iodide in the thyroid gland.

The events of iodide uptake, accumulation, and binding to tyrosine initially were elucidated using radioiodide. Uptake of radioiodide, like that of the normal isotope (^{127}I), is stimulated by TSH from the adenohypophysis, and there is no discrimination among the various radioiodide isotopes in the formation of organically bound

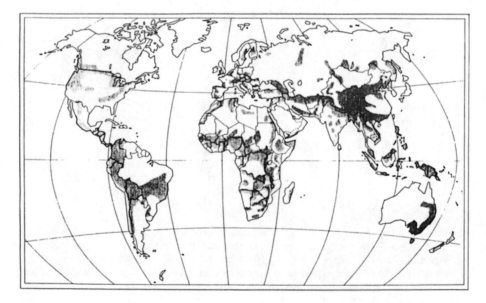

Figure 6-4. **Worldwide location of iodide-poor regions.** The shaded portions indicate the iodide-poor regions. World Health Organization.

iodide associated with thyroid hormone synthesis. For many years, the radioisotope employed most frequently for iodide uptake studies was ^{131}I, a strong beta- and gamma-emitting isotope with a short radiation half-life (about 8 days). This particular isotope could be detected in blood or tissues with relatively unsophisticated detection equipment because of the high-energy gamma radiation it emits. Other isotopes, ^{125}I and ^{123}I, are now employed in most thyroid studies, making use of the lower-energy radiation they produce. These isotopes emit beta and low-energy gamma radiation and are suitable for high-resolution autoradiography at both the level of light and electron microscopes. They also are more suited for metabolic studies and are safer to use than [131]I. However, ^{131}I is still the isotope of choice when attempting to selectively destroy hyperactive follicles (radiothyroidectomy).

Today, radioiodide uptake for clinical imaging and assessment of thyroid gland function in human subjects is often done using **pertechnetate**, a compound containing a radioisotope of technicium, ^{99}Tc. Pertechnetate (^{99}TcO$_4$) is incorporated by thyroid cells like radioiodide but is not incorporated into thyroid hormones and eventually is excreted from the body. It has very low radioactivity compared to radioidide isotopes (Table 6-3). and is much safer to use.

Calculation of a rate for radioisotope accumulation following administration of a given dose provides a quantitative estimate of the degree of TSH stimulation and a reflection of pituitary TSH release. Hence, measurement of radioiodide or pertechnetate uptake and accumulation provides a simple and rapid method for estimating endogenous activities of the HPT axis as well as a means to assess responsiveness of thyroid follicular cells to exogenous TSH. Usually, radioisotope uptake is expressed as percent uptake of the injected dose at some predetermined time (i.e., 24 hours) following administration of the radioisotope (Table 6-4).

Table 6-3. Comparison of Radioiodide Isotopes to Pertechnetate

Isotope	Half-life	Relative damage to tissues (rad[a]/μCi[b])	Common usage
[131]I	8 days	1000	Radiothyroidectomy
[125]I	60 days	650	Radioimmunoassay, synthesis & imaging studies
[123]I	13.3 hr	2	Uptake & imaging
TcO$_4$-		0.2	Uptake & imaging

[a] A rad (radiation absorption dose) is a unit of damage to tissue caused by exposure to radiation. A rad is proportional to the energy level of the gamma ray emitted by the isotope.
[b] A curie (Ci) is a unit of radiation emission concerned with the number of atomic nuclei that disintegrate per second and release gamma rays.

Table 6-4. Comparison of Thyroid Function in a Monotreme (Echidna), Marsupial (Bandicoot), and Placental Mammal (Rabbit)[a]

	Euthyroid parameters			Effect of thyroidectomy	
	Iodide uptake (% injected dose)	Plasma T$_4$ (nmol/liter)	Plasma T$_3$ (nmol/liter)	BMR[b]	Body temperature
Echidna, *Tachyglossus aculeatus*	6.4	15.7	0.7	No effect	No effect
Bandicoot, *Perameles nasuta*	13.7	22.0	1.5	Decrease	No effect
Rabbit, *Oryctolagus cuniculus*	22.9	57.9	6.9	Decrease	No effect

[a] Data from Hurlbert and Augee (1982). *Physiol. Zool.* **55**, 220–228.
[b] BMR, basal metabolic rate.

It is important to understand that the ability to accumulate and bind iodide organically is not a feature unique to thyroid follicular cells, and many cell types will accumulate some iodide. Pigment cells such as melanophores and melanocytes, pigmented retinal cells, and the epithelial cells found in sweat glands, salivary glands, lactating mammary glands, and kidney tubules readily accumulate radioiodide following injection of any radioactive isotope and may add radioiodide to their secretions. Furthermore, oocytes of many oviparous (egg-laying) vertebrates readily accumulate large amounts of radioiodide. This ovarian accumulation is associated with the normal process of ensuring a source of iodide in the egg that can be used by the young animal for early synthesis of thyroid hormones until an adequate dietary source becomes available. In addition, thyroid hormones, presumably of maternal origin, have been found in the oocytes of several teleosts and at least one amphibian. Marsupials, placental mammals, and other live-bearing vertebrates are known to transfer iodide and thyroid hormones to the developing young from the maternal blood or via the milk to suckling newborns.

Thyroid hormones may not be released into the circulation in proportion to the uptake and binding of radioiodide, however. Uptake, binding, and release of thyroid hormones are separate events independently influenced by a variety of factors, as evidenced in the following discussions. Nevertheless, measurement of the uptake of radioiodide isotopes is a rapid and convenient method to assay for TSH activity with respect to endogenous levels or exogenous treatments, and it is widely employed in thyroid diagnosis and research in animals.

B. Biosynthesis of Thyroid Hormones

As described in Chapter 3, the synthesis of thyroid hormones in the follicular cells involves the synthesis of Tgb containing tyrosine followed by the binding of accumulated inorganic iodide to some of these tyrosines. The final step is the linking together (coupling) of two iodinated tyrosines contained within Tgb to form the iodinated hormone T_4. The use of radioiodide, polarized monolayer cultures of porcine thyroid cells, and a clone of normal rat thyroid cells called FRTL-5, has been instrumental in the elucidation of the following events considered typical for mammalian thyroid cells.

1. Synthesis of Thyroglobulin (Tgb)

The protein we call Tgb may occur in more than one molecular form. Tgbs occur in several sizes, ranging from 12S to 27S. ("S" stands for Svedberg sedimentation coefficient, which is related to size, shape, and, to a lesser degree, electrostatic charge of a molecule. These parameters determine the migration and final position of molecules in a molecular gradient following high-speed centrifugation.) The basic monomer is the 12S form. Comparative analysis of Tgbs from different vertebrates indicates different proportions of oligomers of Tgbs (Table 6-5). Most mammalian Tgb preparations exhibit a predominant 19S component (87–100% of the total iodinated protein in thyroid preparations) with a small proportion of larger 27S and occasionally a small quantity of 12S Tgb (rabbit, rat, and especially the guinea pig). The 19S form consists of two 12S-subunits, and the 27S form is composed of four subunits. Regardless of its actual form, Tgb will be treated in the following discussions as though it were a single molecular species.

Tgb synthesis occurs at the rough endoplasmic reticulum and it is packaged into membrane-bound secretion granules in the Golgi apparatus. It appears that noniodinated tyrosines are incorporated into Tgbs first. There are no transfer-RNAs for iodinated tyrosines in follicular cells, and studies show that iodination occurs at the cell-colloid interface after Tgb synthesis. Apparently, the tyrosines in Tgb are sulfated prior to iodination. However, relatively few of the tyrosine residues are iodinated, and the number of thyroid hormone molecules formed within a Tgb molecule is estimated at between 4 and 8.

2. Iodination of Tyrosine Residues in Thyroglobulin

Organic binding of iodine begins with conversion of inorganic iodide to **active iodide**, a form of inorganic iodide that readily is incorporated into the phenolic ring of the amino acid tyrosine. Active iodide apparently is formed in the colloid compartment through the action of an enzymatic **thyroid peroxidase**

Table 6-5. Sedimentation Coefficients for Mammalian Iodoproteins (Thyroglobulins)

Species	Percent		
	12S	19S	27S
Cavia porcellus (guinea pig)	14	83	3
Rattus rattus (rat)	Trace	93	7
Mus musculus (mouse)	—	94	6
Oryctolagus cuniculus (rabbit)	Trace	98	2
Canis familiaris (dog)	—	94	6
Felis catus (cat)	—	92	8
Bos taurus (ox)	—	91	9
Bulbalus bulalis (brahma)	—	93	7
Capra hircus (goat)	—	90	10
Ovis aries (sheep)	—	88	12
Sus scrofa (pig)	—	88	12
Equus caballus (horse)	—	100	—
Equus asinus (donkey)	—	100	—
E. caballus × *E. asinus* (mule)	—	100	—
Homo sapiens (human)	—	92	8
Macaca mulatta (rhesus monkey)	—	92	8

(TPO) system located on the extracellular side of the apical membrane of the follicular cell. TPO catalyzes glucose oxidation and reduction of pyridine nucleotides to form **hydrogen peroxide**, H_2O_2. Inorganic iodide reacts with H_2O_2 to form active iodide, which in turn is attached to tyrosine residues in Tgb.

The binding of one iodide to tyrosine at position 3 on the phenolic ring yields **3-monoiodotyrosine** or **MIT**. A second iodide attaches at position 5 of the same tyrosine residue, resulting in conversion of MIT to **3,5-diiodotyrosine** or **DIT**. In reality, there is no difference between the 3-position and the 5-position due to the symmetry of the phenolic ring and the numbering is arbitrary. Hence, by convention, the first one iodinated always yields a 3-monoiodotyrosine but never a 5-monoiodotyrosine. Unless iodide is in very short supply, all of the MIT will be converted to DIT. The structures of MIT and DIT and their coupling to form T_4 are illustrated in Chapter 3 (Figure 3-36).

3. Coupling of Iodinated Tyrosines

Combination of adjacent DITs in the folded, globular Tgb molecule and the peptide fragment accomplishes the coupling (Figure 6-5). Coupling appears to be an enzymatically controlled process that involves two DITs. The alanine side chain on one of the iodinated tyrosines is cleaved off, and the remaining iodinated phenolic ring is joined to the other iodinated tyrosine through formation of an ether (-O-) linkage. The resultant structure is known as an iodinated **thyronine**. The remains of the tyrosine that donated its phenolic ring is converted to a variant of alanine called **dehydroalanine** (missing one hydrogen). Coupling of DIT and DIT to yield T_4 follows hydrolysis of some peptide bonds to release smaller peptides of 15 to 20 kDa from Tgb. Only a fraction of the DITs are actually coupled, and iodinated thyronines are formed from only about 10% of the iodinated tyrosine residues present in Tgb. Consequently, most of the extractable organic iodide is still in the form of DIT.

4. Hormone Release: Hydrolysis of Thyroglobulin

Release of thyroid hormones following administration of TSH is not linked directly to iodide uptake and iodothyronine synthesis. Thyrotropin independently stimulates engulfment of colloid by the follicular cell and its intracellular hydrolysis (Figure 6-3). Autoradiographic studies indicate that the first event observed following TSH administration is the engulfment of colloid through a process of endocytosis. As these colloid

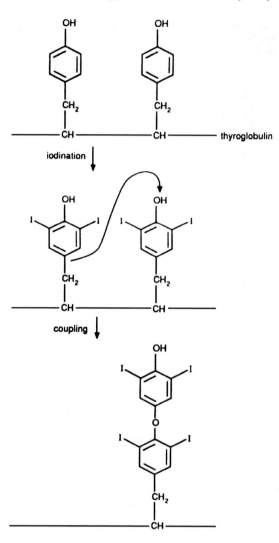

Figure 6-5. **Synthesis of a thyronine.** In this example, the iodinated ring of one molecule of DIT is removed and linked to the oxygen on a second DIT nearby. This coupling is a result of the activity of the thyroid peroxidase system (TPO). The resultant molecule is called a thyronine. This particular thyronine would be thyroxine. From Bolander, F. F. (1989). "Molecular Endocrinology," Academic Press, Inc.

droplets or **endosomes** migrate from the apical portion of the cells toward the basal portion, they become associated with lysosomes that contain a number of hydrolytic enzymes. Fusion of endosomes with lysosomes results in formation of "fusion droplets" or **endolysosomes**. As the endolysosomes continue migrating toward the basal portion of the cell, they become progressively de-granulated, presumably because of hydrolysis of thyroglobulin and diffusion of the hydrolysis products into the cytosol. Tgb hydrolysis within the endolysosome releases DIT, T_4, dehydroalanine, and other amino acids.

A **type I deiodinase** present in the cytosol of thyroid follicular cells plays an important role in iodide metabolism (Table 6-6). This enzyme can deiodinate both the inner and outer rings of a thyronine and can deiodinate iodotyrosines as well. Most of the T_4 released from Tgb rapidly exits from the follicular cell, but a small number of T_4 molecules may be partially deiodinated to form T_3 or **reverse $T_3(rT_3)$**. The amount of deiodination depends on the species. DIT is also deiodinated leading progressively to formation of MIT and tyrosine plus free iodide. Hence, this enzyme is sometimes called an iodotyrosine dehalogenase (iodine is one of a group of elements called halogens). Because iodinated tyrosines cannot be used in Tgb synthesis, they must be either deiodinated or allowed to diffuse from the cell. Thus, deiodination is in part a conservation mechanism to reuse inorganic iodide and tyrosine. Approximately 85–90% of the iodide released through

Table 6-6. Types of Deiodinase Activity

Characteristic	Type of deiodinase		
	I	II	III
Location	Liver, kidney, thyroid	Brain, pituitary, placenta, brown adipose tissue (BAT)	Brain, skin, placenta
Substrate preference	Inner or outer ring	Outer ring	Inner ring
Effect of PTU[a]	Inhibition	No effect	No effect
Reactions catalyzed	$T_4 \rightarrow T_3$	$T_4 \rightarrow T_3$	$T_3 \rightarrow T_2$
	$T_4 \rightarrow rT_3$	$rT_3 \rightarrow T_2$	$T_4 \rightarrow rT_3$
	$rT_3 \rightarrow T_2$		
	$T_3 \rightarrow T_2$		

[a] PTU, propylthiouracil; rT_3, reverse T_3.

deiodination of MIT, DIT, and T_4 enters a "second iodide pool" within the follicular cell, which is then available for diffusion into the colloid and reused for iodination of tyrosines in newly synthesized Tgb.

C. Peripheral Deiodination and Metabolism of Thyroid Hormones

Only about one-seventh to one-half of the circulating T_3, however, is of thyroid origin (depending on the species and/or physiological parameters), and the remainder is produced through peripheral deiodination of T_4. This deiodination is accomplished primarily in the liver by the same type I deiodinase that was present in thyroid cells. Some additional deiodination occurs in kidneys and skeletal muscle. T_4 is deiodinated to either T_3 or rT_3. Approximately one-half of the T_4 deiodinated by the liver is converted to rT_3 by deiodination. However, because rT_3 doesn't bind to plasma proteins as do T_3 and T_4, it is rapidly removed from the blood by the kidney, and rT_3 levels in the blood are extremely low. Type I deiodinase also has a strong preference for rT_3 and some rT_3 is rapidly deiodinated to **diiodothyronine (T_2)**, which has no biological activity. In most mammals, the majority of circulating T_3 has its origin from peripheral deiodination of T_4 in the liver. Type I deiodinase is strongly inhibited by the anti-thyroid drug, **propylthiouracil, PTU** (see ahead). A **type II deiodinase** occurs primarily in the brain, pituitary, brown adipose tissue (rodents), and placenta. It prefers T_4 over rT_3 as a substrate, deiodinates only the outer ring, and is responsible for production of intracellular levels of T_3 in these target tissues. **Type III deiodinase** also is found in the brain and placenta as well as in the intestine and fetal skin. This enzyme attacks only the inner ring, preferring T_3 as a substrate although it can convert T_4 into rT_3 as well and hence inactivates thyroid hormones. Neither type II nor type III deiodinase is affected by PTU.

A second pathway for T_4 metabolism in liver involves conversion of T_4 to **tetraiodothyroacetate (TETRAC)**, which has no significant physiological activity and is excreted rapidly in urine or bile. Some T_3 similarly is converted to **triiodothyroacetate (TRIAC)**, but the majority of nondeiodinated T_3 is conjugated to sulfate for excretion in humans. Some T_3 and T_4 molecules are eliminated intact via the feces as a result of hormone loss through the hepatic-intestinal route. Thyroid hormone metabolites are illustrated in Chapter 3, Figure 3-40.

1. Transport of Thyroid Hormones in the Blood

Under normal conditions, circulating T_4 levels are much greater than T_3 levels. Most of the circulating thyroid hormones are bound reversibly to serum proteins. Serum binding and transporting of thyroid hormones are essential, because T_3 and T_4 are somewhat hydrophobic and are not very soluble in blood. Serum-bound hormones provide a ready reservoir to quickly replenish the levels of free hormones in the blood. Free thyroid hormones appear to enter cells readily and are rapidly removed from the blood and metabolized, especially by the liver and kidneys. Several different serum proteins are capable of binding and transporting thyroid hormones, and binding prevents rapid loss of thyroid hormones via the urine.

About 75–85% of the bound hormones are linked to the α_2-globulins called **thyroid-binding globulin (TBG)**. Only a very small fraction (<0.1%) is transported free in the blood, and the remainder is bound to **prealbumin (TBPA)** and **albumin (TBA)**. Prealbumin is also known as **transthyretin (TTR)**.

Thyroxine is more tightly bound than T_3 to the serum proteins, and consequently T_3 is more rapidly eliminated from the blood. The biological half-life for circulating T_3 in humans is about 24 hours, whereas T_4 has a much longer biological half-life (about 7 days), attributable to the greater affinity of T_4 for the serum-binding proteins. The reduced serum protein binding and more rapid clearance of T_3 from the circulation and binding to target cell receptors are responsible for the observed greater effectiveness of T_3 over T_4 when administered to humans or rats. The nuclear thyroid hormone receptors also have a greater affinity for T_3 than T_4. Many consider T_4 to be only a storage reservoir (a prohormone) from which T_3, the active hormone, is synthesized peripherally. Tgb, then, can be considered a preprophormone.

Low levels of Tgb have been reported in the circulation of several mammals under normal conditions. Levels of about 4-ng Tgb/ml have been found in healthy humans. Elevated plasma Tgb often occurs when carcinomas are present in the thyroid.

D. Mechanism of Action of Thyroid Hormones

Thyroid hormones, because of their somewhat hydrophobic nature, were originally thought to enter target cells by simple diffusion. However, in recent years the presence of a number of **organic anion transporter polypeptides (oatps)** have been discovered in different target cells that transport thyroid hormones across cell membranes. In solution, T_3 and T_4 lose a hydrogen ion from their carboxyl group and hence exist as organic anions.

Once T_4 enters a target cell, it is converted rapidly to T_3 by a cytoplasmic type III deiodinase. T_3 diffuses into the nucleus and binds to a nuclear **thyroid receptor (TR)**. The most effective receptor complex for interacting with a **thyroid receptor element (TRE)** involves a heterodimer of occupied TR plus a **retinoid X receptor protein (RXR)**. Homodimers of TR are less effective in activating and binding to the TRE. Occupied receptors influence the synthesis of new proteins by regulating gene transcription. Nuclear TRs have greater affinity for T_3 than for T_4, supporting the hypothesis that T_3 is the active form of thyroid hormone. Mitochondrial receptor proteins for thyroid hormones also have been demonstrated, and these mitochondrial receptors may be associated with observed effects of thyroid hormones on mitochondrial protein synthesis and oxidative metabolism. Unoccupied receptors for thyroid hormones have not been demonstrated in the cytosol.

Some permissive actions of thyroid hormones may be a consequence of effects of thyroid hormones on nuclear-directed synthesis of adenylyl cyclase or on availability of ATP through their actions on mitochondria or on both. The levels of adenylyl cyclase and ATP would influence the effects of hormones that normally produce their actions through some cAMP-dependent mechanism (see Chapter 3). Another mechanism for their permissive actions could be related to thyroid hormone-induced synthesis of receptor proteins for other regulators.

IV. Factors That Influence Thyroid Function in Mammals

The hypothalamus and pituitary exert direct control over thyroid gland functions but in turn are influenced by environmental factors working through the nervous system. Other hormones (e.g., melatonin) may alter thyroid function. Many additional factors (e.g., diet) influence thyroid state in mammals and hence may influence processes controlled by other hormones by altering permissive roles.

A. Endocrine Factors Affecting Thyroid Gland Function

The hypothalamus exerts regulatory control over release of TSH from the pars distalis via secretion of TRH (see Chapter 4). Thyroid hormones themselves play important roles through negative feedback on the thyroid axis. In addition, the pineal gland may have a negative influence on thyroid function under certain conditions.

1. TRH and TSH

The hypothalamus is the source of TRH that is released from the median eminence and travels to the pituitary thyrotrope via the hypothalamo-hypophysial portal system. Thyrotropin release is stimulated by TRH that in turn produces an increase in circulating thyroid hormones. Both synthesis and release of TSH are regulated through an IP_3 second messenger system (see Chapters 3 and 4). Calcium ions also are involved in release of TSH from the thyrotropic cell. Sensitivity of the thyrotrope to TRH may be affected by paracrines secreted from other pituitary cells (e.g., the pituitary adenylate cyclase-activating peptide, PACAP).

TSH enhances uptake of radioiodide and the synthesis of thyroglobulin and thyroid hormones. In addition, TSH induces endocytosis and subsequent hydrolysis of thyroglobulin, causing thyroid hormones to be released into the blood. Continued stimulation by TSH causes structural changes in the follicular cells that are related to thyroid hormone synthesis and release. The follicular cells in an inactive or unstimulated follicle are usually flat or squamous cells. Thyrotropin can cause such flat cells to assume a cuboidal or even columnar shape, resulting in visible thickening of the follicular epithelium and even increasing the size of the entire gland. Much of this enlargement of the follicular cells is due to an increase in rough endoplasmic reticulum and Golgi apparatus for Tgb synthesis. This increase in cellular size due to increased cellular growth is referred to as **hypertrophy**. Chronically stimulated thyroid glands may exhibit hypertrophy as well as **hyperplasia** (an increase in cellular numbers due to mitotic divisions by the stimulated cells). Hypertrophy or hyperplasia or both can lead to formation of a goiter.

The increase in the cellular portion of the follicle due to hypertrophy and the concomitant reduction in colloid are reflected in a change in the diameter of the follicle with respect to the thickness of the epithelium or to the volume of the lumen. The ratio of follicle diameter to thickness of the epithelium or diameter of the follicular lumen changes predictably with TSH levels and frequently has been used as a measure of the degree of stimulation by TSH. Generally, a "stimulated" histology is indicative of thyroid hormone deficiencies and enhanced TSH secretion to compensate for these deficiencies. Other factors, such as cold stress, may be operating at the hypothalamus, however, to elevate TSH secretion above that normally maintained through negative feedback by the thyroid hormones. This effect also may cause follicular cell hypertrophy.

One of the first cellular events that occurs in follicular cells following administration of TSH is activation of adenylyl cyclase and resultant increase in the intracellular levels of cAMP. Coincident with increased iodide uptake, formation of organic iodide, and endocytosis of colloid is an increase in glucose oxidation that may be caused by cAMP. Glucose oxidation is thought to be the "driving force" for endocytosis and iodination, the latter involving oxidation of pyridine nucleotides and formation of H_2O_2. By controlling reactions such as glucose oxidation, cAMP could mediate several different cellular events associated with the action of TSH on the follicular cells.

2. T_3 and T_4 Feedback Effects

The release of TSH is regulated by negative feedback produced by thyroid hormones, and the administration of exogenous thyroid hormones decreases circulating TSH and associated thyroid gland activities. The major site for negative feedback is on the thyrotropic cells directly and not the hypothalamic thyrotropic center responsible for TRH production. Thyrotropes contain receptors that bind T_3 more effectively than T_4. Occupied thyroid hormone receptors interfere with the cAMP-dependent releasing mechanism such as that stimulated by VIP. Type II deiodinase present in thyrotropes converts most of the T_4 that enters the thyrotrope to T_3 that enhances action with receptors in target cells and feedback in pituitary cells. Thyrotropin levels seem to be maintained by direct negative feedback, and the role of TRH may be to override the system during times of increased demand for thyroid hormones. In other words, thyroid hormones determine the level of TSH secretion that regulates daily thyroid gland activities whereas the hypothalamus adjusts that level through TRH secretion as dictated by other neural factors and/or by environmental cues.

Evidence has been reported for a stimulatory role by thyroid hormones on hypothalamic TRH release. These experimental observations have not established this as a major regulatory pathway in mammals, but they do provide the basis for further investigation into the mechanism whereby hypothalamic control can override the adenohypophysial set point under conditions of increased demand for thyroid hormones.

3. The Epiphysial Complex

The pineal gland of the epiphysial complex in mammals (see Chapter 4) has been implicated as a factor regulating thyroid function. This action on thyroid function is probably mediated through inhibitory effects of melatonin on hypothalamic TRH release. Numerous studies have demonstrated an inhibitory action on the thyroid gland by melatonin. Photoperiodic influences on thyroid activity also may be mediated through inhibition or stimulation of the pineal gland.

B. Non-Endocrine Factors Affecting Thyroid Gland Function

Thyroid activity is affected by a number of chemicals in the diet that block one or more biochemical steps in thyroid hormone synthesis. In addition, a number of environmental factors, such as photoperiod and temperature, can influence the activity of this system through the brain, pineal gland, and pituitary.

1. Diet

Low iodide availability reduces the synthesis of thyroid hormones and leads to development of hypothyroid conditions. Most seriously affected by the reduction in iodide is the synthesis of DIT, which in turn reduces the proportion of T_4 that can be synthesized. Hypothyroidism and goiter formation was once common in certain areas of the world where environmental iodide was is low supply, especially mountainous regions and places distant from the ocean. The introduction of iodide in milk and salt has alleviated this condition in developed countries. Thyroid deficiencies due to low-iodide diets are still the major causes of thyroid dysfunction in Asia and Africa, resulting in widespread incidence of goiter. Furthermore, such iodide deficiencies during pregnancy can result in children with depressed neural function and/or mental retardation. Iodide supplementation could easily and inexpensively eliminate iodide deficiency consequences, and developed countries should adopt a goal to eliminate iodide deficiencies around the world. Paradoxically, there has been a reduction in the use of iodized salt in developed countries and a reduction in the iodide content of milk at the beginning of the 21st century, and we can expect to see increased thyroid dysfunction in countries like Australia and the USA.

An excessive level of blood iodide may inhibit uptake and accumulation of iodide by the follicular cells, presumably by inhibiting the iodide-pumping mechanism. In nature, it would be most unusual for a mammal to be subjected to an excess of iodide, but several instances of excessive iodide are known for humans. Ingestion by Japanese fisherman of large quantities of seaweed, which is naturally rich in iodide, induces a hypothyroid state. In the early 1980s, occurrence of high levels of iodide in milk and fast foods due to artificial additives or contaminants raised medical concerns of potential induction of hypothyroidism, especially in children whose nervous systems would be especially sensitive to insufficient thyroid hormone. However, the low levels of iodide added to commercial salt preparations or those in milk do not pose a threat but are an important deterrent to prevent hypothyroidism from insufficient iodide availability in both children and adults.

Reduced caloric intake or fasting depresses circulating T_3 with (in rats) or without (in humans) depression of T_4 levels. This is an adaptive response that limits growth or metabolic rate when energy sources are low. Studies in rats suggest that overfeeding (especially of carbohydrates) elevates T_3 levels and might be related to hyperactivity in children.

2. Chemical Inhibitors of Iodide Uptake

Certain anions are effective in blocking accumulation of iodide by follicular cells through competitive inhibition of iodide transport. **Thiocyanate (SCN⁻)**, **perchlorate ions (HClO₃₋)**, and pertechnetate (TcO₄₋) are particularly effective at blocking iodide uptake. These agents can be used to block thyroid function and particularly to block iodide uptake mechanisms. Because of its ability to compete with iodide for uptake by thyroid cells, small doses of radioactive pertechnetate may be used in place of radioiodide for determining thyroid activity. High levels of pertechnetate may be useful as a blocking agent since it is less toxic than some other agents, especially SCN⁻. Elevated perchlorate levels in drinking water may be of concern for normal fetal thyroid function (see ahead).

3. Chemical Inhibitors of Iodination

Compounds that interfere with thyroid hormone synthesis by inhibiting iodination of tyrosines are called **goitrogens**. The resultant reduction in circulating hormones causes increased TSH secretion as a consequence of reduced negative feedback. Continuous stimulation of the thyroid gland by TSH results in enlargement of the thyroid and production of a goiter. Typically, goitrogens block formation of active iodide and hence prevent iodination of tyrosines. Intracellular accummulation of iodide secondarily inhibits iodide uptake. Because agents that selectively inhibit iodide uptake secondarily block thyroid hormone synthesis and also can lead to goiter formation, the inhibitory anions, such as perchlorate, are often called goitrogens.

Several anti-thyroid drugs are capable of blocking formation of active iodide, including the classically used drugs PTU and **thiourea (TU)**, as well as newer drugs such as **methimazole** (Figure 6-6). These drugs are not as toxic as some of the anions described earlier. They interfere with the peroxidase system responsible for generation of H_2O_2. Treatment with such drugs can be used to "chemically thyroidectomize" an animal reversibly. Certain reduced compounds such as ascorbic acid, reduced glutathione, and reduced pyrimidines also remove H_2O_2 from the system and can block formation of active iodide.

Many flowering plants of the family *Brassicae* (e.g., cabbage, brussel sprouts, rutabaga, and turnips) naturally contain a compound known as **progoitrin** that can be converted by a specific enzyme to a goitrogenic compound called **goitrin** (Figure 6-6). If sufficient quantities of goitrin are absorbed from the intestine into the general circulation, the synthesis of thyroid hormones is impaired and a hypothyroid state ensues. People or animals that consume large quantities of these plants are at risk for hypothyroidism that may be accentuated if coupled with an iodide-poor diet. Cooking these plants normally destroys the enzyme that converts progoitrin to goitrin, but progoitrin itself is not affected by the quantity of heat applied in cooking the vegetables. Bacteria that are part of the human intestinal flora are capable of converting ingested progoitrin into goitrin, thus reversing the protective effect of cooking.

Some vascular plants such as cauliflower contain a glycoside of thiocyanate that can be converted to free thiocyanate in the body. However, one would have to ingest about 10 kg of cauliflower per day to produce any serious effects on thyroid function unless dietary iodide was extremely low.

4. Specific Inhibitors of Deiodination and of Receptor Binding

Deiodination of T_4 to T_3 can be prevented by treatment with drugs such as **iopanoate** or **ipodate** (Figure 6-6). These drugs were injected initially as radio-opaque agents that were removed from the blood by the liver and secreted into bile where they aided visual examination of the gallbladder in which they accumulated. They later were discovered to be very potent blockers of deiodinating enzymes. It is also possible to block thyroid hormone action with the drug **amiodarone** (Figure 6-6) that binds to thyroid receptors and blocks binding of thyroid hormones. This drug was first used to treat cardiac arrhythmia before its anti-thyroid role was discovered. We now know that amiodarone also is an inhibitor of deiodinase activity, giving it another mechanism for reducing thyroid functioning. As previously mentioned, the type I deiodinase found in the thyroid gland and in the liver is inhibited by PTU although type II and III deiodinases are unaffected by this drug. Hence, PTU not only blocks T_4 synthesis but also blocks conversion of T_4 to T_3.

5. Environmental Factors

Environmental factors such as photoperiod and temperature may affect thyroid hormone secretion rates through nervous or endocrine agents. Such factors may influence synthesis and release of hypothalamic and hypophysial hormones or may alter thyroid function through innervation of the thyroid gland itself.

Internal biological clocks may be related to the actions of environmental factors in regulating thyroid cycles. Cyclical variations have been reported for thyroid hormones on both a diurnal and seasonal basis. Internal secretory rhythms of hypothalamic regulators might be influenced by environmental factors or might regulate the sensitivity of other effectors to external factors. Feedback by thyroid hormones or other hormones in the internal environment may alter sensitivity as well.

Polychlorinated biphenyls (PCBs) that have accumulated in the environment have been shown to be endocrine-disrupting chemicals (EDCs) in that they inhibit thyroid function. Fishes in the Great Lakes area

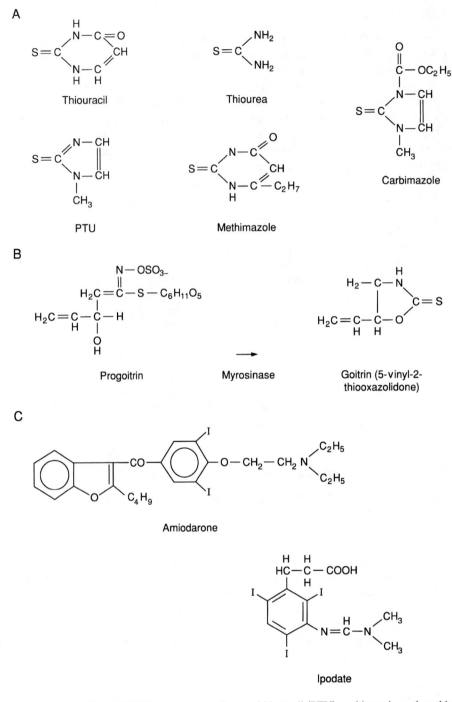

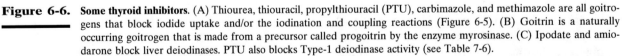

Figure 6-6. **Some thyroid inhibitors.** (A) Thiourea, thiouracil, propylthiouracil (PTU), carbimazole, and methimazole are all goitrogens that block iodide uptake and/or the iodination and coupling reactions (Figure 6-5). (B) Goitrin is a naturally occurring goitrogen that is made from a precursor called progoitrin by the enzyme myrosinase. (C) Ipodate and amiodarone block liver deiodinases. PTU also blocks Type-1 deiodinase activity (see Table 7-6).

of the US have accumulated sufficient PCBs to affect thyroid function in humans consuming them on a regular basis. Exposure of pregnant women to high dietary levels of PCBs produce children with reduced learning capabilities, presumably due to effects of a hypothyroid condition during development of the nervous system. Contamination of water supplies by **ammonium perchlorate** poses another threat to animals and humans due to its accumulation in drinking water. The most common sources of ammonium perchlorate are from military activities and automobiles, and contamination of the environment with perchlorate ions is most prevalent around military installations. Areas of heaviest contamination in the US include southern California and western Texas. Perchlorate ions, as indicated earlier, have a goitrogenic action and block thyroid function. The increasing concentration of perchlorate ions in drinking water are of special concern, especially for pregnant women with the possible effects of thyroid deficiency on fetal nervous system development.

V. Biological Actions of Thyroid Hormones in Mammals

Thyroid hormones affect many diverse tissues and influence major processes such as metabolism, growth, differentiation, and reproduction. They are responsible for maintaining a general state of well-being for many cells so that they are capable of maximal responses to other stimuli.

A. Metabolic Actions

The effects produced by thyroid hormones on mammalian metabolism include a calorigenic or **thermogenic action** (heat-generating) as well as specific effects related to carbohydrate, lipid, and protein metabolism. In general, thyroid activity in mammals is greater during prolonged periods of cold stress (winter) than during warmer periods. Thermogenic actions of thyroid hormones become more meaningful when considered together with the actions of other hormones on metabolism (see Chapter 12). Many of these metabolic actions are possibly permissive actions occurring in cooperation with other hormones such as epinephrine and growth hormone.

Thermogenic actions of thyroid hormones are restricted to certain tissues and are involved in physiological responses to cold stress. They can accelerate the rate at which glucose is oxidized in these tissues and thus increase the amount of metabolic heat produced in a given time. This elevated heat production can be used to warm the body. Accelerated glucose oxidation is reflected in an increased basal metabolic rate (BMR) as measured by an increase in rate of oxygen consumption. In contrast, decreased nutrient intake operates through neural mechanisms that reduce thyroid hormone secretion and lower metabolic rate. As mentioned earlier, there is evidence for thyroid hormone receptors in mitochondria, and thyroid hormones induce increased synthesis of several mitochondrial respiratory proteins, especially cytochrome C, cytochrome oxidase, and succinoxidase. In brown adipose tissue, a tissue especially important for thermogenesis, T_3 but not T_4 stimulates production of a unique mitochondrial protein known as **uncoupling protein 1 (UCP-1)** in a dose-dependent manner. UCP-1 is one of a group of mitochondrial proteins that are up-regulated by thyroid hormones in several tissues, but only UCP-1 has been linked to uncoupling oxidative phosphorylation and heat production. This mitochondrial action to augment oxidative metabolism would be advantageous in adapting to chronic cold stress. Long before the discovery of UCP-1, thyroid hormones were postulated to "uncouple" oxidative phosphorylation, which would decrease the efficiency of ATP synthesis in the mitochondria and increase the quantity of heat released per mole of glucose oxidized. It is not clear if the ability of thyroid hormones to increase the total rate of glucose oxidation or the postulated uncoupling is more important in heat production, but it definitely contributes to chronic cold stress adaptation. Acute cold responses are thought to be mediated primarily by epinephrine from the adrenal medulla (Chapter 8) rather than by thyroid hormones. TSH receptors also have been identified in rat brown adipose cells, and treatment of warm acclimated rats with TSH results in an up-regulation of mRNA levels for both type II deiodinase and UCP-1. Whereas acute cold exposure also caused up-regulation of type II deiodinase and UCP-1, it caused down-regulation of TSH receptors supporting the failure of the HPT axis to regulate acute cold stress homeostasis.

In addition to increasing glucose oxidation, thyroid hormones cause hyperglycemia and may secondarily stimulate lipolysis (hydrolysis of fats). These actions may in part be associated with potentiation of the hyperglycemic and lipolytic actions of epinephrine and/or glucocorticoids (see Chapters 8 and 12). Thyroid hormones may alter nitrogen balance and can be either protein anabolic (through enhancement of GH actions) or catabolic, depending on the tissue being examined and under what experimental conditions it is examined.

In many non-hibernating mammals such as the beaver and muskrat, thyroid activity is depressed during the winter months. Hypothyroidism has been described for hibernating ground squirrels and badgers, but there does not appear to be a causal relationship between reduced thyroid function and the onset of hibernation. Additional field studies employing sophisticated methods for assessing thyroid functions are needed before the endocrine factors related to either onset or termination of hibernation will be established.

B. Growth and Differentiation

Thyroid hormones are essential for normal growth and differentiation in mammals as evidenced in cretinism and juvenile myxedema in humans (see ahead). These growth-promoting actions of thyroid hormones are closely related to the role of pituitary growth hormone (GH), and they probably represent a permissive action on GH secretion and on GH-sensitive target cells. Thyroid hormones also may stimulate insulin-like growth factor (IGF) production and hence augment the actions of GH on its target tissues.

Nervous tissue development is markedly affected by reduced thyroid hormones during differentiation of the nervous system. Normal development of the nervous system as well as attainment of normal mental capacities is dependent on normal levels of thyroid hormones throughout development. Hypothyroidism during gestation and early childhood in humans seriously impairs differentiation and functioning of the nervous system. Similar observations have been made in other mammals as well. Furthermore, a reduction in mental activity can occur in hypothyroid adults, too, emphasizing the continued importance of thyroid hormones in normal nervous system function. Exposure of pregnant women to endocrine-disrupting anti-thyroid chemicals such as polychlorinated biphenyls (PCBs) and perchlorate can have devastating effects on the fetus that are carried into adulthood. The early fetus depends on maternal thyroid hormones as well as for iodide throughout development and is thus critically dependent on the mother's thyroid condition (Figure 6-7).

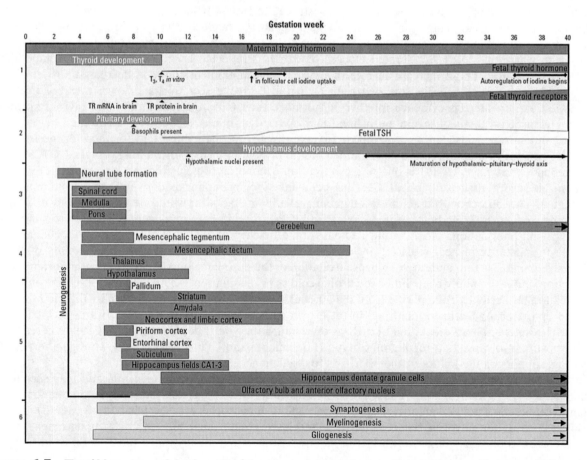

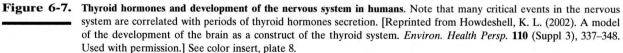

Figure 6-7.   **Thyroid hormones and development of the nervous system in humans.** Note that many critical events in the nervous system are correlated with periods of thyroid hormones secretion. [Reprinted from Howdeshell, K. L. (2002). A model of the development of the brain as a construct of the thyroid system. *Environ. Health Persp.* **110** (Suppl 3), 337–348. Used with permission.] See color insert, plate 8.

Thyroid hormones can affect differentiation processes in adults, too. For example, replacement of hair in adult mammals is stimulated by thyroid hormones. The postnuptial molt cycle in harbor seals, *Phoca vitulina*, involves thyroid hormones and cortisol from the adrenal cortex. Hair loss is correlated with low thyroid function and high cortisol levels, whereas resumption of hair growth is correlated with increased T_4 and return of cortisol to basal levels. Thyroid activity also is related to molting of hair in other mammals including red fox and mink. Changes in hair are seen in hypothyroid humans as well.

C. Reproduction

Another cooperative role for thyroid hormones occurs with respect to gonadal development and function (see Chapter 10). In general, sexual maturation is delayed in hypothyroid mammals. In hypothyroid males, spermatogenesis may occur, but androgen synthesis is low. Similarly, ovarian weight is reduced and ovarian cycles become irregular in hypothyroid females. These reproductive correlations to hypothyroidism have been attributed to reduced GTH levels and can be alleviated by treatment with GTHs or thyroid hormones. Experimental studies also support the notion that thyroid hormones influence GTH release through an effect at the level of the hypothalamus.

VI. Clinical Aspects of Thyroid Function

Although thyroid disorders are among the most common of human endocrine problems (second only to diabetes mellitus), most of these disorders are underactive thyroid conditions and include inherited disorders as well as environmentally induced disorders (e.g., dietary deficiencies and EDCs such as PCBs and perchlorate). In general, thyroid function declines with advancing age, making the elderly more at risk for hypothyroidism. Hyperactive thyroid disorders are less common, and thyroid carcinomas are rare. Either hypothyroid or hyperthyroid conditions may be associated with goiter formation, although their occurrence is more common with hypothyroidism. Generalized symptoms of thyroid disorders are listed in Table 6-1. Although only human disorders are described here, similar conditions can develop in other mammals including domestic dogs and cats.

A. Thyrotoxicosis and Hyperthyroidism

Thyrotoxicosis is a general term referring to an excess of thyroid hormone. If this condition results from thyroid hypersecretion, it is known as **hyperthyroidism**. Primary hyperthyroidism may be due to toxic multinodular goiters consisting of multiple aggregates of small, hyperactive follicles (**Marine-Lenhart syndrome**), or several large TSH-dependent hyperactive follicles (**Plummer's disease**). Follicular adenomas are sometimes autonomously hyperactive as well. Circulating TSH levels typically are low when autonomously hyperactive multinodular goiter or adenomas are present.

Hyperthyroidism may be of a secondary nature caused by a rare pituitary adenoma of TSH-secreting cells. Certain cancerous tumors such as choriocarcinomas of the placenta may elaborate TRH-like or TSH-like molecules that stimulate thyroid activity. Secretory tumors of these types typically are insensitive to any feedback by thyroid hormones.

Graves' disease is a secondary hyperthyroid state that occurs in less than 0.25% of the human population but is much more common in women than men (8 to 1). It appears to be mediated by an immunoglobulin known as **LATS: long-acting thyroid stimulator**. Evidence from studies of twins suggests susceptibility to Graves' disease has a genetic basis. The symptoms of Graves' disease include protruding eyes (exophthalmus), weight loss, increased appetite, restlessness, heat intolerance, fatigue, muscle cramps, tremors, frequent bowel movements, menstrual irregularities, goiter, rapid heartbeat, changes in sex drive, heart palpitations, and blurred or double vision. The basis for production of LATS by the immune system is not understood, but it is an antibody that binds to TSH receptors in the thyroid cell membrane and activates them even in the absence of circulating TSH. These individuals present a hyperthyroid state with very low circulating TSH. The favored treatment, especially in children and adolescents, is to use anti-thyroid drugs such as PTU or methimazole. However, long-term remission occurs in only 20–30% of the patients, and PTU can cause severe hepatitis. Reduction of thyroid tissue by treatment with large doses of radioiodide (^{131}I) is the next approach for treating Graves' disease, and it is much more effective than anti-thyroid drug therapy (80–90% long-term remission). The resultant reduction in thyroid tissue reduces thyroid hormone production. Finally, surgical removal of a portion of the thyroid is sometimes employed. It is as effective as radioiodide treatment (90–95% remission) All of these approaches reduce thyroid hormone production and alleviate the symptoms of hyperthyroidism, but none addresses the cause of the disorder: LATS production by the immune system.

Rarely, hyperthyroidism is due to an ectopic source of thyroid hormones. For example, ovarian dermoid tumors can synthesize sufficient thyroid hormones to bring about hyperthyroidism.

Juvenile thyrotoxicosis is characterized by elevated thyroid hormones, and these patients exhibit nervousness, tremor, accelerated heart rate, and goiter. This syndrome usually occurs in children beyond age 10 (80% of the cases). Exophthalmus is present in about half of these children, and normal weight gain usually is retarded.

A somewhat rare but dramatic hyperthyroid condition is **thyrotoxic crisis** or **thyroid storm**. This disorder involves a sudden increase in thyroid secretion, severe hypermetabolism, fever, and some other, more variable symptoms. It only occurs in hyperthyroid patients and may be precipitated following incomplete thyroidectomy, interruption of anti-thyroid therapy, or even as a reaction to an infection or tooth extraction. It also may be induced by periods of excessive summer heat. The actual cause of thyroid storm is not certain and the condition could encompass a variety of different causes. Perhaps increased levels of UCP-1 contribute to this apparent uncoupling of oxidative processes.

Thyroid hormone resistance is caused by mutation of genes responsible for synthesis of nuclear thyroid receptors, usually the TRβ gene. Mutated receptors result in reduced tissue responses to thyroid hormones.

B. Myxedema and Hypothyroidism

Myxedema is the extreme clinical condition in adults where no thyroid hormones are secreted. In these patients, there is swelling of the skin and subcutaneous tissues caused by the extracellular accumulation of a high-protein fluid. Hypothyroidism refers to any condition where levels of thyroid hormones are insufficient due to defects of primary (at the thyroid) or secondary (hypothalamus or pituitary) origin. It is especially serious in children because of marked effects on both general growth and neural development. The term **juvenile hypothyroidism** refers to cases of hypothyroidism in children that do not lead to severe retardation in somatic and intellectual development. When growth and development are markedly retarded, it is called **cretinism**. This syndrome is remarkably common: 1 in every 8500 births exhibits cretinism. However, if hypothyroidism in the neonate is detected at birth by using a simple thyroid test, it can be alleviated with thyroid hormone therapy so that growth and development from that time are normal. However, because of poor medical care and widespread dietary iodide deficiency, cretinism is a serious, crippling disorder in many developing countries.

Juvenile hypothyroidism does not refer to the fetus that is dependent upon the thyroid state of the mother. It is possible that hypothyroidism during pregnancy can reduce neural development and that can be further affected by hypothyroidism in the neonate.

There are a number of symptoms characteristic of hypothyroidism including rough and dry skin, yellow pallor, coarse scalp hair, hoarse voice, and slow thought and action (Table 6-1). However, sometimes the hypothyroid person exhibits none or only a few of these symptoms. Obesity is often listed as a characteristic but it does not always accompany hypothyroidism and occasionally occurs in patients presenting hyperthyroidism. Conversely, persons suffering from secondary hypothyroidism are often thin as is frequently the case for hyperthyroid patients. Exophthalmus, usually correlated with hyperthyroid states, may occur occasionally in primary myxedema. The fact that these changes are progressive and that they can occur very gradually makes it difficult to diagnose early stages of hypothyroidism using these criteria. However, reduced circulating thyroid hormones, especially if accompanied by elevated TSH levels, is indicative.

C. Goiters

Any enlarged thyroid is referred to as a goiter regardless of the cause or nature of the enlargement. There are actually four kinds of clinical goiters. The first and most common kind is a **hypothyroid goiter** caused by failing thyroid hormone production resulting in a shortage of T_3 and T_4. Circulating TSH levels are elevated because of reduced negative feedback, and this increased TSH causes enlargement of the thyroid gland and formation of a goiter.

The second type is the **hyperfunctioning goiter**. They are not as common as hypothyroid goiters. Typically, circulating thyroid hormones are high due to spontaneously active follicular cells, and TSH levels are low due to feedback. Diffuse thyrotoxic goiter is often termed Graves' disease whereas toxic nodular goiters are associated with Plummer's or Marine-Lenhart syndromes (see above).

The third goiter type is the **hyperfunctioning goiter of pregnancy.** During normal pregnancy, there is an increase in thyroxine-binding globulins and a consequent decrease in free T_4 and T_3 in maternal plasma. This results in elevated TSH through decreased negative feedback and in a slight thyroid enlargement to maintain normal functional levels of thyroid hormones during pregnancy. This condition usually has no serious consequences during pregnancy for either mother or fetus, and typically returns to normal in women after birth.

The fourth kind of goiter develops in people with otherwise normal thyroid function. Such enlargements have many different causes including infiltration of the gland with tuberculosis bacteria, syphilitic bacteria, or parasites as well as by the presence of adenomas or carcinomas. Inflammation due to autoimmune disease (thyroiditis; see below) can also cause enlargement of the thyroid.

D. Thyroiditis

Thyroiditis is a general term often applied to a collection of gene-linked autoimmune disorders involving production of antibodies that attack thyroid proteins, especially the peroxidase enzyme and sometimes Tgb. Thyroid cells also may be attacked by lymphocytes, which in some cases are attracted by the actions of antibodies with thyroid antigens. As with all thyroid disorders, thyroiditis is more prevalent in women than in men. It is sometimes the cause of hypothyroidism that follows pregnancy due to a rebound in immune activity following suppression during pregnancy.

The most common types are **Hashimoto's thyroiditis** (struma lymphomatosa) and **Reidel's thyroiditis** (struma fibrosa). Unlike Graves' disease, a hyperthyroid autoimmune disease, thyroiditis disorders all are associated with hypothyroidism. It is one of the most common causes for goiter among adolescents and is characterized by the presence of numerous lymphoid follicles, diffuse infiltration of the thyroid by lymphocytes, extensive increase in the connective tissue components of the thyroid gland, some changes in follicular structure, and a marked reduction in production of thyroid hormones. In Reidel's thyroiditis, the gland is progressively replaced by fibrous connective tissue. In either type of thyroiditis, a gradual reduction in circulating thyroid hormones brings about an elevation of TSH secretion (negative feedback), which causes goiter formation. Antibodies produced against thyroid iodoproteins and peroxidase are demonstrable in the blood of these patients.

E. Inherited Disorders

More than 20 hereditary defects in thyroid gland metabolism are known and may be classified according to the type of causative metabolic defect. For example, there are several defects related to unresponsiveness of thyroid cells to TSH including insufficient numbers of receptors or abnormal receptors. There also have been numerous mutations discovered in the gene responsible for synthesis of a particular thyroid hormone receptor, TRβ-1. These mutations are linked to generalized resistance to thyroid hormones. In a number of these cases, resistance to thyroid hormones has been correlated with **attention-deficit hyperactivity disorder (ADHD)** in children.

Inherited defects also occur in iodide transport mechanisms, iodination, and coupling of iodinated tyrosines. Several defects have been identified in relation to synthesis of abnormal thyroglobulins. Deficiencies in thyroid deiodinase and total body deiodinaseas as well as the presence of abnormal plasma transport proteins sometimes occur as inheritable errors.

F. Euthyroid Sick Syndrome

Many non-thyroid conditions can alter thyroid function, so that even though the person is actually euthyroid, he/she may appear to be hyper- or hypothyroid. For example, fasting, anorexia nervosa, protein-calorie malnutrition, and untreated diabetes mellitus are all metabolic disturbances that bring about marked decreases in circulating T_3 and increases in rT_3. Thyroid hormones also are altered in a variety of liver and renal diseases as a consequence of numerous infections and following myocardial infarctions. Some conditions may alter levels of T_4, TSH, T_3, and/or rT_3. These alterations in thyroid parameters by peripheral disorders constitute the **euthyroid sick syndrome**, reflecting normal responses of the euthyroid person to the generalized disease states that present superficially as abnormal thyroid function.

VII. Summary

The functional unit of the vertebrate thyroid gland is the thyroid follicle that is unique for storing thyroxine (T_4) extracellularly in the colloid of the follicular lumen. Normal thyroid gland functioning depends upon a constant supply of iodide in the diet as well as upon regulatory stimuli from the hypothalamus (TRH) and the adenohypophysis (TSH). Iodide is accumulated by the follicular cells, and at the apical cell surface is incorporated into tyrosine residues of large glycoproteins collectively referred to as thyroglobulin (Tgb). Iodide is added to tyrosine by thyroid peroxidase (TPO) to form DIT. Two DITs within the Tgb are coupled by thyroid peroxidase to form T_4, and the iodinated Tgb is stored in the follicular lumen. Endocytosis of colloid droplets followed by intracellular hydrolysis of Tgb in endolysosomes frees T_4 to enter the circulation. Some T_4 is degraded to T_3 and rT_3 by a type I deiodinase present in thyroid cells, and these products also may enter the blood. The same deiodinase converts DIT back to tyrosine and inorganic iodide for new synthesis of Tgb and subsequent iodination of its tyrosine residues. Both synthesis and release of thyroid hormones are stimulated by TSH. Anti-thyroid drugs, including certain anions (SCN^-, $HClO_3^-$, TcO_4^-) and the "traditional" goitrogens (e.g., PTU, TU, methimazole) interfere with iodide uptake or the iodination process or both, causing thyroid deficiencies that may lead to goiter formation.

Thyroid hormones are transported in the circulation bound to plasma proteins (TBG, TBPA, TBA), and only a small proportion of free hormones is present. T_4 is more tightly bound to plasma proteins than T_3, and this greater affinity of T_4 for plasma proteins is partly responsible for its much longer biological half-life. Free T_3 apparently enters cells more rapidly than does T_4. Metabolism of most of the T_4 to T_3 and rT_3 occurs in the liver by the action of a type I deiodinase. Most of the circulating T_3 arises peripherally by Type 1 deiodinase action in liver cells on T_4, and it has been suggested that T_4 acts as a circulating reservoir for T_3, which is the "active form" of the hormone. Mitochondrial and nuclear receptors have been prepared from target tissues. These receptors have greater affinity for T_3 than for T_4, which supports the hypothesis that deiodination of T_4 to T_3 may be the important first step in its mechanism of action.

It is difficult to characterize the actions of thyroid hormones with respect to their functions. In addition to their direct actions on development and oxidative metabolism, thyroid hormones play numerous permissive roles. They maintain "responsiveness" in many cells that allows these cells to become more sensitive to other endocrine or neural stimuli. Thyroid hormones also enhance the secretion and actions of other hormones. Processes that are affected by permissive or cooperative actions include growth, metabolism, and reproduction.

The action of thyroid hormones on peripheral tissues following specific binding of the hormone to nuclear receptors (TRs) is followed by activation or inhibition of mRNA transcription and eventual enzyme syntheses. Occupied TRs commonly form heterodimers with RXRs prior to interacting with the TRE in the DNA. The permissive actions of thyroid hormones may be related to such events as the stimulation of the synthesis of components of second messenger systems, up-regulation of receptors for another regulator, effects on structural components, etc. Binding of thyroid hormones to mitochondrial receptors or indirect actions on mitochondria, especially in liver and kidney, may be important in the thermogenic and oxidative actions of thyroid hormones on BMR and in chronic cold stress.

Suggested Reading

Books

Abe, Y., Suzuki, T., Unno, M., Tokui, T., and Ito, S. (2002). Thyroid hormone transporters: Recent advances. *Trends Endocr. Metab.* **13**, 215–220.

Braverman, L. E., and Utiger, R. D. (1996). "Werner and Ingbar's the Thyroid: A Fundamental and Clinic Text," 7th Ed. Lippincott-Raven, Hagerstown, MD.

Fisher, D. A. (2002). Fetal-perinatal thyroid physiology. *In* (E. A. Eugster and O. H. Pescovitzs, Eds.) "Developmental Endocrinology: From Research to Clinical Practice," Humana Press, Totowa, NJ, pp. 135–149.

Greer, M. A. (1990). "The Thyroid Gland. Comprehensive Endocrinology." Rev. Ser. Raven, New York.

McNabb, F. M. A. (1993). "Thyroid Hormones." Prentice-Hall, Englewood Cliffs, NJ.

General Articles

Benvenga, S., and Robbins, J. (1993). Lipoprotein–thyroid hormone interactions. *Trends Endocr. Metab.* 194–198.

Carrasco, N. (1993). Iodide transport in the thyroid gland. *Biochim. Biophys. Acta* **1154**, 65–82.

Christophe, D., and Vassart, G. (1990). The thyroglobulin gene: Evolutionary and regulatory issues. *Trends Endocr. Metab.* **1**, 356–362.

Dumont, J. E., Maenhaut, C., and Lamy, F. (1992). Control of thyroid cell proliferation and goitrogenesis. *Trends Endocr. Metab.* **3**, 12–17.

Franklyn, J. A., and Sheppard, M. C. (1994). Amiodarone and thyroid function. *Trends Endocr. Metab.* **5**, 128–131.

Hafner, R. P. (1987). Thyroid hormone uptake into the cell and its subsequent localisation to the mitochondria. *FEBS Lett.* **224**, 251–256.

Howdeshell, K. L. (2002). A model of the development of the brain as a construct of the thyroid system. *Environ. Health Persp.* **110**, (Suppl 3), 337–348.

Kohn, L. D., Suzuki, K., Nakazato, M., Royaux, I., and Green, E. D. (2001). Effects of thyroglobulin and pendrin on iodide flux through the thyrocyte. *Trends Endocr. Metab.* **12**, 10–16.

König, S., and Neto, V. M. (2002). Thyroid hormone actions on neural cells. *Cell. Mol. Neurobiol.* **22**, 517–544.

Maayan, M. L., Volpert, E. M., and Debons, A. F. (1987). Neurotransmitter regulation of thyroid activity. *Endocr. Rev.* **13**, 199–214.

Rodriguez-Arnao, J., Miell, J. P., and Rosa, R. J. M. (1993). Influence of thyroid hormones on the GH–IGF-l axis. *Trends Endocr. Metab.* **4**, 169–173.

St. Germain, D. L. (1994). Iodothyronine deiodinases. *Trends Endocr. Metab.* **5**, 36–42.

Silva, J. E. (1993). Hormonal control of thermogenesis and energy dissipation. *Trends Endocr. Metab.* **4**, 25–32.

Studer, H., and Gerber, H. (1991). Intrathyroidal iodine: Heterogeneity of iodocompounds and kinetic compartmentalization. *Trends Endocr. Metab.* **2**, 29–34.

Zoeller, R. T., Dowling, A. L. S., Herzig, C. T. A., Iannacone, E. A., Gauger, K. J., and Bansal, R. (2002). Thyroid hormone, brain development, and the environment. *Environ. Health Persp.* **110** (Suppl 3), 355–361.

Clinical Articles

Edwins, D. L., and McGregor, A. M. (1990). Pregnancy and autoimmune thyroid disease. *Trends Endocr. Metab.* **1**, 296–300.

Fisfalen, M.-E., and DeGroot, L. J. (1995). Graves' disease and autoimmune thyroiditis. *In* "Molecular Endocrinology: Basic Concepts and Clinical Implications" (B. D. Weintraub, Ed.), pp. 319–370. Raven, New York.

Gaitau, E., and Dunn, J. T. (1992). Epidemiology of iodine deficiency. *Trends Endocr. Metab.* **3**, 170–175.

Hauser, P., Zametkin, A. J., Martinez, P., Vitiello, B., Matochik, J. A., Mixson, A. J., and Weintraub, B. D. (1993). Attention-deficit-hyperactivity disorder in people with generalized resistance to thyroid hormone. *N. Engl. J. Med.* **328**, 997–1040.

O'Connor, G., and Davies, T. F. (1990). Human autoimmune thyroid disease: A mechanistic update. *Trends Endocr. Metab.* **1**, 266–274.

Usala, S. J., and Weintraub, B. D. (1991). Thyroid hormone resistance syndromes. *Trends Endocr. Metab.* **2**, 140–144.

Wong, T. K., and Hershman, J. M. (1992). Changes in thyroid function in nonthyroid illness. *Trends Endocr. Metab.* **3**, 8–12.

7

The Hypothalamus-Pituitary-Thyroid (HPT) Axis of Non-Mammalian Vertebrates

The functions of the HPT axis in non-mammalian vertebrates are discussed in this chapter, with some emphasis on the evolution of the thyroid and thyroid functions in vertebrates. The reader first should examine Chapter 6 for an understanding of mammalian thyroid functions at the cellular and organismic levels before attempting this chapter since all basic definitions and explanations of thyroid function are provided in Chapter 6 and will not be repeated here.

I. Evolution of the Thyroid Gland and Its Functions

The thyroid gland structurally is a conservative endocrine gland in vertebrates and has a direct connection to an invertebrate chordate structure. In vertebrates, the thyroid is generally found as one or two masses of highly vascularized follicles surrounded by a connective tissue capsule or as scattered follicles throughout the pharyngeal region, as is the case for most fishes (Figures 7-1 and 7-2). Regardless of any gross morphological differences, follicle structure and function are mammalian-like in all the gnathostomes with respect to iodide metabolism (Table 7-1), hormone synthesis, production and storage of thyroglobulin (Tgb)

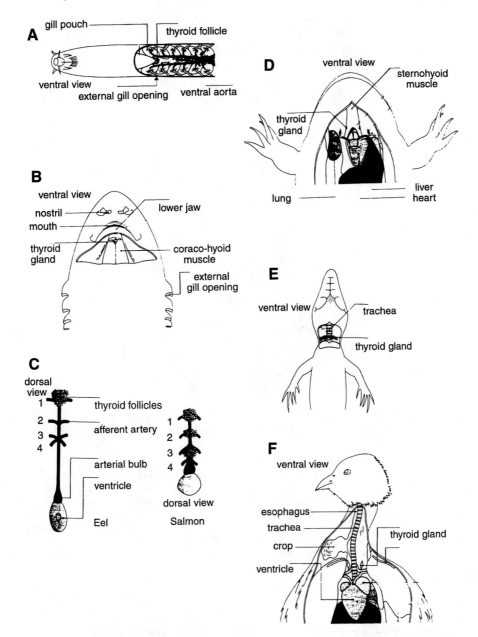

Figure 7-1. **Location of thyroid tissue in non-mammalian vertebrates**. (A) Scattered thyroid follicles in a hagfish (*Eptatretus burgeri*). (B) Discrete thyroid gland of the shark, *Triakis scyllium*. (C) Diffuse thyroids of the eel, *Anguilla japonica* (left) and the Pacific salmon, *Oncorhynchus masou* (right). (D) Paired thyroids in the bullfrog, *Rana catesbeiana*. (E) Medial thyroid gland in neck of the lizard, *Takydromos tachydromoides*. (F) Paired thyroid glands in a bird, the Japanese quail, *Coturnix coturnix japonicus*. [Dissections of thyroid regions modified from Matsumoto and Ishii (1989). "Atlas of Endocrine Organs." Springer-Verlag, Berlin.]

(Table 7-2), hormone release, and responsiveness to thyrotropin (TSH). Biochemical differences are quantitative and not qualitative, and the same thyroid hormones, triiodothyronine (T_3) and thyroxine (T_4), and their metabolites are present in all vertebrates (Table 7-3) and are found in some invertebrates as well (Table 7-4).

The most primitive thyroid condition is considered to be that found in the adult cyclostomes in which only scattered follicles may be present. Extracellular storage of thyroid hormones does not occur in the cyclostome follicle, and iodoproteins are retained in the follicular cells of these primitive fishes. The follicles of all other vertebrates are organized and appear to function like those of mammals (see Chapter 6).

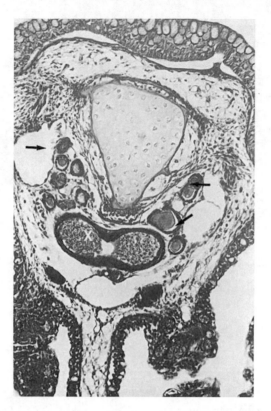

Figure 7-2. **Salmon thyroid follicles**. Cross-section through the lower jaw of a fingerling chinook salmon, *Oncorhynchus tshawytscha*, through the second arotic arch (x). Thyroid follicles (arrows) appear dorsal to the arch on either side.

Table 7-1. Some Effects of Thyrotropin and Thyroid Inhibitors on
^{131}I Uptake[a] by Thyroids of Larval Salamanders, *Ambystoma tigrinum*

N	Mean body weight (g ± SEM)	Daily injections; pretreatment for 7 days	Mean thyroid uptake (% injected dose ± SEM)
6	11 ± 0.5	None	4.6 ± 1.6
6	8 ± 0.6	0.25 μg TSH[b]	12.4 ± 2.5
6	11 ± 0.6	2.5 μg TSH	29.2 ± 4.7
6	17 ± 1.6	25 μg TSH	38.3 ± 1.0
6	9 ± 0.6	2.5 μg TSH + 10 μg PTU[c]	10.2 ± 2.9
6	7 ± 1.0	2.5 μg TSH + 0.5 mg NaSCN[d]	3.9 ± 0.7

[a] Radioiodide uptake was determined 24 hr after intraperitoneal injection of 5 μCi of ^{131}I.
[b] Ovine TSH (NIH-TSH-S6).
[c] PTU, propylthiouracil.
[d] Sodium thiocyanate.

A. The Origin of the Thyroid Gland

Although many biochemical aspects of the synthesis of thyroid hormones are well known in vertebrates, the evolutionary origin of the vertebrate thyroid and acquisition of functional significance for these iodinated compounds are uncertain. The first evidence in chordates of formation of thyroid hormones comes from studies of the **endostyle** of protochordates such as the tunicates and especially the cephalochordate, amphioxus. The endostyle is a mucus-secreting gland located in the pharyngeal region. This mucus, a glycoprotein mixture, is involved in the feeding mechanisms that traps food particles brought into the pharynx by water currents created by movements of pharyngeal cilia. These cilia then move the mucus with trapped food into the digestive tract. Specialized cells near the opening of the endostyle of protochordates accumulate iodide from sea water and use

Table 7-2. Sedimentation Coefficients for Chordate Iodoproteins (Thyroglobulins)

Species	Percent iodoproteins found			
	< 12S	12S	19S	27S
Urochordata				
Ciona intestinalis (tunicate)	100	—	—	—
Vertebrata				
Agnatha				
Lampetra fluviatilis (river lamprey)	32	68	—	—
Chondrichthyes				
Scyliorhinus stellaris (dogfish shark)	—	16	80	4
Osteichthyes				
Conger conger (Congo eel; teleost)	—	6	73	6
Reptilia				
Thalassochelis caretta (sea turtle)	—	11	84	5
Testudo hermanni (land turtle)	—	12	84	4
Aves				
Anas platyrhynchos (domestic duck)	—	Trace	94	6
Gallus gallus (domestic chicken)	—	Trace	94	5

Table 7-3. Levels of Thyroid Hormones for Selected Vertebrate Species

Class/order	Species	Conditions	T_3	T_4
Agnatha/Cyclostomata	*Petromyzon marinus* (sea lamprey)	Mature females	0.5–1.77 nM	69.5–139 nM
		Ammocetes	—	4.9–18.5 μg/dL
		Adults	—	0.46 μg/dL
	Eptatretus stouti (Pacific hagfish)		—	2.2–10.5 μg/dL
Osteichthyes/Teleostei	*Salvelinus fontinalis* (brook trout)			0.15–3.36 μg/dL
	Paralichthys olivaceus (flounder)	Eggs	6–7 ng/g	1 ng/g
		At metamorphic climax	1–1.5 ng/g	10–15 ng/g
	Marone saxatilis (striped bass)	Eggs	4.5 ng/g	5.3 ng/g
		6 weeks postlarvae	6.5 ng/g	7.0 ng/g
Amphibia/Anura	*Bufo marinus* (cane toad)	Fertilized eggs	3.1 ng/g	0.44 ng/g
		At metamorphic climax	5.3 ng/g	8.4 ng/g
Amphibia/Caudata	*Ambystoma tigrinum* (tiger salamander)	Sexually mature larvae	0.07–0.73 ng/ml	0.25–9.0 ng/ml
Reptilia/Squamata	*Naja naja* (cobra)		—	1.25–1.55 μg/dL
	Trachydosaurus ragosus (shingleback lizard)	At preferred temperature	0.28 M	2.6 nM
	Calotes versicolor (garden lizard)	Prior to hibernation	1.2 ng/ml	4.3 ng/ml
		During hibernation	0.6 ng/ml	1 ng/ml
Reptilia/Crocodilia	*Crocodylus johnstoni* (freshwater crocodile)	At preferred temperature	0.51 nM	3.24 nM
Reptilia/Chelonia	*Chelodina longicollis* (long-necked tortoise)	At preferred temperature	0.28 nM	0.55 nM
Aves/Galliformes	*Gallus gallus* (domestic chicks, 1 day to 6 weeks old)		—	1.45–3.0 μg/dL
Mammalia	*Axis axis* (axis deer)	March	115 ng/dL	12.1 μg/dL
		April	70 ng/dL	4.5 μg/dL

Table 7-4. Occurrence of Thyroid Hormones and Their Precursors in Animals and Algae

Organism	MIT	DIT	T_3	T_4
Algae	+	+		
Nereis (Annelida)	+	+	+	+
Sponge (Porifera)	+	+		
Coral (Cnidaria)	+	+		
Periplaneta (Arthropoda: cockroach)	+	+		+
Musca (Arthropoda: fly)	+	+		+
Planorbis (Mollusca: snail)	+	+	+	+
Tunicates	+	+	+	+
Amphioxus (Cephalochordata)	+	+	+	+
Hagfish (Agnatha: Cyclostome)	+	+	+	+
All other vertebrates	+	+	+	+

it to iodinate tyrosines incorporated into the glycoproteins secreted by the endostyle cells. Furthermore, some of those tyrosines are coupled to form the iodinated thyronines, T_3 and T_4. The enzyme thyroid peroxidase (TPO), responsible for iodination of tyrosine and coupling them to form T_4, is present in tunicates.

Acceptance of the simple notion that the thyroid cells evolved from specialized cells of the endostyle of protochordates leaves some basic questions unanswered. For example, why were these iodinated compounds first synthesized? What was their primitive role? What selective forces were responsible for adoption of these iodinated compounds as metabolic regulators? Certainly the ability of iodide to be incorporated into tyrosine residues in a protein and even formation of 3-monoiodotyrosine (MIT), 3,5-diiodotyrosine (DIT), and iodinated thyronines occurs repeatedly among the invertebrate phyla (Table 7-4). However, relatively few studies have examined these iodinated molecules and their functions among invertebrates. In the primitive cnidarians, thyroid hormones are associated with a dramatic developmental change known as **metamorphosis**. The metamorphosis of larvae of the tunicate *Ciona intestinalis* is blocked by exposure to the potential goitrogen, thiourea. Metamorphosis in vertebrates (see below) includes specific gene activation by thyroid hormones resulting in biochemical, physiological, structural, and behavioral changes as well as a major revision of the ecological role of the organism.

One hypothesis for the origin of these primitive iodoproteins is that they first served some enzymatic or structural function and that the basic mechanism became modified into a hormonal synthetic pathway. A more plausible hypothesis may be that these iodine-containing compounds were obtained originally from feeding activities by protochordates and later were utilized opportunistically as regulatory substances following digestion in the gut that liberated the enclosed thyronines. Absorption of T_4 liberated during digestion of these glycoproteins and deiodination of T_4 to T_3 might have been important prerequisites for development of a regulatory role. Later, the retention of these glycoproteins, the ability to accumulate iodide, and the formation of iodinated thyronines were acquired by certain cells of the endostyle (Figure 7-3). These specialized cells later became the follicular cells of the thyroid gland as evidenced from studies in lampreys. Iodide-concentrating cells of the endostyle in the ammocetes larva of the lamprey are reformed into follicles of the thyroid gland during metamorphosis into the adult body form. The production of extracellular colloid and its resultant accumulation in the follicular lumen do not occur in modern cyclostomes and may have been acquired after the cyclostomes branched from the mainline of vertebrate evolution.

There is a basic similarity among thyroid iodoproteins in all vertebrates. They occur as distinct size classes of Tgbs most likely representing monomers, dimers, trimers, and tetramers. Tgbs from birds are similar to those of rats with a trace of 12S Tgb, and about 94% as 19S, and about 5% as 27S (Table 7-2). Turtles, teleost fishes, and elasmobranchs exhibit lower amounts of 19S (73%–84%), but a significant quantity of 12S thyroglobulin is present (6%–16%). Cyclostomes are the most primitive living vertebrates, and they exhibit what may be considered the most primitive condition. Lampreys produce mainly a 12S component (68%), and the remainder of the iodinated protein is in the form of a much smaller component (5.4S monomer). Iodoproteins of about 7.6S have been isolated from urochordates, and hydrolysis of these proteins yields MIT, DIT, T_3, and T_4. These data suggest that Tgb most commonly exists as 12S entities (or an even smaller unit) that aggregate to form 19S and 27S complexes under certain conditions. These data also may be interpreted as reflecting degrees of disruption of the intact Tgb during the extraction procedures from different vertebrates.

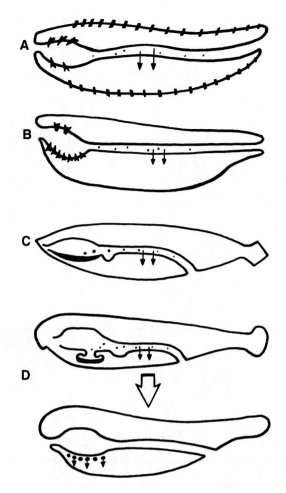

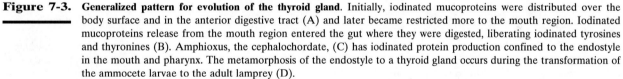

Figure 7-3. **Generalized pattern for evolution of the thyroid gland.** Initially, iodinated mucoproteins were distributed over the body surface and in the anterior digestive tract (A) and later became restricted more to the mouth region. Iodinated mucoproteins release from the mouth region entered the gut where they were digested, liberating iodinated tyrosines and thyronines (B). Amphioxus, the cephalochordate, (C) has iodinated protein production confined to the endostyle in the mouth and pharynx. The metamorphosis of the endostyle to a thyroid gland occurs during the transformation of the ammocete larvae to the adult lamprey (D).

Tgb has been reported in the circulation of chickens and frogs as it has been seen in mammals on occasion. Increases in circulating Tgb occur in obese chicks and during metamorphosis of bullfrogs (see Table 7-5).

B. Regulation of Vertebrate Thyroids

In Chapters 4 and 5, we described the regulation of thyroid function by the HPT axis and its hormones (thyrotropin-releasing hormone, TRH, and TSH). The focus for feedback regulation in the HPT axis is at both the hypothalamus and pituitary. This system maintains a sufficient level of bound and free T_4 that can be converted peripherally by a Type 1 deiodinase to T_3 in liver and kidney or by a Type 2 deiodinase in target cells (see Chapter 6).

C. The Origin of Thyroid Function

There appears to be no consistency in the actions of thyroid hormones when the entire subphylum Vertebrata is surveyed, although in part the inconsistency may be due to lack of thorough investigation in lower vertebrates, especially the fishes and amphibians. It was proposed by Martin Sage in 1973 that thyroid function evolved hand

Table 7-5. Plasma Levels of Thyroglobulin in Bullfrogs and Chickens[a]

Species: stage/strain	Thyroglobulin (ng/ml)
Rana catesbeiana	
Premetamorphic (stage XX)	56
Prometamorphic (stage XV)	179
Metamorphic (stages XVIII–XXV)	347–477
Froglet	154
Adults	267
Chickens	
Newly hatched (three normal strains)	44–73
Newly hatched, obese strain[b]	140–186

[a] Chicks of the obese strain are highly susceptible to autoimmune thyroiditis.

[b] Data from Suzuki, S., and Fujikura, K. (1994). Circulating thyroglobulin levels in tadpoles and adult frogs of *Rana catesbeiana. Gen. Comp. Endocr.* **94**, 72–77; Sanker, A.J., Sundick, R. S., and Brown, T. R. (1983). Analysis of the serum concentration and antigenic determinants of thyroglobulin in chickens susceptible to autoimmune thyroiditis. *J. Immunol.* **131**, 1252–1256.

in hand with endocrine control of reproduction and that the basic function for thyroid hormones is associated primitively with gonadal maturation (Table 7-6). This hypothesis is supported by a variety of observations, including the close parallel of thyroid activity and reproductive cycles in elasmobranchs and bony fishes.

Pituitary thyrotropes and TSH are apparently absent in agnathans, and these cells may have evolved later from gonadotropes. This proposed origin for thyrotropes is supported by their cytological similarity to

Table 7-6. Selected Experimental Results Relating Thyroid and Reproduction in Subavian Vertebrates

Vertebrate	Treatment/observation	Effect on reproduction
Agnathan fishes		
Sea lamprey	Elevated thyroid hormones	Occurs during spermiation and at ovulation
Jawed fishes		
Sharks	Thyroidectomy	Prevents annual onadal recrudescence[a] by blocking vitellogenesis or incorporation of yolk into oocytes
	Stimulated thyroid histology	Coincides with sexual maturation
Teleosts	Elevated thyroid hormones in blood	During gonadal development
	Decreased thyroid hormones in blood	At spawning
	Goitrogen exposure	Inhibits gonadal recrudescence; can cause gonadal atrophy in both sexes
	Presence of goiters in salmon from Great Lakes	Associated with low egg production; low gonadal steroid levels in blood
	Thyroid hormone treatments	No effect or mild enhancement of gonadal maturation
Amphibians	Surgical or chemical thyroidectomy of frogs	Prevents ovulation
	Treatment with thyroxine of thyroidectomized frogs	Permits ovulation
	Treatment of anuran liver with thyroid hormones	Enhances action of estrogen on vitellogenesis
	Thyroid histology	Not correlated with reproductive activities
	Goitrogen treatment of tadpoles of some anurans	Prevents testicular development; may allow sex reversal to females
	Elevated thyroxine in the blood of salamanders	Corresponds to period of gonadal growth in males and females
Reptiles	Excess or insufficient thyroid hormones	Impaired ovarian growth; loss of steroid-secreting cells in testes
	Thyroxine treatment	Causes atrophy of steroid-secreting cells in testes
	Decreased thyroid hormones in blood and thyroid gland histology	Correlated with peak reproductive activity and high androgen levels
	Elevated thyroxine levels in blood	Decreased androgen levels in males

[a] Normal regrowth of the gonad during the next breeding season.

gonadotropes, by their location in the adenohypophysis of elasmobranchs (pars ventralis) and teleosts (proximal pars distalis), and by the biochemical similarity of TSH β-subunit genes to those for the gonadotropins (GTHs; see Chapters 4 and 5). Exogenous thyroid hormones and gonadal steroids both have inhibitory actions on thyrotropes as well as on gonadotropes in teleosts. Similar influences of thyroid hormones on gonadal function and, reciprocally, gonadal steroids on thyroid function have been reported in amphibians, reptiles, and birds. The observations that mammalian luteinizing hormone (LH) stimulates thyroid function in fishes may be interpreted as supportive of this relationship or it may be due simply to a chance similarity in the structures of mammalian LH and teleost TSH or absence of teleost TSH receptor specificity. These same GTHs are ineffective when tested on mammalian thyroids. The effects of thyroid hormones that modify behavior through actions on the central nervous system presumably evolved from the general feedback effects on the hypothalamus originally associated with the gonadal axis. According to Sage, the actions of thyroid hormones related to growth, metabolism, development, and the integument would be later evolutionary events. Location of the major feedback of thyroid hormones on TSH release in the adenohypophysis rather than at the hypothalamus might be a consequence of this evolutionary sequence.

An alternative view to Sage's proposal is to focus on the basic developmental role for thyroid hormones that has been described in all vertebrates. General morphological events as well as development of the central nervous are seen as thyroid hormone-dependent from fishes to mammals. These observations suggest that the reproductive role for thyroid hormones and/or the acquisition of hypothalamic and pituitary control over thyroid function in vertebrates were a later occurrence. The inhibitory role of thyroid hormones on metamorphosis in agnathans may represent a secondary adaptation.

D. Prolactin and Its Interactions with the Thyroid Axis

A general antagonism has been reported between **prolactin (PRL)** and the thyroid axis of amphibians, reptiles, and birds. Studies have demonstrated what appears to be a goitrogenic action of PRL directly on thyroids of teleosts, amphibians, lizards, and birds, but the peripheral antagonism between thyroxine and PRL in certain tissues of larval amphibians is best known. Isolated reports of enhancement of thyroid secretion following treatment with mammalian PRL require further investigation to verify the general applicability of this effect to vertebrates. The significance of an antagonistic interaction between thyroid hormones and PRL in fish, reptiles, birds, and mammals is not clear. In amphibians, the administration of anti-PRL agents (PRL antibodies or ergot derivatives) enhances responses of larval amphibians to endogenous and exogenous thyroid hormones. These observations support an endogenous role for PRL in preventing premature metamorphosis (see ahead). Numerous investigations suggest that high levels of PRL are anti-metamorphic but that lower levels are possibly essential for successful metamorphosis in amphibians.

Synthetic mammalian TRH causes PRL release from pituitaries of bullfrogs, turtles, birds, and mammals but not from the pituitaries of red-spotted newts (see Chapter 5). These observations further complicate the picture and raise some important questions concerning the biological significance, if any, of demonstrations that PRL produces anti-thyroid effects. It also suggests the role of the TRH tripeptide, which is present abundantly in the amphibian brain, is that of a PRL-releasing agent, especially in light of many failed attempts to demonstrate a role for TRH in the activation of the amphibian thyroid axis.

E. Surgical and Chemical Thyroidectomy and Radiothyroidectomy

A basic approach employed in thyroid studies involves hypophysectomy or thyroidectomy or a combination of the two followed by classical replacement therapy. Sometimes, however, it is desirable to make an animal only slightly hypothyroid or reversibly hypothyroid or both. Chemical thyroidectomy involves administration of a chemical goitrogen (see Chapter 6) such as propylthiouracil (PTU) or thiourea (TU) at a predetermined dose for a given period. Withdrawal of the goitrogen may then allow the animal to return to a euthyroid condition for comparisons. With this approach, changes in thyroid function before, during, and after treatment may be examined in each individual. Caution must be exercised in that some goitrogens (e.g., TU) have been shown to produce effects on other tissues (especially the liver) that do not appear following surgical thyroidectomy. Such "nonspecific" actions of chemical inhibitors are well known to investigators, and, when possible, other approaches should be used.

Large doses of radioiodide often are employed as therapeutic agents in humans to destroy excessive amounts of thyroid tissue in certain hyperthyroid conditions. Accumulated radioiodide destroys cells because of the destructive effects of radiation on the cell that has incorporated it. Very large doses can be used to completely destroy thyroid tissue. This approach is especially useful in most species of teleost fishes where it is impossible to surgically remove thyroid tissue that occurs as diffuse follicles. Radiothyroidectomy, however, must be interpreted with caution since radioiodide accumulation may occur in other tissues (see Table 7-7, Figure 7-4) and result in destructive changes that may not be thyroid-related. The general effects of whole-body radiation from this powerful gamma emitter could be a concern as well.

Table 7-7. Accumulation of Radioiodide by Thyroids and Gonads of Sexually Mature Vertebrates

Class	Species	Sex	Radioiodide uptake Gonad/thyroid
Osteichthyes[a]	*Micropterus dolomieu* (smallmouth bass)	M	0.012
		F	3.780
Amphibia[a]	*Ambystoma tigrinum* (tiger salamander, neotene)	M	0.045
		F	0.512
Aves	*Coturnix coturnix japonica* (Japanese quail)	F	4 to 10

[a] Norris, unpublished data (1966).

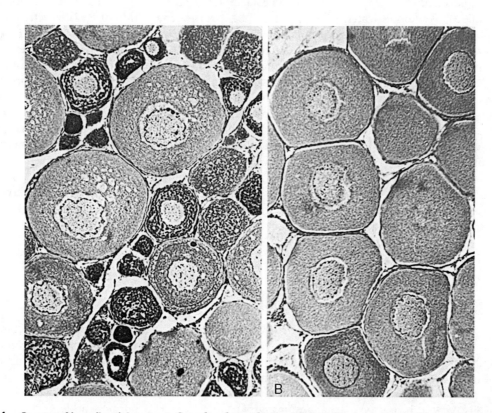

Figure 7-4. **Oocytes of juvenile rainbow trout,** *Oncorhynchus mykiss,* **and radioiodide accumulation**. The ovaries of non-mammalian vertebrates readily concentrate iodide as efficiently as the thyroid and store it in the oocytes. The control ovary at the left exhibits a range of occytes. The ovary at the right accumulated radiodide shortly after hatching. Although the radioactivity quickly decays to undetectable levels, the ovary at the right contains only the largest class of oocytes when examined a year later.

II. Comparative Thyroid Physiology

The following account and Table 7-8 emphasize the biological actions of thyroid hormones on vertebrate target tissues. The secretion of TSH and the effects of various hypothalamic hormones on TSH secretion were discussed in Chapter 5, and the focus here is on the functions of T_3 and T_4.

A. Agnathan Fishes: Cyclostomes

No stimulatory role for thyroid hormones has been verified in cyclostome fishes, although in lampreys the binding of iodide by the larval endostyle increases following administration of T_4. Circulating levels of T_4 decrease markedly as free-living, filter-feeding ammocetes larvae of sea lampreys, *Petromyzon marinus*, undergo metamorphosis to the ectoparasitic adult lampreys.

Hormone synthesis in agnathans differs from other vertebrates in that organic binding of iodide and storage of the iodinated proteins occur intracellularly. Hypophysectomy does not alter thyroid function in adult lampreys or in hagfishes, and TSH has not been demonstrated in an agnathan pituitary. These observations suggest that evolution of thyrotropes and TSH either occurred first in jawed fishes, possibly in the placoderms, or in another agnathan group that gave rise to jawed fishes and has persisted in all other extant vertebrates. T_4 is present in serum from mature female sea lampreys comparable to levels reported for ammocetes of this species. Much lower levels of T_4 are reported for mature male sea lampreys. T_3 occurs in the serum of both immature and mature sea lampreys, but the levels are higher in the mature individuals. These data suggest a relationship to reproductive maturation, but definitive data are needed before a firm relationship can be accepted.

B. Chondrichthyean Fishes

Only limited data are available with respect to thyroid function in sharks, in which the HPT axis appears to be well established. Most studies on sharks are related to effects of thyroid hormones on reproduction or oxygen consumption, and the thyroid systems of other chondrichthyean fishes are virtually unknown.

1. Thyroid and Reproduction in Elasmobranchs

Thyroid cycles are positively correlated with reproductive cycles in sharks. However, increased thyroid activity observed in at least one species is correlated with migratory behavior related to reproduction rather than with reproduction or gonadal maturation *per se*. This area requires further investigation.

Table 7-8. Some Major Actions of Thyroid Hormones in Vertebrates[a]

Vertebrate group	Development	Molting	Growth	Metabolism	Reproduction	Neural behavior	Neural differentiation	Thermogenesis
Sharks					+	+		
Bony fishes	+		+		+	+		
Amphibians	+	+[b]	−[c]		−	+	+	
Reptiles		+	+	?	+			
Birds	+	+	+	+	+/−	+		+
Mammals	+	+	+	+	+	+	+	+

[a] +, stimulatory; −, inhibitory. The stimulatory action of thyroid hormones on metabolism seems to be associated with the evolution of homeothermy.
[b] Urodeles only. Molting in anurans is controlled by corticosteroids.
[c] Prevents growth in larval amphibians by inducing metamorphosis.

2. Thyroid and Oxygen Consumption in Elasmobranchs

Late embryos of *Squalus suckleyi* exhibit a transient increase in oxygen consumption following treatment with T_3 or T_4, but this response cannot be maintained by continued treatment with thyroid hormones. Treatment with PTU has no effect on oxygen consumption in this species. These observations do not provide strong support of a role for thyroid hormones in oxidative metabolism.

3. Thyroid and Neural Differentiation in Elasmobranchs

Differentiation of hypothalamic neurosecretory centers is accelerated in the embryos of the oviparous shark, *S. suckleyi*, following treatment with T_3 or T_4. This effect of thyroid hormones is manifested in both the preoptico-hypophysial fiber tracts and the neurohypophysis. These data are suggestive of a role for thyroid hormones in nervous tissue differentiation and maturation of the HP system.

C. Bony Fishes: Chondrosteans

Some limited data for sturgeons indicate peak thyroid activity coincides with spawning behavior. Although thyroid hormone levels were extremely low in cultured lake sturgeon (0.3 and 0.2 ng/ml for T_4 and T_3, respectively), wild spawning sturgeon had much higher levels (0.83 and 1.31, respectively). Furthermore, thyroid treatments can reverse the degenerative changes that occur in gonads of captive lake sturgeon, suggesting a direct relationship between thyroid hormones and reproduction. Curiously, lake sturgeon thyroid glands contain 10X more T_3 than T_4 suggesting considerable thyroid deiodination compared to other vertebrates. Additional studies are needed in chondrostean fishes to examine other possible roles of thyroid hormones and to confirm this suggestive relationship with reproduction.

D. Bony Fishes: Teleosts

Thyroid function has been studied intensively in teleost fishes and considerable information is available with respect to iodide uptake, hormone synthesis, secretion rates, clearance rates, and metabolism of thyroid hormones. Most of this knowledge about teleost thyroids stems from the work of J. G. Eales and his colleagues working principally with the rainbow trout, *Oncorhynchus mykiss*.

Several features of teleost thyroid function differ markedly from what we know about mammals. Probably the most striking difference is that neuroglandular hypothalamic control in all species studied is inhibitory, with both TRH and somatostatin (SST) capable of preventing TSH release, except in salmonids where both TRH and catecholamines are stimulatory. Teleosts readily accumulate iodide from the surrounding water through their gills, and some species maintain high circulating levels of protein-bound inorganic iodide. Consequently, these fish rarely show iodide deficiencies in nature, and their thyroid iodide metabolism is resistant to excessive iodide inhibition. There is negligible enterohepatic circulation of thyroid hormones or their metabolites in teleosts, and thyroid hormones are readily lost in urine, too. The active form of thyroid hormone is T_3, but its level is apparently controlled through the activity of deiodinases. Administration of T_4 generally has no effect on circulating levels of T_3. Although some species have been shown to metabolize T_4 to reverse T_3 (rT_3), in rainbow trout the production rT_3 is curiously absent (Figure 7-5) unless the fish is treated first with T_3. This is an interesting observation since regulation of the type III deiodinase that causes this conversion is implicated in the occurrence of T_3 surges in other vertebrates.

Thyroid hormones travel through the blood mostly bound to plasma proteins. Studies with sea bream show binding to albumin as well as to a binding protein, transthyretin (TTR).

Thyroid hormones are implicated in reproduction and aspects of behavior in teleost fishes. Their role with respect to oxygen consumption is not so clear, however. Thyroid hormones are essential for normal development and growth and may be involved in metamorphosis of young fishes and in the parr-smolt transformation of salmonid fishes, another metamorphosis-like change. Although thyroid hormones have been implicated in osmoregulation, carbohydrate metabolism, nitrogen metabolism, and growth, other hormones are known to play more direct roles. In fact, some effects of thyroid hormones may be permissive actions similar to those described for mammals (Chapter 6).

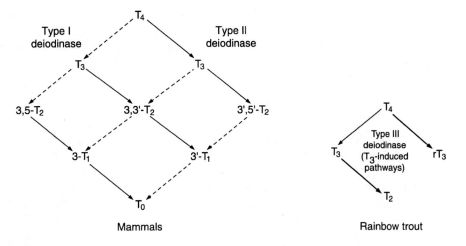

Figure 7-5. **Comparison of the deiodinase pathways in mammals and rainbow trout.** Untreated trout show only conversion of T_4 to T_3, but treatment with exogenous T_3 can induce or augment type-II deiodinase activity so that sufficient rT_3 and T_2 are produced in detectable amounts. [Based on Eales, J. G., and Brown, S. B. (1993). Measurements and regulation of thyroidal status in teleost fish. *Revs. Fish Biol. Fisher.* **3**, 299–347.]

1. Heterotopic Thyroid Tissue in Teleosts

The teleost thyroid consists of scattered thyroid follicles throughout the pharyngeal region. The diffuse nature of the teleost thyroid gland, with only a few exceptions (for example, the tuna and the Bermuda parrot fish), makes assessment of thyroid gland function difficult and renders surgical thyroidectomy impossible. Most of the thyroid tissue is located in the pharyngeal area where follicles are usually found between the second and fourth aortic arches (Figure 7-6). Because of the absence of a covering connective tissue sheath that holds the follicles into one or more masses, thyroid follicles are frequently found outside this pharyngeal region. These extrapharyngeal thyroid follicles are termed accessory or **heterotopic thyroid** follicles because of their location outside the normal site. Heterotopic thyroid follicles occur commonly in species of some of the more recent

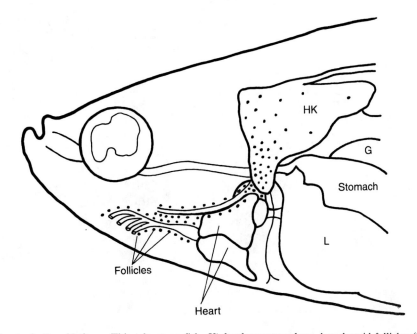

Figure 7-6. **Heterotopic thyroid tissue.** This teleostean fish, *Xiphophorus maculatus*, has thyroid follicles (black dots) located not only throughout the pharyngeal region but also in the heart, head kidney (HK), and sometimes even in the gonads (G) and liver (L).

teleost families (Figure 7-6). Relatively large numbers of thyroid follicles may be found embedded within the head kidney of some species and occasionally in other locations such as the pericardium or ovary. In such species, it may be important to examine the activity of heterotopic thyroid as well as of pharyngeal thyroid when using techniques such as radioiodide uptake.

2. Thyroid and Development in Teleosts

Thyroid hormones are responsible for a posthatching metamorphosis in many species of teleosts. Probably the most dramatic metamorphosis is that of flounders and other flatfishes which involves the migration of the eye and attendant neural structures from one side of the head to the other (Figure 7-7) while the mouth and associated structures migrate to the opposite side. The adult animal then behaves with the left or right side (depending on the species) acting as the ventral surface with the mouth located there for bottom feeding and the other side having both eyes and acting as the dorsal surface. Levels of plasma T_4 rise dramatically during flounder metamorphosis as does cortisol whereas T_3 levels remain low. Measurements of T_3 turnover are lacking, however.

The **parr-smolt transformation** or **smoltification** occurs prior to seaward migration in many salmonids (Figure 7-8). This metamorphosis from a sedentary, cryptically marked fish, the **parr**, with a freshwater physiology to an active, silvery **smolt** that is preadapted for osmoregulation in salt water is accompanied by increased cortisol secretion (see Chapter 10), although surges in T_4, insulin, and PRL also have been reported (Figure 7-9).

Growth in fishes appears to be influenced by thyroid state as described for mammals (see Chapter 6). Retardation of growth is observed in salmonids following radiothyroidectomy. Normal growth is resumed following administration of T_4 (Figure 7-10), suggesting an interaction with GH. Radiothyroidectomy also results in numerous skeletal abnormalities in these fish.

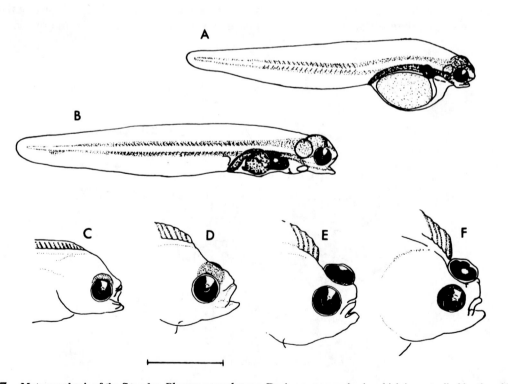

Figure 7-7. **Metamorphosis of the flounder,** *Pleuronectes platessa*. During metamorphosis, which is controlled by thyroid hormones, one eye migrates from one side of the body to the other. [From Blaxter (1988). Pattern and variety in development. *In* "Fish Physiology" (W. S. Hoar and D. J. Randall, Eds.), **11A**, 1–58. Academic Press, San Diego.]

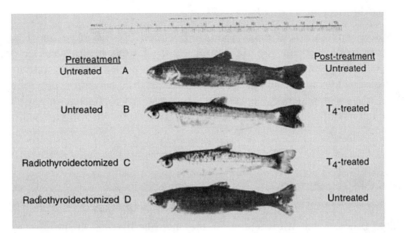

Figure 7-8. **Smolting in rainbow trout.** Thyroid hormone stimulates deposition of guanine in the scales. (A) Normal fingerling. (B) Normal fingerling immersed for 4 weeks in fresh water containing 10^{-8} M T_4. (C) Radiothyroidectomized trout treated as above with T_4. (D) Untreated radiothyroidectomized trout.

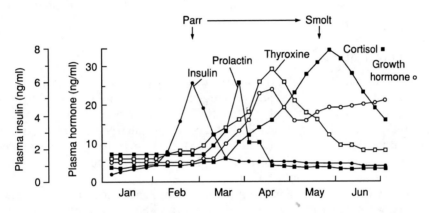

Figure 7-9. **Plasma hormone levels during smoltification of coho salmon.** Prolactin, growth hormone, thyroxine, and cortisol all peak during smoltification. Insulin peaks in the parr and declines as smoltification gets under way. [Reprinted with permission from Fish and amphibian models for developmental endocrinology. Dickhoff, W., Brown, C. L., Sullivan, C. V., and Bern, H. A. *J. Exper. Zool.* © 1990 John Wiley & Sons.]

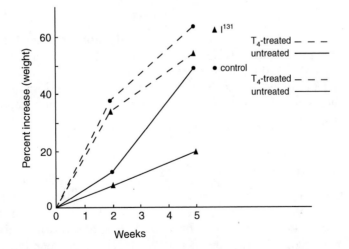

Figure 7-10. **Effect of T_4 treatment on growth of radiothyroidectomized steelhead trout.** [From Norris, D. O. 1969. Depression of growth following radiothyroidectomy of larval chinook salmon and steelhead trout. *Trans. Am. Fisheries Soc.* **97**, 204–206.]

3. Thyroid and Reproduction in Teleosts

There is a strong positive correlation in many teleosts between thyroid state and reproductive cycles. Thyroxine consistently stimulates precocial gonadal maturation, whereas radiothyroidectomy or treatment with goitrogens inhibits or retards gonadal development. In several species, thyroid activity is greatest at spawning. Furthermore, increased thyroid activity as well as glucocorticoid secretion are coincident with migrations and spawning in Pacific salmon and may represent a response to increased metabolic demands. Similarly, this increased thyroid activity appears to be more closely correlated with the spawning migration than with reproductive events.

4. Thyroid and Oxygen Consumption in Teleosts

Observations have yielded opposing results with respect to the importance of thyroid hormones in oxygen consumption by teleost fishes. Most studies suggest that neither thyroid hormones nor goitrogens have any effects on oxygen consumption. A positive correlation has been reported for cyclic seasonal variations in thyroid activity and oxygen consumption by *Heteropneustes fossilis*. Studies of oxygen consumption are difficult to interpret because temperature, changes in behavior, and potential side effects of treatments used to render the fish hypothyroid (goitrogens, radiothyroidectomy) may have direct effects on metabolism.

5. Thyroid and Osmoregulation in Teleosts

The endocrine regulation of osmoregulation is primarily under the control of prolactin and cortisol with respect to maintaining Na^+ balance (see Chapter 9) and with arginine vasotocin (AVT) responsible for water balance (see Chapter 5). Calcium regulation is probably controlled by hormones from the corpuscles of Stannius embedded in the kidney, the ultimobranchial body found in the pharyngeal region (see Chapter 14), and somatolactin (SL) from the pars intermedia (see Chapter 5). Less direct roles in ionic and osmotic regulation are attributable to catecholamines, thyroid hormones, and factors from the pineal gland (see Chapter 5) as well as the caudal neurosecretory system (see Chapter 9).

Thyroid hormones may enhance seawater adaptation and may influence migratory behavior especially in species that migrate between salt and fresh water. These proposed actions may be related to a permissive type of action rather than to a causative role for thyroid hormones or may be only correlated events and not causally related.

6. Behavioral Actions of Thyroid Hormones in Teleosts

Thyroid hormones are elevated in relation to spawning, pre-migratory, and migratory behaviors. Increased thyroid function has been reported for a variety of migrating fishes, and pre-migratory restless behavior has been correlated with increased thyroid function. Thyroid activity is greater in young salmon smolts migrating to the ocean and in adults during their upstream return to freshwater for spawning. Again the action of thyroid hormones may only enhance the sensitivities of neural components to environmental stimuli.

E. Bony Fishes: Sarcopterygians

The function of thyroid hormones in lungfishes has received only a cursory examination. Thyroid hormones have been linked to a particularly fascinating aspect of the life history of African lungfishes: the ability to survive periods of drought while encased in a "cocoon." Awakening of estivating African lungfish *Protopterus annectens* from the cocoon of dried mud when moistened may involve a neuroendocrine mechanism associated with the thyroid axis. One hypothesis, based upon limited experimental data, suggests that increasing humidity activates the HPT axis and stimulates thyroid hormone secretion. Thyroid hormones in turn would increase the sensitivity of olfactory centers that evoke normal feeding behavior as well as other behaviors associated with wakening. Additional studies of thyroid function in these fishes are needed to substantiate this interesting hypothesis.

F. Thyroid Functions in Amphibians

Thyroid hormones influence many processes in both anurans and urodeles, including reproduction, metamorphosis, metabolism, growth, and molting. The most dramatic and best-studied event among amphibians is the endocrine induction of metamorphosis from an aquatic larva to a terrestrial or semi-terrestrial form.

1. Thyroid and Reproduction in Amphibians

Experimental reduction of thyroid function, such as thyroidectomy or administration of goitrogens, accelerates gonadal development in several anurans. In one urodele, *Ambystoma tigrinum*, circulating levels of T_4 are inversely correlated with seasonal gonadal development, although such correlations do not substantiate cause-effect relationships. Some conflicting results with respect to thyroid hormones and seasonal maturation have been reported for some adult anurans, but the general relationship in amphibians appears to be an antagonistic one. All of the data reported to date are circumstantial, and an absolute antagonism by endogenous thyroid hormones in natural populations is yet to be demonstrated.

2. Thyroid and Oxygen Consumption in Amphibians

The relationship between thyroid hormones and metabolism is not clear. Some studies have shown a positive correlation between thyroid state and oxygen consumption, whereas most studies show no effects. Oxygen consumption is not elevated during either spontaneous metamorphosis caused by elevated endogenous thyroid hormones or during induced metamorphosis caused by exogenous thyroid hormones.

Liver slices prepared from T_4-treated adult frogs, *Rana pipiens*, exhibit significantly greater oxygen consumption *in vitro* than appropriate controls at 25°C. Oxygen consumption of treated slices is the same as for controls when observed at 15°C. These data suggest that the respiratory response of amphibian tissues to thyroid hormones may be temperature-dependent and that the response occurs only at higher temperatures. Most studies reporting no effect for thyroid hormones on oxygen consumption were performed below 20°C. What the biological importance is for enhanced oxygen consumption at higher temperatures is open to speculation.

3. Thyroid and Metamorphosis in Amphibians

Thyroid hormones induce metamorphosis, a marked biochemical, physiological, morphological, and behavioral transformation from an aquatic larva to a terrestrial or semiterrestrial form. These events occur in the life history of every amphibian, although the developmental sequence and duration of the various stages may be modified extensively in those species that incubate their eggs on land or are live-bearing.

Amphibian metamorphosis has been studied at all levels of organization and provides an excellent illustration of hormonal interactions of thyroid hormones with other hormones (e.g., PRL, corticosteroids) in a variety of tissues. Furthermore, this process is closely linked to the interaction of complex environmental factors that together with endocrine-related events constitutes the metamorphosis phenomenon.

Metamorphosis in amphibians involves regulation of specific genes, often initiated by an external factor, that orchestrate a programmed sequence of biochemical (see Table 7-9), morphological (e.g., tail and gill resorption; see Figure 7-11 and Table 7-10), physiological (e.g., nitrogen excretion; see Figure 7-12), and behavioral events. Three decades ago, William Etkin proposed a model to explain the then-known stimulatory role of the thyroid axis and observed inhibitory actions of PRL on metamorphosis (see Figure 7-13)

Box 7A. Endocrine Disruption

The presence of the anti-thyroid compound perchlorate ions in drinking water has raised concerns about human health, especially with respect to fetal nervous system development (see Chapter 6). Perchlorate contamination of natural waters also is a concern for wildlife. For example, the presence of perchlorate in natural waters of west Texas is associated with environmental contamination from US military bases. Tree frogs collected from perchlorate-contaminated sites exhibit hypertrophied thyroid epithelia as compared to thyroids of frogs from reference sites (Box Figure 7A-1). Furthermore, frogs exposed to ammonium perchlorate (14 ng /L = 14 parts per trillion) in the laboratory exhibit thyroid follicular hypertrophy compared to controls (Box Figure 7A-2).

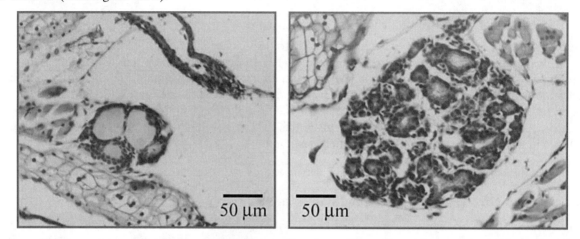

Box Figure 7A-1. **Environmental perchlorate and frog thyroid histology**. Thyroid tissue in a tree frog from a reference site in west Texas appears at the left. On the right is a hyperstimulated thyroid gland from a perchlorate-contaminated site. This goitrous response is typical of the anti-thyroid action of perchlorate resulting in excessive production of thyrotropin and resultant stimulation of the thyroid gland. (Photomicrographs courtesy of Dr. James A. Carr, Texas Tech University.)

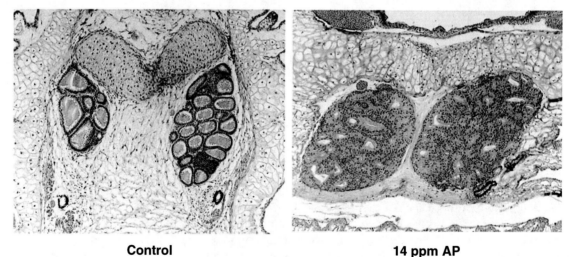

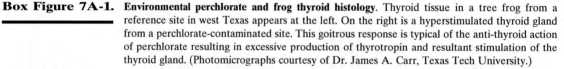

Control   **14 ppm AP**

Box Figure 7A-2. **Effect of perchlorate exposure in the laboratory**. The paired thyroid glands of a control frog can be seen at the left in marked contrast to the goitrous thyroids in the frog exposed to 14 ppm of ammonium perchlorate. This goitrous response is typical of the anti-thyroid action of perchlorate resulting in excessive production of thyrotropin and resultant stimulation of the thyroid gland. (Photomicrograph courtesy of Dr. James A. Carr, Texas Tech University.) See color insert, plate 9.

Table 7-9. Genes Affected by Thyroid Hormones during Amphibian Metamorphosis

Gene	Tissue	Regulation
Early-response genes		
Tail 1 (zinc finger region of SPI)	Tail	Up
TRβ (thyroid hormone receptor)	Tail and intestine	Up
Tail 8/9 (bZIP^F of E4BP4)	Tail and intestine	Up
Tail 14 (stromelysin 3)	Tail and intestine	Up
Tail 15 (type I 5′-deiodinase)	Tail	Up
Late-response genes		
Carbamyl-phosphate synthetase I	Liver	Up
Argininosuccinate synthetase	Liver	Up
Arginase	Liver	Up
Albumin	Liver	Up
Myosin heavy chain	Limb	Up
Keratin	Epidermis	Up
Trypsin	Pancreas	Down
Intestinal fatty acid-binding protein	Intestine	Down

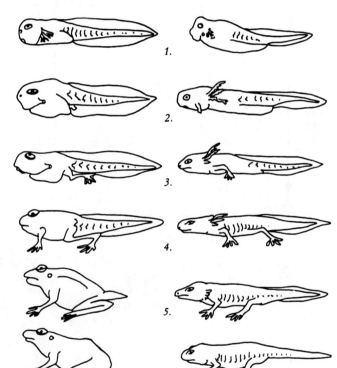

Anuran   *Urodele*

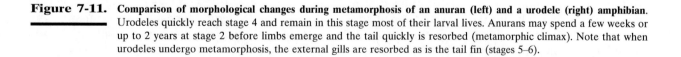

Figure 7-11. Comparison of morphological changes during metamorphosis of an anuran (left) and a urodele (right) amphibian. Urodeles quickly reach stage 4 and remain in this stage most of their larval lives. Anurans may spend a few weeks or up to 2 years at stage 2 before limbs emerge and the tail quickly is resorbed (metamorphic climax). Note that when urodeles undergo metamorphosis, the external gills are resorbed as is the tail fin (stages 5–6).

The **Etkin hypothesis** has necessarily undergone considerable revision since the discoveries that corticosteroids also are involved, that corticotropin-releasing factor (CRH) may release TSH as well as corticotropin (ACTH) from the pituitary, and that TRH may be responsible for the surge of PRL that also accompanies metamorphosis (Figure 7-14). In fact, CRH may be the endogenous hypothalamic stimulator of the

Table 7-10. Life History of *Rana pipiens* at 23°C

Period	Events	Duration
Embryonic	Embryogenesis	8 days
Premetamorphic	Growth	5–6 weeks
Prometamorphic	Accelerated growth of hind limbs; skin changes occur	3 weeks
Metamorphic climax	Forelimbs emerge; tail resorbs; gills resorb; head and gut reconstruction; etc.	1 week
Juvenile	Growth	—
Adult	Reproductive maturation and breeding	—

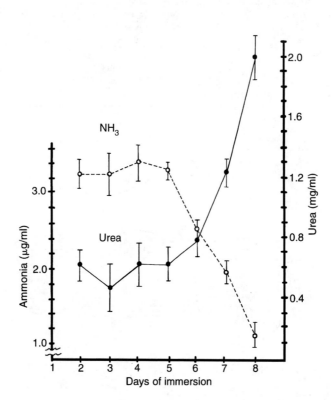

Figure 7-12.   **Urea-ammonia excretion during anuran metamorphosis.** Aquatic animals excrete ammonia as their principal nitroge-nous waste whereas terrestrial amphibians produce urea. Immersion of tadpoles in water containing thyroxine induces a switch from ammonia excretion to urea excretion similar to that observed during normal metamorphosis. A similar pattern to the ammonia change is seen for other metamorphic changes such as regression of tail whereas growth of hind limbs exhibits a urea-like pattern.

thyroid axis in larval amphibians as demonstrated by Robert Denver, and the TRH peptide may be a PRL releaser.

Environmental factors such as photoperiod may operate through catecholaminergic mechanisms in the brain to influence neurohormone release from hypothalamic nuclei (Figure 7-15). The pineal gland may play an important role in mediating the observed stimulatory actions of light on thyroid function and metamorphosis. In part, this is based on inference from observations that long-day photoperiods stimulate thyroid activity and metamorphosis in both salamanders and frogs. However, numerous studies by Mary Wright have demonstrated an inhibition of thyroid secretion and action by melatonin in frog tadpoles.

An important mechanism for induction of metamorphosis involves changes in deiodinase activities. In premetamorphic larvae, type III deiodinase is present, which keeps T_3 levels low by converting T_4 preferentially to rT_3 and hastening deiodination of T_3. During the activation of metamorphosis, there is a measurable increase in type II deiodinase that enhances formation of T_3 from T_4 as well as a decrease in type III deiodinase activity. Patterns of deiodinating activity in liver and target tissues (Figure 7-16) affect the availability of active T_3 and

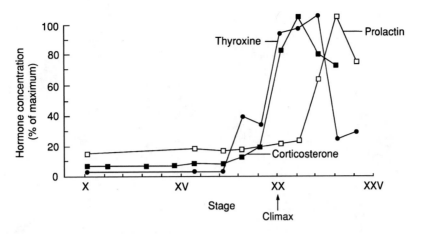

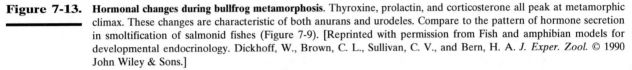

Figure 7-13. **Hormonal changes during bullfrog metamorphosis**. Thyroxine, prolactin, and corticosterone all peak at metamorphic climax. These changes are characteristic of both anurans and urodeles. Compare to the pattern of hormone secretion in smoltification of salmonid fishes (Figure 7-9). [Reprinted with permission from Fish and amphibian models for developmental endocrinology. Dickhoff, W., Brown, C. L., Sullivan, C. V., and Bern, H. A. *J. Exper. Zool.* © 1990 John Wiley & Sons.]

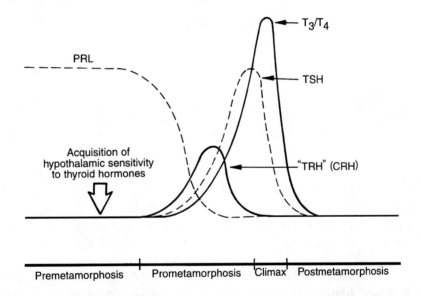

Figure 7-14. **The Etkin hypothesis**. William Etkin proposed that low levels of thyroid hormones secreted autonomously by the thyroid gland mature the hypothalamus to produce a "TRH" that results in TSH secretion and eventually in accelerated thyroid hormone production which causes metamorphosis. He also proposed that prolactin (PRL) levels would be high prior to metamorphosis and then drop off. Later studies have modified various aspects of the original hypothesis with the discovery of involvement of other hormones as well as the role of CRH, timing of the appearance of thyroid receptors, and changes in the type of deiodinase activity. See text for more explanation.

facilitate metamorphosis. Marked changes in tissue thyroid receptor levels also occur during metamorphosis. Changes in both α- and β-type thyroid receptors similar to the mammalian receptors have been demonstrated in different amphibian tissues, but their role in the metamorphosis process is uncertain at this time.

Thyroid hormones influence gene activity in target cells and initiate metamorphic changes (Table 7-9). For example, in the hindlimbs of anurans, thyroid hormones have been shown to activate 14 genes while 5 others are down-regulated, resulting in rapid hindlimb growth characteristic of the later stages of metamorphosis. In tadpole tail fins, researchers have identified 15 genes activated during thyroid hormone-induced tail resorption and 4 others that are down-regulated. Twenty-two genes are activated in the intestine of metamorphosing anurans but only one is down-regulated. Many of these genes are called direct- or **early-response genes** and

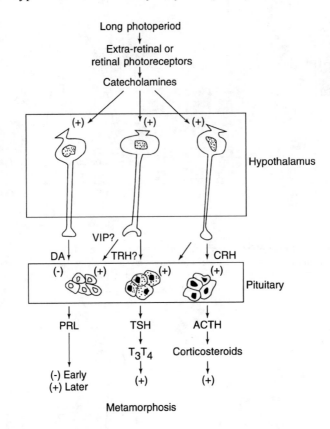

Figure 7-15. **The role of long photoperiod in urodele metamorphosis.** Light working through pineal or retinal photoreceptors activates hypothalamic centers that secrete DA and CRH that initially prevent PRL (DA) release and activate TSH and ACTH release (CRH) causing surges in thyroid hormones and corticosteroids, respectively. Later, a secondary surge of PRL occurs (see Figure 7-13), possibly due to TRH or VIP release.

are activated directly by thyroid hormones whereas **late-response genes** (e.g., urea cycle genes in liver; keratin genes in skin) are not activated until about two days after application of thyroid hormones. This delay implies that synthesis of other molecules including transcription factors is dependent on protein synthesis activated by the original stimulus.

Programmed cell death or **apoptosis** is another component of tail regression that is influenced by thyroid hormones. Induction of **ubiquitin**, a biochemical marker for apoptosis, is caused by T_4 treatment of isolated tadpole tail tips.

Thyroid hormones are also involved in a second metamorphic event, the **water drive** associated with reproduction in newts. Water-drive behavior is a well-known bioassay for PRL activity (see Appendix D). Small quantities of thyroid hormones facilitate the preinduced water drive and associated morphological changes in the integument. Larger amounts of thyroid hormones inhibit water drive, and thyroid hormones appear to be responsible for land-drive behavior of recently metamorphosed amphibians.

4. Thyroid and Growth of Amphibians

The involvement of thyroid hormones in growth of amphibians, like the relationship to reproduction, deviates from the general vertebrate pattern. Growth in natural populations is arrested during metamorphosis. The surge of thyroid activity that initiates metamorphosis in larval amphibians apparently arrests growth for a time. Normal growth resumes in juvenile animals after metamorphosis is complete. Treatment of anuran tadpoles with goitrogens or mammalian PRL accelerates larval growth and blocks metamorphosis. The complicated metamorphic process itself involves many drastic physiological changes and tissue rearrangements that may be

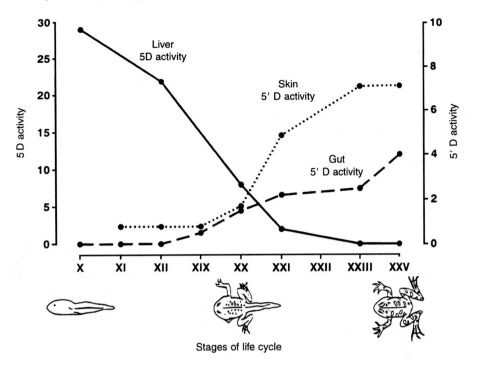

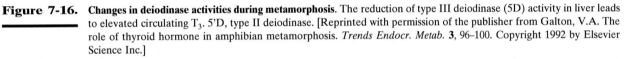

Stages of life cycle

Figure 7-16. **Changes in deiodinase activities during metamorphosis.** The reduction of type III deiodinase (5D) activity in liver leads to elevated circulating T_3. 5'D, type II deiodinase. [Reprinted with permission of the publisher from Galton, V.A. The role of thyroid hormone in amphibian metamorphosis. *Trends Endocr. Metab.* **3**, 96–100. Copyright 1992 by Elsevier Science Inc.]

responsible for arrested growth. These observations associated with larval growth do not eliminate participation of low levels of thyroid hormones in growth of the subadult or post-metamorphic juvenile forms. Such participation for thyroid hormones in the growth of metamorphosed amphibians has not been reported, however.

5. Molting and Other Skin Effects of Thyroid Hormones in Amphibians

Molting or shedding of skin (**ecdysis**) in larval and adult urodeles is under direct stimulatory control by thyroid hormones, and frequent molting accompanies and follows metamorphosis in these animals. Molting in adult anurans, however, does not appear to be influenced by thyroid hormones. Here molting is stimulated by corticosteroids or indirectly by ACTH operating through its action of increasing corticosteroid secretion. The reasons for this marked difference in hormonal control of molting between urodeles and anurans are not known.

Thyroid hormones cause a number of skin changes related to invasion of the terrestrial environment. Both a thickening of the epidermis and keratinization are induced by thyroid hormones in urodeles and anurans. In the newts, thyroid hormones antagonize the effects of PRL on the skin of the eft prior to its return to water. PRL reduces the keratinization and enhances mucus production that helps return the skin to a smooth, moist condition characteristic of aquatic newts.

The large and conspicuous **Leydig skin cells**, which are characteristic of urodele larvae, disappear during metamorphosis, presumably a consequence of thyroid hormone actions. The role of these cells in the larvae is unknown. Histochemical observations suggest a contribution of their contents to formation of a keratinized layer in the skin that probably aids in reducing desiccation following metamorphosis.

G. Thyroid Functions in Reptiles

There are relatively few studies on thyroid function in reptiles. Changes in thyroid state in reptiles are correlated with reproduction, environmental temperature, and activity level, although cause-effect relationships have not been established clearly. Exogenous thyroid hormones also stimulate oxygen consumption, growth, and molting under certain conditions.

The presence of iodinated tyrosines in the blood is a situation unique to reptiles. Blood of the striped racer *Elaphe taeniura* and the cobra *Naja naja* contains MIT and DIT. Thyrotropin stimulates *in-vitro* release of MIT, DIT, and T_4 from chunks of thyroid tissue isolated from a turtle (*Geochemys reevsii*), a lizard (*Gekko gecko*), and a snake (*E. rachiata*). These studies suggest that reptilian thyroid glands may lack any deiodinase to convert MIT and DIT to inorganic iodide and tyrosine. These data, however, are open to other interpretations, and additional research is needed. Evidence for a type I deiodinase (PTU-sensitive) has been reported for the lizard *Sceloporus occidentalis*, and conversion of T_4 to T_3 is blocked in another lizard, *Calotes versicolor*, following treatment with the deiodinase inhibitor, iopodate.

1. Thyroid and Reproduction in Reptiles

Seasonal changes in thyroid function have been correlated positively with a number of reproductive events in lizards, snakes, and turtles. An active thyroid, usually assessed histologically, is associated with spermatogenesis, ovulation, and mating in a number of lizards. Similar observations have been reported in snakes and in at least one turtle. However, negative correlations between thyroid activity and reproduction also have been reported for reptiles (see Table 7-6).

Among live-bearing reptiles, there is no evidence for increased thyroid function during gestation. However, thyroidectomy of pregnant lizards *Lacerta vivipara* six weeks prior to term caused premature discharge of most eggs, and those eggs that were retained failed to hatch.

2. Environmental Temperature and Reptilian Thyroid

In general, thyroid function in reptiles varies proportionally with changes in temperature, although the cause-effect relationships are still obscure. Behaviors such as basking in lizards make it difficult to estimate body temperature when assessing thyroid state. Thyroid activity in temperate lizards is highest during the warmer seasons. Lowering the environmental temperature artificially during the summer months causes reduction in thyroid activity, and lizards maintained in the laboratory at high temperatures (35°C) exhibit greater thyroid activity than when maintained at 15°C. Thyroid activity in snakes is greater during warm periods and lowest during hibernation. The greatest level of thyroid activity, however, correlates with reproductive events in some lizards and snakes and not with temperature. Similar data have been reported for turtles.

An exception to the relationship of thyroid activity and temperature described above is the situation found in several species of lizard inhabiting warmer climates. These lizards do not exhibit depressed thyroid function at lower temperatures. In fact, thyroids of such lizards tend to be more active during cool periods.

There appears to be a positive correlation also between thyroid state and physical activity in lizards and snakes. Increased humidity and activity are correlated with increased thyroid function in the lizard *Agama agama savattieri*, suggesting that a more complex relationship exists among thyroid state, physical activity level of the animal, and environmental factors.

3. Thyroid and Oxygen Consumption in Reptiles

The relationship between thyroid state and oxygen consumption is temperature-dependent. Thyroid hormones, TSH, and thyroidectomy have little effect on lizards maintained at 20°C, but a positive relationship appears between oxygen consumption and thyroid state at 30°C. Heart, brain, liver, muscle, and lung tissues from lizards incubated *in vitro* at 30°C respond to T_4 with increased consumption of oxygen. Homogenates of both liver and skeletal muscles from T_4-treated snakes *Natrix piscator* exhibit higher oxygen consumption at 30°C than do tissues from untreated snakes. Thyroidectomy causes a decrease in oxygen consumption in these animals that is restored to normal by treatment with T_4. Metabolic rate and cytochrome oxidase activity also are stimulated by T_4 at 25°C. These observations suggest that homeothermy in birds and mammals (as well as homeothermy proposed for certain large, extinct reptiles) is an adaptation to maximize some basic features of oxidative metabolism and its stimulation by thyroid hormone.

4. Thyroid and Molting in Reptiles

Shedding of the skin is stimulated in lizards by thyroid hormones and is retarded by thyroidectomy. Implants of thyroid tissue into muscles of thyroidectomized *Lacerta spp.* restore molting that has been interrupted by thyroidectomy. Apparently either mammalian TSH or PRL is capable of restoring molting in some hypophysectomized lizards, and PRL enhances the effect of T_4 on intact animals. Such a relationship between PRL and the thyroid axis in lizards is unlike the role for PRL in premetamorphic amphibians, but fits with the synergistic roles of these hormones observed during late stages of metamorphosis in both urodele and anuran amphibians.

In marked contrast to lizards, thyroidectomy in snakes increases molting frequency, and cessation of molting follows administration of thyroid hormones. No explanation for this contradiction between snakes and lizards has been offered. This situation in snakes is different from that found in amphibians in which thyroid hormones and corticosteroids are stimulators of molting in urodeles and anurans, respectively.

5. Thyroid and Growth of Reptiles

Although detailed studies of the relationship of thyroid state to growth are lacking for reptiles, a variety of studies employing embryonic, juvenile, and adult reptiles suggest a relationship between thyroid hormones and growth that is similar to the mammalian pattern. Thyroidectomy of the lizard *Sceloporus undulatus* retards growth. Other studies in reptiles are needed to substantiate this relationship.

H. Thyroid Functions in Birds

The structural and functional features of avian thyroid glands are similar to those of mammals. Thyroid hormones have been reported to affect reproduction, growth, metabolism, temperature regulation, molting, and various behaviors. Most studies on avian species have concentrated heavily on certain domestic birds (chicken, duck, pigeon, Japanese quail), and few data are available for wild bird species. Nevertheless, with respect to most of these processes, the relationships are similar for those wild and domestic species studied.

1. Development of Thyroid Function in Birds

The thyroid axis develops early in some birds, being functional in the chicken by day 13 of development. The embryonic chick thyroid actually responds to TRH and TSH administration on the 6th day of incubation, indicating that although the thyroid gland's secretory capacity is all ready to go, the endogenous activity of the hypothalamic-pituitary connection is still immature. Plasma levels of T_4 increase steadily after day 13 to maximal levels by day 20. In contrast, levels of T_3 remain low until day 19 when there is a surge of T_3 production during pipping and hatching. This surge corresponds to a rise in type I deiodinase activity in the liver and a marked decrease in type III deiodinase similar to events described in tail tissues during amphibian metamorphosis. Thus, conversion of T_4 to T_3 increases as degradation of T_3 decreases. This relationship continues after hatching. Hypophysectomy of hatchlings, however, causes an increase in type III deiodinase activity which can be prevented by treatment with growth hormone (GH). A similar effect of GH is seen in adult chickens as well, suggesting an additional side to the traditional synergistic actions between thyroid hormones and GH in growth (see Chapters 4 and 5). Type I deiodinase is unaffected by GH. This dramatic change in thyroid activity has been documented in chicken and Japanese quail that are **precocial birds** but not in **altricial birds** such as ring doves. Altricial birds, unlike precocial species, are totally dependent on their parents after hatching. In ring doves, thyroid and deiodinase activity change much more gradually as the birds develop greater independence from their parents.

2. Thyroid and Reproduction in Birds

Domestic birds require thyroid hormones for normal gonadal development. For example, T_4 stimulates testicular growth, whereas thyroidectomy or goitrogen administration impairs testicular function or induces gonadal regression. T_4 can stimulate testicular growth out of season in some wild birds as well. However, exogenous T_4 under some circumstances may exert suppressive actions on gonads. In several wild species, thyroidectomy prior to the time for normal gonadal growth results in precocious gonadal growth and maintenance at maximal condition. Treatment with T_4 results in gonadal regression in thyroidectomized birds at any time of year. In other wild species, thyroidectomy simply prolongs the active gonadal phase and shortens the time during which the gonads are regressed. Obviously, one cannot generalize about the relationships between thyroid hormones and reproductive events in birds since each species may prove to be a special case.

3. Thyroid, Thermogenesis, and Oxygen Consumption in Birds

The role for thyroid hormones in cold adaptation appears for the first time in birds and can be considered a relatively new functional acquisition for thyroid hormones (see Figure 7-17). **Thermogenesis** (heat production) in birds as in mammals is closely linked to oxygen consumption. Some wild birds in temperate regions exhibit heightened thyroid activity in late autumn and early winter as evidenced by histological examination and changes in thyroid gland weight. Thyroidectomy of adult birds depresses their ability to produce heat, and treatment with thyroid hormones increases oxygen consumption.

4. Thyroid, Carbohydrate Metabolism, and Growth in Birds

Thyroid hormones reduce glycogen stores in liver, increase free fatty acid levels, and induce mild hyperglycemia. Thyroidectomy causes a decrease in blood glucose and liver fatty acid levels but an increase in blood cholesterol levels. These effects may not be of primary importance since a number of other hormones, such as glucagon and epinephrine, are known to be more important than thyroid hormones with respect to controlling carbohydrate metabolism in birds (see Chapters 12 and 13). Thyroid hormones may produce a permissive effect with respect to the actions of these other "glucohormones," possibly through an effect on adenylyl cyclase levels in the target tissues. These effects on carbohydrate metabolism may be related to the thermogenic action of thyroid hormones.

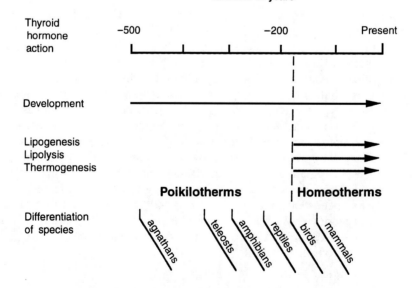

Figure 7-17. **Distribution of developmental and thermogenetic action of thyroid hormones in vertetrates.** Thermogenesis appears with the acquisition of homeothermy possibly in the reptilian ancestors of birds and mammals. [From Oppenheimer, J. H. et al. (1995). An integrated view of thyroid hormone actions *in vivo*. *In* "Molecular Endocrinology: Basic Concepts and Clinical Correlations" (B. D. Weintraub, Ed.) pp. 249–268. Raven Press Ltd., New York.]

Table 7-11. Plasma levels of T_3 and T_4 in Migrating and Post-Migrating Canadian Goose, *Branta canadensis interior*[a]

Sampling time	Plasma T_4 (ng/ml)	Plasma T_3 (ng/ml)	T_3/T_4
Spring pre-migration	11.8	3.5	0.28
Spring post-migration	17.0	2.0	0.10
Fall pre-migration	13.3	1.0	0.05
Fall post-migration	11.8	2.0	0.18

[a] Values estimated from Fig. 27 in George, J. C., and John, T. M. (1990). Canada goose thyroid: Seasonal ultrastructural changes in relation to circulating levels of its hormones. *Cytobios* **61**, 97–115.

There is evidence that thyroid hormones act cooperatively with GH in birds. Thyroidectomy causes depression or retardation of growth in birds and seasonal changes in circulating GH and T_4 are correlated. Release of GH is reduced by elevated thyroid hormones as if this were a normal negative feedback loop for controlling GH release.

5. Thyroid and Molting in Birds

Thyroid hormones produce stimulatory effects on the skin and feathers that are usually associated with the molting process. It is generally accepted, however, that the gonadal axis provides the factors that directly regulate the molting process in birds (see Chapter 11). Unlike the condition for urodele amphibians and lizards, the role for thyroid hormones in the molting process of birds may be permissive rather than causative.

6. Thyroid and Migration in Birds

Migratory birds have been shown to possess active thyroid glands as compared to non-migrating or post-migrating individuals of the same species, suggesting some correspondence between thyroid activity and the migratory process. Although some of the older literature indicates that thyroid hormones may directly influence migratory behavior, the nature of this influence has not been confirmed. Thyroid hormones may alter metabolic patterns associated with energy requirements during migration. Another suggestion is that thyroid hormones "tune" the nervous system so that it is more sensitive to environmental or other endocrine cues or both. In the Canadian goose (*Branta canadensis interior*), thyroid histology appeared activated and plasma T_4 levels increased in association with spring pre-migratory restlessness or **Zugunruhe** as compared to post-migrating birds, but the plasma T_3/T_4 ratio decreased dramatically (Table 7-11). However, in relation to the fall migration, there was a marked increase in T_3 in post-migrants and the T_3/T_4 ratio increased. This latter observation may reflect differences in thermal conditions and the role of thyroid hormones in thermogenesis during the cooler fall.

III. Summary

The thyroid axis of vertebrates shows many parallels with respect to thyroid structure and to the synthesis and metabolism of thyroid hormones as well as to their actions. T_3 appears to be the more active form of thyroid hormones in all vertebrates. Thyroid hormones appear to interact with a variety of other endocrine-regulated systems where they play permissive or possibly synergistic roles especially in development, growth, and reproduction. The systems of deiodinases seem to be responsible for allowing surges in T_3 to occur at critical times. Direct actions of thyroid hormones on development occur in all vertebrates, but their participation in lipid metabolism and thermogenesis is correlated with homeothermy.

Some notable phylogenetic differences stand out with respect to hypothalamic regulation in teleost fishes and amphibians. TRH appears to exert a negative control in many fishes over TSH release, and in amphibians evidence is mounting to identify the CRH peptide as the endogenous TSH-releasing hormone.

Considerable work remains to be done on thyroid systems in non-mammalian vertebrates, especially in elasmobranchs, a greater variety of teleosts, and reptiles. Once this has been accomplished, a clearer pattern of vertebrate thyroid function should appear.

Suggested Reading

Books

Armstrong, J. B., and Malacinski, G. M. (1989). "Developmental Biology of the Axolotl." Oxford Univ. Press, New York.

Balls, M., and Bownes, M. (1985). "Metamorphosis." Oxford Univ. Press, Oxford.

Gilbert, L. I., and Freiden, E. (1981). "Metamorphosis: A Problem in Developmental Biology," 2nd Ed. Plenum, New York.

Gilbert, L. I., Tata, J. R., and Atkinson, B. G. (1996). "Metamorphosis: Postembryonic Reprogramming of Gene Expression in Amphibian and Insect Cells." Academic Press, San Diego.

Matsuda, R. (1987). "Animal Evolution in Changing Environments with Special Reference to Abnormal Metamorphosis." Wiley, New York.

McDiarmid, R. W., and Altig, R. (1999). Tadpoles: The Biology of Anuran Larvae. The University of Chicago Press, Chicago.

Shi, Y-B. (2000). Amphibian Metamorphosis: From Morphology to Molecular Biology. John Wiley & Sons, New York.

General Articles

Dickhoff, W. W., and Darling, D. S. (1983). Evolution of thyroid function and its control in lower vertebrates. *Am. Zool.* **23**, 697–708.

Fritzsch, B. (1990). The evolution of metamorphosis in amphibians. *J. Neurobiol.* **21**, 1011–1021.

Kuhn, E. R., Mol, K. A., and Darras, V. M. (1993). Control strategies of thyroid hormone monodeiodination in vertebrates. *Zool. Sci.* **10**, 873–885.

Norris, D. O. (1999). Thyroid hormones, in subavian vertebrates. *In* "Encyclopedia of Reproduction," (E. Knobil and J. D. Neill, Eds.), Vol. 4, pp. 807–812. Academic Press, New York.

Protochordates

Patricolo, E., Cammarata, M., and D'Agati, P. (2001). Presence of thyroid hormones in ascidian larvae and their involvement in metamorphosis. *J. Exp. Zool.* **290**, 426–430.

Fishes

Blaxter, J. H. S. (1988). Pattern and variety in development. *In* "Fish Physiology, the Physiology of Developing Fish" (W. S. Hoar and D. J. Randall, Eds.), Vol. 11A, pp. 1–58. Academic Press, San Diego.

Eales, J. G., and Brown, S. B. (1993). Measurements and regulation of thyroidal status in teleost fish. *Rev. Fish Biol. Fisher.* **23**, 299–347.

Joss, J. M. P. (2006). Lungfish evolution and development. *Gen. Comp. Endocr.* **148**, 285–289.

Leatherland, J. F. (1988). Endocrine factors affecting thyroid economy of teleost fish. *Am. Zool.* **28**, 319–328.

Leloup, J., and de Luze, A. (1985). Environmental effects of temperature and salinity on thyroid function in teleost fishes. *In* "The Endocrine System and the Environment" (B. K. Follett, S. Ishii, and A. Chandola, Eds.), pp. 23–32. Japan Sci. Soc./Springer-Verlag, Berlin.

Plohman, J. C., Dick, T. A., and Eales, J. G. (2002). Thyroid of lake sturgeon, *Acipenser fulvescens*. I. Hormone levels in blood and tissues. *Gen. Comp. Endocr.* **125**, 47–55.

Power, D. M., Llewellyn, L., Faustino, M., Nowell, M. A., Björnsson, B. Th., Einarsdottir, I. E., Canario, A. V. N., and Sweeny, G. E. (2001). Thyroid hormones in growth and development of fish. *Comp. Biochem. Physio. C* **130**, 447–459.

Sukumar, P., Munro, A. D., Mok, E. Y. M., Subburaju, S., and Lam, T. J. (1997). Hypothalamic regulation of the pituitary-thyroid axis in the tilapia *Oreochromis mossambicus*. *Gen. Comp. Endocr.* **106**, 73–84.

Amphibians

Galton, V. A. (1992). Thyroid hormone receptors and iodothyronine deiodinases in the developing Mexican axolotl, *Ambystoma mexicanum. Gen. Comp. Endocr.* **85**, 62–70.

Galton, V. A. (1992). The role of thyroid hormone in amphibian metamorphosis. *Trends Endocr. Metab.* **3**, 96–100.

Kikuyama, S., Kawamura, K., Tanaka, S., and Yamamoto, K. (1993). Aspects of amphibians metamorphosis: Hormonal control. *Intl. Rev. Cytol.* **145**, 105–148.

Norris, D. O., and Dent, J. N. (1989). Neuroendocrine aspects of amphibian metamorphosis. *In* "Development, Maturation, and Senescence of Neuroendocrine Systems" (M. P. Schreibman and C. G. Scanes, Eds.), pp. 63–90. Academic Press, San Diego.

Sachs, L. M., Damjanovski, S., Jones, P. L., Li, Q., Amano, T., Ueda, S., Shi, Y.-B., and Ishizuya-Oka, A. (2000). Dual functions of thyroid hormone receptors during *Xenopus* development. *Comp. Biochem. Physiol. B* **126**, 199–211.

Safi, R., Vlaeminck-Guillem, V., Duffraisse, M., Seugnet, I., Plateroti, M., Margotat, A., Duterque-Coquillaud, M., Crespi, E. J., Denver, R. J., Demeneux, B., and Laudet, V. (2006). Pedomorphosis revisited: thyroid hormone receptors are functional in *Necturus maculosus. Evol. Dev.* **8**, 284–292.

Shi, Y.-B. (1994). Molecular biology of amphibian metamorphosis: A new approach to an old problem. *Trends Endocr. Metab.* **5**, 14–20.

Wakahara, M., Miyashita, N., Sakamoto, A., and Arai, T. (1994). Several biochemical alterations from larval to adult types are independent of morphological metamorphosis in a salamander, *Hynobius retardatus. Zool. Sci.* **11**, 583–588.

Reptiles

Hulbert, A. J. (1985). A comparative study of thyroid function in reptiles and mammals. *In* "The Endocrine System and the Environment" (B. K. Follett, S. Ishii, and A. Chandola, Eds.), pp. 105–115. Japan Sci. Soc./Springer-Verlag, Berlin.

Birds

May, J. D. (1989). The role of the thyroid in avian species. *Crit. Rev. Poultry Biol.* **2**, 171–186.

McNabb, F. A. M. (2006). Avian thyroid development and adaptive plasticity. *Gen. Comp. Endocrinol.* **147**, 93–101.

Sharp, P. J., and Klandorf, H. (1985). Environmental and physiological factors controlling thyroid function in galliformes. *In* "The Endocrine System and the Environment" (B. K. Follett, S. Ishii, and A. Chandola, Eds.), pp. 175–188. Japan Sci. Soc./Springer-Verlag, Berlin.

8

The Mammalian Adrenal Glands: Cortical and Chromaffin Cells

The responses an animal makes to an adverse or **stressful stimulus** leads to a **stress response** which includes the release of hormones from the adrenal glands and their subsequent effects. These hormones enable the animal to address the stressful stimulus. These responses are controlled largely through the **hypothalamus-pituitary-adrenal (HPA) axis** and secretion of **corticotropin-releasing hormone (CRH)** and **corticotropin (ACTH)**. The

272

adrenal hormones induce changes in metabolism and/or ionic regulation that work to combat physiological and psychological factors and eventually to eliminate or at least neutralize the stressful stimulus. Knowledge of this stress response system contributes to our understanding of how animals adapt physiologically to physical and psychological traumas. In addition, these adrenal hormones play other important roles that are described in this chapter.

Mammals typically possess two adrenal glands, one located superior to each kidney (*ad-renal* or *supra-renal*; Figure 8-1). This anatomical arrangement is responsible for their present name, adrenals or adrenal glands, and for an alternative name in humans, the suprarenal glands.

Each adrenal gland actually consists internally of four almost separate endocrine glands. The outer portion or **adrenal cortex** represents three glandular regions and is composed largely of lipid-containing, steroidogenic **adrenocortical cells**. The adrenal cortex surrounds a fourth endocrine region consisting of an inner mass of **chromaffin cells** called the **adrenal medulla**. Chromaffin cells are so named because they contain intracellular granules containing catecholamines that can be stained by certain chromium compounds (see ahead).

The adrenocortical cells are derived from the coelomic epithelium in the pronephric region of the embryo adjacent to the genital ridge that gives rise to the gonads. These cells produce steroid hormones including **glucocorticoids, mineralocorticoids**, and weak androgens such as **dehydroepiandrosterone, DHEA** (see Chapter 3, Figures 3-29 and 3-30). The first two glandular regions of the adrenals secretes glucocorticoids and DHEA under the direct stimulatory influence of ACTH from the pituitary gland (see Chapter 4) although

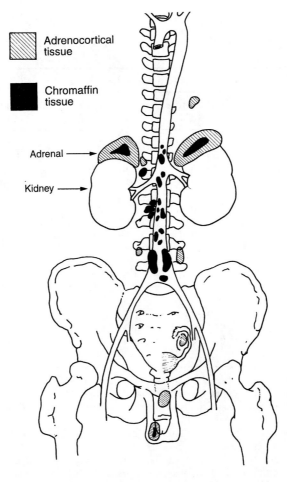

Figure 8-1. **Location of adrenal tissue in the human**. Note that in addition to the expected location of adrenocortical and chromaffin cells in the adrenal gland, heterotopic locations where either tissue may be found in either sex.

DHEA secretion also may be stimulated by LH and LH-like hormones. Mineralocorticoid secretion by the third region, however, is regulated mainly by the **renin-angiotensin system** (see ahead). Glucocorticoids are named for their influences on glucose metabolism and mineralocorticoids for their effects on Na^+ and K^+ balance. The major glucocorticoids synthesize by mammals are **cortisol, corticosterone**, and to some extent **11-deoxycortisol**. The major mineralocorticoids are **aldosterone** and **deoxycorticosterone**. Representative blood levels for glucocorticoids and mineralocorticoids in mammals are provided in Table 8-1. Relative glucocorticoid and mineralocorticoid activities of some common natural and synthetic corticosteroids can be found in Table 8-2.

The chromaffin cells are of neural crest origin, and the medulla functions essentially like a modified sympathetic ganglion. The adrenal medulla is under direct neural control (preganglionic cholinergic sympathetic neurons originating in the hypothalamus) and releases **norepinephrine** and/or **epinephrine** into the blood. These secretions are usually termed "hormones" but, considering the embryonic origin of the medulla, they could be called "neurohormones," too.

At first glance, there seems to be no functional significance for the close anatomical relationship of the adrenocortical and chromaffin cells. Although there is participation of both systems with respect to adaptations to stressful stimuli, the factors controlling release of their secretions are not obviously related nor do their biological actions seem to overlap. The anatomical closeness of the cortex and medulla in mammals as well as relationships of their homologous tissues in non-mammals may simply be a function of the physical closeness of their embryological sites of origin although the progressive evolution of this arrangement is obvious when non-mammals are examined (see Chapter 9). ACTH and glucocorticoids do have effects on catecholamine synthesis by chromaffin cells, and these systems are not entirely independent.

Table 8-1. Circulating Levels of Corticoids in Selected Mammalian Species (Prototheria, Metatheria, and Eutheria)

Species	Mean steroid levels ± SD in peripheral blood				
	Aldosterone (ng/dL)	Corticosterone (μg/dL)	Cortisol (μg/dL)	Deoxycorticosterone (ng/dL)	11-Deoxy-cortisol (μg/dL)
Prototheria					
Echidna[a]	1.5	0.35	0.18	—	—
Echidna[b]	—	0.14 ± 0.07	0.07 ± 0.03	—	—
Echidna + ACTH[b]	—	1.06 ± 0.56	0.42 ± 0.23	—	—
Metatheria					
Black-tailed wallaby	8.2 ± 4.3	0.12 ± 0.02	1.1 ± 0.2	3.3 ± 0.6	0.13 ± 0.08
Common wombat	0.9 ± 1.4	0.06 ± 0.02	0.04 ± 0.04	2.0 ± 1.3	0.14 ± 0.08
Dingo	6.7 ± 4.3	0.04 ± 0.21	1.90 ± 1.90	23.6 ± 23.7	0.19 ± 0.09
Koala	1.6 ± 2.2	0.20 ± 0.05	*[c]	6.0 ± 8.3	0.06 ± 0.11
Eutheria					
Sheep	2.1 ± 1.7	0.09 ± 0.04	0.52 ± 0.50	2.5 ± 2.5	0.05 ± 0.03
Dog	2.1 ± 3.6	0.20 ± 0.13	0.85 ± 0.39	11.3 ± 6.0	0.07 ± 0.05
Fox	13.9 ± 3.2	0.59 ± 0.17	2.30 ± 1.2	37.4 ± 22.7	0.17 ± 0.03
BALB/cfC3H mice[d]	—	12.00 ± 2.16	—	—	—
Sand rat[e]	2.8 ± 13.3	0.20 ± 0.8	10.7 ± 24.9	—	—
Human, male	12.4	0.42	14.4	6.6	0.05
Harbor seals[f]			0.494 ± 0.153		

[a] Oddie, G. J., Blaine, E. H., Bradshaw, J. P., Coghlan, J. P., Denton, D. A., Nelson, J. F., and Scoggins, B. A. (1976). Blood corticosteroids in Australian marsupial and placental mammals and one monotreme. *J. Endocr.* **69**, 341–348.

[b] Sernia, C., and McDonald, I. R. (1977). Adrenocortical function in a prototherian mammal. *J. Endocr.* **72**, 41–52.

[c] *, Undetectable.

[d] Hawkins, E. F., Young, P. N., Hawkins, A. M. C., and Bern, H. A. (1975). Adrenocortical function: Corticosterone levels in female BALB/C and C34 mice under various conditions. *J. Exp. Zool.* **194**, 479–484.

[e] Amirat, Z., Khammar, F., and Brudieux, R. (1980). Seasonal changes in plasma and adrenal concentrations of cortisol, corticosterone, aldosterone, and electrolytes in the adult male sand rat (*Psammomys obesus*). *Gen. Comp. Endocr.* **40**, 36–43.

[f] Oki, C., and Atkinson, S. (2004). Diurnal patterns of cortisol and thyroid hormones in the harbor seal (*Phoca vitulina*) during summer and winter seasons. *Gen. Comp. Endocr.* **136**, 289–297.

Table 8-2. Activities of Corticosteroids

Steroid	Relative activity in assay				
	MR[a]	Na[+b]	GLY[c]	GR[d]	AI[e]
Aldosterone	1	1	0.15	1	—
DOC[f]	0.8	0.03	0.02	1	—
Corticosterone	0.2	0.004	0.36	2	0.3
Cortisol	0.1	0.001	1	1	1
18-OH-DOC[f]	0.015	0.004	—	0.02	—
Dexamethasone	0.05	0.001	17–250	10	25–169

[a] MR, mineralocorticoid; MR receptor assay is based on competition for [^{3}H]aldosterone-binding sites in rat kidney.

[b] Na$^+$ bioassay, normally based on change in urinary Na$^+$/K$^+$ in the adrenalectomized rat.

[c] GLY, glycogen; GLY bioassay is based on glycogen deposition in the adrenalectomized rat liver.

[d] GR, glucocorticoid receptor; GR assay is based on competition with [3H]dexamethasone-binding sites in rat kidney.

[e] AI, anti-inflammatory; AI bioassay is based on anti-inflammatory activity.

[f] DOC, deoxycorticosterone; 18-OH-DOC, 18-hydroxy-DOC.

I. The Mammalian Adrenal Cortex

The adrenal cortex of adult mammals may be subdivided by means of histological criteria into three well-defined regions: **zona glomerulosa, zona fasciculata**, and **zona reticularis** (Figure 8-2). These regions are arranged as concentric shells surrounding the adrenal medulla. In addition, there are inner zones described between the

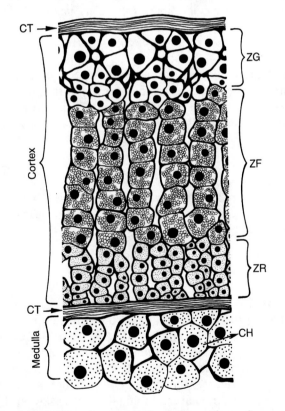

Figure 8-2. **Zonation of the adrenal gland.** The cortex consists of an outermost layer of connective tissue (CT), the zona glomerulosa (ZG) producing aldosterone, the zona fasciculata (ZF) secreting most of the glucocorticoids, and the inner zona reticularis (ZR) specializing in adrenal androgen production. The adrenal medulla is separated from the cortex by another layer of CT and consists primarily of chromaffin cells (CH) that secrete catecholamines and endogenous opiates (EOPs).

outer zones and the medulla in some mammals. These regions may perform unique functions and may be transitory.

A. Zonation of the Adrenal Cortex

The cells of the outermost region of the adrenal cortex, the zona glomerulosa, are smaller, are more rounded, and contain less lipid than those of the more central zona fasciculata. The zona glomerulosa is responsible for synthesis of aldosterone as well as some other corticosteroids. There are few cytological changes in the zona glomerulosa following hypophysectomy or administration of ACTH, suggesting that the secretion of aldosterone is independent of pituitary control. Although ACTH is not necessary for synthesis and release of aldosterone, the responsiveness of the glomerulosal cells to agents that normally elicit these events is reduced in hypophysectomized mammals and is enhanced with ACTH treatment. Consequently, ACTH does have a permissive effect on cells of the zona glomerulosa.

The zona fasciculata is the largest zone in the adrenal cortex. It is located between the zona glomerulosa and the innermost zona reticularis and is histologically distinct from both. It consists of polyhedral (many-sided) cells that are sources of the glucocorticoids. The cells of the zona fasciculata are arranged in narrow columns or cords surrounding blood sinusoids that allow the cells to be bathed directly with blood (i.e., there is no tissue-blood barrier). The proportion of cortisol and corticosterone secreted differs markedly, from secretion of primarily cortisol (human), through mixtures of both (cat, deer), to primarily corticosterone (rat). Thickness of the zona fasciculata is most sensitive to circulating levels of ACTH. It exhibits hypertrophy and hyperplasia in response to prolonged elevation of ACTH secretion caused by stress or treatment with the drug **metyrapone** which blocks the 11-hydroxylation step necessary for glucocorticoid synthesis (see Chapter 3) and hence elevates ACTH in the blood. Unlike the zona glomerulosa, the zona fasciculata atrophies markedly following hypophysectomy and hypertrophies as a result of prolonged glucocorticoid therapy.

The zona reticularis typically borders the adrenal medulla, and it contains numerous thin, extracellular connective tissue elements known as reticular fibers (hence its name). It is a primary source of adrenal androgens, but some glucocorticoids may be synthesized here as well. The zona reticularis also hypertrophies in response to ACTH and atrophies following hypophysectomy, but not so dramatically as the zona fasciculata.

It should be noted that the "typical" anatomical pattern described here within the adrenal cortex and the anatomical relationship of cortex to medulla varies considerably within mammals as a group. Furthermore, ectopic nodules of functional cortical tissue are not uncommon (Figure 8-1), and this accessory adrenocortical tissue may become a source for corticosteroids following surgical adrenalectomy.

B. Additional Zonation

Several unique adrenocortical zones are known only for certain species, but the adrenals of most mammalian species have not been examined in detail. These special zones may be conspicuous only at certain times in the life of an animal or in only one sex.

1. The Fetal Zone

In primates, a very conspicuous zone occupies the bulk of the adrenal gland prior to birth. This region is called the **fetal zone** and is responsible for the relatively large size of the adrenal at birth (Figure 8-3). In humans, the neonate adrenal may be as large as the adrenal gland of a 10- to 13-year-old. During gestation, the fetal zone, which is found between the cortex and the medulla, synthesizes and releases relatively large quantities of DHEA and lesser amounts of its sulfated derivative, **DHEA-S**. These adrenal androgens serve as precursors for the synthesis of estrogens by the placenta (see Chapter 10). Failure of the fetal zone to produce adequate amounts of DHEA/DHEA-S results in premature termination of gestation. Formerly, it was believed that chorionic gonadotropin (CG) from the placenta (see Chapters 4 and 10) was responsible for stimulating fetal adrenal androgen production, but recent studies suggest adrenal androgen secretion is strongly influenced by ACTH and PRL. The fetal adrenal plays important roles in the birth process, too (see Chapter 10).

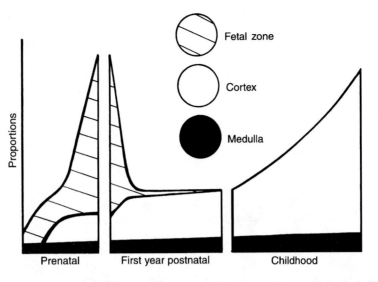

Figure 8-3. **Comparison of fetal zone to remainder of adrenal gland in humans.** Prior to birth, the bulk of the adrenal consists of the androgen-secreting fetal zone that regresses rapidly after birth. Whereas the fetal zone is gone by one year of age, the medulla and cortex continue to grow until puberty. In the actual adrenal gland, the fetal zone appears between the zona reticularis and the medulla but is shown above the cortex here for effect.

Following birth, the fetal zone ceases to function in humans and degenerates rapidly. The fetal zone typically has disappeared completely by one year of age. The zona reticularis begins to synthesize DHEAS/DHEA at about age 5 or 6 (Figure 8-4), and DHEA synthesis accelerates during puberty. Maximal DHEA production is achieved around age 20 after which its production slowly declines. It has been suggested that DHEA may be an anti-tumor substance and/or a precursor for synthesis of other androgens or estrogens, especially in postmenopausal women.

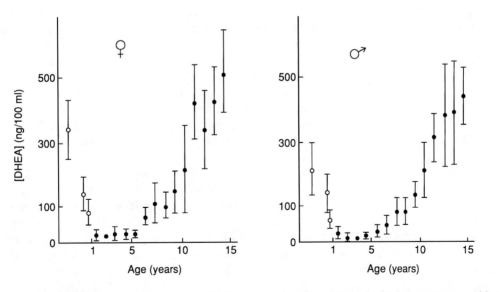

Figure 8-4. **Adrenarche in humans.** After birth, adrenal DHEA (open circles) declines as the fetal zone regresses. Although the fetal zone has regressed completely by age 1, production of the adrenal androgen DHEA continues in the zona reticularis (solid circles). DHEA secretion begins to increase at about age 5 and peaks at puberty. [Modified from de Peretti, E., and Forest, M. G. (1976). Unconjugated dehydroepiandrosterone plasma levels in normal subjects from birth to adolescence in human: The use of a sensitive radioimmunoassay. *J. Clin. Endocr. Metab.* **43**, 982–991.]

2. The Mouse X-Zone

The cortex of the mouse adrenal contains a unique **X-zone** located between the zona reticularis and the medulla. The X-zone appears to be unrelated to the fetal zone of primates although it appears in the same anatomical location. This zone degenerates in males at puberty and in females of most mouse strains during the first pregnancy. Degeneration in the males is correlated with production of androgens by the testes. The function of this X-zone is not known.

3. The "Special Zone"

In at least one marsupial, the brush-tailed possum (*Trichosurus vulpecula*), there is a large inner special zone that appears only in the adult female. Its function has not been elucidated, and it is not known whether it is comparable to either the primate fetal zone or the X-zone of mice.

II. Biosynthesis and Transport of Corticosteroids

Glucocorticoids and mineralocorticoids not only differ in their actions but also in their synthesis and transport in the blood. As outlined in Chapter 3, all of the corticosteroids are derived from conversion of **cholesterol** to **pregnenolone** in the mitochondria by the action of the side chain cleavage enzyme, **P450$_{scc}$**. Pregnenolone is converted into progesterone and then further modified via the Δ^5 pathway (see Chapter 3, Figure 3-30). Cholesterol is readily obtained from circulating **low-density lipoprotein droplets (LDLs;** see Chapter 12) or from stored deposits in the adrenal cells. Synthesis of cholesterol from acetyl groups also can occur in adrenal cells as described in Chapter 3.

A. Synthesis of Corticosteroids

At the membranes of the smooth endoplasmic reticulum, pregnenolone can be metabolized along either the **17α-hydoxysteroid pathway** or the **17-deoxysteroid pathway**. The former pathway leads to **11-deoxycortisol** and is accomplished by the actions of the enzyme **21-hydroxylase**. 11-Deoxycortisol may be secreted or may reenter the mitochondria where the **11β-hydroxylase enzyme (P450$_{11β1}$)** converts it to cortisol. Conversion of pregnenolone to progesterone in the zona fasciculata or glomerulosa, via the 17-deoxysteroid pathway yields **11-deoxycorticosterone** which is converted to corticosterone by employing the same enzymes as did the 17α-hydroxysteroid pathway. Cortisol and/or corticosterone are the major end products of corticosteroidogenesis in the zona fasciculata and to a lesser extent in the zone reticularis.

In the zona glomerulosa, the 17-deoxysteroid pathway is favored and corticosterone is further modified to **18-hydroxycorticosterone** and then to aldosterone. Another mitochondrial enzyme called **aldosterone synthase** (P450$_{11β2}$ or P450$_{aldo}$) is responsible for aldosterone synthesis in rodents and humans. Aldosterone and 18-hydroxycorticosterone have mineralocorticoid activity, but aldosterone is more potent and is typically the dominant secretory product of the zona glomerulosa *in vivo*. However, deoxycorticosterone may be the major secretory product in some species (see Table 8-1).

As mentioned previously, adrenal androgens are synthesized primarily in the zona reticularis or by the fetal zone of primates. Both the Δ^4 and Δ^5 pathways may be utilized (see Chapter 3), but the Δ^5 pathway is more common, resulting in DHEA which is them sulfated to form DHEAS. The primate fetal zone makes little or no **androstenedione**, and this weak Δ^5 androgen is more commonly found in the adult adrenal. DHEA also is a weak androgen and the sulfated form does not penetrate readily into potential target cells, reducing the threat of masculinization to a female fetus or the mother. DHEAS is converted by the placenta into **16α-hydroxyDHEA** and then by the **aromatase** enzyme (P450$_{aro}$) to estriol. Androstenedione is converted by P450$_{aro}$ to estrone that can be processed further to estradiol. These conversions of fetal androgens are essential for maintaining pregnancy. Because the placenta cannot synthesize androgens, it must depend entirely on the fetal adrenal to provide the androgen precursor for estrogen synthesis.

B. Release of Corticosteroids

Circulating corticosteroids reflect synthesis rates since little hormone is stored in the adrenal, and corticosteroids are released as they are made. In adult humans, daily episodic release of cortisol is maximal between 0600 and 0900 hr in the morning, with lower values occurring in the afternoon and minimal levels at night. This daily rhythm can be disrupted by eating lunch, which causes increased cortisol secretion, but is not affected, by eating dinner. In nocturnal animals, such as the rat, the rhythmic pattern of secretion is reversed.

Aldosterone secretion shows a similar rhythm to glucocorticoids in humans with peak levels observed between 0600 and 0900 hr. Unlike the glucocorticoid rhythm, the aldosterone rhythm is independent of ACTH levels. The drug **propranolol**, a β-adrenergic blocker, abolishes the aldosterone rhythm in rats, suggesting that catecholamines from sympathetic neurons are responsible for the rhythm.

In humans, as is generally true for other mammals, adrenal androgen synthesis accelerates at the onset of puberty (**adrenarche**) in both males and females (Figure 8-4) and continues at this level until the early 20s when it begins to decline. Adrenal function in general declines after age 40–50. This age-related decline in adrenal production has been termed **adrenopause**.

Because of the episodic nature of corticosteroid release and the strong diurnal aspect of secretion, measurements to determine appropriate levels of corticosteroids are complicated by the need for repeated sampling of blood or saliva. (Saliva contains corticosteroids in proportion to their concentrations in the blood, and their measurement can be used as an index of blood levels.) Furthermore, sampling itself can evoke corticosteroid secretion causing an overestimate of secretory activity. Analysis of steroid metabolites in 24-hour urine samples can provide an index of integrated secretion over that time period.

C. Transport of Corticosteroids in the Blood

Probably, more than 90% of the glucocorticoids are bound to a specific plasma transport protein called **corticosteroid binding globulin (CBG)** or **transcortin**. Some glucocorticoid also binds nonspecifically to albumin, as was described for thyroid hormones in Chapter 6. Although there is a bias for assuming free hormone is most important for entering target cells and producing effects, there also is evidence to support a role for interaction of occupied CBG with target cell membranes that facilitates dissociation of glucocorticoids from CBG and their entrance into the target cell.

Aldosterone does not bind significantly to CBG or other plasma proteins. Consequently, aldosterone is present only in the free state at much lower concentrations in the blood than are the glucocorticoids. Aldosterone is cleared from the blood much more rapidly because of the lack of binding proteins.

D. Metabolism of Corticosteroids

The liver is the major site for metabolizing corticosteroids (see Chapter 3) although other tissues, such as the kidneys and intestines, also can perform this task. Most corticosteroids are conjugated with sulfates or glucuronides to increase their solubility in water, and they are readily excreted via the urine, bile, or feces. Cortisol, aldosterone, and most adrenal androgens are conjugated as glucuronides, but DHEA is excreted primarily as DHEAS. In humans, the majority of corticosteroid metabolites are excreted via the urine whereas in the rat the biliary and fecal routes are more popular.

One way in which corticosteroids are metabolized is by reduction of the A-ring and addition of hydroxyl groups at C_3 or C_{20} followed by side-chain cleavage to yield C_{19} steroids. Hydroxylation by cytochrome P450 enzymes also occurs at C_6 and C_{16}. In humans, up to a third of the cortisol may be oxidized to corotic acids. Some selected metabolites of corticosteroids are depicted in Chapter 3, Figure 3-38.

III. Secretion and Actions of Glucocorticoids

Secretion of glucocorticoids from the zona fasciculata and zona reticularis is under direct control of the HPA axis involving CRH and ACTH (see Chapter 4). Circulating ACTH levels are depressed by elevated levels of glucocorticoids and are increased following adrenalectomy, establishing the existence of direct negative feedback of corticosteroids on ACTH release. **Arginine vasopressin (AVP)** potentiates the action of CRH on the corticotropic cells of the pars distalis during responses to chronic stress (see Chapter 4). ACTH also may be released by direct neural input to the hypothalamus as a result of such stressful events as physical trauma (injury, surgery), and this response may occur even in the presence of elevated glucocorticoid levels. Thus, stressful stimuli can bring about and maintain a marked increase in glucocorticoid levels. The ability of traumatic stimuli to override the normal negative feedback mechanism verifies the importance of multiple control mechanisms governing ACTH release.

A. Actions of Glucocorticoids

Glucocorticoids produce marked effects on energy metabolism at physiological doses as a result of changes in transport of materials into cells and induction of new enzyme syntheses.

Their major effect is to supplant and conserve the energy normally derived from circulating glucose by (1) inhibiting glucose utilization by peripheral tissues (especially skeletal muscle), (2) stimulating entry of amino acids into liver cells and their conversion to glucose and storage as glycogen, and (3) enhancing the mobilization of fat stores in non-neural tissues. By blocking glucose utilization, glucocorticoids spare blood glucose so that the brain has a preferential source of glucose.

As described in Chapter 3, glucocorticoids can bind to both intracellular glucocorticoid receptors (GR = type II GR) or to intracellular mineralocorticoid receptors (MR = type I GR). However, glucocorticoids usually are inactivated by enzymatic conversion to cortisone in the cytosol of cells involved with mineral balance. Cortisone does not bind to the MR. Some of the glucocorticoid feedback on brain neurons is accomplished through MR receptors, however (see Chapter 4). Membrane GR also have been described in the vertebrate brain and may be associated with behavior.

B. Mechanism of Glucocorticoid Cellular Action

Glucocorticoid effects on target cells are described in Chapter 3, and only a brief summary is provided here. The initial requirement for glucocorticoid action on liver cells is binding to type-II glucocorticoid receptors (GR), translocation of occupied GR into the nucleus, and eventual stimulation of nuclear RNA synthesis (both messenger RNA and ribosomal synthesis). Approximately two to four hours following application of glucocorticoids, there is an increase in new enzymes that bring about the changes in cellular metabolism characteristic of glucocorticoid action.

1. Glucocorticoids and Metabolism

In liver cells, these new enzymes include those associated with the conversion of fatty acids or amino acids into glucose and the polymerization of glucose to form glycogen (see Chapter 12). Amino acid transport into liver cells also is stimulated. In contrast, glucocorticoids inhibit the uptake of amino acids and the metabolism of glucose in peripheral tissues such as skin, skeletal muscle, and adipose cells. This action makes glucose more readily available to the brain during stress.

In the brain, glucocorticoids may act classically through intracellular receptors or may bind to plasma membrane receptors and bring about rapid effects in target cells. These membrane receptors appear to operate through second messenger systems to produce their rapid effects.

Elevated glucocorticoids or excessive doses of glucocorticoids inhibit protein synthesis in certain tissues (heart and diaphragm) and accelerate protein catabolism in others (especially skeletal muscle, bone, and lymphoid tissue). Protein catabolism provides amino acids for glucose synthesis and contributes to hyperglycemia.

Early feedback effects of glucocorticoids on pituitary corticotropes during a stress response reduce the availability of intracellular Ca^{2+} that normally are increased by CRH working through second messengers. Consequently, ACTH release is blocked. Later actions of glucocorticoids involve blocking ACTH synthesis and down-regulation of CRH receptors in corticotropes. However, release of AVP is not affected by glucocorticoid feedback and can sustain elevated ACTH secretion.

The metabolic conversion of amino acids into glucose is termed **gluconeogenesis**, the production of glucose from a noncarbohydrate precursor; in this case, amino acids. Glucocorticoids also enhance the actions of growth hormone on lipolysis in adipose tissue. This causes release of fatty acids and glycerol into the circulation and their conversion by liver cells into glucose, another form of gluconeogenesis. Furthermore, glucocorticoids stimulate liver cells to produce the gluconeogenic enzyme **phosphoenolpyruvate carboxykinase (PEPCK)**.

2. Glucocorticoids and Reproduction

The onset of pubery is correlated with activation of adrenal secretion (adrenarche; see above). Animals with reduced adrenocortical function may exhibit delayed puberty and/or seasonal breeding. Glucocorticoid secretion is always elevated during the breeding season and is considered to be essential for successful reproduction. However, high levels of glucocorticoids can block gonadotropin secretion and delay or prevent reproduction. Interestingly, dominant males exhibit lower glucocorticoid levels than do subordinate males.

In male marsupial mice (e.g., *Antechinus spp.*), high cortisol is associated with aggressive breeding that results in the death of all males by the end of the breeding season. The females exhibit lower levels of cortisol than the males and survive to rear the young. Although stress levels of glucocorticoids typically reduce breeding success, stress does not prevent breeding in male *Antechinus* even though it contributes to their death.

3. Glucocorticoids and Immunity

It is common to observe an increased incidence of disease in stressed animals. In fact, the immune response system is inhibited by the HPA axis at several levels. For example, elevated levels of glucocorticoids inhibit the inflammatory response as well as the production of antibodies. Furthermore, CRH not only stimulates ACTH release but also causes release of somatostatin (SST) and dopamine that reduce secretion of growth hormone (GH) and prolactin (PRL), respectively. Either GH or PRL can restore immune function that is normally depressed following hypophysectomy. The observation that GH and PRL secretion occurs at night with ACTH and glucocorticoid levels normally at their lowest supports these relationships since renewal of immune function also occurs at night.

Recent evidence shows that cytokines influence the HPA axis and this may be part of the mechanisms for homeostatic regulation of the immune response system. A variety of cytokine effects on brain function have been described including effects of interleukins on the blood brain barrier allowing access of other elements into the nervous system. Cytokines may enter the brain through special structures called **circumventricular organs** such as the **organum vasculosum lateralis terminae (OVLT)** of the preoptic area. Circumventricular organs contain fenestrated capillaries that allow access of many blood-borne materials directly into the brain. Other evidence suggests cytokines also can enter at certain sites via carrier-mediated transport. Regardless of how they enter, cytokines such as interleukins and interferons released during increased immune activity can activate CRH release from the hypothalamus that ultimately causes elevated glucocorticoids and suppression of the immune response. Recent studies of cytokine effects on brain function suggest that at least some of their effects are mediated via sensory fibers of the vagus nerve. In rats, vagotomy blocks several responses classically attributed to cytokine effects on the brain including fever, hypothalamic depletion of norepinephrine, and elevated plasma corticosterone.

Not all actions of glucocorticoids are suppressive of immune function. Certain aspects of cellular immunity are enhanced by glucocorticoids at physiological levels even though chronic elevations may be suppressive.

4. Epinephrine, Glucocorticoids, and Stress

The responses characteristic of chronic stress are mediated by glucocorticoids. These responses were demonstrated in rats by Hans Selye and incorporated into a general theory of adaptation to stress termed the **general adaptation syndrome**. According to Selye, there are three stages of adaptation by an organism to stressful stimuli. Furthermore, Selye noted that regardless of the nature of the stressful stimulus he applied, the physiological consequences were the same (gastric ulcers, enlarged adrenals, and shrunken immune tissues). Thus, initially the stress response was defined as an all-encompassing term to include the responses to all stimuli (stressors) that are harmful or potentially harmful to the organism.

The first phase of Selye's general adaptation syndrome is the **alarm reaction**, which includes a generalized increase in sympathetic stimulation involving the adrenal medulla followed closely by increased secretion of

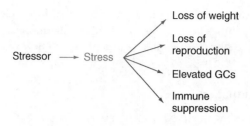

Figure 8-5. **Evidence of chronic stress.** See discussion in text.

glucocorticoids. Because of the activation of glucocorticoid secretion, the alarm reaction is not identical to the "emergency" or "fight-or-flight" response of Cannon that emphasizes only epinephrine release.

The next phase of adaptation is termed the **stage of resistance** and is characterized by prolonged increased secretion of glucocorticoids. During this stage, the organism adapts to the continued presence of the stressful stimuli. The resistance phase is frequently marked by enlargement of the adrenal glands, primarily due to hypertrophy of the zona fasciculata and, to a lesser extent, the zona reticularis in response to elevated ACTH. Finally, under continuation of extremely stressful conditions, the ability of the organism to function normally is impaired. Chronic stress and prolonged glucocorticoid elevation are characterized by loss of body weight, loss of reproductive activity, and immune suppression (Figure 8-5).

The continuous presence of the stressful stimuli causes the organism to enter the final **stage of exhaustion** that leads to death. Although Selye seemed to focus on an exhaustion of the HPA axis as the cause of death, it is the general debilitation of the body (e.g., responses to prolonged hyperglycemia, increased neurodenegeration, immune suppression) that leads to death.

Although Selye envisioned that all stressors evoke an identical stress response, it is clear that all stressors do not affect the animal in precisely the same manner. Careful studies have revealed that the relative impact of various stressors differs with respect to how heavily the HPA axis is involved in contrast to other physiological mechanisms as well as the relative involvements of glucocorticoids, epinephrine, and norepinephrine. Nevertheless, the general physiological pattern of the stress response as originally formulated by Selye is heavily documented and accepted.

The relative roles of the adrenal cortex and the adrenal medulla are not fixed but can vary. For example, humans were examined performing the same task under self-paced conditions or externally paced conditions that challenged their ability to keep up. Plasma epinephrine levels were similar in both groups suggesting an equal intensity of effort, but cortisol levels were much higher in the externally challenged subjects. Social position, especially in species exhibiting a clear dominance hierarchy, also can influence the physiological response to a potentially stressful stimulus. Following establishment of a new laboratory colony, mice becoming subordinate were found to have higher levels of plasma corticosterone whereas mice emerging as dominants had higher levels of catecholamines as evidenced by increased tyrosine hydroxylase activity (see Chapter 3).

Stress of experimental animals is important when attempting to interpret data on corticosteroid levels or nutrient levels (amino acids, glucose, etc.). Laboratory conditions alone can influence the adrenal axis. Stress can also influence the levels of other hormones. For example, the order in which groups of rats were removed from a common holding facility and killed at a remote site influenced the mean levels of PRL that were measured for each group. Since it is not possible to undertake experimental work on animals free from stress, detailed knowledge of how animals were maintained and all procedures involved with an experiment is essential when interpreting results.

Focus on the deleterious effects of prolonged activation of the HPA axis as a consequence of chronic stress has led to a general impression that the stress response is non-adaptive. Instead, one should focus on the adaptive nature of the alarm reaction to immediate survival as well as the resistance phase of the stress response that allows an animal to cope with the continued presence of a stressor. Usually, it is only in extreme cases of prolonged stress that the organism develops pathologies associated with its physiological responses to stress.

5. Permissive Actions of Glucocorticoids

It has been suggested that, in addition to their roles during stress and participation in immune suppression, glucocorticoids may act as "permissive agents" as described earlier for thyroid hormones (see Chapter 6).

Through changes in membrane permeabilities to important metabolites and by stimulating the synthesis of new enzymes or receptors, glucocorticoids may provide the appropriate cellular environment in which other hormones operate.

6. Pharmacological Actions of Glucocorticoids

The glucocorticoids possibly are better known for their pharmacological actions and therapeutic effects than for their biological actions. The tremendous potential for glucocorticoids in the treatment of the rare hypoadrenocorticism described by Thomas Addison in 1885 (Addison's disease) was not recognized for many years. However, the discovery of the **anti-inflammatory effects** of glucocorticoids and their use for treatment of rheumatoid arthritis spurred a tremendous explosion in therapeutic applications of glucocorticoids. The debilitating symptoms of rheumatoid arthritis are the consequence of inflammation associated with an autoimmune response in which the patient produces antibody against his/her own connective tissue. Glucocorticoid therapy alleviates painful inflammation occurring as a result of the immune reaction but does nothing to correct the causative factors.

One mechanism whereby glucocorticoids reduce inflammation is by interfering with the elaboration of histamine or with its actions in mediating the inflammatory response, which includes local hyperemia and resultant edema. One postulated mechanism for this interference is the glucocorticoid-induced inhibition of the **kallikreins**, enzymes which catalyze formation of **kinins** from a plasma precursor protein. Kinins induce inflammation by causing release of histamine normally observed following the combination of antigen and antibody. Another suggestion for glucocorticoid anti-inflammatory activity stems from observations of their effects on lysosomes. Glucocorticoids stabilize lysosomal membranes, thereby reducing release of hydrolytic enzymes following cell injury and hence reducing the spread of the inflammatory reaction. Inhibition by glucocorticoids of the cyclooxygenase enzyme necessary for prostaglandin synthesis reduces prostaglandin induction of inflammation. Glucocorticoids also inhibit the synthesis of leukotrienes and cytokine agents (e.g., interleukins) that mediate inflammation and cell-mediated immune responses.

One of the most recent therapeutic applications of massive doses of synthetic glucocorticoids is to suppress the entire immune response so as to allow tissue and organ transplantations. Although normal therapeutic anti-inflammatory doses of glucocorticoids do not interfere with normal antigen-antibody interactions, very high doses depress new antibody synthesis. Immune suppression prevents the host from producing antibodies against the foreign transplants. However, continuous treatment of the transplant recipient is necessary for retention of the transplanted tissue and can lead to deleterious effects as well as susceptibility to diseases (see above).

IV. Aldosterone: The Principal Mammalian "Mineralocorticoid"

The zona glomerulosa secretes aldosterone independently of direct pituitary control, although, as mentioned earlier, ACTH appears to play a permissive role in maintaining the responsiveness of these cells to other controlling factors. The major action of aldosterone is maintenance of the normal sodium-potassium balance in body fluids, and its secondary action is to regulate extracellular fluid volume. Aldosterone stimulates sodium reabsorption into the blood and potassium secretion into the urine by kidney nephrons. The mechanism controlling secretion of aldosterone involves a most complex and seemingly circuitous series of events involving the lungs, liver, and kidney: **the renin-angiotensin system**.

A. The Renin-Angiotensin System and Aldosterone Secretion

Renin is an enzyme produced in the kidney by the **juxtaglomerular body**, a modified group of smooth muscle cells located in the afferent arteriole carrying blood to the glomerulus (Figure 8-6). This enzyme is a glycoprotein (about 40,000 daltons) possibly secreted as a larger, inactive form or **prorenin** (63,000 daltons). Conversion of prorenin to renin may be accomplished by the activity of kidney kallikrein. Development of renin activity from prorenin also occurs following mild acidification of the plasma. Renin has a plasma biological

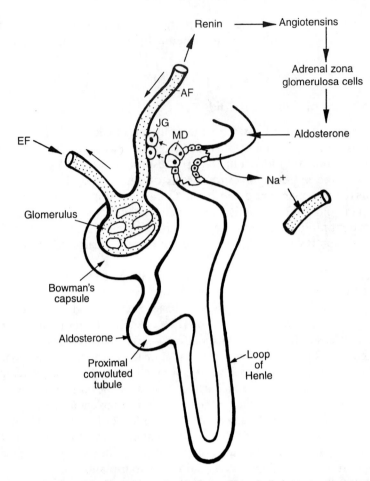

Figure 8-6. **Schematic representation of the juxtaglomerular apparatus.** The stippled structures represent a portion of the vasculature
of the nephron including the afferent arteriole (AF) bringing blood to the glomerulus (a capillary bed) housed in
Bowman's capsule of the nephron and exiting via the efferent arteriole (EF) prior to entering the peritubular capillaries
(not shown). The juxtaglomerular apparatus consists of the renin-secreting juxtaglomerular cells (JG) embedded in the
walls of the afferent arteriole and the macula densa (MD) that consists of modified cells in the distal convoluted portion
of the nephron.

half-life of about 15 minutes and is rapidly degraded. The juxtaglomerular body is intimately associated with
a modified region of the distal convoluted portion of the nephron known as the **macula densa**. Together these
two structures comprise the **juxtaglomerular apparatus**.

Release of renin is controlled by blood volume as reflected in blood pressure within the renal arterioles
and/or by sodium concentration in the glomerular filtrate as it enters the proximal (convoluted) tubule of the
nephron. Intrarenal blood pressure is monitored by stretch receptors in the juxtaglomerular body. Renin is
released in response to a decrease in this pressure. Sodium concentration in the tubular lumen is monitored by
cells of the macula densa, and low sodium levels somehow trigger communication between the macula densa
and the juxtaglomerular cells, resulting in renin release. Changes in either or both parameters influence renin
secretion.

Once renin enters the blood, it comes in contact with a plasma protein termed **renin substrate
(= angiotensinogen)** that was synthesized by the liver. Mammalian renin substrates are large glycoproteins
(mol wt 58,000–110,000) that behave like α_1-globulins, α_3-globulins, or albumin in humans, herbivores, and
rodents, respectively. In venous blood returning to the heart from the kidneys, renin causes the enzymatic
release of a decapeptide known as **angiotensin-I (Ang-I)** from renin substrate. Although Ang-I can facilitate
release of norepinephrine from the adrenal medulla and can produce direct and indirect pressor effects on the
cardiovascular system, it is generally believed to be of little physiological importance due to the pattern of
blood flow and the rapid enzymatic degradation of Ang-I. Venous blood containing Ang-I travels first to the

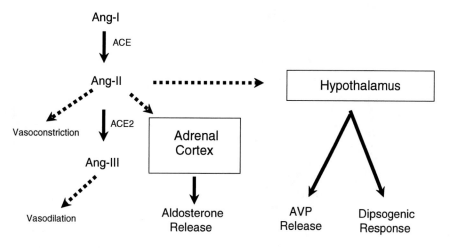

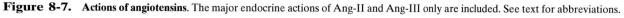

Figure 8-7. **Actions of angiotensins.** The major endocrine actions of Ang-II and Ang-III only are included. See text for abbreviations.

the heart and then directly to the lungs where **angiotensin-converting enzyme (ACE)**, located in the endothelial cells of the lung capillaries, hydrolyzes most of the Ang-I to an octapeptide, **angiotensin-II (Ang-II)**. **Captopril** is a potent synthetic inhibitor of ACE and can be used to block formation of Ang-II.

The actions of the Ang-II are summarized in Figure 8-7. Blood containing mostly Ang-II returns from the lungs to the heart and then is pumped into the general circulation where it produces multiple short-term effects. Ang-II has a biological half-life of only about two minutes. When Ang-II reaches the adrenal cortex, it stimulates synthesis and release of aldosterone from cells of the zona glomerulosa. Aldosterone release appears to be a result of activation of inositol trisphosphate (IP$_3$) and diacylglycerol (DAG) as second messengers and their effects on calcium channels in zona glomerulosa cells (see Chapter 3). Aldosterone travels through the blood to the kidney and stimulates increased reabsorption of sodium and some increased excretion of potassium. This increased sodium reabsorption aids in water retention, reduces urine volume, and helps to restore normal fluid volume.

In addition to stimulating aldosterone release, Ang-II is a potent vasoconstricting agent (about 40X more potent than norepinephrine) and quickly helps restore blood pressure to normal by causing contraction of vascular smooth muscle resulting in a decrease in arteriole diameter. Ang-II also induces hypertrophy of cardiac myocytes as well as mitosis in mesangial cells. This hypertrophic response in cardiac cells is mediated by transcription and synthesis of **transforming growth factor β, TGFβ**. Prolonged elevation of Ang-II can induce significant cardiac hypertrophy and contribute to chronic hypertension. Furthermore, Angi-II causes release of norepinephrine from atrial sympathetic nerve endings causing increased heart rate and/or contraction strength contributing further to increased blood pressure.

Ang-II has two important central nervous system effects that also contribute to an elevation in blood pressure. Through actions on the subfornical organ in the brain, Ang-II stimulates drinking (dipsogenic response), and absorption of ingested water from the gut contributes to increased blood volume and pressure. Furthermore, Ang-II causes release of vasopressin through actions on the hypothalamus. These two effects contribute to the resumption of normal fluid balance.

The levels of an enzyme, **aminopeptidase a**, are increased by actions of Ang-II. This enzyme degrades Ang-II. In addition, a second form of ACE called **ACE2** is present in numerous tissues (especially the kidney, heart, and arteriole smooth muscle) and converts Ang-II into a heptapeptide called **angiotensin-III (Ang-III)** or angiotensin 1–7 (Figure 8-8). Ang-III locally counteracts the effects of A-II by causing vasodilation. In the heart Ang-III is also antihypertrophic. Although Ang-III can bind to the Ang-II receptor, it is much less potent than Ang-II on aldosterone release and on vasoconstriction. However, the vasodilation and hypertrophy effects of Ang-III are mediated via a unique Ang-III receptor. Some conditions of xhypertension are related to the absence of sufficient ACE2 expression. The regulation of blood pressure by the renin-angiotensin system is summarized in Figure 8-9.

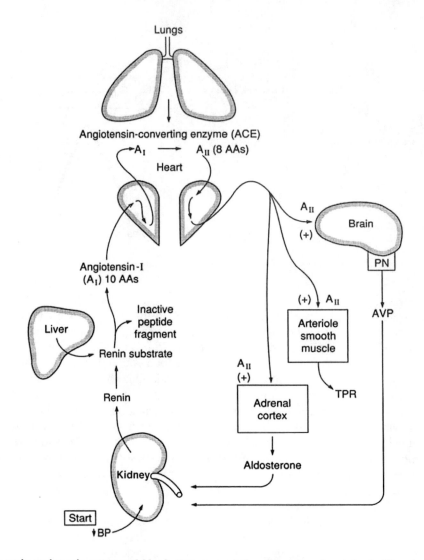

Figure 8-8. **The renin-angiotensin system and blood pressure regulation**. The roles of angiotensin III and natriuretic peptides on blood pressure are not included. See text for explanation. A_I = Ang-I; A_{II} = Ang-II.

B. Independent Renin-Angiotensin Systems

Since the discovery of the renin-angiotensin system involving the cooperative efforts of several organs to regulate blood pressure and sodium/potassium balance, complete renin-angiotensin mechanisms have been demonstrated within the brain, pituitary, gonads, and the adrenal cortex itself. The presence of a complete renin-angiotensin system within the adrenal cortex suggests the possibility of an adrenal paracrine regulatory system for controlling basal secretion of aldosterone. Evidence suggests a more active brain renin-angiotensin system may be present in hypertensive rats. In the pituitary, Ang-II may stimulate proliferation of tropic hormone-secreting cells. There is evidence to support a role for Ang-II in ovulation. In the cow ovary, the number of Ang-II receptors increases with size of the follicle. The amount of prorenin in seminal fluid is proportional to the sperm count, but neither the origin nor the significance of seminal prorenin is known.

C. Additional Factors Controlling Aldosterone Secretion

Aldosterone secretion is influenced by several factors in addition to the renin-angiotensin system. For example, elevated blood potassium levels can stimulate aldosterone release directly. Release of aldosterone can be inhibited by **natriuretic peptides** secreted by the heart during chronic hypertension.

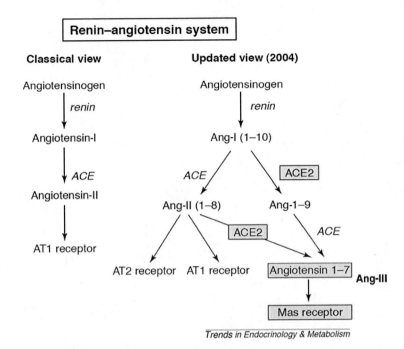

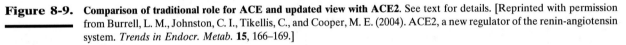

Figure 8-9. **Comparison of traditional role for ACE and updated view with ACE2.** See text for details. [Reprinted with permission from Burrell, L. M., Johnston, C. I., Tikellis, C., and Cooper, M. E. (2004). ACE2, a new regulator of the renin-angiotensin system. *Trends in Endocr. Metab.* **15**, 166–169.]

1. Potassium

High levels of potassium in extracellular fluids directly stimulate aldosterone secretion from cells of the zona glomerulosa which, in turn, promotes renal potassium loss. Potassium may increase the sensitivity of cells in the zona glomerulosa to Ang-II or may directly cause aldosterone release. In contrast, extracellular sodium variations do not directly influence aldosterone secretion unless unusually large variations are produced.

2. Natriuretic Peptides

Two similar peptides are known to inhibit release of aldosterone through direct actions on cells of the zona glomerulosa. The first natriuretic peptide discovered was believed to be secreted by the atria of the heart and was named **atrial natriuretic peptide (ANP)** for its ability to increase sodium excretion via the urine and its presumed origin. A second peptide was discovered in the brain and became known as **brain natriuretic peptide (BNP)**. However, both ANP and BNP are found in the heart (including in the ventricles). A third form (CNP) has been found in the arcuate and paraventricular nuclei of the hypothalamus and within gonadotropes in the pituitary.

In humans, ANP is the predominant circulating form and consists of 28 amino acids (Figure 8-10). BNP occurs in two forms of 26 and 32 amino acids, respectively, both of which are structurally similar to ANP. Peripheral GC-A receptors bind ANP and BNP equally well. CNP has a unique receptor, GC-B, that has high specificity for CNP. All of these peptides activate guanylyl cyclase and produce cGMP as a second messenger. CNP may be the oldest member of this group of related peptides as it is phylogenetically the most conservative of the three natriuretic peptides (Figure 8-10). GC-B receptors occur on hypothalamic GnRH neurons as well as on gonadotropes, and CNP is believed to be a paracrine inhibitor of gonadotropin release. CNP also has been reported to inhibit ACTH release and stimulate GH secretion.

Chronically elevated blood volume and/or blood pressure stretches the atria and causes release of ANP which not only inhibits aldosterone release, but also inhibits vasopressin release and directly promotes sodium excretion and water loss in the kidney. Release of ANP also is stimulated directly by elevated plasma sodium. ANP also lowers renin production in the kidney. All of these effects will reduce blood volume and blood pressure.

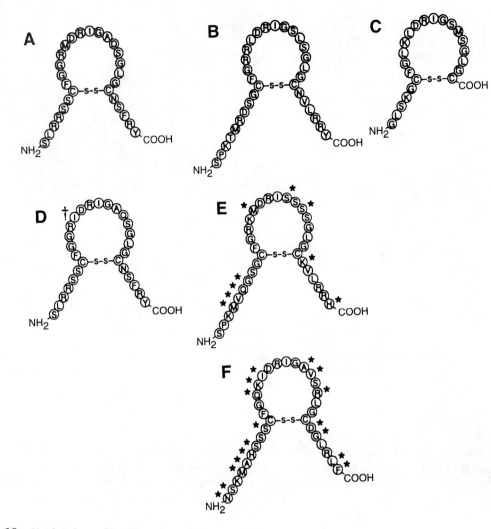

Figure 8-10. **Natriuretic peptides**. Three forms have been identified: ANP (A & D), BNP (B, E & F), and CNP (C). Asterisks denote amino acid substitutions in BNP and the dagger shows the single change in rat ANP. Amino acid designations can be found in Appendix A. (A) Porcine & human α-ANP; (B) porcine BNP; (C) porcine CNP; (D) rat ANP; (E) human BNP; (F) rat BNP. [Reprinted by permission of the publisher from Samson, W. K. Natriuretic peptides. A family of hormones. *Trends Endocr. Metab.* **3**, 86–90. Copyright 1992 Elsevier Science Inc.]

3. Neurotransmitters

The adrenal cortex is well-supplied with neurons employing a variety of neurotransmitters. Serotonin, norepinephrine, acetylcholine, vasoactive intestinal peptide (VIP), vasopressin, and prostaglandins are found in the adrenal cortex and can stimulate aldosterone release. SST may be produced locally and is known to inhibit Ang-II-induced release of aldosterone.

D. Mechanism of Aldosterone Action

Aldosterone stimulates sodium reabsorption and potassium excretion in the distal (convoluted) tubule of the kidney and possibly enhances some sodium reabsorption in the proximal portion as well as in the intestinal mucosa, salivary glands, and sweat glands. Aldosterone produces the typical steroidal pattern of action on target cells following binding to cytoplasmic MRs. Increased nuclear RNA synthesis results in production of a specific protein, **aldosterone-induced protein**, that somehow mediates the movement of sodium across the target cells. This is somewhat reminiscent of the mechanism for movement of Ca^{2+} across cells of the duodenal mucosa by the steroid hormone 1,25-DHC (see Chapter 3).

V. Clinical Aspects of the Adrenal Axis

Glucocorticoid pathologies generally are distinct from those for aldosterone. However, high levels of glucocorticoids can bind to and activate aldosterone receptors and mimic aldosterone effects on Na^+ and K^+ balance as well as on blood pressure. Primary and secondary disorders as well as hypersecretion and hyposecretion pathologies have been described.

A. Glucocorticoid Hypersecretion

The major disorders of glucocorticoid hypersecretion or **hyperadrencorticism** are **Cushing's disease** and **Cushing's syndrome**. The latter term encompasses any adrenal disorder accompanied by elevated glucocorticoids whereas the former refers to the specific condition of hyperadrenocorticism caused by hypersecretion of ACTH by the pituitary.

1. Cushing's Disease

This condition was described by Cushing in 1932 and is the most common cause of Cushing's syndrome. Hypersecretion of ACTH by a basophilic pituitary adenoma is the cause of this condition. Such adenomas are not sensitive to feedback by glucocorticoids. In this secondary adrenal disorder, the adrenal cortices are hypertrophied and plasma cortisol levels also are elevated (hypercortisolism). Hyperpigmentation (excessive darkening of the skin) may occur due to the α-MSH-like actions of chronically elevated ACTH (see Chapter 4). Excessive cortisol levels have adverse effects on metabolism of many tissues including the brain, muscles, skin, vascular tissue, kidney, liver, and skeleton. Hypophysectomy alleviates the symptoms (see Table 8-3) but necessitates extensive replacement therapies since all of the tropic hormones are removed by this procedure whereas adrenalectomy requires only corticosteroid therapy. Cushing's disease is three to four times more common in women than in men.

2. Cushing's Syndrome

The symptoms of this disorder are due to production of an excess of glucocorticoids, and the cause usually is due to excessive secretion of ACTH by pituitary cells (i.e., Cushing's disease) but may be due to elevated cortisol from adrenal adenomas or adrenal carcinomas or due to ACTH secreted by non-pituitary tumors (e.g.,

Table 8-3. Some Symptoms Commonly Presented with Cushing's Disorders

Symptom	Percentage of cases
Obesity or weight gain	80
Thin skin	80
Hypertension	75
Purple skin striae	65
Hirsutism	65
Amenorrhea (women only)	60
Abnormal glucose tolerance test	55
Acne	45
Osteoporosis	40
Hyperpigmentation	20

bronchial carcinoid tumor, pancreatic carcinoid tumor, or medullary thyroid carcinoma). Such corticosteroid-secreting tumors suppress CRH and ACTH and bring about atrophy of normal adrenal cortical cells. Consequently, hyperpigmentation only occurs in the pituitary-dependent form of hyperadrenocorticism, Cushing's disease. Cushing's syndrome may occur in a small percentage of diabetic patients as well. Excessive glucocorticoid secretion can be associated with obesity-related diabetes and escape diagnosis as an adrenal disorder.

B. Glucocorticoid Hyposecretion

The best-known examples of **hypoadrenocorticism** are the primary disorders called **Addison's disease** and **congenital adrenal hyperplasia (CAH)**. Secondary hypoadrenocorticism is not so common.

1. Addison's Disease

This disease is characterized by a shortage or absence of cortisol resulting in hypersecretion of ACTH. Hyperpigmentation occurs in most cases due to elevated ACTH and its ability to bind to α-MSH receptors on melanocytes. A person with Addison's disease is usually hypoglycemic due to lack of cortisol and a reduced capacity for gluconeogenesis. Concomitant glucocorticoid therapy typically employs sufficient glucocorticoids that also stimulates MR receptors. Absence of aldosterone causes other symptoms including muscle weakness, water losses, hypotension, and salt-craving.

Although Addison's disease once was commonly associated with tuberculosis infections, today the most common cause of Addison's disease is bilateral atrophy of the adrenals resulting from an autoimmune attack. It also may occur as a result of drug-induced or congenital deficiencies in steroidogenetic enzymes or as a complication in AIDS.

2. Congenital Adrenal Hyperplasia (CAH)

A genetic defect in one or more genes coding for steroidogenic enzymes involved in corticosteroid synthesis can cause reduced glucocorticoid synthesis and hence excessive ACTH secretion due to the absence of normal feedback. Hypersecretion of ACTH, in turn, causes hypertrophy and hyperplasia of the adrenal cortex, principally the zona fasciculata and zona reticularis. This condition is known as **congenital adrenal hyperplasia (CAH)**. Depending upon what enzymes are affected, there usually is an increase in adrenal androgen production caused by the elevated levels of ACTH.

The most common form of CAH is caused by the absence of the enzyme 21-hydroxylase ($P450_{c21}$) that blocks synthesis of cortisol, corticosterone, and aldosterone. This disorder is responsible for 90%–95% of the cases of CAH, with the remaining cases being attributed mainly to the absence of enzymes such as 11β-hydroxylase ($P450_{c11}$) and $P450_{scc}$. Failure to convert progesterone to deoxycorticosterone in the absence of a functional C_{21}-hydroxylase causes a buildup of 17α-hydroxypregnenolone and 17α-hydroxyprogesterone that are consequently converted into DHEA (Δ^5 pathway) and androstenedione (Δ^4 pathway). These weak androgens may be converted by peripheral tissues into testosterone causing virilization. Newborn males with CAH may not be readily recognized, but a newborn female with CAH may be diagnosed as an ambiguous sex or as a male depending on the extent of masculinization of the external genitalia. Early diagnosis is important because both sexes suffering from CAH tend to exhibit rapid somatic growth associated with early cessation of long bone growth and attainment of short stature. The penis and clitoris also show continuous growth. Aldosterone synthesis is impaired in about two-thirds of these cases due to the unavailability of suitable precursors resulting in loss of sodium and elevation of plasma potassium. Hence, these subjects also are said to suffer from salt-losing or **salt-wasting disease** because they cannot retain sodium ions.

There is a much milder form called **cryptic CAH** in which excessive androgen production does not occur until puberty. Subjects with cryptic CAH caused by C_{21}-hydroxylase deficiency can be identified by a simple test that shows elevated 17α-hydroxyprogesterone levels in the blood following a 60-minute challenge with exogenous ACTH.

3. Secondary Hypoadrenocorticism

Hypothalamic or pituitary lesions that block production of CRH or ACTH can produce the symptoms of hypoadrenocorticism. People with secondary hypoadrenocorticism lack the hyperpigmentation that usually accompanies Addison's disease but have the other symptoms. This condition can develop as a result of hypophysectomy, autoimmune disorders, viral illnesses, prolonged morphine administration, and other causes. The most common origin of this disorder is a consequence of prolonged therapy with cortisol or related steroids (e.g., dexamethasone) chronically employed as anti-inflammatory agents or immune suppressants that block the HPA axis through feedback effects.

C. Disorders of Aldosterone Secretion

Hyperaldosteronism is characterized by low blood potassium, high blood sodium, and muscle weakness. Elevated plasma sodium levels bring about water retention and may produce hypertension. Hyperaldosteronism may result from an adenoma or carcinoma in the zona glomerulosa that autonomously secretes excessive amounts of aldosterone. These symptoms also develop when ACTH or ACTH-like peptides are elevated chronically. Treatment with aldosterone inhibitors can reduce these symptoms until the source of the excessive aldosterone is removed.

Loss of the zona glomerulosa through adrenalectomy or Addison's disease, congenital (e.g., CAH) or drug-induced depression of aldosterone production, and defects in the renin-angiotensin system can induce **hypoaldosteronism**. Potassium excretion is reduced, sodium is lost in the urine, and water retention is impaired. Imbalances in sodium/potassium ratios can alter muscle and nerve function. These conditions can be alleviated by treatment with aldosterone therapy.

D. Adrenal Excesses in Androgen Production

Adrenal androgen production may be elevated in several hyperadrenocorticoid conditions such as Cushing's syndrome or with hypoadrenocorticism as in the case of CAH. Adrenal tumors may secrete excessive quantities of adrenal androgens. Symptoms of excessive production of adrenal androgens in adult women include hirsutism (excessive body hair production), acne, seborrhea (dandruff), irregular menses, reduced fertility, lowered voice pitch, atrophy of the breasts, possible thinning of hair and recession of the scalp in the temporal region, clitoral enlargement, and hypertrophy of skeletal muscles. These same symptoms may be present in males but are not as noticeable since many of the symptoms bear a similarity to normal male features. Young adult women that exhibit anorexia nervosa (a disorder characterized by greatly reduced food intake and an elevated adrenal axis) may develop facial hair (hirsutism) as a result of ACTH-induced secretion of adrenal androgens.

E. Side Effects of Corticosteroid Therapy

Corticosteroids typically are administered in high doses to achieve their therapeutic effects. This is especially true of glucocorticoid use for treating inflammations that vary in their intensity from skin rashes to muscle injuries or arthritis. Adverse side effects on metabolism and/or osmotic and ionic balance that occur as a consequence of prolonged glucocorticoid therapy are predictable from a simple knowledge of glucocorticoid actions.

1. Adverse Effects of Glucocorticoid Therapy

The beneficial therapeutic effects of glucocorticoids are manifest only when applied at doses two to three times physiological levels. Consequently, a number of adverse side effects occur with prolonged administration of glucocorticoids, including mild diabetes mellitus as a consequence of a prolonged hyperglycemic antagonism induced by glucocorticoids (see Chapter 12). Subjects also experience muscle weakness due to extensive protein catabolism (an effect that does not occur with physiological doses), osteoporosis due to destruction of bone substance, reduced activity of the immunological response system, and mental depression. Glucocorticoids also produce mineralocorticoid-like effects on Na^+ and K^+ balance due to high levels that operate through saturation of the mineralocorticoid receptor (MR) and/or of the mechanisms for intracellular inactivation of cortisol and corticosterone (see Chapter 3).

2. Adverse Effects of Aldosterone Therapy

Excessive doses of mineralocorticoids cause sodium retention and consequent accumulation of fluids (edema), as evidenced by rapid weight gain following their administration. However, an "escape" phenomenon due to unknown factors usually occurs, and the condition is alleviated before serious complications arise and irreparable damage has occurred. In cases of cardiac failure, the escape mechanism also fails.

Aldosterone therapy results in decreased blood potassium and increased urine potassium. Excessive aldosterone can cause severe potassium losses that can induce muscle cramps and muscle weakness. These events occur primarily because of adverse effects on cell membrane characteristics and resultant alterations of normal muscle cell physiology. Because pharmacological doses of glucocorticoids result in increased binding to the MR, excess glucocorticoids can mimic the effects of excess aldosterone.

VI. The Mammalian Adrenal Medulla

The medullary portion of the mammalian adrenal consists of sympathetic preganglionic neuronal endings (cholinergic) and modified cells derived from neural crest and homologous to postganglionic sympathetic neurons (adrenergic). In other words, the adrenal medulla is a modified sympathetic ganglion that secretes either norepinephrine or epinephrine directly into the blood. Both epinephrine and norepinephrine (as well as small quantities of dopamine) can be extracted from the adrenal medulla, but the ratio in most adult mammals strongly favors epinephrine (Table 8-4). The proportion of norepinephrine to epinephrine may vary throughout life, however. Fetal and neonatal adrenals secrete predominantly norepinephrine followed by a gradual increase for most species in the proportion of epinephrine so that eventually epinephrine dominates in adults. Whales are an apparent exception in that the adult whale adrenal consists of about 83% norepinephrine.

Treatment of adrenal medullary cells with potassium dichromate or chromic acid results in formation of a yellowish or brown oxidation product, the **chromaffin reaction**. Cells that exhibit a positive chromaffin reaction are termed chromaffin cells. The catecholamine-secreting cells of the adrenal medulla show a positive chromaffin reaction, but so do other catecholamine-secreting cells in the body (for example, in the brain, intestinal epithelium, and skin). Cells containing the tryptophan derivative serotonin also exhibit a positive chromaffin reaction. However, the term "chromaffin cell" is usually applied only to catecholamine-secreting cells of the adrenal medulla.

Table 8-4. Percentage of Catecholamines in Adult Adrenal Medulla Represented by Norepinephrine

Vertebrate group/species	Percent NE
Whale	83[a]
Ungulates	15–50[a]
Carnivores	27–60[a]
Rodents	2–50[a]
Lagomorphs	0–12[a]
Rabbit (*Oryctolagus cuniculus*)	8–13[b]
Primates	0–20[a]

[a] Data from Gorbman, A., and Bern, H. A. (1962). "A Textbook of Comparative Endocrinology." Wiley, New York.
[b] Data from Coupland, R. E. (1953). On the morphology and adrenaline-noradrenaline content of chromaffin tissue. *J. Endocr.* **9**, 194–203.

Norepinephrine-secreting cells can be distinguished from epinephrine-secreting cells by the formaldehyde treatment devised by Hillarp and Falck. Formaldehyde combines chemically with norepinephrine storage granules and the resulting complex will fluoresce. Today, we can readily separate epinephrine- and norepinephrine-secreting cells using immunohistochemical techniques to localize either the specific catecholamine or the enzyme responsible for synthesis of epinephrine (see ahead).

A. Synthesis and Metabolism of Adrenal Catecholamines

Two distinct cellular types in the mammalian adrenal medulla are related to production of norepinephrine and epinephrine, respectively. Both epinephrine and norepinephrine are synthesized from the amino acid tyrosine and employ the same biochemical pathway (see Chapter 3, Figure 3-3). However, only the epinephrine-secreting cell possesses the critical enzyme **phenylethanolamine N-methyltransferase (PNMT)** necessary for converting norepinephrine to epinephrine through addition of a methyl group donated by S-adenosylmethionine.

Norepinephrine and epinephrine may be found circulating free in the plasma or as conjugates with sulfate or glucuronide. Most of the circulating epinephrine is bound to plasma proteins, especially albumin. Norepinephrine binds to plasma proteins to a much lesser degree than does epinephrine.

Circulating catecholamines have a short biological half-life and are rapidly excreted via the urine in either free or conjugated forms. The biological half-life for epinephrine is about five minutes. The most common metabolic pathway for inactivation of catecholamines involves liver monoamine oxidase (MAO) followed by aldehyde oxidase to produce inactive metabolites that appear in the urine. The most common urinary metabolites of chromaffin cell cartecholamines are **3-methoxy-4-hydroxymandelic acid, metanephrine**, and **normetanephrine** (see Chapter 3, Figure 3-5).

B. Regulation of Catecholamine Secretion

Primary control of secretion by the adrenal medulla is by the sympathetic nervous system. Environmental stimuli operate through the sympathetic system under emergency conditions or stress. In addition, some control of medullary secretion is exerted directly by ACTH and by glucocorticoids.

1. The Central Nervous Pathway

Stimulation of the cholinergic sympathetic fibers innervating the medulla causes local release of acetylcholine (ACh), which in turn stimulates release of norepinephrine, epinephrine, or both from the chromaffin cells. This action of ACh involves Ca^{2+} uptake by the chromaffin cells. Apparently separate control centers for release of epinephrine and norepinephrine are located in the anterior and medial hypothalamus, and selective release of these medullary hormones occurs through neural pathways. Norepinephrine and epinephrine may be released separately under differing physiological conditions, and these two catecholamines have independent physiological roles in homeostasis.

2. Environmental Factors and Catecholamine Release

Walter B. Cannon first formulated an **emergency reaction** hypothesis involving secretions of the adrenal medulla and activity of other portions of the sympathetic nervous system. These emergency responses include increased heart rate, vasodilation of arterioles in skeletal muscle, general venoconstriction, relaxation of bronchiolar muscles, pupillary dilatation, piloerection (elevation of hair), and mobilization of liver glycogen and free fatty acids. All of these responses contribute to increased efficiency of operation so that the organism can best respond to whatever emergency has arisen. This type of response to short-term stress may be distinguished from the response to chronic stress associated with the glucocorticoids and the General Adaptation Syndrome of Selye described earlier. However, the emergency reaction of Cannon may be thought of as being similar to the adrenal medulla component in the alarm reaction of the Seyle hypothesis.

The major physiological actions of adrenal medullary hormones are their effects on metabolism in response to emotional stress (anxiety, apprehension), physical stress (injury, exercise), or what has been distinguished as physiological stress (temperature, pH, oxygen availability, hypotension, and hypoglycemia). The actions of adrenal catecholamines on cardiovascular events other than the acceleration of heart rate (which is due to metabolic effects of epinephrine on cardiac muscle) are probably secondary to the effects of norepinephrine released from postganglionic sympathetic fibers or, in the case of the skeletal muscle arterioles, the release of ACh from postganglionic fibers. This secondary role for adrenal catecholamines is further supported by the relatively low percentages of norepinephrine in the adrenals of most adult mammals. Sympathetic control mechanisms are not well developed in fetal and neonatal mammals, and this observation could be linked to the high proportion of norepinephrine in their adrenals.

Epinephrine stimulates hydrolysis of liver glycogen to glucose by a cAMP-dependent activation of phosphorylase a (see Chapter 3) and production of lactate from muscle glycogen stores. Circulating norepinephrine produces a similar effect on liver glycogen, but muscle glycogen stores are not affected by norepinephrine. This would explain the ineffectiveness of exogenous norepinephrine as a cardioacceleratory drug, whereas epinephrine is very potent. The mobilization of lipids and release of free fatty acids from adipose tissue is largely under neural sympathetic control and is not influenced appreciably by adrenal catecholamines.

Emotional and severe physical stress increase circulatory levels of catecholamines via hypothalamus-adrenal neural pathways. Response to emotional stress such as fear of written or oral examinations involves an increase only in epinephrine, whereas the adrenal response to positive anticipation involves primarily norepinephrine. Exercise causes an increase in norepinephrine levels, presumably from both adrenal and neural sources. Epinephrine secretion is not influenced by moderate exercise, but it is markedly increased during long-distance running. Several physiological factors such as cold and heat stress, alkalosis or acidosis, and hypotension do not appear to involve primary actions of adrenal medulla hormones. However, responses to asphyxia or anoxia and to hypoglycemia are major factors influencing epinephrine release from the adrenal medulla in adult mammals. Asphyxia causes an increase in epinephrine release, probably through direct actions of oxygen deprivation on the nervous system. In fetal or neonatal animals, asphyxia directly evokes catecholamine release from the adrenal.

Insulin-induced hypoglycemia results in cardiac acceleration through increased epinephrine release. Hypoglycemia induces epinephrine release primarily through direct effects on glucose-sensitive centers in the hypothalamus. Epinephrine also retards the insulin-induced decrease in blood sugar through its antagonistic actions on liver glycogen. Release of insulin can be inhibited by epinephrine.

3. ACTH and Glucocorticoids on Catecholamine Secretion

Development of a close anatomical association between adrenocortical and chromaffin tissues during vertebrate evolution has suggested a concomitant development of a functional relationship as well. Extensive studies by Wurtman and his coworkers have demonstrated that ACTH exerts a stimulatory effect on epinephrine secretion through the action of ACTH on circulating glucocorticoid levels. Hypophysectomy reduces adrenal epinephrine levels, and treatment with either ACTH or glucocorticoids restores adrenal levels of epinephrine to normal. Furthermore, glucocorticoids increase the activity of adrenal medullary PNMT, the enzyme responsible for conversion (methylation) of norepinephrine to epinephrine. Some studies indicate that ACTH may have a direct action on the medulla as well. Levels of both **tyrosine hydroxylase** (rate-limiting enzyme for catecholamine synthesis) and **dopamine-β-hydroxylase** but not PNMT are increased by ACTH treatment. These observations indicate that chronic stress may influence epinephrine secretion not only during the alarm reaction but also in the later stages of the response. It has been reported that epinephrine can cause release of ACTH through actions at either the hypothalamic or adenohypophysial level, but the physiological significance of these observations is not clear.

C. Mechanism of Action for Adrenal Catecholamines

The presence of specific receptors for epinephrine was first postulated in 1906 by Sir Henry Dale, who showed that ergot alkaloids (drugs such as ergocornine and ergocryptine) blocked some of the actions of epinephrine. Later studies suggested there are two kinds of adrenergic receptors in target cells that are capable of binding

Table 8-5. Some Catecholamine Agonists and Antagonists and the Receptor Type to Which They Preferentially Bind

Adrenal catecholamine	Receptor type			
	α_1	α_2	β_1	β_2
Agonists				
Clonidine		×		
Isoproterenol			×	×
Phenylephrine	×			
Ritodrine				×
Antagonists				
Butoxamine				×
Metoprolol			×	
Propranolol			×	×
Phentolamine	+	×		
Yohimbine	×	+		

[a] Epinephrine binds to all types, but best to β-receptors. Norepinephrine binds best to α-receptors, but will bind β_1-receptors (although not as well as epinephrine).
×, binding; +, weak binding compared to other receptor types.

adrenal catecholamines: α- and β-receptors. These receptors also respond to a number of epinephrine-like drugs that have been termed sympathomimetic drugs since they mimic actions of sympathetic catecholamines (see Table 8-5; also Table 3-2). Two common sympathomimetic drugs are **isoproterenol** and **phenylephrine**. Norepinephrine binds mainly to α-receptors, whereas epinephrine binds to both. When both α- and β-receptors are present on a target cell that binds epinephrine, the α-effect predominates unless epinephrine is administered with an α-blocking agent (for example, **phentolamine**).

Detailed studies of the mechanism of adrenal catecholamine actions on target cells have concentrated on the effects of epinephrine in cardiac muscle and liver cells. In fact, it was studies in cardiac cells that led Earl Sutherland and his coworkers to the discovery of the second messenger role for cyclic adenosine 3',5' monophosphate (cAMP) and an eventual Nobel Prize in Physiology or Medicine (see Chapter 3). Epinephrine stimulates the breakdown of glycogen to glucose in both liver and muscle cells by first stimulating an increase in intracellular cAMP. The glucose released from liver glycogen tends to enter the general circulation, whereas the glucose liberated from muscle glycogen is utilized for rapid ATP synthesis and production of lactate. For a further explanation of this difference, see Chapter 12.

VII. Summary

The mammalian adrenal gland consists of an outer region (cortex) of adrenocortical cells (steroidogenic) and an inner region (medulla) of chromaffin cells (adrenergic). The cortex consists of a zona glomerulosa that secretes primarily the mineralocorticoid aldosterone and two inner zones, zona fasciculata and zona reticularis. The zona fasciculata secretes primarily glucocorticoids (typically cortisol or corticosterone). Adrenal androgens (DHEA and DHEAS) are produced primarily in the zona reticularis. The medulla contains two chromaffin cellular types that secrete the two catecholamine hormones, norepinephrine and epinephrine, respectively.

The synthesis and release of aldosterone are controlled by the renin-angiotensin system. Renin is released from the juxtaglomerular apparatus in the kidney in response to reduction in sodium levels of extracellular fluids or reduction in blood pressure. Renin acts on a protein substrate (renin substrate or angiotensinogen) in the blood to release ang-I. Angiotensin-converting enzyme (ACE) in lung capillaries transforms ang-I to ang-II that in turn stimulates aldosterone release. Ang-II may be converted to ang-III by ACE2. Ang-III may function locally as a vasodilator. ACTH plays only a permissive role in aldosterone secretion. Aldosterone regulates sodium levels by increasing sodium reabsorption by the kidney. This response of the cells of certain regions in the nephron to aldosterone involves the synthesis of a specific protein that is responsible for sodium reabsorption.

Aldosterone plays a secondary role in regulating volume of the extracellular fluids through its action on sodium reabsorption. It also regulates potassium excretion. Ang-II may stimulate hypertension, drinking, and vasopressin release to aid in fluid volume regulation. The renin-angiotensin system may have evolved to regulate blood pressure and secondarily acquired control of aldosterone secretion. Natriuretic peptides (ANP and BNP) oppose the actions of the renin-angiotensin system and aldosterone on blood pressure. Pharmacological levels of cortisol or corticosterone also can bind effectively to the MR and mimic aldosterone actions.

Secretion of cortisol or corticosterone is under direct pituitary control through ACTH, and these hormones produce their effects after binding to intracellular or membrane GRs. The main physiological actions of these glucocorticoids are related to their effects on transport of materials into cells and the induction of new cellular enzymes. Glucocorticoids inhibit glucose utilization by peripheral tissues, stimulate amino acid uptake and conversion to glucose and storage as glycogen, and stimulate mobilization of fat stores. They are also anti-inflammatory and may produce immunosupression. Cytokines from immune responses may also activate adrenal activity. Another important contribution may be the permissive action whereby glucocorticoids create an intracellular environment favorable to the actions of many other hormones. Glucocorticoids certainly are important in the adaptive mechanisms whereby an organism combats chronic stress (general adaptation syndrome of Selye). Some important pharmacological actions of glucocorticoids include anti-inflammatory properties, a diabetogenic action, and excessive catabolism of body proteins.

Release of epinephrine and norepinephrine in mammals is directed by separate centers in the hypothalamus that innervate the medulla through preganglionic sympathetic neurons. Glucocorticoids and ACTH may also influence the ability of the medulla to secrete catecholamines by stimulating the synthesis of key enzymes. Epinephrine is primarily a metabolic hormone. For example, it stimulates hydrolysis of glycogen in liver and skeletal muscle to provide glucose for combating hypoglycemia (liver) or for use as an immediate energy source (in skeletal muscle). Epinephrine is responsible for the emergency response of Cannon and is also involved in the alarm reaction of the general adaptation syndrome of Selye. Administration of epinephrine causes increased glucose metabolism and ATP availability within cardiac cells leading to cardiac acceleration. Epinephrine binds to either α- or β-receptors in target cell membranes. Norepinephrine binds significantly only to α-receptors, and its major physiological action is venoconstriction. Circulating norepinephrine is not a cardiac stimulator since cardiac muscle cells possess predominantly β-receptors on their exposed surfaces. In most adult mammals, circulating norepinephrine appears to be of secondary importance to the sympathetic postganglionic neurons for control of vascular tone.

Suggested Reading

Books

Brown, M. R., Koob, G. F., and Rivier, C. (1990). "Stress: Neurobiology and Neuroendocrinology." Dekker, New York.
Fink, G. (2000). "The Encyclopedia of Stress, Vols. 1–3." Academic Press, Inc. San Diego.
Vinson, G. P., Whitehouse, B., and Hinson, J. (1993). "The Adrenal Cortex." Prentice-Hall, Englewood Cliffs, NJ.

Articles

Black, P. H. (1995). Psychoneuroimmunology: Brain and immunity. *Sci. Med.* **2**, 16–25.
Burrell, L. M., Johnston, C. I., Tikellis, C., and Cooper, M. E. (2004). ACE2, a new regulator of the renin-angiotensin system. *Trends Endocr. Metab.* **15**, 166–169.
Celander, M. (1999). Impact of stress on animal toxicology. In P. H. M. Balm (Ed.), "Stress Physiology in Animals." CRC Press, Boca Raton, FL, pp. 246–279.
Charmandari, E., Tsigos, C., and Chrouros, G. (2005). Endocrinology of the stress response. *Ann. Rev. Physiol.* **67**, 259–284.
Dallman, M. F. (1993). Stress update: Adaptation of the hypothalamic–pituitary–adrenal axis to chronic stress. *Trends Endocr. Metab.* **4**, 62–69.
Fuller, R. W. (1992). The involvement of serotonin in regulation of pituitary–adrenocortical function. *Front. Neuroendocri.* **13**, 250–270.
Funder, J. W. (1993). Aldosterone action. *Ann. Rev. Physiol.* **55**, 115–130.
Gabriel, L. Pang, S. C., and Ackermann, U. (2000). Atrial natriuretic peptide: Regulator of chronic Atrial blood pressure. *News Physiol. Sci.* **15**, 143–149.
Gaillard, R. C. (1994). Neuroendocrine–immune system interactions: The immune–hypothalamo–pituitary adrenal axis. *Trends Endocr. Metab.* **5**, 303–309.
Henry, J. P. (1993). Biological basis of the stress response. *NIPS* **8**, 69–73.

Jacobson, L., and Sapolsky, R. (1991). The role of the hippocampus in feedback regulation of the hypothalmic-pituitary–adrenocortical axis. *Endocr. Rev.* **12**, 118–134.

Labrie, F., Luu-The, V., Labrie, C., and Simard, J. (2001). DHEA and its transformation into androgens and estrogens in peripheral target tissues: Intacrinology. *Frontiers in Neuroendoc.* **22**, 185–212.

Sapolsky, R. M., Romero, L. M., and Munck, A. U. (2000). How do glucocorticoids influence stress responses? Integrating permissive, suppressive, stimulatory, and preparative actions. *Endocrine Rev.* **21**, 55–89.

Shipston, M. J. (1995). Mechanism(s) of early glucocorticoid inhibition of adrenocorticotropin secretion from anterior pituitary corticotropes. *Trends Endocr. Metab.* **6**, 261–266.

Vinson, G. P., Pudney, J., and Whitehouse, B. J. (1985). The mammalian adrenal circulation and the relationship between adrenal blood flow and steroidogenesis. *J. Endocr.* **105**, 285–294.

Watkins, L. R., Maier, S., and Goehler, L. E. (1995). Cytokine-to-brain communication: A review and analysis of alternative mechanisms. *Life Sci.* **57**, 1011–1026.

Wong, P. C. (1992). Angiotensin II receptor antagonists and receptor subtypes. *Trends Endocr. Metab.* **3**, 211–217.

Clinical Articles

Magiakou, M.-A., and Chrousos, G. P. (1995). Diagnosis and treatment of Cushing's disease. *In* "The Pituitary Gland" (H. Imura, Ed.), 2nd ed., pp. 491–508. Raven, New York.

Malchoff, C. D., and Malchoff, D. M. (1995). Glucocorticoid resistance in humans. *Trends Endocr. Metab.* **6**, 89–94.

Newell-Price, J., Jorgensen, J. O. L., and Grossman, A. (1999). The diagnosis and differential diagnosis of Cushing's syndrome. *Human Res.* **51** (suppl 3), 81–94.

Pang, S., and Clark, A. (1990). Newborn screening, prenatal diagnosis, and prenatal treatment of congenital hyperplasia due to 21-hydroxylase deficiency. *Trends Endocr. Metab.* **1**, 300–307.

Trainer, P. J., and Besser, M. (1990). Cushing's syndrome. Difficulties in diagnosis. *Trends Endocr. Metab,* **1**, 292–295.

White, P. C., and Pascoe, L. (1992). Disorders of steroid 11β-hydroxylase isozymes. *Trends Endocr. Metab.* **3**, 229–234.

9

Comparative Aspects of Vertebrate Adrenals

The anatomical organization of the adrenocortical homologues and chromaffin cells in non-mammalian vertebrates differs markedly, with the only obvious uniformity being a tendency in amniotes for combining both cellular types into one organ, the adrenal gland (Figure 9-1). Although the term "chromaffin" may be used to designate the catecholamine-secreting cells responsible for elaborating epinephrine and norepinephrine in all vertebrates, several terminologies have been proposed in attempting to deal with the diverse character of the adrenocortical homologues, including interrenal, corticosteroidogenic, and adrenocortical. Although the adrenals of non-mammals lack the anatomical cortex-medulla relationship of mammals (and in many cases no

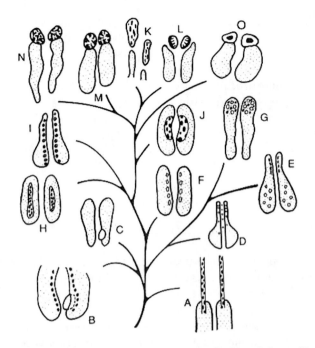

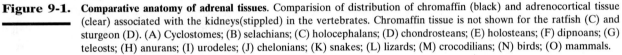

Figure 9-1. **Comparative anatomy of adrenal tissues**. Comparision of distribution of chromaffin (black) and adrenocortical tissue (clear) associated with the kidneys(stippled) in the vertebrates. Chromaffin tissue is not shown for the ratfish (C) and sturgeon (D). (A) Cyclostomes; (B) selachians; (C) holocephalans; (D) chondrosteans; (E) holosteans; (F) dipnoans; (G) teleosts; (H) anurans; (I) urodeles; (J) chelonians; (K) snakes; (L) lizards; (M) crocodilians; (N) birds; (O) mammals.

distinctly separate adrenal gland is present), the term "adrenocortical" will be used here to designate these cells because it denotes the functional and evolutionary relationship of this cellular type to those of the mammalian adrenal cortex.

The structures of the more common corticosteroids and the catecholamines and details about their synthesis and metabolism as well as the mechanism of corticosteroid action on target cells are provided in Chapter 3. The hypothalamus-pituitary-adrenal (HPA) axis is described in Chapters 4, 5, and 8, and the chromaffin cells are described in Chapter 8. The reader is referred to those chapters for basic definitions that are not repeated here.

I. Comparative Aspects of Adrenocortical Tissue

Cytologically, the adrenocortical cells of non-mammals resemble the steroidogenic cells of the mammalian zona fasciculata. Adrenocortical cellular types of cyclostomes, teleosts, and non-mammalian tetrapods possess well-developed smooth endoplasmic reticula, mitochondria with tubular cristae, and numerous osmiophilic (lipoidal) inclusions. Following stimulation with corticotropin (ACTH), pituitary extracts, or appropriate environmental stimuli, these cells exhibit increased basophilia, increased activity of Δ^5, 3β-hydroxysteroid dehydrogenase (3β-HSD), and decreased lipid content. Nuclear and cellular enlargement and hyperplasia occur as a consequence of chronically elevated ACTH or treatment with the drug metyrapone (SU4885), which blocks the 11β-hydroxylation step catalyzed by $P450_{11\beta}$. This prevents glucocorticoid synthesis and causes elevation of plasma ACTH. As in the zona fasciculata of mammalian adrenals, atrophy of non-mammalian adrenocortical cells follows hypophysectomy.

Zonation of adrenocortical cells is suggested cytologically in some anurans, reptiles, and birds, and two separate cellular types have been claimed for the bullfrog *Rana catesbeiana* and for birds. However, little work has been done to establish firmly the existence of more than one functional type of adrenocortical cell in fishes and most other non-mammals.

Adrenocortical cells of fishes differ most from the general mammalian pattern of corticosteroidogenesis with respect to some of the hormones produced. However, the general sequences for corticosteroidogenesis are similar in all the vertebrates with respect to precursor-product relationships, with many of the same enzymes being involved (Chapter 3). Among non-mammalian tetrapods, the nature of corticosteroid secretion is nearly identical, and the pattern of secretion is very similar to that described for cells of the mammalian zona fasciculata.

Daily rhythms and seasonal variations in corticosteroid secretory patterns occur in non-mammals as well as in mammals. Peak seasonal adrenocortical activity is roughly correlated to periods of reproductive activity, although a cause-effect relationship cannot be categorically applied. Some studies suggest that "stress" may be the critical factor and that stressors associated with reproduction may be only one of the components involved in stimulating adrenocortical function (albeit a major one). The responses of non-mammals to stressors such as surgery, forced exercise, and handling are very much like those described for mammals.

II. Adrenocortical Tissue in Non-Mammals

A. Agnathan Fishes: Cyclostomes

In lampreys, presumed adrenocortical cells have been identified as islands of cells above the pronephric funnels in the kidney as well as in the walls of the large dorsal blood vessels (postcardinal veins) in this same region. However, *in-vitro* studies employing radioactively labeled steroidal precursors (pregnenolone, progesterone, or both) have not demonstrated the ability of these presumed adrenocortical cells in lampreys or hagfishes to produce corticosteroids. Nevertheless, cortisol, cortisone, corticosterone, and 11-deoxycortisol have been isolated from hagfish and lamprey plasma and are believed to be of adrenal origin (Table 9-1). Steroidogenic enzymes, such as 3β-HSD, have not been demonstrated in cyclostome adrenocortical cells, however. The site for corticosteroidogenesis has not been established in cyclostomes, and more studies of this group are needed.

B. Chondrichthyean Fishes

Some elasmobranchs and holocephalans have one large unpaired adrenal gland. Since this gland consists exclusively of adrenocortical cells and is located between the posterior ends of the kidneys, it is truly interrenal in position. In others, the adrenocortical tissue may occur as paired strands along the medial border of the posterior kidney. In addition, small islands or islets of adrenocortical cells may be found on the surface of the kidneys extending anteriorly. Chromaffin tissue occurs as small masses along the medial border of each kidney.

Table 9-1. Plasma Levels[a] of Corticosteroids[b] in Fishes

Source	Cortisol	Corticosterone	DOC	11-DOC	1α-OHB	Aldosterone
Agnathans						
Myxine glutinosa	70	20				
Eptatretus stouti		8		27		
Petromyzon marinus	5	2				
Selachians						
Raja laevis		160	420	30	940	
Squalus acanthias		2500		160	2800	
Chondrosteans						
Acipenser oxyrhynchus	1.8	0.7	0.8	0.7		
Holosteans						
Amia calva	7.6					
Teleosteans						
Salmo trutta	24	0.22				
Carassius auratus	440	72	8			1.1
Clupea harengus	750	0.6		0.3		
Dipnoans						
Lepidosiren paradoxa	60	1.6		0.3		5.8

[a] In nanograms per milliliter.
[b] DOC, deoxycorticosterone; 11-DOC, 11-deoxycorticosterone; 1α-OHB, 1α-hydroxycorticosterone.

In 1934, Grollman and coworkers used extracts of the interrenal glands from three skates (*Raja* species) to maintain adrenalectomized rats, demonstrating the presence of corticosteroids in these glands. Soon afterwards, elasmobranchs were shown to produce a unique corticosteroid, 1α-hydroxycorticosterone (1α-OHB). The enzyme necessary for synthesizing this unique steroid, 1α-hydroxylase, is found only in the elasmobranch interrenal gland and nowhere else. Even holocephalans, such as the ratfish *Hydrolagus colliei*, lack 1α-hydroxylase and secrete primarily cortisol.

Shark interrenals (*Scyliorhinus canicula*) incubated *in vitro* with exogenous pregnenolone as a substrate synthesize primarily corticosterone and 11-deoxycorticosterone with lesser amounts of 1α-OHB. When endogenous precursors only are involved, the primary product *in-vitro* becomes the expected 1α-OHB. There are no 18- or 17α-hydroxylases present in the shark interrenal, and consequently aldosterone, cortisol, cortisone, and 11-deoxycorticosterone are not synthesized. Data from plasma analyses, however, indicate that not only is 1α-OHB secreted in the dogfish shark, *Squalus acanthias*, but also cortisol, corticosterone, and 11-deoxycortisol (Table 9-1). Rays and skates produce 11-deoxycorticosterone as well. Such discrepancies between *in-vivo* plasma levels and *in-vitro* synthesis occur in other vertebrate classes as well, and one should be extremely cautious in extrapolating from *in-vitro* capabilities (in which various intermediates and products accumulate) to *in-vivo* situations in which the final products are removed rapidly from the site of synthesis (secreted into the blood). Accumulation of intermediates and products in the vicinity of the secretory cells under *in-vitro* conditions may upset chemical equilibria so that unusual ratios of steroids are observed.

C. Ray-Finned Osteichthyean Fishes: Actinopterygians

The anatomical arrangement of adrenocortical cells in the actinopterygian fishes differs markedly from that described for all other fish groups and could be described anatomically as "intrarenal." In the sturgeons and polypterine fishes (chondrosteans) and in the ganoids (holosteans), the adrenocortical cells are scattered in small clumps throughout the kidney. The identification of these cells is hampered in the ganoids (*Amia, Lepisosteus*) by the presence in the kidney of large numbers of corpuscles of Stannius, which although not steroidogenic do resemble cytologically the adrenocortical cells. The corpuscles of Stannius may play a role in calcium metabolism (see Chapter 14). The teleost adrenocortical cells are embedded in the most anterior portion of the kidney, known as the head kidney (Figure 9-2). Frequently, these cells are associated with the dorsal posterior cardinal veins as described for cyclostomes. The head kidney has lost its renal function and

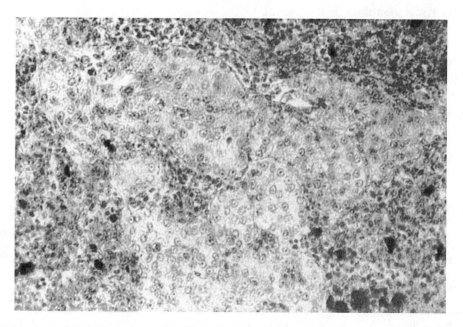

Figure 9-2. **Adrenocortical tissue in a teleost.** The larger, clear cells are adrenocortical (interrenal) cells located in clumps among the much smaller lymphoid cells of the head kidney of a brown trout, *Salmo trutta*.

consists mostly of lymphoid tissue, nonfunctional pronephric tubules, and small islands of adrenocortical cells. In a few species, all of the adrenocortical cells surround the posterior cardinal veins, and none are associated with kidney elements (Figure 9-1). Because of the diffuse nature of the adrenocortical tissue in teleosts, it is not possible to remove these cells surgically, and one must resort to the use of selective inhibitors of corticosteroid synthesis such as metyrapone, which blocks the synthesis of corticosteroids (see Chapter 9).

The principal circulating steroid in the chondrostean, holostean, and teleost fishes is cortisol, with corticosterone, aldosterone, and some others present in lesser quantities in the teleosts (Table 9-1). Bony fishes lack the 1α-hydroxylase of elasmobranchs and consequently do not synthesize 1α-OHB. *In-vitro* studies with teleost adrenocortical cells indicate that they convert pregnenolone preferentially to cortisol. When progesterone is supplied as a precursor, the principal product is corticosterone. *In-vivo*, cortisol primarily is produced.

Teleosts respond rapidly to ACTH and to acute or chronic stress with markedly elevated corticosteroids within 5 to 10 minutes (Table 9-2). Treatment with metyrapone elevates ACTH secretion causing adrenocortical hypertrophy and hyperplasia. Chronically stimulated adrenocortical cells also exhibit enlarged nuclei. The adrenocortical cells respond to treatment with ACTH by secreting more cortisol, and ACTH levels as well as cortisol levels are elevated under conditions of stress. Release of ACTH is direct through innervation by neurons containing corticotropin-releasing hormone (CRH) that enter the adenohypophysis where the corticotropes reside. Immunoreactive CRH cells in the preoptic nucleus (PON) of the common white sucker also contain arginine vasotocin (AVT), but those in the nucleus lateralis tuberis (NLT) that send fibers into the adenohypophysis contain only CRH. Studies in the goldfish suggest that the PON regulates release of ACTH whereas the NLT controls synthesis of ACTH. The peptides sauvagine and urotensin I are chemically similar to CRH and also are effective ACTH releasers. It remains to be proven that they play an endogenous role in ACTH release, but the CRH-like activity in the NLT may be due to either urotensin I or a urotensin-like peptide.

D. Lobe-Finned Osteichthyean Fishes: Sarcopterygians

The lungfishes *(Dipnoi)* have been of special interest to comparative endocrinologists seeking to understand the evolution of corticosteroids since they represent close relatives to both the fish and tetrapod lines. In dipnoan fishes, the adrenocortical cells are found as small cords located between renal and perirenal tissues adjacent to branches of the postcardinal veins.

Adrenocortical cells from estivating *Protopterus* synthesize corticosterone *in vitro* from progesterone. However, only cortisol was identified in the plasma of the aquatic phase, suggesting a tetrapod-like secretion (corticosterone) occurs during its moist, air-breathing phase and a teleost-like secretion (cortisol) during its aquatic phase. Although it is tempting to speculate on the evolutionary significance of these data, it would be premature to do so without further investigation.

Table 9-2. Effects of Stress on Plasma Cortisol Levels in Fishes

Species	Treatment	Unstressed (ng of cortisol/ml)	Stressed (ng of cortisol/ml)
Salmo trutta (brown trout)	Mild confinement, 1 hr	20	75
	Severe confinement, 1 hr	—	150
Salmo salar (Atlantic salmon)	Mild confinement, 30 min	—	200 (50–600)
Salvelinus namaycush (lake trout)	Acute handling and examined 1 hr later	20	270
Oncorhynchus mykiss (rainbow trout)	Acute handling and examined 1 hr later	2–25	300
Perca flavescens (yellow perch)	Acute exposure to air	8	90
Stizostedon vitreum (walleye)	Acute exposure to air	11	229
Anoplopoma fimbria (Sablefish)	Chronic confinement	8	170
Gadus morhua (cod)	Chronic chasing	3	27
Rutilus rutilus (roach)	Chronic confinement	1.4	600

Aldosterone, cortisol, corticosterone, and a trace of 11-deoxycortisol (Table 9-1) circulate in the blood of the predominently aquatic South American lungfish, *Lepidosiren paradoxa*. Recent studies show that the obligate aquatic Australian lungfish, *Neoceratodus fosteri*, secretes only corticosterone and 11-deoxycorticosterone. It would be interesting to know which corticosteroids are secreted by adrenocortical cells of the crossopterygian coelacanths, *Latimeria chalumnae* and *L. menadoensis*.

E. Amphibians

The adrenocortical cells of amphibians are extrarenal and extremely variable with respect to their location. The anatomical pattern of anurans generally differs markedly from that of apodans and urodeles. However, the specific adrenal secretions correlate more to habitat than to anatomy or phylogeny. Adrenal corticosteroid secretion is stimulated by ACTH, which in turn is controlled by CRH. Evidence suggests that CRH also causes release of thyrotropin (TSH) from the adenohypophysis of larval amphibians (see Chapter 7).

1. Anatomical Features of Amphibian Adrenocortical Tissue

In anurans, adrenocortical tissue is found in irregular nodules organized loosely into a pair of interrenal glands on the ventral surface of the kidneys (Figure 9-1). In most anurans, some chromaffin cells are associated with the interrenal glands, and in one anuran, *Rana hexadactyla*, there are more chromaffin cells than adrenocortical cells in the interrenal glands. In addition to the adrenocortical cells and chromaffin cells, a third cellular type, the summer or Stilling cell, has been found in ranid frogs (Figure 9-3). This Stilling cell appears in summer and regresses in winter frogs. It is an eosinophilic cell and resembles a mast cell (histamine-producing cell). The functional significance of the Stilling cell is unknown.

Adrenocortical cells of both apodans and urodeles occur in scattered islands on the ventral surface of the kidney (Figure 9-1). This anatomical arrangement in part explains the virtual absence of studies employing apodan or urodele adrenocortical cells *in vitro*. Curiously, in one anuran, *Xenopus laevis*, the adrenocortical tissue also is organized as small islets on the ventral surface of the kidney. Each of these adrenocortical islets contains two or three chromaffin cells as well.

2. Amphibian Adrenocortical Secretions

Studies with adult anuran adrenocortical tissue *in-vitro* have shown that the major corticosteroids synthesized are aldosterone and corticosterone, and both hormones have been identified in adult amphibian plasma (Table 9-3). In addition, *in-vitro* syntheses result in production of a large quantity of 18-hydroxycorticosterone, which can function as a precursor for the synthesis of aldosterone. The ratio of aldosterone to 18-hydroxycorticosterone to corticosterone *in-vitro* is 6:3:1. However, corticosterone is the predominant circulating corticosteroid, and the high levels of corticosterone (an aldosterone precursor) and aldosterone may simply be an artifact of *in-vitro* conditions (see Chapter 8). Ovarian production of significant quantities of 11-deoxycorticosterone has been reported, and this may be an important source for circulating corticosteroids in sexually mature females. It is not clear if these ovarian corticosteroids play a reproductive role in ovulation as suggested in certain teleosts.

Although corticosterone is the dominant corticosteroid reported for terrestrial amphibians, cortisol has been reported to be the major corticosteroid in metamorphosing ranid tadpoles, in the permanently aquatic frog *X. laevis*, and in some permanently aquatic urodeles. Aquatic-phase, adult red-spotted newts, *Notophthalmus viridescens*, produce substantial amounts of cortisol whereas the terrestrial efts produce primarily corticosterone. These observations would support the hypothesis that cortisol is important for maintaining sodium balance in freshwater amphibians, as reported for fishes, and that corticosterone becomes more important following metamorphosis to a terrestrial-phase amphibian. Corticosterone is also the major corticosteroid in reptiles, birds, and many mammals. It may be that there is a transition from cortisol to corticosterone secretion that takes place during or immediately following metamorphosis (see Chapter 7).

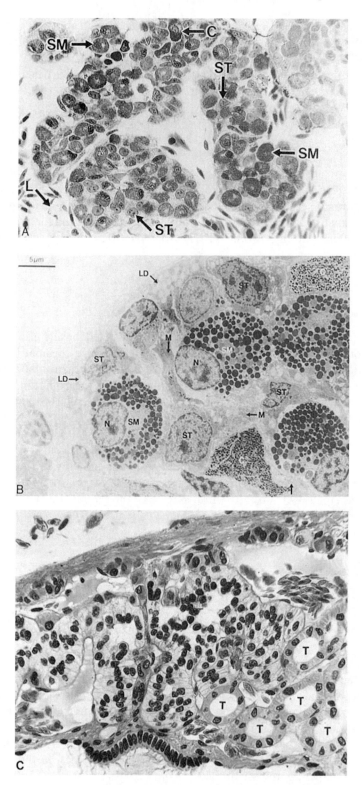

Figure 9-3. **Amphibian adrenal tissue**. (A) Light micrograph from the bullfrog, *Rana catesbeiana*, showing adrenocortical (ST),
chromaffin (C), and summer or Stilling cells (SM). (B) Electron micrograph from the bullfrog, *Rana catesbeiana*.
The cells with the large secretory granules are Stilling cells (SM). The steroidogenic cells contain lipid droplets (LD)
and mitochondria with tubular cristae. N., nucleus. (C) Adrenocortical cells in a salamander are located close to
kidney tubules [(T).] (A) and (B) from Matsumoto, A., and Ishii, S. (1989). "Atlas of Endocrine Organs." Springer-
Verlag. (C) from Vinson, G. P., Whitehouse, B., and Hinson, J. (1993). "The Adrenal Cortex," Prentice Hall, Upper
Saddle River, NJ.

Table 9-3. Circulating Corticosteroids[a] in Amphibian Species (Order Anura)

Species	Corticosterone	Aldosterone
Rana catesbeiana control	8.8	1.8–50.2
ACTH treated	18.0	0.2
Freshly collected	0.2–1.6	
Hypophysectomized	1.3	0.15
Rana esculenta	—	0.82
Bufo marinus		
In distilled water	380.6	54.7
Saline adapted	66.2	15.2
Bufo americanus		
October animals	1.4	—

[a] In micrograms per deciliter.

3. Direct Regulation by AVT in Amphibians

AVT directly stimulates secretion of corticosterone (*X. laevis*) and aldosterone (*X. laevis, Rana catesbeiana*) by adrenocortical cells. Recall that in mammals, AVT also has a positive influence on the adrenal axis but does so by increasing ACTH release.

F. Reptiles

Chelonians, crocodilians, and most snakes have paired suprarenally positioned adrenal glands similar to mammals. There is a variable degree of intermingling of chromaffin cell cords within a mass of adrenocortical cells which may show evidence of zonation (Figure 9-4). In lizards and some snakes, the adrenocortical cells are partially encapsulated by chromaffin cells, resulting in a "cortex" homologous to the mammalian medulla. Some chromaffin cells also are found within the central mass of adrenocortical cells. The chromaffin cells of *Sphenodon* (the primitive rhynchocephalian reptile) surround the dorsal aspect of the gland as well as form islets within the mass of adrenocortical cells. For the first time in vertebrates, the interrenals of reptiles have attained their own vascular supply and venous drainage, no longer relying on the kidney and a renal portal system for distribution of their secretory products. The metanephric kidney appears first in reptiles and has its own blood supply.

Although very few species have been studied, all of those examined under *in-vitro* conditions (including turtles, lizards, snakes, and the American alligator) synthesize aldosterone and corticosterone as the major corticosteroids and what appears to be 18-hydroxycorticosterone. Corticosterone synthesis predominates *in-vitro* with the amounts of 18-hydroxycorticosterone exceeding the levels of aldosterone.

Adrenocortical cells from turtles (*C. picta*) secrete corticosterone *in-vitro* following addition of mACTH or crude extracts of avian, chelonian, or anuran pituitaries to the culture medium. Adrenocorticoid synthesis in the cobra, *Naja naja*, also is stimulated by mACTH. Corticosterone levels *in-vivo* (Table 9-4) and *in-vitro* are elevated following administration of ACTH to *Caimen crocodilus* or *Caimen sclerops*. ACTH also elevates corticosterone levels in lizards but does not influence aldosterone levels. Hypophysectomy causes a reduction in adrenal weight of reptiles whereas treatment with metyrapone elevates ACTH levels and causes adrenal hypertrophy and hyperplasia.

One extra-adrenalocortical source of corticosteroids has been reported for reptiles. As in fishes and amphibians, isolated ovaries from the night lizard, *Xantusia vigilis*, synthesize 11-deoxycorticosterone, but the importance of this observation to either corticosteroid physiology or to reproductive function in reptiles is uncertain.

G. Birds

The adrenal glands of birds are organized in the same manner as described for turtles, crocodilians, and most snakes. The relative quantities of chromaffin with respect to adrenocortical cells vary, however. There appears

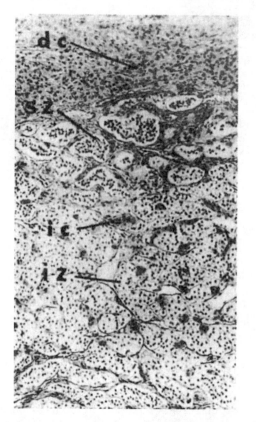

Figure 9-4. **Adrenal gland of the cobra**, *Naja naja*. The dorsal band of chromaffin tissue is prominent. The steroidogenic tissue appears as two distinct zones. [From Lofts, B., Phillips, J. G., and Tam, W. H. (1971). Seasonal changes in the histology of the adrenal gland of the cobra, *Naja naja. Gen. Comp. Endocri.* **16**, 121–131.]

Table 9-4. Plasma Corticosteroids in Reptiles

	Corticosterone (ng/ml)	Aldosterone (ng/ml)
Turtles		
Caretta caretta	1.19 ± 0.8	
Crocodilians		
Caiman crocodiles	220 ± 47	
Crocodylus johnstoni		
Basal levels	4 ± 0.50	
Capture stress (10 hr)	~ 40	
Snakes & lizards		
Sceloporus cyanogenys		
Control	596 ± 113	
ACTH-treated	1292 ± 117	
Boiga irregularis		
Basal	4.4 ± 0.77	
Confined in bag (2 hr)	49.3 ± 6.16	
Varnus gouldi		
Hydrated		4200 ± 700
Salt-loaded		1830 ± 600

to be some zonation of cell types on histochemical and cytological bases similar to that seen in mammals (Figures 9-5 and 9-6).

The major corticosteroids synthesized by adrenocortical cells taken from domestic species and incubated *in vitro* are predictably corticosterone, aldosterone, and 18-hydroxycorticosterone. This sequence of

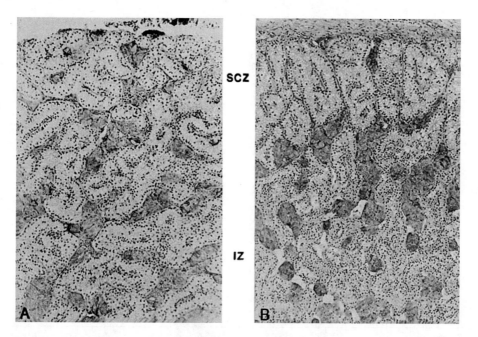

Figure 9-5. **Adrenal glands from normal (A) and hypophysectomized (B) ducks.** There is no apparent zonation in the normal gland but, following hypophysectomy, the cells of the subcapsular zone (SCZ) are larger and contain numerous lipid droplets. The cells of the inner zone (IZ) are smaller and contain less lipid. [From Pearce, R. B., Cronshaw, J., and Holmes, W. N. (1978). Evidence for the zonation of interrenal tissue in the adrenal gland of the duck (*Anas platyrhynchos*). *Cell Tissue Res.* **192**, 363–379.]

steroidogenesis (corticosterone–18-hydroxycorticosterone–aldosterone) is characteristic of birds as well as anuran amphibians and reptiles and is essentially the same pattern found in cells of the mammalian zona glomerulosa.

Studies with duck adrenal slices *in vitro* suggest that corticosterone is the immediate precursor for 18-hydroxycorticosterone and that the latter is converted to aldosterone. However, only corticosterone and aldosterone have been found in avian plasma (Table 9-5). The absence of 18-hydroxycorticosterone in plasma further supports the conclusion that it is only a precursor for aldosterone synthesis, and its accumulation *in vitro* is an artifact. In addition to corticosterone and aldosterone, 11-deoxycorticosterone has been reported in the herring gull. The biological half-lives for corticosteroids in avian plasma are provided in Table 9-6.

Although mACTH stimulates adrenocorticoid secretion (corticosterone) in chickens, hypophysectomy does not cause complete cessation of corticosteroidogenesis (Table 9-5). Thus, there may be a basal level of secretion that does not require ACTH. It also has been proposed that melanophore-stimulating hormone (α-MSH) produced and released by the hypothalamus maintains corticosteroidogenesis in hypophysectomized chickens. Apparently, bird adrenals also secrete corticosteroids in response to PRL, hGH, serotonin, or parathyroid hormone. The response to ACTH is also enhanced by exposure to parathyroid hormone-related peptide (PTHrP) although the physiological significance of this observation is not clear.

III. Physiological Roles for Corticosteroids in Non-Mammalian Vertebrates

Many of the studies of corticosteroid function in non-mammals have focused on their effects on salt transport, particularly sodium; that is, mineralocorticoid activity. Unlike the mammalian condition, aldosterone, cortisol, or corticosterone may possess strong mineralocorticoid activity when tested in non-mammals. The effects of glucocorticoids on metabolic activities have not been studied extensively, but considerable effort has been made to examine the response of glucocorticoid secretion to various natural and artifical stressors. In this regard, one must distinguish between natural events (reproduction, migration, feeding, etc.) and unpredictable events (storms, droughts, reduction in food supply) that can result in elevated corticosteroids. Whereas the

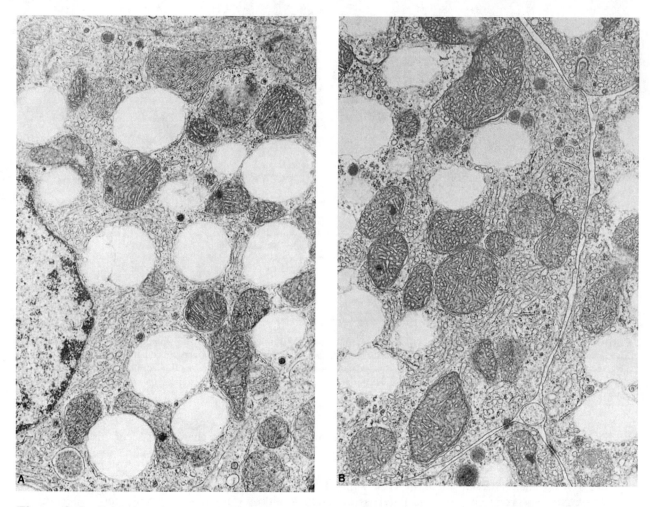

Figure 9-6. **Comparison of adrenocortical cells from the subcapsular (A) and inner zones (B) of the duck interrenal.** Subcapsular zone (SCZ) cells have mitochondria with platelike cristae and many free ribsomes in the cytoplasm. Cells of the inner zone (IZ) have mitochondria with tubular cristae and occasional paracrystalline inclusions. [From Pearce, R. B., Cronshaw, J., and Holmes, W. N. (1978). Evidence for the zonation of interrenal tissue in the adrenal gland of the duck (*Anas platyrhynchos*). *Cell Tissue Res.* **192**, 363–379.]

Table 9-5. Plasma Corticosteroids in Birds Following Stress

	Corticosterone (ng/ml)
Starling[a]	
(*Sturnus vulgaris*)	
Basal	~ 10
Handling restraint (45 min)	~ 40
White-crowned sparrows[b]	
(*Zonotrichia leucophrys gambelii*)	
Basal	~ 15
Handling restraint	~ 27

[a] Romero, L. M., and Remago-Healey, L. (2000). Daily and seasonal variation in response to stress in captive starlings (*Sturnus vulgaris*): corticosterone. *Gen. Comp. Endocri.* **119**, 52–59.

[b] Breuner, C. W., Wingfield, J. C., and Romero, L. M. (1999). Daily rhythms of basal and stress-induced corticosterone in a wild, seasonal vertebgrate, Gambel's white-crowned sparrow. *J. Exp. Zool.* **284**, 334–342.

Table 9-6. Biological Half-Life of Adrenocorticosteroids in Avian Species[a]

Species	Corticosterone half-life (min ± SE)	Aldosterone half-life (min ± SE)
Duck	7.5 ± 0.6	6.2 ± 0.6
Pigeon	18.4 ± 0.1	12.8 ± 1.6

[a] Modified from Holmes, W. N., and Phillips, J. G. (1976). The adrenal cortex of birds. *In* "General, Comparative and Clinical Endocrinology of the Adrenal Cortex" (I. Chester Jones and I. W. Henderson, Eds.), pp. 293–420. Academic Press, New York.

natural events may result in elevated corticosteroids, typically there is no disruption of normal reproductive activities. The unpredictable events would result in a greater secretion of corticosteroids and may even shut down reproductive function. Such severe stressor effects often are observed in captive populations, but these responses may be abnormal in the sense that placing the animal in the laboratory has severly limited the repertoire of activities in which it might engage to eliminate the stressor.

A. Agnathan Fishes: Cyclostomes

The blood of myxinoids (hagfishes) is isosmotic to sea water, but there are some minor differences in concentrations of specific ions. Therefore, although osmotic balance *per se* is no problem, the differential distribution of certain ions must be maintained actively. Injections of aldosterone or deoxycorticosterone acetate alter electrolyte composition of the body fluids with respect to sodium ions, but cortisone has no effect.

Lampreys are either freshwater organisms or migrate between fresh water and the sea. While lampreys are in fresh water, their body fluids are hyperosmotic to their surroundings, and they produce a large quantity of dilute urine. Sea lampreys (*Petromyzon marinus*) do not secrete corticosteroids when in sea water, but, when they are in fresh water, corticosteroids can be identified in the circulation. Aldosterone treatment can reduce renal and extrarenal sodium losses from lampreys held in fresh water. The significance of this latter observation to osmoregulatory control in lampreys must await demonstration of aldosterone in lampreys.

B. Chondrichthyean Fishes

Elasmobranchs have plasma that is hyperosmotic to sea water and hence do not have the osmoregulatory problems exhibited by most marine fishes. This hyperosmotic condition is achieved by maintaining high circulating levels of urea and trimethylamine oxide. There is no clearly defined role for any corticosteroids, including 1α-OHB, in elasmobranchs. However, 1α-OHB does bind to cells in the gills, rectal gland, and nephrons of the kidney. Although corticosteroids stimulate salt excretion by the rectal gland, this salt-secreting gland reportedly plays only a minor role in iono-osmotic homeostasis. Interrenalectomy of the skate, *Raja radiata*, had no effect on plasma osmolarity or on the concentrations of Na^+, Cl^-, Mg^{2+}, K^+, or urea. Exogenous angiotensin stimulates release of 1α-OHB, and suggests a mammalian-like regulatory pattern for corticosteroid secretion. A possible role for corticosteroids in carbohydrate metabolism of elasmobranchs has been suggested. There are no reports of corticosteroid actions in holocephalans.

C. Bony Fishes

Among the bony fishes, corticosteroids have been investigated with respect to function only in the teleosts. In general, corticosteroids (especially cortisol) stimulate sodium transport across gills (both influx and efflux), across the mucosa of the gut, and in the kidney of fresh water fish. Cortisol appears to be the major corticosteroid in bony fishes (Table 9-1), and it appears to regulate sodium fluxes. The most complete studies have been conducted on freshwater- and seawater-adapted eels, *Anguilla spp.* Seawater-adapted eels exhibit a marked turnover of Na$^+$ (50–60%/hour), but ion flux is very low in freshwater-adapted eels (<1%/hour). Eels in sea water are faced with an influx of Na$^+$ that they must eliminate, whereas fresh water eels must conserve body Na$^+$ that readily can be lost to their Na$^+$-poor surroundings. Cortisol treatment increases the activity of Na$^+$/K$^+$-dependent adenosine triphosphatase (Na$^+$/K$^+$-ATPase) in gills, gut epithelial cells, and kidneys. Circulating levels of cortisol are similar in freshwater-adapted and seawater-adapted eels, suggesting cortisol is not important. However, other studies show that elevated cortisol occurs during the initial process of adapting to fresh water and later drops back to a basal level. Neither cortisol nor ACTH is completely effective in maintaining normal Na$^+$ balance in hypophysectomized freshwater eels, and PRL, another osmoregulatory hormone in fishes, may be important as well.

Cortisol also has been reported in several species to maintain gluconeogenesis and increase levels of PEPCK to provide a balance between lipid, carbohydrate, and protein metabolism. A comprehensive study of rainbow trout with chronically elevated cortisol, however, did not increase plasma glucose. Feeding results in elevated cortisol as does starvation, implying an important role for cortisol in the management of energy stores. It may be premature to draw any conclusions about possible actions of corticosteroids on metabolism of bony fishes until more species are examined in a similar manner.

Stressors produce marked elevations of corticosteroids in fishes (Table 9-2). Comparisons of absolute corticosteroid levels cannot be made among different species, or in some cases even within the same species, since it is not possible to assess the role of stressors in most case. Capture and confinement of wild trout cause a marked elevation in cortisol over time, and bringing wild trout into the laboratory can induce sustained increases in levels of plasma cortisol. Elevated corticosteroids in migrating juvenile and adult Pacific salmon (genus *Oncorhynchus*) probably reflect a response of the HPA axis to chronic stress. This condition leads to pathological changes similar to those described for Cushing's disease in humans (see Chapter 8) and what appears to be adrenal exhaustion after spawning that contributes to the death of the spawned fish (Table 9-7).

Cortisol or 11-deoxycorticosterone is elevated during spawning in a number of species, but it is not clear whether this is a stress response or part of the reproductive scenario. Extensive protein catabolism observed in spawning Pacific salmon may be due to high circulating levels of cortisol. In the killifish, cortisol peaks along with estradiol at ovulation. Secretion of ovarian 11-deoxycorticosterone in the Indian catfish, *Heteropneustes fossilis*, may be responsible for induction of ovulation.

Seasonal and daily rhythms in circulating levels of cortisol have been reported for several species. Maximal levels of corticosteroids in rainbow trout maintained on long photoperiod are observed at night (2400 hours). In the spring, plasma corticosteroids rise markedly in juvenile salmonid fishes prior to their migration from fresh water to the ocean or while adapting to sea water. Part of the osmoregulatory stress prior to migration may be due to decreased PRL secretion, a hormone considered necessary for freshwater adaptation. Adult

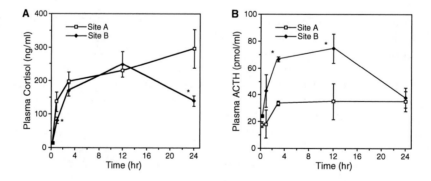

Figure 9-7. **Effects of cadmium exposure on HPA axis of brown trout. (A)** Fish living in cadmium contaminated water exhibit a delayed response in cortisol secretion in response to confinement stress but catch up to trout from an uncontaminated reference site by three hours. However, after 12 hours of confinement, cadmium exposed trout can no longer maintain a high level of cortisol secretion. **(B)** A significantly greater amount of ACTH secretion is necessary for trout chronically exposed to cadmium to maintain normal cortisol secretion in response to confinement stress. After 12 h, these fish can no longer maintain ACTH secretion and cortisol scretion also decreases. [Reprinted with permission from **Norris, D.O.**, Donahue, S., Dores, R.M., Lee, J.K., Maldonado, T.A., Ruth, T., and Woodling, J.D. 1999. Impaired adrenocortical response to stress by brown trout, *Salmo trutta*, living in metal-contaminated waters of the Eagle River, Colorado. General and Comparative Endocrinology 113, 1–8.

Table 9-7. Comparison of Cushing's Syndrome with Experimental Hyperadrenocorticism and with Natural Hyperadrenocorticism of Spawning Salmon

Tissue	Spawning salmon	Cushing's syndrome	Experimental hyperadrenocorticism
Adrenal	Hyperplasia and degeneration	Hyperplasia and tumors	Hyperplasia
Pituitary	Degeneration	Hyaline change in basophils	Minimal degeneration
Spleen	Depletion of lymphocytes, fibrosis	No reported change	Depletion of lymphocytes
Thymus	Involution, depletion of thymocytes	Involution, occasional tumor	Depletion of thymocytes
Liver	Degeneration	Occasional fatty degeneration	No change
Kidney	Degeneration	Degeneration	Degeneration
Pancreas	Hypertrophy of islets	Hypertrophy of islets; variable	Hypertrophy of islets
Stomach	Atrophy and generation	Occasional ulcers	Atrophy of epithelium and occasional ulcers
Thyroid	Atrophy and generation	Atrophy of follicular epithelium	Atrophy of follicular epithelium
Gonads	Degeneration of testes	Atrophy	Degeneration
Muscle	Degeneration of masseter	Atrophy	No change
Cardiovascular system	Degeneration and beginning arteriosclerosis	Arteriosclerosis	Arteriosclerosis
Skin		Hypertrophy	Atrophy

[a] Adapted from Robertson, O. H., and Wexler, B. C. (1960). Histological changes in the organs and tissues of migrating and spawning Pacific salmon (genus *Oncorhynchus*). *Endocri.* **66**, 222–239.

salmonids exhibit adrenocortical cell hyperplasia and elevated corticosteroid levels during their spawning migration from the ocean to fresh water. This increase in corticosteroid levels is accompanied by accelerated catabolism of protein, suggesting a major metabolic role for corticosteroids. Chronically elevated cortisol in reproducing Pacific salmon is correlated with accelerated and extensive neurodegeneration in the brain followed by extensive deposition of β-amyloid peptide (Figure 9-8). Distribution of β-amyloid closely parallels the distribution of glucocorticoid receptors in the salmon brain.

D. Amphibians

Hypophysectomy or exposure of ranid frogs to sea water induces atrophy of the adrenocortical tissue, presumably because of reduced requirements for corticosteroids. Adrenalectomy of these frogs causes a decrease in plasma sodium and an increase in plasma potassium similar to that observed in mammals. Winter ranid frogs usually survive adrenalectomy, but summer frogs die; possibly, death is related to the Stilling cells whose role in unknown in summer frogs.

Aldosterone seems to be the important salt-regulating hormone (mineralocorticoid) acting on the skin and urinary bladder, increasing sodium influx and retention, respectively. The action of aldosterone on the urinary bladder involves synthesis of new protein and would appear to be analogous to the production of aldosterone-induced protein in the mammalian distal convoluted tubule (see Chapter 8). ACTH elevates aldosterone levels in *Rana esculenta*, implying a direct action of ACTH on aldosterone, a condition very different from that described for mammals. Aldosterone treatment reverses the depression of plasma sodium caused by treatment with amino-glutethamide in the tiger salamander. Higher doses of corticosterone than aldosterone were needed to bring plasma sodium back to normal, supporting a physiological role for aldosterone principally as a mineralocorticoid in urodele amphibians. Both aldosterone and corticosterone induce marked hyperglycemia as well as some increase in liver and muscle glycogen levels, but it is not certain that both molecules function as physiological glucocorticoids.

Seasonal and daily rhythms of cortisol levels have been reported in plasma samples from *R. esculenta* and *Bufo americanus*. The time of the daily maximum varied in *R. esculenta* from 2400 hours in May to 1900 hours in July and 0800 hours in November. Greatest secretion of corticosteroids coincided with reproduction in the spring. Two peaks of corticosteroid secretion were observed in captive and free *B. americanus*. One peak coincided with reproduction in the spring but the second peak occurred in the fall at the time of pre-hibernating migrations. Daily maxima corresponded to increased locomotor activity.

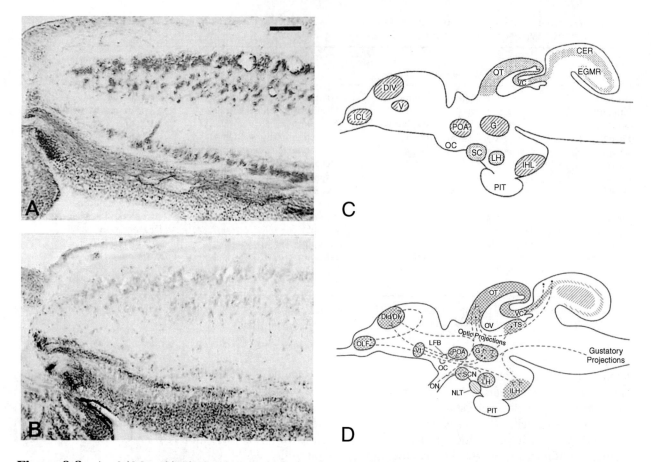

Figure 9-8. **Amyloid deposition in the salmon brain.** Brains of spawning Pacific salmon are characterized by extensive neurodegeneration and the deposition of immunoreactive β-amyloid as shown in the optic tectum (A) compared to an adjacent section of the same brain that was pretreated with immune serum (B) Staining in the optic tectum of a prespawning animal would resemble the immune control. (C) Distribution of immunoreactive glucocorticoid receptors in the brain of kokanee salmon. Compare to D. (D) Distribution of immunoreactive β-amyloid in the brain of kokanee salmon. Compare to the distribution of glucocorticoid receptors in C. [A, B, and D reprinted from Maldonado, T.A., Jones, R.E., and Norris, D.O. (2000). Distribution of β-amyloid and amyloid precursor protein in the brain of spawning (senescent) salmon: a natural brain-aging model. *Brain Research* **858**, 237–251. C reprinted with permission from Carruth, L.L., Jones, R.E., and Norris, D.O. 2000. Cell density and intracellular translocation of the glucocorticoid receptor in the kokanee salmon (*Oncorhynchus nerka kennerlyi*) brain, with an emphasis on the olfactory system. *Gen. Comp. Endocr.* **117**, 66–76.] See color insert, plate 10.

Stressors cause elevation in plasma corticosteroids in amphibians. Placing freshly collected bullfrogs in sacks for up to 24 hours doubles their corticosterone levels. Stress also can alter secretion of other hormones. The secretion of PRL, GTHs, and androgen all decrease in some species of stressed amphibians following capture. The failure of certain species to breed in captivity and the stimulus for some larvae to undergo metamorphosis (see Chapter 7) following capture and laboratory confinement may be consequences of stress. Other species, however, breed readily in captivity and should be examined more closely in this regard.

Extensive studies by Frank Moore and associates at Oregon State University of male rough-skinned newts (*Taricha granulosa*) have implicated CRH and corticosterone in the inhibition of amphibian reproductive behavior. Corticosterone, operating through neural membrane receptors in male newts, blocks clasping behavior that is stimulated by AVT (see Chapter 11).

E. Reptiles

The roles of corticosteroids in ionic regulation by reptiles have not been studied extensively, but effects on Na$^+$ balance have been shown. Like the situtation in the non-mammalian vertebrate groups discussed previously, there does not seem to be any clear distinction between mineralocorticoids and glucocorticoids, with both aldosterone and corticosterone producing similar effects. Reptiles have nasal (orbital) salt-excreting glands similar to those found in aquatic birds. Corticosterone increases Na^+ secretion by these glands, and aldosterone decreases Na^+ excretion while stimulating Na^+ reabsorption in the kidneys and urinary bladder. Injections of concentrated sodium chloride solutions (salt-loading) depress plasma aldosterone levels in several species of lizards. Similar observations are reported for the tortoise, *Testudo hermanni*. Salt-loaded lizards also have elevated levels of AVT that is consistent with its antidiuretic role (see Chapter 5).

In the lizard *Dipsosaurus dorsalis*, it appears that corticosterone does not play much of a role in lactate utilization by skeletal muscles during recovery from exercise. Epinephrine, however, produces a marked stimulation of lactate incorporation into glycogen under similar conditions. Both hormones are elevated in the blood after five minutes of exhaustive exercise in the laboratory. Following aggressive bouts in the American chameleon, *Anolis carolinensis*, winners had much higher levels of epinephrine and norepinephrine than did losers that may relate to this metabolic action. In comparing dominant to subordinate male *A. carolinensis*, corticosterone plasma levels were greater in the subordinate animal.

F. Birds

Corticosteroids cause the nasal salt-excreting glands of certain aquatic birds to secrete a hypertonic NaCl solution. This salt secretion is enhanced by treatment with ACTH or corticosterone, and corticosterone uptake by nasal salt glands is followed by an increase in salt excretion. Adrenalectomized ducks cannot excrete a salt load, but corticosteroid therapy restores this salt-excreting ability. Metyrapone treatment blocks nasal gland secretion. Aldosterone also stimulates nasal salt excretion, unlike the situation in reptiles where aldosterone diminishes excretion of Na^+ as it normally does in the kidney. However, due to aldosterone's powerful action on Na^+ reabsorption in the kidney, there is a net positive effect on Na^+ retention in spite of what occurs locally at the salt glands. Both aldosterone and corticosterone promote Na^+ retention in the lower intestine (copradeum).

Increases in environmental salinity are correlated with increases in Na^+/K^+-ATPase in salt gland cells, and this event is possibly related to increased protein synthesis caused by corticosteroids. Marine birds have larger adrenal glands than do freshwater or terrestrial birds, supporting the role for corticosterone in nasal salt gland regulation. Predictably, birds inhabiting brackish water have intermediate-sized adrenals.

In addition to mineralocorticoid effects, corticosterone causes metabolic effects in birds including weight loss, which probably is a reflection of changes in protein catabolism. In addition, chronic treatment with corticosterone elevates blood glucose and liver glycogen probably through gluconeogenesis.

Circadian rhythms for corticosteroids have been described in some birds, usually peaking early in the morning and exhibiting lowest levels at dusk. The time of the daily corticosteroid peak is believed to determine the behavioral response following injection of PRL into migratory white-crowned sparrows. These observations have led to hypotheses concerning the control of migratory behavior by the phase relationships between rhythms of corticosterone and PRL secretion. North American migratory birds exposed to a day-night cycle with a long photophase release PRL, which induces pre-migratory fattening. Seasonal PRL and corticosteroid rhythms differ markedly throughout the year, and fattening can be altered experimentally simply by changing the timing of the corticosteroid peak with respect to the pattern in timing of the daily PRL peak.

Stress activates the HPA axis in birds. However, this effect is blunted under laboratory conditions as compared to free-ranging birds (Figure 9-9). This also involves release of epinephrine from the adrenal medulla. The HPA axis is responsive to stress and is critical in determining how birds will respond to stress. Migratory birds are more sensitive to environmental stress prior to breeding when the decision is made to breed or not to breed. Nesting birds exhibit a markedly reduced HPA response to stress. The factors involved and the mechanisms whereby sensitivity is controlled are under investigation.

Activation of the endocrine stress mechanism influences other endocrine glands. Corticosterone is added to eggs by the female and, although its role in early development is not known, the amount deposited in the egg may influence the time of hatching. In 10- to 14-day-old chicken embryos, there is a surge of catecholamines (dopamine and epinephrine) in the face of short-term stress. Profound effects of stress are noted in adult birds, too. For example, chasing (the stressor) of male zebra finches for 15 minutes results in a significant depression in plasma androgens measured 2 hours later. Isolation of males in small cages for 12 hours virtually obliterates testosterone in the circulation.

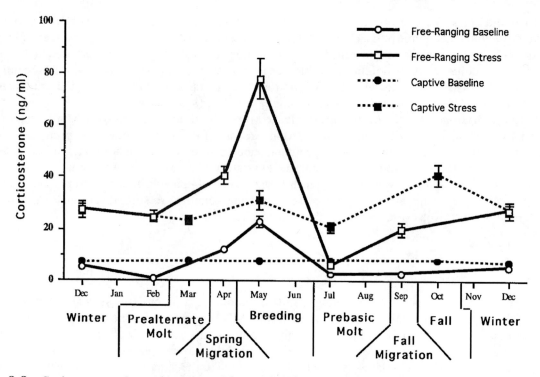

Figure 9-9. **Corticosterone and stress in captive and free-ranging birds**. Resting plasma corticosterone levels and the response to stress in captive birds are blunted as compared to free-ranging birds. [Reprinted with permission from Romero, L.M., and Wingfield, J.C. (1998). Alterations in hypothalamic-pituitary-adrenal function associated with captivity in Gambel's white-crowned sparrows (*Zonotrichia leucophrys gambelii*). *Comp. Biochem. Physiol. Part B*, **12**, 13–20.]

IV. Renin-Angiotensin System in Non-Mammals

The renin-angiotensin system discussed in Chapter 8 involves the enzyme renin secreted into the blood by the kidney in response to lowered blood pressure or lowered blood Na^+. Renin acts upon renin substrate to generate the decapeptide angiotensin-I (Ang-I). In the lung capillaries, Ang-I is converted by angiotensin-converting enzyme (ACE) into the octapeptide angiotensin-II (Ang-II). Ang-II is a stimulator of aldosterone release from the adrenal cortex (zona glomerulosa) and in turn stimulates Na^+ and water reabsorption that increases blood pressure. Ang-II also stimulates contraction of arteriole smooth muscle, secretion of arginine vasopressin (AVP), and drinking behavior, which all contribute to an elevation of blood pressure. It has been hypothesized that the renin-angiotensin system evolved as a mechanism for regulating blood pressure. Control over mineralocorticoid synthesis and regulation of sodium/potassium balance presumably were acquired later.

A. Renin-Angiotensin System in Agnathan Fishes

No evidence of either renin or a juxtaglomerular apparatus has been found in cyclostomes. This kidney specialization may not have evolved until later in the chondrichthyean and bony fishes or in their immediate common ancestor.

B. Renin-Angiotensin System in Chondrichthyean Fishes

Although it has been reported repeatedly that the renin-angiotensin system is absent in chondrichthyean fishes and that attempts to demonstrate the presence of renin have been unsuccessful, careful cytological and histological studies have shown otherwise. Examination of four selachian species (2 sharks, 1 ray, 1 skate) reveals that definite modified smooth muscle cells containing renin-like secretion granules are associated with the afferent arterioles and form juxtaglomerular-like structures in the kidneys. Furthermore, a distinct macula densa-like modification of the distal tubule where it passes between the afferent and efferent arterioles is present. Angiotensin-coverting enzyme-like action (ACELA) is present in gills and spleen as well as in lesser amounts in brain and kidney of *S. canalicula*. Ang-II stimulates production of 1α-OHB by shark interrenals. Although ACTH stimulated steroidogenesis in the Atlantic stingray, *Dasyatis sabina*, this action was not altered by aplication of hAng-II. Additional physiological studies are still needed, but it seems likely that a mammalian-like renin-angiotensin system is present in these primitive fishes.

C. Actinopterygian Renin-Angiotensin System

Renin activity is present in all of the spiny-rayed fish groups and juxtaglomerular-like cells have been identified in several teleosts (Figure 9-10). Histological and cytological identification of renal cells exhibiting

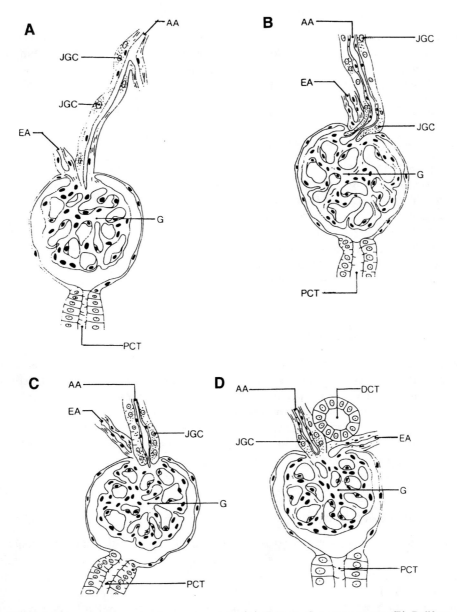

Figure 9-10. **The juxtaglomerular apparatus in non-mammals.** (A) Teleost, *Carassius auratus*. (B) Bullfrog, *Rana catesbeiana*. (C) Snake, *Elpahe quadrivirgata*. (D) Domestic chicken. JGC, juxtaglomerular cells; G, glomerulus, PCT, proximal convoluted tubule; DCT, distal convoluted tubule; AA, afferent arteriole; EA, efferent arteriole; MD, macula densa. [Modified from Matsumoto, A., and Ishii, S. (1989). "Atlas of Endocrine Organs." Springer-Verlag, Berlin.]

renin granules has not been verified in any of the non-teleost actinopterygian fishes, however. No macula densa-like structure has been reported for any bony fish. Ang-II stimulates secretion of cortisol that is the principal salt-regulating corticosteroid in these fishes with actions at both the gills and kidney.

The renin-angiotensin system appears to regulate osmotic and ionic adaptation in teleosts. Freshwater-adapted eels exhibit greater renin activity in sea water than in fresh water. Furthermore, there are gradual changes in plasma renin activity during adaptation of eels to either fresh water or sea water. Administration of either ACTH or renin causes elevation of circulating cortisol levels in eels. Treatment of freshwater-adapted eels with captopril, an inhibitor of ACE, lowers the secretory response of corticosterone following a seawater challenge.

D. Sarcopterygian Renin-Angiotensin System and ANP

Renin activity and the presence of renal cells containing renin granules have been observed in the coelacanth and in two genera of lungfishes. Infusion of isosmotic sodium chloride solution into the lungfish *Neoceratodus fosteri* causes reduction in plasma renin activity, suggesting the involvement of a renin mechanism in osmotic adaptation Ang-II causes secretion of corticosteroids in *N. fosteri*.

E. Amphibian Renin-Angiotensin System

Renin activity is present in amphibian renal tissue, although the secretory renin-containing granules differ morphologically from those of mammals. Several studies report no macula densa in amphibians (Figure 9-10), but a macula densa-like structure has been reported for one toad. This report is of considerable interest since a macula densa appears to be absent in reptiles.

Salt-depleted frogs exhibit elevated kidney levels of renin, suggesting the presence of both mechanisms for regulating aldosterone production, although plasma renin levels do not appear to differ between distilled water-adapted toads and saline-adapted toads. Ang-II stimulates both corticosterone and aldosterone synthesis *in vitro* by adrenocortical fragments from *Rana ridibunda*.

F. Reptilian Renin-Angiotensin System

Renin activity has been reported for kidneys of turtles, lizards, and snakes, but no macula densa has been described (Figure 9-10). This is curious considering the possibility of a macula-like structure in amphibians and evidence for a distinct macula in elasmobranchs, birds, and mammals. Ang-II stimulates corticosterone release in both turtles and lizards. No data are available on other reptilian groups.

Ang-II stimulates corticosterone and aldosterone secretion in lizards but only corticosterone secretion in turtles. However, sodium depletion apparently does not affect renin activity in turtles. Whether or not there is a role for the renin-angiotensin system *in vivo* is not clear.

G. Avian Renin-Angiotensin System

Renin activity is present in birds, and both the juxtaglomerular apparatus and a macula densa have been described. Cells of the avian macula densa are similar to those of mammals, with only some minor differences.

Renin activity and angiotensin activity in blood plasma of ducks and pigeons increase following hemorrhage, establishing a physiological role for the renin-angiotensin system that is similar to mammals. Furthermore, elevated dietary Na^+ causes a reduction in circulating aldosterone without affecting corticosterone levels. Conversely, a reduction in dietary Na^+ raises aldosterone levels. Ang-II stimulation of aldosterone secretion is reduced by administration of ANP. However, in turkeys, ANP stimulates aldosterone release as it does in teleosts.

V. Natriuretic Peptides in Non-Mammals

In mammals, three naturiuretic peptides (NPs) are established with ANP and BNP occurring in the general circulation and CNP limited mainly to the brain (see Chapter 8). NPs have been discovered in all non-mammalian groups and an even greater variety of NPs occurs among the fishes.

Early studies reported that extracts prepared from atria and ventricles of the hagfish, *Myxine glutinosa*, produce relaxation of the precontracted rabbit aorta, a standard bioassay for the hypotensive action of ANP. In addition, ANP binding sites were identified in gills and kidney of this species, suggesting an osmoregulatory role for ANP-like peptides. A unique NP has been discovered in the hagfish *Eptatretus burgeri* that is called **EbuNP**. Its amino acid sequence differs equally from all three mammalian forms. Chondrichthyean fishes also have a single form of NP, but this one most closely resembles mammalian CNP that, because of its conservative sequence throughout mammals, has been suggested to be the most primitive form of NPs (Figure 9-11). Most of the NP activity resides in the atria of the heart. Radiolabelled ANP binds to the secondary lamellae of gill filaments and to kidney glomeruli in the shark *Scyliorhinus canicula*. hANP causes release of 1α-OHB from elasmobranch adrenals that is not consistent with ANP's inhibitory action on corticoid release described in tetrapod vertebrates.

In addition to ANP, BNP, and CNP, teleosts have been shown to produce a unique NP called **ventricular NP (VNP)** although most of the bioassayable NP resides in the atria of the heart. Binding of ANP to secondary lamellae of gills occurs in both chondrosteans and teleosts and it is clear that the gill is a major target for ANP in seawater-adapted fish whereas CNP is more important in freshwater-adapted fish. Data on osmoregulatory effects by NP on the kidney are contradictory. Furthermore, it is difficult to study this in seawater-adapted

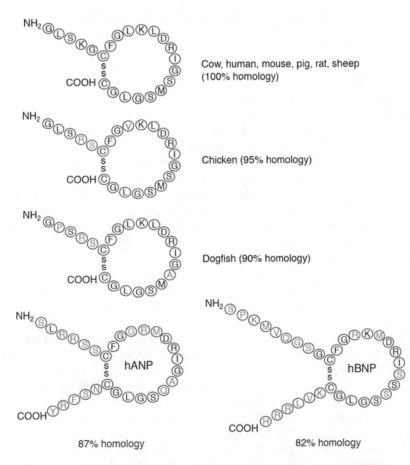

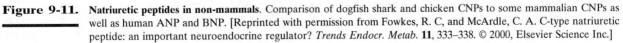

Figure 9-11. **Natriuretic peptides in non-mammals.** Comparison of dogfish shark and chicken CNPs to some mammalian CNPs as well as human ANP and BNP. [Reprinted with permission from Fowkes, R. C, and McArdle, C. A. C-type natriuretic peptide: an important neuroendocrine regulator? *Trends Endocr. Metab.* **11**, 333–338. © 2000, Elsevier Science Inc.]

fish that produce little urine. Data on effects of NPs in stenohaline fish are scarce indeed. Several studies have shown that NPs stimulate cortisol secretion that in turn stimulates gill Na^+/K^+ ATPase to excrete Na^+ and Cl^- through the gills. This is similar to observations in elasmobranches. ANP is present in myocardial tissue of the African lungfish, *Protopterus aethipicus*, and may play a role in controlling corticosteroid release.

ANP, BNP, and CNP are secreted by amphibians. Amphibian NPs are potent vasodilators and cause diuresis and natriuresis. Like mammals, NPs inhibit the actions of ACTH or Ang-II stimulation of corticosterone secretion. However, in *X. laevis*, ANP blocked aldosterone release but did not affect corticosterone secretion. Effects of NPs on the amphibian urinary bladder have yielded conflicting results, and their role if any on this important osmoregulatory site need clarification.

In reptiles, cDNA has been isolated from a crocodilian and a turtle for BNP but not for ANP. A CNP precursor protein has been demonstrated in the venom gland of snakes. ANP-like binding sites have been described for turtle kidney, brain, gastrointestinal tract, adrenal gland, and epididymis. Rat ANP blocks basal and Ang-II induced secretion of aldosterone and corticosterone in cultured adrenocortical cells from the eastern fence lizard, *Sceloporus undulatus*. In general, although the reptiles are the most poorly studied group with respect to NPs, they appear to have similar response to NPs as described for birds and amphibians.

Both ANP and ANP receptors have been described for birds. Birds also produce BNP and CNP (Figure 9-11). ANP binds to bird BNP receptors, and ANP has been shown to lower blood pressure in some species. Nasal salt glands have NP receptors and NPs have been shown to stimulate their secretion of salt. BNP also blocks Ang-II stimulated aldosterone secretion in birds with the exception of the domestic turkey where it stimulates aldosterone secretion.

VI. Evolution of Chromaffin Tissue and Adrenal Medullary Hormones

Morphologically, there has been a general trend to develop a close anatomical relationship between chromaffin tissues homologous to the mammalian adrenal medullary cells and the adrenocortical cells. Chromaffin tissue in agnathans is found in association with the posterior cardinal veins as are the separate clusters of adrenocortical cells. In the cartilaginous fishes, the chromaffin tissue is intrarenal and is more widely separated from the "interrenal" adrenocortical cells than in any other vertebrate group. Although some chromaffin cells have been described in association with the cardinal veins of lungfishes, chromaffin cells are found mostly in the heart. These cardiac chromaffin cells are claimed to represent the homologue of the adrenal medulla in lungfishes. There is considerable anatomical variation among the adrenals of teleosts, but no species are known to exhibit cardiac chromaffin tissue. The chromaffin cells may form clumps entirely separate from the adrenocortical cell clusters in the head kidney or may be intermingled with adrenocortical cells. In some species, both conditions may be found (i.e., separate and mixed clusters of cell types). Clusters of adrenocortical cells (islets) in amphibians typically contain only a few chromaffin cells, and the latter usually are separated from adrenocortical cells. The anatomical distribution of chromaffin cells in reptiles is varied. The adrenal glands of squamates and the tuatara *Sphenodon punctatus* have peripherally located norepinephrine-secreting chromaffin cells and central islets of epinephrine-secreting cells intermingled among the adrenocortical cells. The avian adrenal glands consist of such a mixture of cortical and chromaffin cells that no distinction of "cortex" and "medulla" is possible.

Early studies on the proportion of adrenal catecholamines in non-mammals suggest that the mammalian fetal pattern of high norepinephrine production with increasing production of epinephrine following birth (see Chapter 8) is an example of the old principle that ontogeny recapitulates phylogeny. Analysis of extractable catecholamines from the shark *S. acanthias* (which has entirely separate chromaffin tissue), the frog *Rana temporaria* (which exhibits some mixing of chromaffin and adrenocortical cells), and the rabbit *Oryctolagus cuniculus* suggests an evolutionary change from reliance on norepinephrine to the progressive reliance on epinephrine (see Table 9-8). Although it seems logical to assume that the methylation step (norepinephrine to epinephrine) was a later evolutionary event, the picture is even more complex. Histochemical and chromatographic procedures indicate that norepinephrine predominates in some bird species whereas others produce mainly epinephrine. Still other groups show only a slight preference for producing one catecholamine over the other. Although norepinephrine predominates in extracts of adrenals prepared from chickens, turkeys,

Table 9-8. Proportion of Norepinephrine of Total Catecholamines in Adult Adrenal Extracts

Species	Percent norepinephrine
Elasmobranchs	66–73[a]
Dogfish shark (*Squalus acanthias*)	100[b]
Amphibians	40–60[a]
Frog (*Rana temporaria*)	55–69[b]
Reptiles	60[a]
Snake (*Xenodon merremii*)	
Peripheral chromaffin cells	97[c]
Central chromaffin islets	15[c]
Birds	55–80[a]
Some passerine birds	0[a]

[a] Data from Gorbman, A., and Bern, H. A. (1962). "A Text-book of Comparative Endocrinology." Wiley, New York.
[b] Data from Coupland, R. E. (1953). On the morphology of adrenaline-nonadrenaline content of chromaffin tissue. *J. Endocri.* **9**, 194–203.
[c] Data from Gabe, M. (1970). The adrenal. *In* "The Biology of the Reptilia" (C. Gans, Ed.), Vol. 3, pp. 263–318. Academic Press, New York.

and pigeons, the major circulating catecholamine in these species is epinephrine. These data point out the dangers of extrapolating too broadly from gland content to secretory activities, especially with respect to substrate-production relationships.

Few comparative studies of adrenal catecholamines on carbohydrate metabolism have been reported. The hyperglycemic action of epinephrine seems to be a primitive action in non-mammalian vertebrates although the mechanisms involved are not clear. In chinook salmon, for example, both epinephrine and norepinephrine stimulate glycogen utilization in the liver and release of glucose. Incorporation of lactate into glycogen also is stimulated by epinephrine in carp liver, but this effect is overshadowed by a general breakdown of glycogen that occurs concomitantly. Epinephrine produces glycogen breakdown in the liver of all birds examined. Norepinephrine, on the other hand, produces hypoglycemia in the ratfish and in 6- to 9-week-old Japanese quail. The bases for these unusual observations on norepinephrine action are unknown.

Studies of catecholamine effects on lipid metabolism are less common than studies of catecholamines on carbohydrate metabolism in lower vertebrates, although numerous studies of effects by other hormones have been reported (e.g., GH, PRL, thyroxine). One of the more thorough studies shows that while acting through β-adrenergic receptors, norepinephrine stimulates, in a dose-dependent manner, a triglyceride lipase that causes lipolysis in liver slices from coho salmon. Epinephrine has no lipolytic action in this system although it has been shown to have lipolytic effects in other fishes. More work in this area clearly is needed.

VII. Summary

Non-mammalian vertebrates do not exhibit the anatomical cortex-medullary relationship like mammals for the homologous adrenocortical cells and chromaffin cells. However, there is a general trend for a closer anatomical relationship between these tissues from being entirely separate in ancient fishes with direct associations with the kidneys to the evolution of discrete, separate glands in reptiles and birds.

The synthesis of corticosteroids is the same as in mammals with the exception of elasmobranchs that produce a unique corticosteroid, 1α-OHB. Teleosts rely on cortisol as the principal mineralocorticoid and glucocorticoid. Amphibians, reptiles, and birds secrete corticosterone and aldosterone as their glucocorticoid and mineralocorticoid, respectively. The roles of cortisol and corticosterone in gluconeogenesis, the stress response, and aging are similar to mammals. Aldosterone secretion is regulated by a renin-angiotensin system in non-mammalian tetrapods. Blood pressure regulation involves the renin-angiotensin system in non-mammals similar to that of mammals and natriuretic peptides antagonize Ang-II actions.

Chromaffin cells participate in the emergency reactions and the stress response as described for mammals. In non-mammals, chromaffin cells generally secrete more norepinephrine than epinephrine.

Suggested Reading

Books

Chester-Jones, I., and Henderson, I. W. (1976–1980). "General, Comparative, and Clinical Endocrinology of Adrenal Cortex." Academic Press, New York.

Delrio, G., and Brachet, J. (1984). "Steroids and Their Mechanism of Action in Nonmammalian Vertebrates." Raven, New York.

Pickering, A. D. (1981). "Stress and Fish." Academic Press, New York.

Vinson, G. P. (1993). "The Adrenal Cortex." Prentice-Hall, Englewood Cliffs, NJ.

General Articles

Chan, D. K. O., and Wong, C. K. C. (1996). The adrenal cortex and the renin-angiotensin system of lower vertebrates. *In* G. P. Vinson and D. C. Anderson, Eds. "Adrenal Glands, Vascular System and Hypertension," *J. Endocr. Bristol*, pp. 23–35.

Chester-Jones, I. (1987). Structure of the adrenal and interrenal glands. *In* "Fundamentals of Comparative Vertebrate Endocrinology" (I. Chester Jones, P. M. Ingleton, and J. G. Phillips, Eds.), pp. 95–121. Plenum, New York.

Chester-Jones, I., and Phillips, J. G. (1986). The adrenal and interrenal glands. *In* "Vertebrate Endocrinology: Vol. I, Fundamentals and Biomedical Implications" (P. K. T. Pang and M. P. Schreibman, Eds.), pp. 319–349. Academic Press, San Diego.

Fowkes, R. C., and McArdle, C. A. (2000). C-type natriuretic peptide: An important neuroendocrine regulator? *Trends Endocr. Metab.* **11**, 333–338.

Greenberg, N., and Wingfield, J. C. (1987). Stress and reproduction: Reciprocal relationships. *In* "Reproduction in Fishes, Amphibians, and Reptiles" (D. O. Norris and R. E. Jones, Eds.), pp. 461–503. Plenum, New York.

Henderson, I. W., and Kime, D. E. (1987). The adrenal cortical steroids. *In* "Vertebrate Endocrinology: Fundamental and Biomedical Implications" (P. K. T. Pang and M. P. Schreibman, Eds.), Vol. 2, pp. 121–142. Academic Press, San Diego.

Romero, L. M. (2002). Seasonal changes in plasma glucocorticoid concentrations in free-living vertebrates. *Gen. Comp. Endocr.* **128**, 1–24. (tetrapods only).

Fishes

Barton, B. A. (2002). Stress in fishes: A diversity of responses with particular reference to changes in circulating corticosteroids. *Integrative Comp. Biol.* **42**, 517–525.

Hanke, W., Hegab, S. A., Assem, H., Berkowsky, B., Gerhard, A., Gupta, O., and Reiter, S. (1993). Mechanisms of hormonal action on osmotic adaptation in teleost fish. *In* "Fish Ecotoxicity and Ecophysiology" (T. Branbeck, W. Hanke, and H. Segner, Eds.), pp. 315–326. VCH, Weinheim.

Holloway, A. C., Reddy, P. K., Sheridan, M. A., and Leatherland, J. F. (1994). Diurnal rhythms of plasma growth hormone, somatostatin, thyroid hormones, cortisol and glucose concentrations in rainbow trout *Oncorhynchus mykiss*, during progressive food deprivation. *Biol. Rhythm Res.* **25**, 415–432.

Hontela, A., Rasmussen, J. B., Audet, C., and Chevalier, G. (1992). Impaired cortisol stress response in fish from environments polluted by PAHs, PCBs, and mercury. *Arch. Environ. Contam. Toxicol.* **22**, 278–283.

Iger, Y., Balm, P. H. M., and Wendelaar Bonga, S. E. (1994). Cellular responses of the skin and changes in plasma cortisol levels of trout (*Oncorhynchus mykiss*) exposed to acidified water. *Cell Tissue Res.* **278**, 535–542.

McCormick, S. D. (1995). Hormonal control of gill Na^+, K^+-ATPase and chloride cell function. *In* "Fish Physiology, Vol. 14, Cellular and Molecular Approaches to Fish Ionic Regulation" (C. M. Wood and T. J. Suttle-Worth, Eds.), pp. 285–315. Academic Press, San Diego.

Norris, D. O. (2000). Endocrine disruptors of the stress axis in natural populations: How can we tell? *Amer. Zool.* **40**, 393–401.

Norris, D. O., and Hobbs, S. L. (2006). The HPA axis and functions of corticosteroids in fishes. In M. Reinecke, G. Zaccone and B. G. Kapoor (Eds.). "Fish Endocrinology." Oxford and Science Publishers, Enfield, NH, pp. 721–765.

Toop, T., and Donald, J. A. (2004). Comparative aspects of natriuretic peptide physiology in non-mammalian vertebrates: A review. *J. Comp. Physiol. [B]* **174**, 189–204.

Wedemeyer, G. A., Barton, B. A., and McLeay, D. J. (1990). Stress and acclimation. *In* "Methods in Fish Biology" (C. B. Schreck and P. B. Moyle, Eds.), pp. 451–489. Amer. Fish Soc., Bethesda, MD.

Amphibians

Ceballos, N. R., Shackleton, C. H., Harnik, M., Cozza, E. N., and Gros, E. G. (1993). Corticosteroidogenesis in the toad *Bufo arenarum* H. Evidence for a precursor role for an aldosterone 3β-hydroxy-5-ene gene analogue (3β, 11β, 21-trihydroxy-20-oxo-5-pregnen-18-al). *Biochem. J.* **292**, 143–147.

Donald, J. A., and Trajanovska, S. (2006). A perspective on the role of natriuretic peptides in amphibian osmoregulation. *Gen. Comp. Endocr.* **147**, 47–53.

Guardabassi, A., Muccioli, G., Andreoletti, G. E., Pattono, P., and Usai, P. (1991). Prolactin and interrenal hormone balance in *Xenopus laevis* adult specimens adapted to brackish water. *Atti. Acad. Sci. Torino* **125**, 55–69.

Iwamuro, S., Hayashi, H., Yamashita, M., and Kikuyama, S. (1991). Arginine vasotocin (AVT) and AVT-related peptide are major aldosterone-releasing factors in the bullfrog intermediate lobe. *Gen. Comp. Endocr.* **84**, 412–418.

LaForgia, V., and Capaldo, A. (1992). The interrenal gland of *Triturus cristatus* after insulin administration during the annual cycle. *J. Morphol.* **211**, 87–93.

Lihrmann, I., Netchitailo, P., Feuilloley, M., Cantin, M., Delarue, C., Leboulenger, F., De Lean, A., and Vaudry, H. (1988). Effect of atrial natriuretic factor on corticosteroid production by perifused frog interrenal slices. *Gen. Comp. Endocr.* **71**, 55–62.

Moore, I. T., and Jessop, T. S. (2003). Stress, reproduction and adrenocortical modulation in amphibians and reptiles. *Hormones and Behavior* **43**, 39–47.

Zerani, M., and Gobetti, A. (1991). Effects of β-endorphin and naloxone on corticosterone and cortisol release in the newt (*Triturus carnifex*): Studies *in vivo* and *in vitro*. *J. Endocr.* **131**, 295–302.

Reptiles

Carsia, R. V., and John-Alder, H. B. (2006). Natriuretic peptides are negative modulators of adrenocortical cell function of the eastern fence lizard (Sceloporus undulates). *Gen. Comp. Endocr.* **145**, 1457–1461.

Dauphin-Villement, C., and Xavier, F. (1987). Nychthemeral variations of plasma corticosteroids in captive female *Lacerta vivipara* Jacquin: Influence of stress and reproductive state. *Gen. Comp. Endocr.* **67**, 292–302.

Gabe, M. (1970). The adrenal. *In* "Biology of the Reptilia, Vol. 3, Morphology C" (C. Gans, Ed.), pp. 263–318. Academic Press, New York.

Gleeson, T. T. (1993). Plasma catecholamine and corticosterone and their *in vitro* effects on lizard skeletal muscle lactate metabolism. *Am. J. Physiol.* **265**, R632–R639.

Mahapatra, M. S., Mahata, S. K., and Maiti, B. R. (1987). Influence of age on diurnal rhythms of adrenal norepinephrine, epinephrine, and corticosterone levels in soft-shelled turtles (*Lyssemys punctata punctata*). *Gen. Comp. Endocr.* **67**, 279–281.

Reinhart, G. A., and Zehr, J. E. (1994). Atrial natriuretic factor in the freshwater turtle *Pseudemys scripta*: A partial characterization, *Gen. Comp. Endocr.* **96**, 259–269.

Summers, C. H. (2002). Social interactions over time: Implications for stress responsiveness. *Integrative and Comparative Biology* **42**, 591–599.

Summers, C. H., Watt, M. J., Ling, T. L., Forster, G. L., Carpenter, R. E., Korzan, W. J., Lukkes, J. L., and Overli, O. (2005). Glucocorticoid interaction with aggression in non-mammalian vertebrates: Reciprocal action. *European Journal of Pharmacology* **526**, 21–35.

Birds

Gray, D. A., Schutz, H., and Gerstberger, R. (1991). Interaction of atrial natriuretic factor and osmoregulatory hormone in the Peking duck. *Gen. Comp. Endocr.* **81**, 246–255.

Kocsis, J. F., McIlroy, P. J., and Carsia, R. V. (1995). Atrial natriuretic peptide stimulates aldosterone production by turkey (*Meleagris gallopavo*) adrenal steroidogenic cells. *Gen. Comp. Endocr.* **99**, 364–372.

Wingfield, J. C. (2005). Modulation of the adrenocortical response to acute stress in breeding birds. In A. Dawson and P. J. Sharp (eds) "Functional Avian Endocrinology", Narosa Publishing House, New Delhi, PP. 225–256.

10

The Endocrinology of Mammalian Reproduction

Reproduction is the process that perpetuates a species through evolutionary time. It includes the process of sex determination and sexual differentiation (conversion of the indifferent gonads into testes or ovaries), embryonic development and birth, sexual maturation or puberty, development of gametes, physiological and behavioral aspects of mating, fusion of gametes, and development of the resulting zygote. In addition, a period of complex parental care is intercalated between birth and sexual maturation and possibly extends longer, such as in the case of humans. Every step in this complicated reproductive process is controlled directly or is modified by chemical regulators secreted within the body or by pheromones from other members of the species.

The "reproductive system" includes the complex **hypothalamus-pituitary-gonad (HPG)** axis as well as the targets of steroid hormones secreted by the gonads. Environmental factors (chemical, visual, photic, thermal, and tactile stimuli) operating through effects on neural and endocrine factors frequently determine the timing of many reproductive events. Regulators of other endocrine axes, such as the thyroid (HPT) and adrenal (HPA) axes, have important effects on reproductive events, too.

Reproductive mechanisms are of central importance to survival of a species and hence are under intense evolutionary selection. Consequently, the reproductive system has been highly responsive to selective forces throughout the long evolutionary history of vertebrates. Because the same selective forces in the environment act upon all animal species, it should not come as a surprise that similar mechanisms have evolved in diverse vertebrates to achieve reproductive success in the face of similar pressures. Progressive "improvements" in the endocrine mechanisms regulating reproduction may not show progressive "development" from fishes to mammals but instead we see specific adaptations to solve common environmental problems appearing in diverse groups of vertebrates. A case in point would be the achievement of viviparity in all but two extant vertebrate groups, the agnathans and birds, as specific adaptations that, when coupled with varying degrees of parental care, result in a greater percentage survival of a small number of offspring. Viviparity represents only one solution, however, to similar selective pressures that confront all species. In birds, extensive and complicated parental behavior serves the evolutionary role that viviparity does in mammals to ensure reproductive success. In spite of the problems of environmental adaptations that tend to confuse evolutionary relationships, there remain numerous conservative features in the regulatory mechanisms of reproductive biology, and it is these that are emphasized in this chapter and in Chapter 11, where reproduction of non-mammalian vertebrates is discussed.

I. General Features of Mammalian Reproduction

Mammals can be separated into three, distinct taxonomic groups: the Prototheria (monotremes), the Metatheria (marsupials), and the Eutheria (placentals). All possess **mammary glands**, specialized skin glands that are employed in secretion of milk to feed their young. The egg-laying monotremes comprise the most ancient group of mammals of which only a handful of species are extant. The marsupials or pouched mammals (**marsupium** = pouch) are confined mostly to Australia with a few species in North, Central, and South America. The marsupials are evolutionarily intermediate between the prototherians and the placental mammals, and there are about 230 extant species of marsupials. Their survival in Australia is due largely to the late arrival of eutherian mammals to that continent whereas competition with eutherians have limited them in North and South America. The placental mammals are the dominant group of living mammals in number of species (about 4600), distribution over the earth, and abundance. The **placenta** is a specialized structure that develops through interactions of zygote-derived extra-embryonic tissues and maternal uterine tissues. It provides nutritional, respiratory, excretory, and endocrine support for the offspring developing within the uterus. Although a placenta is present in marsupials, it is very short-lived and the marsupial fetus soon exits the uterus via the vagina and finds its way into the pouch. Most development for this exteriorized fetus takes place within the pouch rather than in utero with the mammary glands providing the nutrition for continued development.

Reproduction is closely regulated primarily through the HPG axis that coordinates specific gonadal events through regulation by circulating **gonadotropins (GTHs)**. This gonadal axis is modified by other systems, especially the HPT axis (Chapter 6) and the HPA axis (Chapter 8). Factors influencing GTH release and hence gonadal functions were discussed in Chapter 4 and are summarized only briefly below (see also Table 10-1).

Reproductive events in mammals are controlled through the release of **luteinizing hormone (LH)** and **follicle-stimulating hormone (FSH)** from the adenohypophysis under the control of a hypothalamic hormone, **gonadotropin-releasing hormone, GnRH** and possibly a **gonadotropin inhibitory hormone (GnIH)**. Pulsatile release is an innate feature of GnRH neurons. The **tonic center**, occuring in both males and females, maintains a relatively constant pattern of pulsatile release of GnRH and produces rather static circulating levels of both LH and FSH. The **surge center** found only in females is responsible for the midcycle **LH surge** observed

Table 10-1. Summary of Generalized Hormone Actions in Mammalian Reproduction (Eutheria)

Hormone	Action in: Females	Action in: Males
GnRH	Stimulates FSH and LH secretion	Stimulates FSH and LH secretion
FSH	Initiates follicle growth; conversion of androgen to estrogen; synthesis of inhibin, P450$_{aro}$	Initiates spermatogenesis; secretion of androgen-binding protein, STP, and inhibin by Sertoli cells; conversion of androgen to estrogen by Sertoli cell
LH	Androgen synthesis; ovulation; formation of corpus luteum from granulosa; secretion of progesterone initiated in corpus luteum	Androgen secretion by interstitial cell (Leydig)
Prolactin	Synthesis of milk	Stimulates certain sex accessory structures (with androgen)
Oxytocin	Contraction of uterine smooth muscle; menstrual sloughing; birth; orgasm; milk ejection from mammary	Ejaculation of sperm; orgasm
Androgens	Precursors for estrogen synthesis; stimulates sexual behavior	Completes FSH-initiated spermatogenesis; stimulates prostate gland, other sex accessory structures; stimulates secondary sexual characters, such as beard growth in man
Estrogens	Stimulates proliferation of endometrium; induces LH surge; sensitizes uterus to oxytocin; negative feedback on pituitary release; may be primate luteolytic factor (estrone); may induce PRL surge; maintains pregnancy	Converted from androgens; induces male hypothalamus; stimulates sexual behavior
Progesterone	Maintains secretory phase of uterus; inhibits release of gonadotropins from adenohypophysis; maintains pregnancy	
Prostaglandins	Causes corpus luteum to degenerate at end of luteal phase (not in primate); may be involved in birth initiation (induction of labor)	Ejaculation
Relaxin	Softens pelvic ligaments and cervix; possible role in lactation	
Chorionic gonadotropin	Stimulates corpus luteum to produce progesterone	
Chorionic somatomammotropin	Stimulates mammary to synthesize milk during late pregnancy; growth hormone-like (somatotropin) actions on metabolism	
Inhibin (Sertoli cell factor, folliculostatin)	Inhibits FSH secretion from pituitary	Inhibits FSH secretion from pituitary

in mature females in response to elevated estrogen. In some species, these centers are distinctly separated in females (e.g., the rat) and in others there is no obvious anatomical separation (e.g., human). Pulsatile secretion of GnRH is under stimulatory control by catecholaminergic neurons (e.g., norepinephrine, NE) and is inhibited by endogenous opioid peptides (EOPs). Positive feedback of estrogens on GnRH release in females is mediated by GABA (γ-amino butyric acid) neurons. Elevation of estrogens prior to ovulation also is responsible for the induction of **estrus**, a period of receptivity for copulation with a male.

Gonadotropins stimulate gamete maturation in males and females as well as steroidogenesis and release of **estrogens, androgens** and **progestogens** (=progestins) into the general circulation. **Gametogenesis** (oogenesis in females and spermatogenesis in males) is controlled primarily by FSH, whereas LH is mainly responsible for controlling steroidogenesis as well as release of gametes in both sexes. Steroidogenesis also can be influenced by FSH in both males and females. In some species, **prolactin (PRL)** may play a role in regulating ovarian steroidogenesis. The details of these events are discussed later. GTHs may be responsible for synthesis of a variety of paracrine or autocrine factors by the gonads. These factors may play roles in steroidogenesis or gametogenesis.

Induction of ovulation and formation of corpora lutea from the remnants of the ovulated follicle in the ovaries are due to LH. Surges in both LH and FSH occur in response to elevated GnRH prior to ovulation, but the magnitude of the LH surge greatly exceeds the FSH surge. LH release is enhanced selectively by the neuropeptide **galanin**, a peptide that is co-released with GnRH just prior to the midcycle LH surge. Galanin has no effect on FSH release. Under the influence of FSH, the ovaries secrete a peptide called **inhibin** that selectively blocks FSH release from the pituitary and contributes to the reduced FSH surge. In polyestrous species, the importance of the FSH surge may be related to initiation of follicle development in the next cycle.

The gonadal steroids, secreted as a result of the action of GTHs on special cells in the ovaries and testes, control differentiation and maintenance of many **primary sexual characters** (such as the uterus or vas deferens) and **secondary sexual characters** (such as muscle development and beard growth in men). These gonadal actions were recognized hundreds of years ago by the Chinese who used gonadal (and placental) preparations routinely to treat conditions ranging from impotence in men to the inability of a woman to bear sons. The hypothalamic centers regulating GnRH release are sensitive to circulating steroids that generally produce negative feedback on GnRH release, the exception to this pattern being the positive feedback effect by estrogens on release of GnRH and subsequent stimulation of LH release from the pituitary.

Several other hormones are involved in mammalian reproduction in addition to those of the HPG axis. The HPT and HPA axes as well as PRL have already been mentioned. In addition, nonapeptides from the pars nervosa influence reproductive events including courtship, birth, and parental behavior. The placenta of eutherian mammals assumes an endocrine role in pregnant females, producing steroids (primarily estrogens and progesterone) and polypeptide hormones (**chorionic gonadotropins** or **CG, chorionic somatomammotropin** or **CS, corticotropin-releasing hormone** or **CRH**, GnRH, PRL, etc.). In addition, the endocrine glands of the fetus may influence reproductive events; for example, contribution of the adrenal cortex to steroidogenesis by the placenta. The **pineal gland** may be a modulator of photoperiod and a source of antigonadotropic factors that influence gonadal function and prevent early onset of puberty (see Chapter 4). Finally, there are numerous reports of chemical agents termed **pheromones** that are produced by one sex to influence reproductive physiology, behavior, or both in the opposite sex.

A. Embryogenesis of Gonads and Their Accessory Ducts

The gonads, ducts, and associated glands are often termed the primary sexual characters because of their essential roles and direct participation in reproduction. Primary sexual characters include the vagina, uterus, and oviducts of the female and the penis, vasa deferentia, and prostate gland of the male. Secondary sexual characters are often dependent on gonadal hormones and usually enhance mating success but are not necessarily required for physically mating and producing offspring. For example, the male physique and beard growth are secondary sexual characters in humans.

1. The Gonads

The paired gonadal primordia arise from the intermediate mesoderm of the mammalian embryo as a genital ridge on either side of the midline in close association with the transitory mesonephric kidney of the embryo. Numerous derivatives of the mesonephric kidney and its duct system are retained as functional portions of the adult reproductive system although the bulk of the mesonephric kidney degenerates. A gonadal primordium consists of an outer **cortex** derived from peritoneum and an inner **medulla** (Figures 10-1 and 10-2). Germ

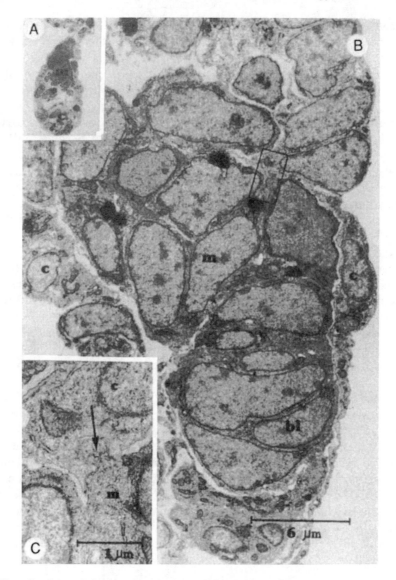

Figure 10-1. **Undifferentiated gonad.** Section of gonad from 25-mm tadpole of *Rana pipiens* showing cortical (c) and medullary (m) cells separated by a basal lamina (bl = basement membrane). 4, total gonad (upper left); 5, enlargement; 6, further enlargement showing contact between cortical and medullary cells (arrow). [From Merchant-Larios, M. (1978). Ovarian differentiation. *In* "The Vertebrate Ovary" (R.E. Jones, Ed.), pp. 47–81. Plenum Publishing Corp., NY.]

cells do not arise within the gonadal primordium itself but migrate from their site of origin in the yolk sac endoderm to either cortex (female) or medulla (male) depending upon the genetic sex.

Initially, the medullary component in males and females differentiates into **primary sex cords**. Differentiation of the primary sex cords and regression of the cortex results in a testis. Each testis consists of seminiferous tubules derived from the primary sex cords. The seminiferous tubules contain the **germ cells** that eventually will produce sperm and the **Sertoli** or **sustentacular cells** that support sperm development. Steroidogenic **interstitial cells** or **Leydig cells** are located between the seminiferous tubules. These interstitial cells arise from medullary tissue surrounding the primary sex cords and become sources of androgens. Germ cells that have migrated into the primary sex cords give rise to spermatogonia that eventually will give rise to gametes.

In females, the primary sex cords degenerate, and **secondary sex cords** differentiate from the cortical region. These secondary sex cords become the definitive ovary. In the ovary, the germ cells give rise to **oogonia** that

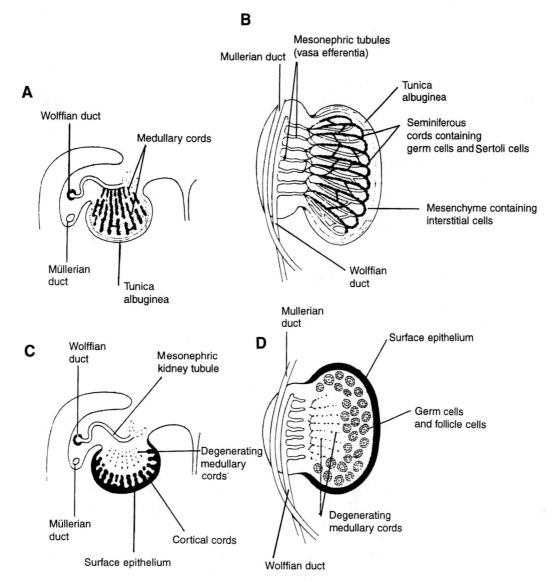

Figure 10-2.   **Development of primitive testis and ovary**. In the male, the medullary tissue develops into the testis cords (a) which give rise to the seminiferous tubules including the Sertoli cells. Mesonephric tubules give rise to the vas deferens and the vasa efferentia. In the female (c), the medullary cords degenerate and the cortical cords give rise to an ovary (d). Some mesonephric elements remain in the female as well. The vasa deferentia are retained in amphibians but eventually they degenerate in reptiles, birds, and mammals in which the ureters develop to drain the metanephric kidneys (not found in anamniotes). [Modified from Johnson, M., and Everitt, B. (1988). "Essential Reproduction," 3rd ed. Blackwell, Oxford.]

soon enter meiosis to form **primary oocytes**. The ovaries contain **follicles** that consist of one or more layers of **follicular cells** surrounding a primary oocyte.

2. Accessory Ducts

In males, the central portion of each differentiating testis forms a network of tubules, known as the **rete testis**, that do not contain seminiferous elements. The rete testis forms a connection between the seminiferous tubules and a surviving portion of the primitive mesonephric kidney duct called the **wolffian duct**, which, under the influence of testosterone, differentiates into the vas deferens and conducts sperm from the testis to the urethra. Most of the mesonephric kidney in mammals degenerates, with the exception of some of the anterior

Box 10A.   Vertebrate Kidney Evolution

The first kidney in vertebrates was the pronephros. It appears only as a transitory structure during early development, and the only remaining example is the anteriormost part of the fish kidney, known as the "head kidney." This structure consists largely of lymphoid tissue as well as adrenocortical cells. The duct that drained the pronephros to the cloaca is retained. It is called the pronephric or archinephric duct. Posterior to the pronephros develops a second kidney, the mesonephros that co-opts the pronephric duct as its conduit to drain urine to the cloaca. Developmentally, this mesonephric duct is called the wolffian duct in the embryo. The mesonephros becomes the definitive kidney of fishes and amphibians where it is often designated as the opistonephric kidney. The wolffian duct is retained in both male and female fishes as a kidney duct and may also be used as a sperm duct in male elasmobranchs as well as in amphibians. In amniote vertebrates, a third kidney develops posterior to the opistonephros and is called the metanephric kidney. A new urinary duct, the ureter, develops to connect the metanephric kidney to the urogenital sinus. The wolffian duct is retained as the epididymis and the vas deferens in males. A portion of the wolffian duct also gives rise to the seminal vesicles that retain a connection to the vas deferens. In addition, some of the mesonephric kidney tubules form the rete testis that connects the seminiferous tubules of the testes to the epididymis. In female amniotes, the wolffian duct degenerates. Some mesonephric tubules also are retained in females and become associated with the ovaries. In elasmobranchs, amphibians, and amniotes, a pair of müllerian ducts develop adjacent to the wolffian ducts. In females, these ducts give rise to the oviducts and uteri but usually degenerate in males. The utricle of the prostate gland in male mammals actually is a müllerian remnant. It is the stimulation of this female remnant by estrogens that is responsible for most prostate cancer.

mesonephric kidney tubules (see Box 10A). In the presence of testosterone, this tissue together with a portion of the wolffian duct forms two glandular structures, the **epididymis** and the **seminal vesicle** (Figures 10-2 and 10-3).

A second pair of longitudinal ducts develops in the embryo from the mesial wall of each wolffian duct and lie parallel to them. These structures are known as the **müllerian ducts**. In genetic females, the müllerian ducts develop into the oviducts, the uterus, and the upper part of the vagina (Figure 10-3), usually fusing together to form a common vagina and, in some species, a single uterus as well. The wolffian ducts degenerate in female mammals. In males, it is the müllerian ducts that are suppressed in favor of wolffian duct development.

Mullerian-inhibiting substance (MIS) was first proposed by Jost in the 1940s to explain the inhibitory effect of the testes on development of müllerian ducts in rabbit embryos. It also has been called the **anti-mullerian hormone** or AMH. Implantation of a testis into a female embryo results in sufficient MIS secretion to prevent development of the müllerian ducts. MIS not only blocks müllerian duct development but is capable of inhibiting growth of tumors from ovaries and müllerian duct derivatives. It appears that MIS acts cooperatively with testosterone in producing these effects on the müllerian ducts. The ovary also makes MIS, but the müllerian ducts are protected by local estradiol secreted by the ovary.

Maleness in eutherian mammals is dependent upon secretion of androgens from the testis. In the absence of androgens, the male animal (genotype XY) will develop a female phenotype. Similarly, exposure of developing males to estrogens will result in female development to a degree proportional to the amount of estrogen and the timing of the exposure (see Table 10-2). Conversely, treatment of newborn females with androgens destroys the cyclical secretory pattern of the HPG axis and replaces it with a noncyclical or tonic pattern like that of males (see Box 10B). Becoming a male mammal, then, involves overcoming the basic tendency for mammalian embryos to develop as females. A gene seemingly responsible for male sex determination called **SRY** has been localized on the short arm of the Y-chromosome that is characteristic of genetic males. In mice, the SRY gene is activated in gonads of genetic males before they begin to differentiate into testes. Insertion of the SRY gene into XX mice followed by its activation leads to formation of male-specific structures and regression of female ducts. The activated gonad secretes MIS that causes regression of the müllerian ducts. Presumably, the SRY gene produces a factor that activates the MIS gene. Androgens secreted by the transformed gonad cause male-like differentiation of the external genitalia and the wolffian ducts as well as changes in the hypothalamus

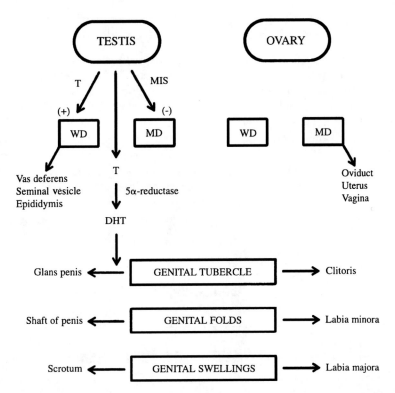

Figure 10-3. **Patterns of development for ducts and genitalia.** In males, the testis secretes testosterone (T), that stimulates differentiation of wolffian ducts, and mullerian-inhibitory substance (MIS), that causes regression of mullerian ducts. Dihydrotestosterone (DHT) is converted from T in the gential tubercle, genital folds, or gential swellings causing them to differentiate in the male direction. Estradiol from the ovary prevents MIS (also secreted by ovary) from causing mullerian duct regression, and the absence of sufficient androgens determines the fate of the other structures.

Table 10-2. Critical Periods for Sexual Differentiation of the Brain in Mammals

Species	Gestation period (days)	Critical period (days)
Hamster	16	16–21
Laboratory rat	21–22	18–28
Laboratory mouse	19–20	20
Guinea pig	68	30–35
Human	270	84–126

to suppress development of the surge center. This establishes the tonic secretory pattern for GnRH and GTHs that characterizes males. Studies with estrogen receptor β knockout (βERKO) mice verify that defeminization of the male brain requires conversion of androgens to estradiol. Genetically male βERKO mice will exhibit female behavior whereas wild-type males do not.

Although the female has been called the default sex in mammals, becoming a female is not just the absence of androgens. For example, studies have shown that estrogens are necessary for development of the female difference in the corpus callosum of the brain.

Androgens and estrogens may alter basic traits through what are termed **organizational effects**. Stimulation of the development of male genitalia by androgens is an example of an organizational effect. Organizational effects are permanent and can not be reversed later by exposure to other gonadal steroids. In contrast, **activational effects** can be induced by gonadal steroids, for example, by inducing a specific behavior in adults. The type of behavior induced depends on the steroid applied, not on the genetic sex of the individual.

Box 10B.   Changes in Sexual Differentiation Caused by Exposure to Gonadal Steroids

Exposure of developing mammals to external (exogenous) sources of either androgens or estrogens can alter the sexual phenotype regardless of the genetic sex. The most elegant demonstration of subtle effects of exposure to exogenous steroids by Frederick vom Saal, who observed that the position of the mouse embryo *in utero* could determine anatomical, physiological, and behavioral traits in the offspring (Box Figure 10-B1). Thus, a genetic female that developed between two males could be influenced by male hormones. When examined as newborns or adults, such females exhibited male traits (see Box Table 10-B1). Similarly, a male developing between two females will later exhibit some degree of feminization. In cattle, when male and female twins share a common blood supply, the female will be masculinized to such a degree that it will be born as an intersex incapable of reproduction (called a freemartin). Similarly, recent studies of human dizygotic twins of opposite sexes provide evidence for masculinization in the female presumably as a result of *in utero* exposure to androgens.

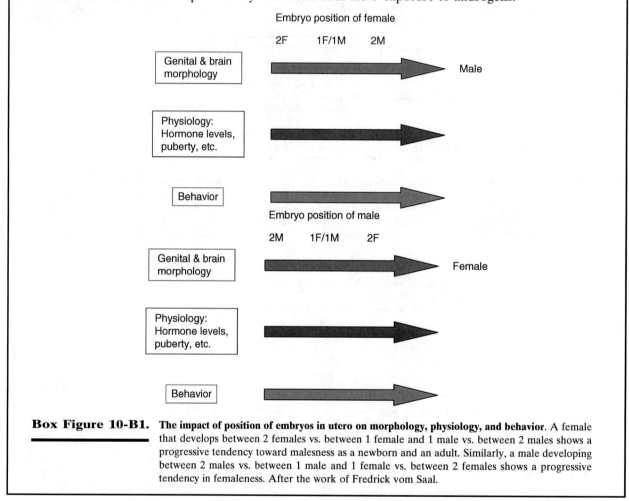

Box Figure 10-B1.   **The impact of position of embryos in utero on morphology, physiology, and behavior**. A female that develops between 2 females vs. between 1 female and 1 male vs. between 2 males shows a progressive tendency toward malesness as a newborn and an adult. Similarly, a male developing between 2 males vs. between 1 male and 1 female vs. between 2 females shows a progressive tendency in femaleness. After the work of Fredrick vom Saal.

II. Reproduction in Monotremes and Marsupials

A. Monotremes

The monotremes have retained the reptilian feature of laying eggs but have mammary glands for feeding the young after they hatch. Unlike the eggs of reptiles and birds, monotreme eggs contain little yolk and embryonic nutrition is supplied through uterine secretions that pass through the porous leathery egg shell as the egg passes through the female genital tract. Upon hatching, the new monotreme appears as a tiny, fetus-like creature with only a few well-developed features that enable it to attach itself to its mother's mammary gland and obtain nourishment. The mammary glands of monotremes lack external teats. Consequently, milk is secreted onto a special common area, the **areola**. The newly hatched monotreme must attach itself to its mother with its forelimbs and suck or lick milk from the areola. Development continues and the offspring, because of its primitive nature, can be considered an exteriorized fetus until it has completed development.

1. Monotreme Reproductive Patterns

Seasonally breeding monotremes are difficult to study because they are largely nocturnal animals and are carefully protected in nature. Furthermore, they do not breed readily in captivity. The duckbill platypus lays its eggs in a nest, but the female spiny echidna places her freshly layed eggs in a brood pouch that develops seasonally on her ventral surface. Formation of the pouch is probably dependent upon estrogens, although no experimental data are available to confirm this. The eggs develop and hatch within the pouch, and after the breeding season the pouch regresses.

Echindnas enter a period of torpor and inactivity prior to the breeding season when they arouse to mate. Attempts to measure circulating estrogens by radioimmunoassay in platypus and echindnas have been unsuccessful as plasma levels are below the detectable level (<1 ng/ml). Examination of steroid metabolite levels in feces employed with chromatographic and mass spectrophotometry methods (see Chapter 2) would provide the sensitive noninvasive approach needed for these species. Measurable progesterone levels in female echidnas rise after mating as the pouch undergoes development and peak just prior to the appearance of an egg in the pouch (Figure 10-4). When males are in breeding groups with females, they exhibit elevated testosterone levels (Figure 10-4).

B. Marsupials

The marsupial placenta is rather primitive and apparently has no major endocrine function when compared to the eutherian placenta. The period of pregnancy or gestation is very short in marsupials (Table 10-3), and the young marsupial is born in an extremely immature condition. For example, among the macropodid marsupials (kangaroos, wallabies), the **joey** must find its way essentially unaided to the mother's pouch where it permanently attaches to the nipple of a mammary gland. The attached joey, like the newly hatched monotreme, continues its development as an exteriorized fetus. After a long period of pouch development (about 200 days in the red kangaroo), the young marsupial disengages itself from the teat and ventures outside the pouch, returning first at regular and later at irregular intervals for milk.

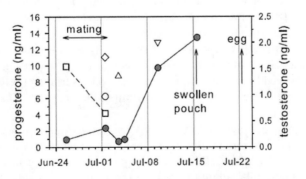

Figure 10-4. **Progesterone and egg laying in the echidna.** Progesterone levels (shaded circles) rise following mating and prior to the appearance of an egg. Testosterone levels in five attendant males are indicated by the open symbols. [Reprinted with permission from Nicol, S., Anderson, N. A., and Jones, S. M. (2005). Seasonal variations in reproductive hormones in free-ranging echidnas (*Tachyglossus aculeatus*): Interaction between reproduction and hibernation. *Gen. Comp. Endocr.* **144**, 204–210.]

Table 10-3. Comparison of Length of Estrous Cycle, Gestation Period, and Ratio of Body Weight of Neonate to Body Weight of Mother in Metatherian and Eutherian Mammals

Species	Length of estrous cycle[a] (days)	Length of gestation period (days)	Neonate: mother body weight ratio
Eutherial			
Rat	4–5	22	—
Sheep	16	148	1:14
Metatheria			
Virginia opossum	29	12	1:8,300
Long-nosed bandicoot	26	12	1:4,250
Brush possum	26	17	1:7,250
Dama wallaby	30	29	1:10,000
Swamp wallaby	31	37	—
Red kangaroo	35	33	1:33,400
Western gray kangaroo	35	30	—

[a] The estrous cycles are similar to the gestation period in metatherians and may not require a pregnancy-recognition mechanism. Based on Sharman, G. B. (1976). Evolution of viviparity in mammals. *In* "Reproduction in Mammals" (C. R. Austin and R. V. Short, Eds.), Vol. 6, pp. 32–70. Cambridge University Press.

1. Marsupial Reproductive Patterns

Follicular enlargement, estrogen-dependent uterine proliferation, and enlargement of elements of the vaginal complex precedes estrus in females. Peak uterine and vaginal development coincides with estrus and copulation. Ovulation occurs spontaneously one to several days after the onset of estrus, and postovulatory follicles transform into corpora lutea that maintain a short secretory uterine condition. Progesterone continues the secretory uterine phase in castrates and is undoubtedly the hormone responsible for maintaining gestation as it is in eutherian mammals.

The post-ovulatory phase is the same in mated and unmated females, and no "pregnancy-recognition signal" is necessary. Pregnancy does not affect ovarian function, and both pregnant and unmated females begin a new cycle at about the same time in most species. Equivalent mammary gland development occurs during post-estrus in both pregnant and non-pregnant females, and newborn foster young will develop normally if attached to virgin or non-lactating females at the equivalent post-estrous state in relation to the time of birth (**parturition**) or cycle cessation. Circulating progesterone and urinary pregnanediol levels are similar in pregnant, unmated, and luteal-phase females. There are no endocrine differences between the pregnant and non-pregnant post-estrous phase that support the conclusion that the marsupial placenta is not an endocrine organ.

A number of rodent-like marsupials have a reproductive cycle in which all of the males die after a single breeding. For example, in the brown antechinus, *Antechinus stuartii*, annual reproduction is controlled strictly by photoperiod. Mating is restricted to the same two-week period each year with the males exhibiting extreme aggression to one another and mating vigorously and frequently with females. This mating frenzy is accompanied by elevated cortisol levels in the males that are associated with neural, gastrointestinal, and kidney degeneration, and is soon followed by death. The females generally survive breeding and rear their young with no help from the departed males. In years of good environmental conditions, the females may live to breed a second year.

Another unusual feature of marsupials is the ability to simultaneously produce two kinds of milk. As in eutherian mammals, the first milk differs markedly in composition from that produced later during lactation. However, macropodids, which may have both a newborn **joey** and one that has already detached itself from a teat, will produce early and late milk simultaneously in the respective glands. The developmental state of a particular mammary gland would seem to be independent of endocrine conditions and strongly influenced by external conditions; that is, the joey.

A major developmental difference between eutherians and marsupials has had a profound influence on reproductive patterns in the latter group. Marsupials exhibit a primitive reptilian pattern of wolffian and mullerian duct origins. Instead of developing medially to the kidneys and ureters as in eutherians, these ducts develop laterally. Consequently, it is not possible for left and right mullerian ducts of females to fuse in the midline without placing considerable strain on the ureters. It is believed that the short gestation period of marsupials is a consequence of separate uteri and vaginas and limited space for uterine hypertrophy. A special birth canal must be formed so that parturition can occur, and in some species it forms anew each season. This development of separate vaginas has influenced evolution of the male reproductive system as well. Males of some species have a bifid penis, with left and right prongs apparently being inserted into the separate vaginas of the female during copulation.

III. Reproduction in Eutherian Mammals

Eutherian mammals employ the placenta not only as an endocrine organ to maintain gestation but also as a replacement for the mammary glands to supply early nutrition to the fetus. Consequently, parturition is delayed considerably, and the newborn or **neonate** of most placental mammals is at a comparable stage of development to the young joey when it first ventures out of the pouch. Like the juvenile marsupial, the placental neonate relies at first on the mammary gland as the exclusive source of nourishment but gradually abandons it for other foods.

Three distinct reproductive patterns occur in sexually mature eutherians: one typical for all males and two among females. Males of some domesticated species and humans are characterized by continuous secretion of GTHs and occasionally continuous spermatogenesis, and these males are capable of siring offspring at any time of year. Most eutherian species, however, exhibit seasonal episodes of spermatogenesis, sexual activity, or both such as displayed by most non-mammalian vertebrates (see Chapter 11).

Although considered a continuous breeder, humans show some dramatic seasonal patterns of breeding activity correlated with photoperiod and lattitude (based on the past 30–50 years of birth records). In Europe and Japan, there are more births in the early spring (March-April) with the amplitude of the birth peak increasing in a south-to-north gradient. In South Africa, Australia, India, and New Zealand, the birth peak is associated with September-November. The amplitude of the birth peak decreases from North to South, which is opposite to the latitudinal change observed in the northern hemisphere. However, in North America, the greatest number of births for both white and non-white people (many having their origins as transplants from Europe and Africa, respectively, in the past 300 years) occurs in August-October with a decrease in amplitude from warmer to colder latitudes as occurs in countries of the southern hemisphere of the Old World. It has been proposed that North American patterns are a response to environmental temperature superimposed over the Old World patterns that correlate more strongly with photoperiod. These variations with latitude are less obvious for the northern hemisphere in the Old World which are opposite to that observed in the New World and the southern hemisphere of the Old World. In spite of these differences, it is clear that humans show seasonal tendencies in reproductive activity that resemble those of other eutherians.

Females exhibit cyclic patterns of GTH secretion that can be traced to a basic rhythmicity probably residing within the hypothalamus. There are two types of female cycles: the ovarian-based estrous cycle and the uterine-based menstrual cycle. The **estrous cycle** is typical for mammals (except possibly humans) and consists of a series of precisely regulated endocrine events repeated in each cycle. **Proestrus** is characterized by hormonal changes that bring about follicular development and ovulation. Estrus, a short period when the female is receptive to the male and during which mating can occur, immediately follows proestrus and coincides with ovulation. Estrus represents the time when fertilization is most likely to lead to pregnancy and successful birth of offspring. The interim between estrus and the onset of hormonal changes characteristic of proestrus in cases in which pregnancy did not result is termed **diestrus** and usually is associated with ovarian inactivity and uterine regression. Carnivores and some other mammals may be classified as **monestrous**. If mating does not occur in a monestrous species or if mating occurs but fertilization and implantation are unsuccessful, the female will not return to estrus until the next breeding season (mono = one). Hence, these species have a long diestrous phase. Many mammalian species are **polyestrous**, however, and will return immediately to proestrus if mating does not occur or if mating is unsuccessful (poly = many; i.e., a very short diestrous phase). Eventually, the female will enter a prolonged diestrus if pregnancy does not occur. In some mammals (e.g., certain rodents), mating without successful fertilization and implantation may result in a short period of simulated or false pregnancy, termed **pseudopregnancy**, after which the female re-enters proestrus without experiencing diestrus.

Some mammals exhibit a sequence of uterine events, known as a **menstrual cycle** that is characterized by one phase in which rapid sloughing of the uterine epithelium (**menses**) occurs if fertilization does not lead to pregnancy rather than the slow regression seen in diestrus. Often, these animals do not experience diestrus and may breed continuously whereas others are seasonal breeders. Menstrual cycles are found in humans, monkeys, gibbons, the slender loris, marmosets, zebras, and several shrews and bats. The sloughing of the uterine epithelial lining often results in a vaginal discharge (**menstruation**) of uterine epithelial cells and trapped blood. The blood is trapped due to constriction of special spiral-shaped arteries that supply most of the blood flow to the uterine epithelium. The lack of blood flow to the outer portion of the epithelium results in cell death and hastens sloughing. A few of these mammals with menstrual cycles are known to exhibit **covert menstruation** where the sloughed tissues are resorbed and there is no uterine discharge. The onset of menses marks the end of one cycle and the beginning of the next. Although reproductive endocrinologists consistently focus upon the cyclic nature of estrous and menstrual cycles and their restarting with the failure of pregnancy to occur, it is important to remember that the normal sequel to ovulation is pregnancy. In nature, it is probably unusual for a female to enter estrus and not become pregnant.

Most primates exhibit estrous behavior to some degree at about the time of ovulation, including species characterized as having menstrual cycles, although a well-defined estrus is not observed in the human female. Exhibition of menstrual or estrous cycles should not be considered as alternative strategies, but that, with the possible exception of humans, the menstrual cycle is one variation within the estrous cycle.

Although there have been numerous hypotheses developed as to why menstrual cycles evolved, most are discounted because they cannot be generalized to all mammals exhibiting menses. Some, for example, relate menstruation to a placental type common to menstruating mammals yet other species with this same type of placental anatomy do not have menstrual cycles. If it is simply a byproduct of endometrial function, then it is a costly one in terms of nutrient losses. One intriguing hypothesis suggests that menstruation evolved as an adaptation in mammals to neutralize and eliminate pathogens introduced during copulation and/or by sperm deposited in the vagina. However, this doesn't explain the scarcity of menstrual cycles among eutherian species. Perhaps the menstrual cycle is simply another adaptation in favorable climates that allows for continuous breeding activity to ensure pregnancy will occur at some point but so that not all females in the population are pregnant at the same time.

Uterine bleeding and discharge occur at other times in the estrous cycles of some mammals. For example, the cow, domestic dog, and coyote discharge blood prior to ovulation and the onset of estrous behavior. This discharge is estrogen-induced and does not involve degeneration of the uterine lining. Periovulatory bleeding also occurs either overtly or covertly in several primates including humans, Sykes and vervet monkeys, and possibly in the cottontop tamarin.

A. Puberty

The achievement by the gonads of their full hormonal and gametogenic capacity for reproduction is termed **puberty**. This process may be gradual or rather sudden, depending on the species, and may be accompanied by a variety of morphological changes as well. In rats, monkeys, and humans, puberty is associated with a marked increase in GnRH release from the hypothalamus resulting in elevated GTH secretion. In children, the frequency of these GTH pulses increases two-fold at night and later during the day as puberty progresses. The amplitude of the GTH pulses also increases as the sensitivity of pituitary gonadotropes to GnRH is enhanced. Experimental studies suggest that the most critical factor in the induction of puberty is the increase in the frequency of GnRH pulses.

These changes in the HPG axis are paralleled in other endocrine systems. Nocturnal release of PRL also is elevated along with FSH and LH although its role in puberty is uncertain. Adrenal androgens increase in boys and girls prior to the onset of puberty and continue to rise during puberty. This process is called adrenarche (see Chapter 8). These events are independent of the changes in the gonadal axis but are important contributions to puberty. For example, adrenal androgens stimulate the prepubertal growth spurt and the appearance of axillary and pubic hair.

GnRH mRNA in the hypothalamus rises markedly prior to the onset of puberty. The GnRH neurons are interconnected so that release of their products is synchronous in a self-regulated rhythmic pattern (pulses). Thus, they are often called **pacemaker neurons**, analogous to the pacemaker cells of the heart.

There are several hypotheses concerning the mechanism(s) for the normal onset of puberty. The **gonadostat hypothesis** suggests that there is a development of decreased feedback sensitivity in the hypothalamus to gonadal steroids that brings about increased release of GnRH. Accelerated gonadotropin release from the pituitary activates gonadal steroidogenesis and gametogenesis or **gonadarche**. Gonadal responses also may involve receptor synthesis. For example, receptors for FSH are present in early ovarian follicles but not LH receptors. FSH stimulates production of LH receptors and increases the levels of aromatase enzyme. Now, the ovary can respond to both GTHs. The **missing link hypothesis** implies that some factor is missing and that it is the brain and not the gonads that is functionally incompetent prior to puberty. Data obtained from experimental and clinical observations that support these hypotheses also support the **active inhibition hypothesis** that currently is in favor. This hypothesis states that puberty occurs because of a progressive decrease in physiological inhibition. The well-known actions of the pineal gland and melatonin on inhibiting reproductive function (see Chapter 4), and the observed reduction in melatonin secretion with precocial puberty, offer strong support to the inhibitory hypothesis (see below). Early puberty events in humans also have been linked to exposures to endocrine-disrupting chemicals.

A separate hypothesis has been formulated to explain puberty and **menarche**, the onset of menstruation in girls. This **lipostat hypothesis** or **critical weight hypothesis** implies that attainment of puberty is in part a function of fat storage in the body. Consequently, girls who have more body fat reach menarche sooner than leaner girls. Furthermore, chronic strenuous exercise reduces body fat and may prevent young girls from reaching menarche just as it can block menstruation in women. Once the excessively lean girls are placed on a less severe regimen so that body fat increases, menarche usually is achieved. This mechanism probably is not related to puberty *per se* but rather may be an evolutionary mechanism to ensure that there is evidence of sufficient environmental resources (as evidenced in body fat) to support the energy demands of pregnancy and lactation for successful rearing of young. Recent studies suggest that the peptide **leptin** secreted by adipose cells may influence GnRH release in the brain. Higher levels of leptin occur when lipid stores are greater, and leptin may provide a signal to the brain of the extent of fat storage in addition to suppressing appetite (see Chapter 12).

IV. Endocrine Regulation in Eutherian Males

In some species, mature males are capable of copulating with a female whenever she is receptive. Secretion of GnRH and hence of GTHs is more or less continuous in these males but with daily fluctuations occurring in circulating levels of some GTHs. Daily secretory patterns for GTHs show considerable variation among different species. Hourly fluctuations of LH have been reported in bulls, and these variations in LH are correlated with following increases in circulating testosterone (Figure 10-5). However, in human males, FSH shows no cyclic variation in blood levels although LH and testosterone exhibit obvious daily patterns with peak levels occurring during early morning hours and minimum values reported for the afternoon. Most wild mammals exhibit distinct seasonal breeding, and active spermatogenesis may be restricted to only a few months of the year or less.

A. Spermatogenesis

Each testis develops primarily from the medullary portion of an embryonic gonadal blastema as described above (see Figure 10-2). Differentiation of the medullary portion with concomitant regression of the cortical components (progenitor of the ovary) appears to be controlled by local embryonic androgen secretion activated by the SRY gene. The medullary region differentiates into seminiferous tubules and interspersed masses of

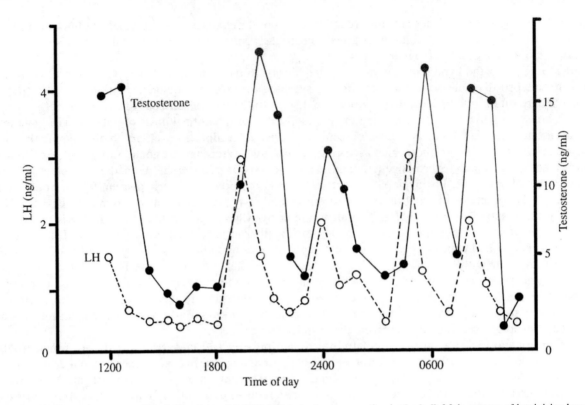

Figure 10-5. **Male pattern of luteinizing hormone (LH) and testosterone secretion in the bull.** Male pattern of luteinizing hormone (LH) and testosterone secretion in a bull. Pulsatile release of GnRH (not shown) would precede each LH peak that precedes each testosterone peak.

interstitial cells. These interstitial cells are located between the seminiferous tubules and synthesize and release androgens into the general circulation.

The seminiferous tubules consist of large Sertoli cells, germ cells, spermatogonia, and cells derived from the spermatogonia (Figures 10-6 and 10-7). Each tubule is surrounded by a thin layer of connective tissue. Under the influence of androgens, **peritubular myoid cells** develop in this connective tissue layer during puberty. They surround and provide support for the seminiferous tubules and are believed to be responsible for contractile activity of the tubules that propels sperm to the epididymis. The Sertoli cell has an extensive cytoplasm extending from the outer edge to the lumen of the tubule. The angular nucleus of the Sertoli cell is located at the outer edge of the tubule. Sertoli cells form tight junctions with the peritubular myoid cells, and together they secrete the components that form the basement membrane. This basement membrane is the blood/testis barrier that isolates the seminiferous tubules from the blood and requires all chemical signals to pass through the Sertoli cells in order to reach the spermatogenetic cells.

Germ cells are present along the outer margins of the seminiferous tubules and differentiate into **spermatogonia**. Spermatogonial cells proliferate mitotically under the influence of FSH to produce more spermatogonia. Eventually some of these spermatogonia will undergo differentiation characterized by nuclear enlargement and will become **primary spermatocytes** that are capable of entering spermatogenesis (Figure 10-8). Testicular androgens are somehow necessary for initiation of meiosis in primary spermatocytes that undergo the first meiotic division to give rise to two smaller **secondary spermatocytes**. These latter cells are infrequently observed in histological preparations because, once formed, they quickly enter the second meiotic division to yield four haploid **spermatids** which are transformed to sperm (spermatozoa) by concentrating the chromatin material into the sperm head and by elimination of the majority of the cytoplasm. The process of transformation of spermatids to sperm is termed **spermiogenesis**.

A given histological section of a seminiferous tubule may show varying numbers of spermatogonia, primary spermatocytes, possibly a few secondary spermatocytes, spermatids, and sperm in sequence from the outer

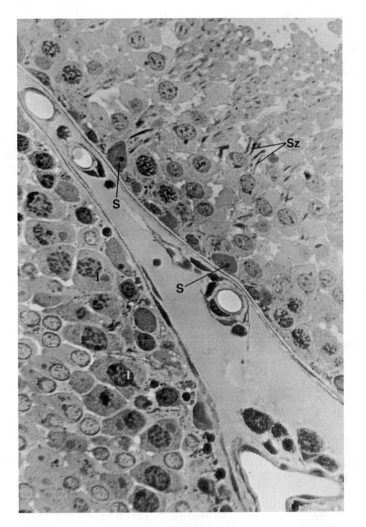

Figure 10-6. **Spermatogenesis in rat testis.** Section of rat testis showing edges of adjacent seminiferous tubules. S, nuclei of Sertoli cells; I, primary spermatocytes; Sz, heads of sperm. [Courtesy of Dr. C. H. Muller, University of Washington.]

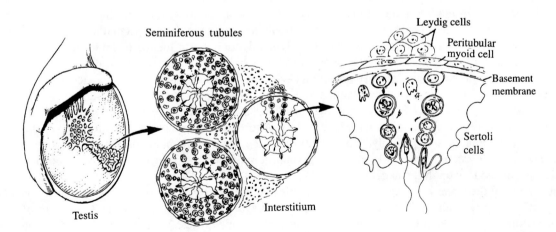

Figure 10-7. **Organization of mammalian testis.** Detail at right shows events of spermatogenesis and spermiogenesis in relation to three Sertoli cells. The endocrine roles of interstitial (Leydig) cells, peritubular myoid cells, and Sertoli cells are described in the text. [Reprinted with permission from Skinner, M. K. *Endocr. Rev.* **12**, 45–77 (1991). © The Endocrine Society.]

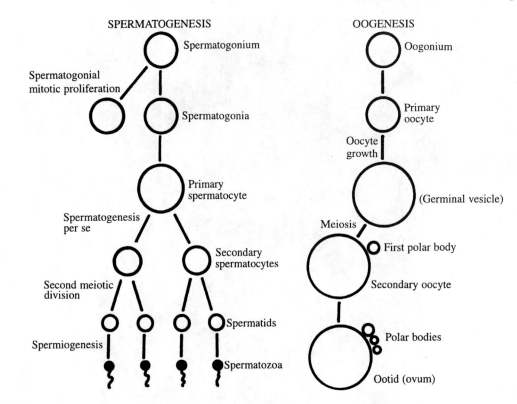

Figure 10-8. **Comparison of spermatogenesis and oogenesis.** A major difference between males and females is the mitotic proliferation of gonial cells after birth in males whereas the germ cells have all progressed to the primary oocyte stage in females and no new oocytes appear after birth. The primary spermatocyte undergoes meiosis to produce 4 spermatids whereas meiotic division of the primary oocyte with unequal distribution of cytoplasm produces only 1 oocyte plus up to 3 polar bodies. The first polar body (a secondary oocyte with very little cytoplasm) often does not undergo the second division.

margin (gonia) to the lumen (sperm). The tails of the spermatozoa extend into the lumen, and the heads of the sperm typically are still surrounded by highly folded margins of Sertoli cells (Figure 10-7).

Millions of mature sperm may be sloughed off into the lumina of the seminiferous tubules each day. This process is termed **spermiation** and is stimulated by LH. These sperm pass through the tubules that eventually coalesce into larger ducts of the rete testis that eventually join the epididymis associated with each testis. Vast numbers of maturing sperm are stored in the epididymis. Under the influence of androgens, the epididymis secretes materials into its lumen where the sperm are being held. Included in this secretion are protein-bound **sialic acids** (sialomucoproteins), **glycerylphosphoryl-choline**, and **carnitine**. These particular substances are involved directly in maturing and maintaining sperm in viable condition until ejaculation. Androgens and **androgen-binding protein (ABP)** produced by Sertoli cells in the seminiferous tubules are released along with sperm and travel to the epididymis (Figure 10-7). Androgen molecules freed from ABP in the lumen or androgen-ABP complexes or possibly both are absorbed by the epididymal cells. These androgens stimulate epididymal cells to secrete materials involved in maintenance of the sperm. PRL from the pituitary also stimulates secretion by epididymal cells.

Contraction of the smooth muscles of the epdidiymis and vas deferens causes ejection of sperm (ejaculation). The sperm leave the epididymis, enter the vas deferens, travel to the urethra, traverse the length of the penis via the urethra, and are deposited in the female's vagina during coitus. Various glands such as the **prostate gland** add their fluid secretions to the sperm and epididymal secretions to form a watery mixture of sperm and various organic and inorganic substances known as **semen**. The entire ejaculatory event may be induced by the release of oxytocin (OXY) from the pars nervosa in response to a neural reflex initiated by mechanical stimulation of the penis.

B. Endocrine Regulation of Testicular Functions

Spermatogenesis is a temperature-sensitive process, and high temperatures such as found within the body cavity of terrestrial eutherians can impair normal spermatogenesis and produce temporary sterility. Consequently, at some time prior to the attainment of sexual maturity or prior to the annual breeding season, the testes descend into the scrotum where spermatogenesis can proceed at a slightly lower temperature. The failure of the testes to descend, a condition known as **cryptorchidism** (*crypto-*, hidden, *orchi*, testis), may cause irreparable damage to the seminiferous epithelium in most species. Some mammals lack a scrotum (for example, elephants, whales, seals), and the testes are permanently located within the abdominal cavity. Male elephants, however, are capable of producing viable sperm and copulating with a female at any time of year. In such species, spermatogenesis either does not exhibit the same temperature sensitivity characteristic for scrotal species or these animals possess other mechanisms to reduce testicular temperature.

GTHs and a number of paracrine factors including testosterone (Table 10-4) control production of sperm. Many of the details of the endocrine regulation of these processes are not clear, but a generalized picture is emerging. Relatively separate roles have been defined for LH and FSH in males although FSH and testosterone work cooperatively in some cases. Spermatogenesis is initiated indirectly by FSH through mitotic proliferation of spermatogonia and formation of primary spermatocytes. Spermatogonia lack FSH receptors and the mechanism of spermatogonial activation is mediated by paracrine factors from the Sertoli cells that do have FSH receptors. This intermediary role of the Sertoli cell is supported by observations that FSH stimulates mitosis in Sertoli cells whose number in the adult testis is directly proportional to sperm abundance. Testosterone may initiate meiotic divisions of primary spermatocytes that differentiate from spermatogonia, resulting eventually in formation of spermatids. The production of ABP and cytoskeletal proteins (**actin, vinculin**) by the Sertoli cell also is stimulated by FSH. **Aromatase (P450$_{aro}$)** synthesis in the Sertoli cell is also stimulated by FSH.

The synthesis and release of circulating androgens by the interstitial cells are controlled primarily by LH. Steroidogenesis by the Leydig cell is enhanced by another action of FSH on the Sertoli cell where FSH causes secretion of a protein complex called **steroidogenesis-stimulating protein (STP)**. STP is a paracrine regulator that enhances steroidogenesis in the Leydig cell in response to stimulation by LH.

Testosterone is the major circulating androgen in mammals, although other androgens such as **androstenedione** or **5α-dihydrotestosterone (DHT)** may circulate in significant amounts (Table 10-5). Some **5β-dihydrotestosterone** also is produced and stimulates red blood cell production in bone marrow and contributes to the higher hematocrit found in males as compared to females. Prior to attainment of puberty in bulls, androstenedione is the principal circulating androgen, but it is gradually replaced by testosterone at puberty. Testosterone within the testis, however, seems to be the most important androgen influencing sperm production.

Testosterone has several important paracrine effects on spermatogenesis and spermiogenesis. These actions probably are indirect since testosterone receptors appear to be absent or occur in very low numbers on germ cells. However, estrogen receptors, ERβ, are present on germ cells that also possess aromatase activity. Furthermore, at least in rodents, the local metabolism of DHT to an androgen metabolite **3β-diol** (see Chapter 3) has been reported in brain, prostate, and testes. 3β-diol binds and activates ERβ. Furthermore, aromatase knockout male mice exhibit disruption of spermatogenesis, supporting a local role for estrogen receptor-binding regulators. The attachment of Sertoli cells to spermatids involves cytoskeletal actin and vinculin interactions with the spermatids, as well as indirect effects of testosterone. Peritubular myoid cells (Figure 10-7) are stimulated by testosterone to release two proteins, **P-Mod-SA** and **P-Mod-SB**, that cause Sertoli cells to secrete additional paracrine regulators that may alter spermiogenesis (Table 10-4).

The Leydig cells of the testis also synthesize and release small quantities of estrogens. Testicular estrogens reach dramatic levels in the stallion, and estrogens may have definite physiological roles in males. Locally, estradiol can block androgen synthesis by interstitial cells and can influence the responsiveness of these cells to GTHs. Estradiol also binds to receptors in the epididymis where it regulates resorption of excess testicular fluid that was used to conduct sperm to the epididymis. The ratio of testosterone to estradiol in the general circulation may alter the ratios of FSH and LH being released from the pituitary through negative feedback. Finally, conversion of androgens to estrogen occurs in certain brain cells, and circulating estrogens themselves may influence male sexual behavior.

Table 10-4. Possible Local Actions for Gonadal Secretions

Factor	Source	Proposed action
Gonadotropin-releasing hormone (GnRH)	Ovary	Working through IP$_3$ second messenger, GnRH alters steroidogenesis by granulosa cells in certain follicular stages; may signal atresia
	Sertoli cell	Alters androgen synthesis by interstitial cells; increases local permeability of capillaries
Testosterone	Interstitial cell	Regulates functions of Seroli cells; stimulates meiosis in primary spermatocytes
Estradiol	Interstitial cells in male	Blocks androgen synthesis
	Epididymis	Stimulates fluid resorption
Transforming growth factor α (TGF-α)	Thecal cells	Facilitates proliferation of thecal and granulosa cells but slows their GTH-induced differentiation
	Sertoli and peritubular myoid cells	Causes EGF-like growth stimulation in interstitial cells; decreases steroidogenesis
Fibroblast growth factor (FGF)	Granulosa cell	Causes epithelial proliferation in early follicular development and conversion of thecal cells to ovarian interstitial cells after ovulation
	Testicular germ cells	Binds to receptors on Sertoli cell; function unknown
Nerve growth factor (NGF)	Ovarian cells	Stimulates follicular formation and organization as well as differentiation of ovarian interstitial cells
Epidermal growth factor (EGF)	Thecal/interstitial cells of ovary	Stimulates granulosa cell proliferation
Insulin-like growth factor I (IGF-I)	Granulosa cells	Increases number of LDL receptors on granulosa cells; stimulates cholesterol and inhibin synthesis
Activin	Granulosa cells	Unknown
	Sertoli and interstitial cells	Specific receptors shown on germ cells
Growth hormone-releasing hormone (GHRH)	Corpora lutea, oocyte	Promotes follicular development and ovulation
	Germ cells of testes	Stimulates Sertoli cells to make stem cell factor
Interleukin 6 (IL-6)	Ovarian T cells	Suppresses response of granulosa cells to FSH, i.e., decreased progesterone synthesis; induces apoptosis and atresia of granulosa cells
Interleukin 1 (IL-1)	Sertoli cells	Decreases steroidogenesis in interstitial cells
P-Mod-S protein	Peritubular myoid cells	Non-mitogenic factor that regulates differentiation and function of Sertoli cells

C. Actions and Metabolism of Androgens in Males

Circulating androgens influence development and maintenance of several glands and related structures associated with the male genital tract, such as the prostate gland and seminal vesicles, and induce development of certain secondary sexual characters such as growth of the beard and development of skeletal muscles in men. Androgens also exert a negative feedback effect upon the secretion of GTHs primarily through actions at the level of the hypothalamus (see Chapter 4).

The action of testosterone in some of its target cells involves its cytosolic conversion to DHT by the enzyme **5α-reductase**. DHT has a greater affinity for the androgen receptor than does testosterone and hence is more potent than testosterone. Timely development of prostate and bulbourethral glands, the penis and scrotum, are dependent upon conversion of testosterone to DHT by target cells in these structures. This conversion of testosterone to the stronger androgen DHT is necessary due to the low circulating level of testosterone that is insufficient to activate these tissues. Brain tissue also employs 5α-reductase in some neurons, and some effects of testosterone on behavior may involve prior conversion to DHT.

Table 10-5. Plasma Levels of Reproductive Steroid in Mammals

Species	Testosterone (ng/ml)	Dihydrotestosterone (ng/ml)	Estradiol (pg/ml)	Progesterone (ng/ml)
Mustela ermina (stoat)				
Male (annual range)	4.5–26			
Ursus americanus (black bear)				
Female				
Nonpregnant			35–71	17.8
Pregnant			32–35,000	29,40
Elaphus maximus (Asian elephant)				
Male (annual range)	0.7–45			
Female				
Not pregnant (peak)			26	0.153–0.195
Pregnant (peak)			26	4
Macaca fuscata (Japanese monkey)				
Male (annual range)	0.2–19.8			
Female				
Follicular phase (peak)			150	2
Luteal phase (peak)			250	5.3
Homo sapiens				
Male (mean)	7.9	0.4	50	
Female				
Follicular phase (range)	0.6	0.3	60–600	0.3–1.5
Luteal phase (range)	0.6	0.3	200	3–20
Pregnant (range)			5,500–30,000	45–210

Many androgenic responses, however, are not mediated by DHT, and this conversion is not necessary for testosterone to produce these effects. For example, development of wolffian duct derivatives (the epididymis, vas deferens, and seminal vesicles) is accomplished by a low level of testosterone that is sufficiently large to activate receptors without prior conversion to DHT. (The testes generally do not synthesize DHT until puberty.) This effect may occur because local testosterone levels from the developing testes are sufficiently high to effectively activate androgen receptors in these structures. In some target tissues, androgens have been shown to undergo conversion to estrogens through aromatization of the A-ring and removal of the C19 carbon atom (see Chapter 3). Conversion of androgens to estrogens also occurs in both Sertoli and Leydig cells. This process also occurs in the central nervous system where aromatization may be essential to some androgen actions. Induction of some male behaviors in castrates requires aromatization and cannot be induced by essentially non-aromatizable androgens such as DHT, whereas others may be induced by either aromatizable androgens or DHT.

The Sertoli cells, under the influence of FSH, secrete two forms of inhibin that selectively block FSH release from the adenohypophysis. Inhibin activity also has been found in rete testis fluid, seminal plasma, testicular extracts, and ejaculate, suggesting local actions (see Table 10-4). Two forms of inhibin have been isolated: **inhibin A** and **inhibin B** (Figure 10-9) with the latter form being more active. These molecules are glycoprotein heterodimers of 31–35 kDa that possess a common α-subunit combined with one of two β-subunits (βA or βB). Inhibins are believed to be the major factor responsible for negative feedback in the selective regulation of FSH release in both males and females. In addition, a β-subunit heterodimer called **activin** has been isolated from gonads. Activin composed of one βA-subunit and one βB-subunit is a potent releaser of FSH from the pituitary gland in laboratory experiments, although its physiological role is still undetermined. It may be a local regulator since activin receptors occur on spermatogenetic cells in the testis. Alternative forms of activin also have been reported (βA-βA and βB-βB homodimers), but their importance is not established.

V. Endocrine Regulation in Eutherian Females

Regardless of whether an animal exhibits a menstrual cycle in addition to an estrous cycle or not, there are numerous distinctive features that characterize reproduction in all female mammals. In addition to the

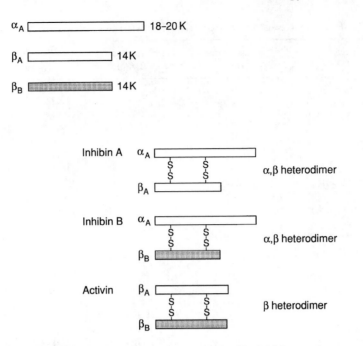

Figure 10-9. **Gonadal proteins of the transforming growth factor β family.** The inhibin proteins are each heterodimers composed of one copy of αA and one copy of either βA (inhibin A) or βB (inhibin B). Activin is a heterodimer composed of one βA-subunit and one βB-subunit. Other activin combinations are known but their biological importance, if any, is unclear. MIS is also a member of this family of bioregulators. See Table 10-4 for descriptions of their local actions.

roles of GTHs and gonadal steroids described below, numerous other regulators (including GnRH, inhibins, prostaglandins, and growth factors) are synthesized in the ovaries and are suspected of playing important paracrine roles in ovarian events. A partial listing and some demonstrated autocrine and paracrine ovarian regulators are provided in Table 10-4. One of those, **growth differentiation factor 9 (GDF-9)** is produced by the oocyte and is responsible for proliferation of follicular cells and subsequent ovarian follicle development. Ovarian and uterine cyclical events during reproduction are similar. The ovarian events are discussed first followed by the uterine events that are linked to the ovarian cycle.

For sexually mature mammals in nature, fertilization and pregnancy are normal events, and coitus occurs frequently during estrus. The character of the ovarian cycle, with its rapid resumption in polyestrous species (or following a short menses as in primates if fertilization and successful implantation do not occur) enhances the chances for successful reproduction. Either rapid reentry into estrus or rapid appearance of one or more new ova or both can occur and a second opportunity to produce offspring is made possible during that season. In some cases, polyestrous animals (especially rodents) produce more than one litter in a single breeding season.

A. The Ovarian Cycle

The basis for the cyclical nature of female reproductive events resides in the hypothalamus and is a genetically determined female characteristic. The ovary undergoes cyclical development in response to GTHs. The duration of the ovarian cycle is characteristic for each species. During proestrous, the growth of one or more follicle occurs in the ovaries. This portion of the ovarian cycle is the **follicular phase**. The follicular phase results in development of one or more mature follicles, each containing one oocyte. Following ovulation, which ends the follicular phase, the remains of a ruptured follicle are transformed into a corpus luteum. Thus, ovulation also marks the onset of the **luteal phase** of the ovarian cycle. The luteal phase may last from a few days to weeks, depending upon the species. Some species, like humans, may begin another follicular phase during the latter portion of the luteal phase whereas others may enter an inactive period (diestrus) that may last until the next breeding season when a new follicular phase is initiated.

1. The Follicular Phase of the Ovarian Cycle

During the follicular phase of the ovarian cycle (Figures 10-10 and 10-11), the tonic hypothalamic center releases small quantities of GnRH into the portal circulation, and relatively low but rather constant circulating levels of FSH, LH, or both are maintained. Prior to puberty, which is characterized by increased GTH levels, the ovary contains **primordial follicles** consisting of **primary oocytes** invested with an additional layer of flattened follicle cells derived from the germinal epithelium that surrounds the ovary. In most mammals, it is assumed that there are no oogonia in the ovary because all of them entered meiosis and became primary oocytes prior to or shortly after birth. However, recent studies in mice have demonstrated new follicle development occurs after birth, and production of new oocytes has been described among certain primates as well.

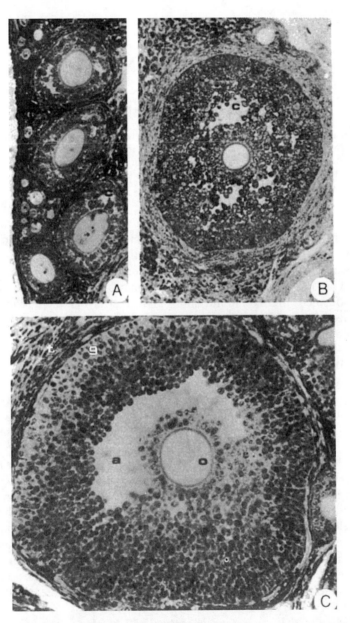

Figure 10-10. **Ovarian follicule stages**. Sections of mouse ovary showing stages of follicular development. (A) Naked oocytes, primary follicles, and four growing follicles. (B) A later follicle with proliferated granulosa and the beginnings of an antral cavity (c). (C) A young antral follicle. a, antrum; g, granulosa; o, oocyte; t, theca. [From K. P. Natty (1978). Follicular fluid. *In* "The Vertebrate Ovary" (R. E. Jones, Ed.), pp. 215–259. Plenum Publishing Corp., New York.]

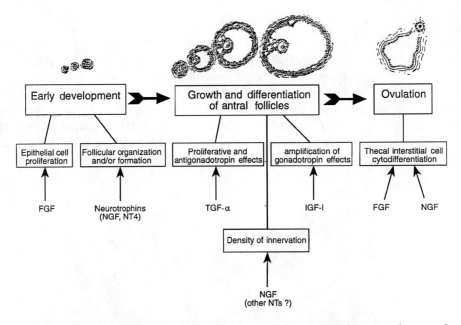

Figure 10-11.   **Follicular phase and growth factors.** Summary of ovarian developmental stages and proposed paracrine actions of certain growth factors and neurotransmitters. FGF, fibroblast growth factor; TGFα, transforming growth factor-α; NGF, nerve growth factor; NT, neurotropins; NT4, neurotropin 4. [Reprinted by permission of the publishers from Ojeda, S. R., and Dissen, G. A. Developmental regulation of the ovary via growth factor tyrosine kinase receptors. *Trends Endocr. Metab.* **5**, 317–323. Copyright 1994 by Elsevier Science Inc.]

The arrival of FSH at the ovary stimulates a number of primordial follicles to begin to enlarge and differentiate into **primary follicles**. The follicle cells surrounding the growing oocyte develop into **granulosa cells** that are in contact with the oocyte. The granulosa cells secrete a basement membrane along their outermost surfaces. A second layer of **thecal cells** derived from the ovarian stroma surrounds the granulosa outside the basement membrane. Thecal cells further differentiate into inner and outer layers: the endocrine **theca interna** and the connective tissue-like **theca externa**. The rich supply of capillaries in the thecal layer do not cross the basement membrane and penetrate the granulose layer. The presence of FSH receptors on the granulosa cells and their ability to proliferate mitotically is initiated by the oocyte through production of GDF-9 (Figure 10-12). In GDF-9-knockout mice, the ovary develops normally but follicle formation is blocked by the failure of follicle cells to respond to FSH.

As the follicle grows, the granulosa cells secrete the **liquor folliculi** or **antral fluid** that is primarily an ultrafiltrate of blood plasma. Increasing production of antral fluid results in formation and progressive enlargement of a fluid-filled cavity within the follicle, the **antrum**. The follicle is now called a **secondary follicle** or an **antral follicle**.

Under the influence of LH and FSH as well as a variety of paracrine factors (see Table 10-4, Figure 10-11), growing ovarian follicles synthesize and release estrogens, predominantly estradiol (= 17β-estradiol), into the general circulation. The synthesis of estrogens in the ovary appears to be a cooperative effort between cells of the theca interna and the granulosa (Figure 10-13). Recent studies support the interpretation that LH stimulates the thecal cells to produce androgens (principally androstenedione) that are aromatized by the granulosa cells to form estradiol. Conversion of androgens to estradiol by the granulosa cells is stimulated by FSH. In turn, FSH increases P450$_{aro}$ levels in these cells. In addition, FSH causes the granulosa cells to produce inhibins which feed back on the pituitary to selectively inhibit FSH release, as was described earlier for males. Inhibin also inhibits P450$_{aro}$ activity locally in granulosa cells whereas the related peptide activin increases P450$_{aro}$ activity.

The final stage of follicle growth is the **tertiary** or **mature follicle** (also called a Graafian follicle). This follicle has reached maximal size and often is characterized by a single large antrum surrounded by a relatively thin layer of granulosa cells with the oocyte relegated to and surrounded by a small mass of granulosa cells, the **cumulus oophorus**. The final meiotic maturation of the oocyte apparently is influenced by paracrine factors

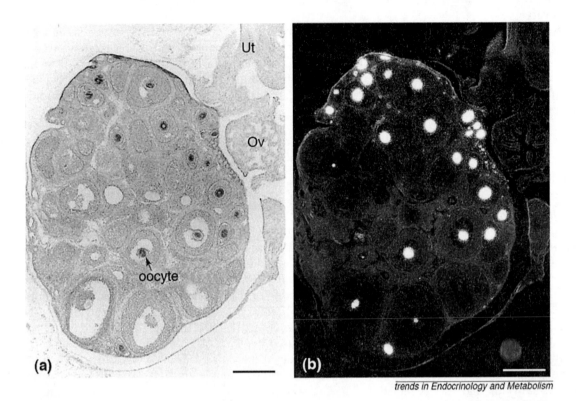

Figure 10-12. **Location of GDF-9 within oocytes**. Mouse ovary showing follicle histology (a) and autoradiography showing location GDF-9 within oocytes only (b). [Reprinted with permission from Erickson, G. F., and Shimasaki, S. The role of the oocyte in folliculogenesis. *Trends Endocr. Metab.* **11**, 193–198. Copyright 2000 by Elsevier Science Ltd.]

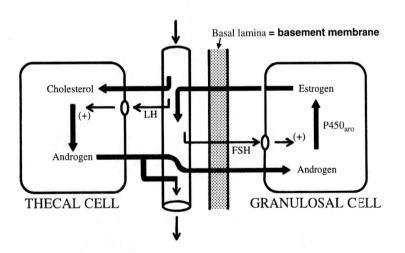

Figure 10-13. **Two-cell model for steroidogenesis**. Binding of LH to receptors found only on thecal cells (or ovarian interstitial cells) stimulates androgen synthesis, most of which diffuses through the basal lamina (basement membrane) to the granulosa cell. FSH stimulates aromatase ($P450_{aro}$) production that transforms androgens into estrogens. A similar two-cell system is present in the testis but with both FSH and LH receptors associated with the interstitial cells (Leydig cells) and FSH receptors on the Sertoli cells. Androgens reach the Sertoli cell by diffusion through the basal lamina surrounding the seminiferous tubule.

from cells of the cumulus oophorus following ovulation. The mature follicle is located just beneath the surface of the ovary.

Most of the follicles that begin to grow during a given ovarian cycle will exhibit apoptosis and degenerate, a process called **atresia**. These degenerating follicles are called **corpora atretica**. Atresia can occur at any stage of follicle development. Some of the steroidogenic cells from these atretic follicles will remain active and contribute to what has been called the **interstitial gland** of the ovary. Androstenedione produced in the interstitial gland by LH stimulation supplements thecal cell contributions for synthesis of estradiol by the granulosa cells.

2. Ovulation

The process of ovulation involves the rupture of the mature follicle and release of the oocyte from the ovary into the body cavity. This event marks the end of the follicular phase and the beginning of the luteal phase in the ovary and is correlated with estrus. Ovulation occurs as a result of the progressive increase in circulating estradiol that occurs with the growth of the follicles. Increased estradiol also is responsible for estrous behavior in the female and the enhanced attractiveness of the female to the male at this time. A maximal or critical estrogen level in the blood in most cases activates the surge center in the hypothalamus, which releases a large pulse of GnRH as described in Chapter 4. The pulse of GnRH released results in the LH surge (Figure 10-14) that causes ovulation of one or more follicles within a matter of hours (usually 12 to 24 hr regardless of the species). The number of follicles that reach maturity and ovulate is species-specific, varying from a norm of one in women to a dozen or more in the sow. The determining factors appear to be the amount of GTH available, and increased numbers of mature follicles are produced following supplementation with exogenous GTHs. The physical mechanism by which LH causes the mature follicle to rupture and release the mature oocyte is not understood completely. It apparently involves changes in the follicular wall that can be attributed to the LH surge and the action of LH on the mature follicle (see Box 10C).

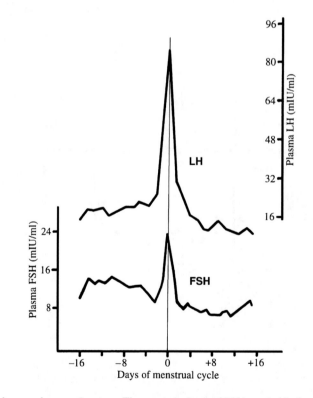

Figure 10-14. **Gonadotropin surge in normal women.** The greater release of LH is probably due to the presence of galanin released with GnRH at this time as well as negative feedback effects of inhibins on FSH release at the pituitary level.

Box 10C. Mechanism of Ovulation

Ovulation occurs as a consequence of a series of events (Box Figure 10-C1) that take place in the follicular wall at an avascular site called the **stigma**. At this location, a locally produced prostaglandin (PGF_2) induces the thecal cells to produce an enzyme, **collagenase**, that digests the intracellular matrix protein, **collagen**. This weakens the follicular wall. Enzymatic breakdown products bring about an inflammatory response and release of another prostaglandin (PGE_2) that causes local blood vessels to constrict, leading to local ischemia and cell death. These events weaken the follicular wall further. Pressure in the antral cavity causes the follicular wall to rupture at its weakest point, the stigma, and the ovum and surround cells of the cumulus oophorus (now called the **corona radiata**) is expelled along with the antral fluid. It is speculated that the smooth muscle-like cells located in the follicular wall may be responsible for producing the increased antral pressure that triggers ovulation. Another hypothesis suggests the increased pressure results from water influx into the antral fluid.

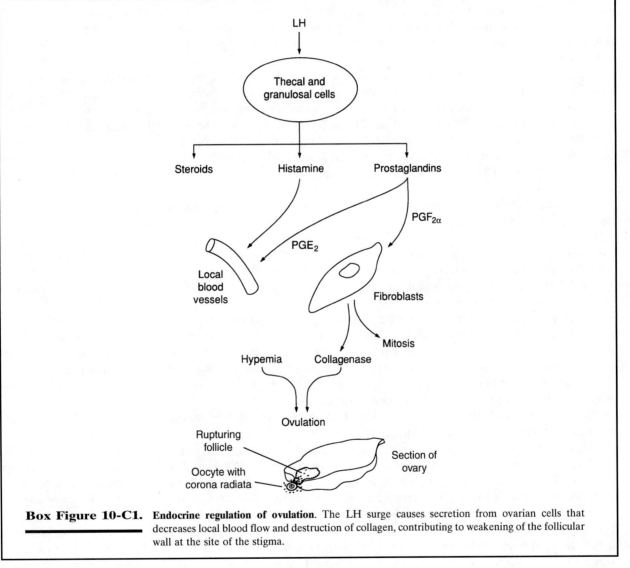

Box Figure 10-C1. **Endocrine regulation of ovulation.** The LH surge causes secretion from ovarian cells that decreases local blood flow and destruction of collagen, contributing to weakening of the follicular wall at the site of the stigma.

In some species, meiosis in the oocyte is not completed until after fertilization. Prior to fertilization, the ovulated cell is an arrested oocyte. If meiosis were completed prior to ovulation, this cell would be termed an ovum. The situation in mammals apparently varies from ovulation of oocytes to ova, but in the following discussions, the ovulated cell in every case will be referred to as an ovum to simplify terminology.

Some mammals ovulate following coitus and are termed **induced ovulators**. Several carnivores (for example, ferrets, minks, raccoons, cats), rodents (for example, *Microtus californicus*), lagomorphs (for example, cottontail and domestic rabbits), at least one bat (the lump-nosed bat), and several insectivores (for example, hedgehogs, common shrews) are confirmed induced ovulators. Some other species are suspected to be induced ovulators including the elephant seal, the nutria, and the long-nosed kangaroo rat (a marsupial). Most mammals are believed to be **spontaneous ovulators** in that the LH surge and ovulation are independent of coitus. However, even some spontaneous ovulators can be induced to ovulate following copulation under special conditions. Evidence from humans suggests ovulation may be induced in rape cases especially if the female is very young.

3. The Luteal Phase of the Ovarian Cycle

Ovulation marks the onset of the **luteal phase** of the ovarian cycle as well as the end of the follicular phase. In addition to causing ovulation, the LH surge induces granulosa cells as well as some theca interna cells to differentiate into the **corpus luteum**. This process, known as **luteinization**, results in the corpus luteum, which functions as an endocrine gland, secreting both estrogens and progesterone into the general circulation. One corpus luteum will form from each ovulated follicle. In addition, other developing follicles may undergo premature luteinization and function as **accessory corpora lutea** during pregnancy. The corpus luteum begins secreting large quantities of progesterone, along with lesser amounts of estradiol as well as other other estrogens and progestogens. Circulating progesterone and estrogens inhibit both the tonic and cyclic hypothalamic GnRH centers during the luteal phase so that additional follicular development is arrested and a second ovulatory episode is prevented. All developing follicles that do not ovulate undergo atresia or form accessory corpora lutea. Some of the follicular cells from the atretic follicles will persist as part of the ovarian interstitial gland that is responsive to LH and synthesizes androstenedione that can be used as a substrate by the corpus luteum to form estradiol.

Depending on the species, regulation of corpora lutea function may require LH or be independent of LH once it has formed. In sheep, PRL together with LH apparently stimulates steroid secretion by the corpus luteum. However, only PRL is necessary to maintain the activity of the rat corpus luteum. Preovulatory estradiol can produce a surge of PRL release in several species and might be related to corpora lutea function. These actions of PRL on the corpus luteum were the basis for the older name of luteotropic hormone for this molecule. However, PRL has no role in corpus luteum functions in primates and most other mammals, and the older name should not be used.

The corpus luteum secretes steroids for only a relatively short period in many species (five to eight days in humans) after which it begins to degenerate. As the corpus luteum undergoes degeneration, steroidogenesis declines, and the uterus enters a regressive phase unless the animal becomes pregnant. In some species, the corpus luteum is relatively long-lived, especially in carnivorous species like the dog, which will not reenter estrus until the next breeding season. Corpora lutea in the bitch are active for about 63 days after ovulation, which is equivalent to the normal gestation period.

The predetermined life span for the functional corpus luteum has provided one of the most intriguing mysteries of the ovarian cycle. Apparently, the corpus luteum sows the seeds of its own destruction. In female rats, mice, hamsters, rabbits, guinea pigs, and ewes, progesterone from the corpora lutea stimulates the synthesis and release of prostaglandins of the F series (PGFs, see Chapter 3) from the uterine endometrium. These PGFs, especially $PGF_{2\alpha}$, are **luteolytic factors**, that is, they cause destruction of the corpus luteum and cessation of steroidogenesis. The mechanism of their luteolytic activity is not clear, although it may relate to an influence on the integrity of the blood vascular supply to the corpus luteum. In primates, the destruction of the corpus luteum toward the end of the luteal phase is not influenced by the uterus but appears to be caused locally by a luteolytic factor (e.g., estrone), produced by the corpus luteum itself. Once fertilization has taken place, there are several mechanisms by which corpus luteum degeneration may be prevented and the life of the corpus luteum prolonged (see below).

Degeneration of the corpora lutea frees the hypothalamic GnRH centers from the inhibitory influence of estrogens and progesterone, resulting in a moderate increase in circulating GTHs and consequently renewal of follicular development. In fact, increased FSH release occurs in many species during the later stages of the luteal phase so that follicular growth may resume even before regressive uterine events become obvious.

The importance of the corpus luteum in maintaining pregnancy varies considerably as does the role of pituitary hormones in stimulating corpus luteum function. For example, in rats, PRL is necessary for maintaining the first half of gestation through actions on the corpus luteum. However, in pigs, the corpora lutea secrete progesterone to maintain the uterine secretory phase during the early portion of the gestation period without aid of any pituitary hormones. In ewes, both LH and PRL are necessary for maintaining corpus luteum function during the first third of pregnancy, but maintenance of pregnancy actually resides in the ability of the conceptus to neutralize the uterine luteolytic factor $PGF_{2\alpha}$. Estrogens of placental origin apparently are responsible for prolonging the life span of corpora lutea in rabbits as well as promoting progesterone synthesis. If the estrogen-secreting placental cells are damaged (for example, by X-rays), pregnancy is abruptly terminated.

B. The Uterine Cycle

The uterine cycle can be separated into a **proliferative phase** corresponding to the ovarian follicular phase, a **secretory phase** corresponding roughly to the ovarian luteal phase, and a **post-luteal phase** (Figure 10-15). The proliferative phase is separated from the secretory phase by the occurrence of ovulation. The end of the luteal phase marks the entrance into the post-luteal phase that is a quiescent period of slow regression of the uterine eopitheium in most mammals and is termed the **menses** in mammals that exhibit menstrual cycles.

The wall of the uterus consists of an outermost connective tissue covering, a thick intermediate layer of smooth muscle called the **myometrium**, and an innermost epithelium, the **endometrium**, that contacts the uterine lumen. The endometrium can be further separated into an outer **basal layer** that proliferates during each uterine cycle to produce an inner **functional layer** that later regresses or is shed.

1. The Proliferative Phase of the Uterine Cycle

Estradiol produced during the follicular phase by the ovary stimulates differentiation and proliferation of the endometrium in preparation for implantation of the **blastocyst**, an embryonic stage formed from the first series of cellular divisions following fertilization. The blastocyst consists of an outer extraembryonic layer of cells, the **trophoblast**, which will form the fetal component of the placenta, and an **inner cell mass**, which will become the embryo proper. The proliferative phase of the uterine cycle is characterized by hyperplasia of the basal layer of the endometrium to form the functional layer in response to estrogens secreted by the growing ovarian follicles. In addition, there is a marked increase in the vasculature (hyperemia) of the functional layer

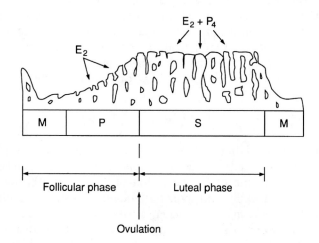

Figure 10-15. **The uterine cycle with menses.** The menses (M) occupies the first 5 days of the human cycle. The endometrium is stimulated by estradiol (E_2) during the proliferative stage (P). The follicular phase in the ovary corresponds to M + P. Following ovulation the corpus luteum secretes E_2 and progesterone (P_4) during the luteal phase which maintain the vascularity of the endometrium as well as secretion by exocrine glands during the secretory phase (S). Following the death of the corpus luteum, the uterine lining degenerates and the uterus reenters menses.

as a result of estradiol stimulation. In higher primates, this hyperemia response includes the development of special **spiral arteries** that play an important role in the menstrual cycle of these mammals.

There may be two independent targets for estradiol in the uterus. One target is the basal epithelial cell that responds to estrogens with new protein synthesis and mitosis. This results in an increase in the functional layer as well as in the development of tubular uterine exocrine glands. A second target for estrogens is the uterine eosinophil, which is a white blood cell that has infiltrated the uterine lining. These eosinophils possess specific receptors for estradiol and appear to be responsible for the rapid uptake of water and release of histamine that causes local hyperemia.

2. The Secretory Phase of the Uterine Cycle

Progesterone and estradiol secreted by the corpora lutea in the ovary are the hormones controlling this phase that is characterized by secretion of the exocrine glands in the functional layer of the endometrium. During the secretory phase, estradiol maintains the proliferated uterine endometrium and increased hyperemia that were initiated during the proliferative phase. Progesterone stimulates the uterine glands to secrete a fluid called **uterine milk** or **embryotroph**. Uterine milk is believed to be a source of nourishment for unimplanted blastocysts. The endometrium of both eutherian and marsupial mammals produces uterine milk. Progesterone and estradiol also maintain the highly vascularized state of the uterus necessary for implantation and development of the embryo. Uterine muscle becomes desensitized by progesterone and reduces the chance that rhythmic contractions of the uterine smooth muscle might dislodge an implanting or recently implanted blastocyst.

3. The Post-Luteal Phase of the Uterine Cycle

If fertilization is successful and implantation occurs, the secretory phase will continue throughout pregnancy. Should implantation not occur, the corpus luteum of many eutherian mammals will rapidly degenerate, resulting in a marked decrease in circulating levels of progesterone and estrogens. This decrease in circulating ovarian steroids causes regressive changes in the endometrium following steroid withdrawal. The endometrium becomes less vascular and secretion by the uterine glands is reduced. Thus, the uterus becomes less capable of supporting implantation of a blastocyst. In monoestrous species such as carnivores, the uterus would enter the quiescent post-luteal phase called diestrus during which the functional layer would be slowly resorbed. In polyestrous species, however, the female may quickly reenter proestrus, resulting in the resumption of endocrine secretions that would prevent uterine regression.

Instead of a quiescent post-luteal phase, animals with a menstrual cycle exhibit a rapid regression and actual sloughing of the outer portion of the endometrium during the menses if implantation is not successful. In higher primates, the spiral blood vessels constrict, preventing flow of blood to the functional layer of the endometrium and causing extensive cell death. The degenerating tissue and trapped blood are sloughed into the uterine lumen where it is resorbed or discharged as the menstrual flow. Following the menses, considerable rebuilding of the endometrium (another proliferative phase) must occur during the next follicular ovarian phase to prepare for implantation of blastocysts resulting from the next ovulation.

C. The Pregnancy Cycle

Estrus usually occurs just prior to ovulation and normally leads to mating. The recently ovulated ovum still surrounded by some of the granulosa cells, the **corona radiata**, enters the open upper end of the fluid-filled oviduct and is propelled toward the uterus by the action of cilia lining the oviduct. The possible role of muscular contractions of the oviduct wall in transport of the ovum has been suggested but not verified. Sperm deposited in the vagina by the copulating male during estrus are transported at least in part by peristalsis through the uterus and ascend into an oviduct in which recently ovulated ova are descending. Fertilization leading to successful implantation typically occurs in the upper third of the oviduct. Cleavage begins soon after fertilization, and the **zygote** or fertilized egg rapidly becomes a minute, multicellular blastocyst. The outer layer of the blastocyst, the trophoblast, will give rise to the extraembryonic membrane called the **chorion**. The trophoblast produces enzymes that enable the blastocyst to implant; i.e., erode the highly vascularized, secretory uterine endometrium and settle in for development.

Implantation marks the beginning of gestation or pregnancy. In some species, the blastocyst may not implant immediately into the endometrium but may remain in the uterine lumen for a period of time before implanting. This **delayed implantation** (see Box 10D) allows species with a short developmental period to prolong the time before birth will take place after mating. The gestation period is specific for each species and may be as short as 12 days in the opossum (a marsupial) or as long as 22 months in an elephant (eutherian).

Box 10D. Delayed Implantation

Several eutherian mammals, such as mink, bats, and skunks, have evolved a mechanism known as delayed implantation whereby development of the blastocyst is arrested and the unimplanted blastocyst remains in the oviduct or uterus for an extended period prior to implantation. Among some eutherian mammals, delayed implantation appears to be an adaptation allowing copulation to occur at a particular time that is especially advantageous to the parent while ensuring that the young are born at the most favorable time for their survival. Neither the basis for causing the blastocyst to remain in a healthy, arrested state nor the stimulus to bring about implantation is known.

Macropodid marsupials have developed a form of delayed implantation called embryonic diapause. Embryonic diapause has been reported for 14 macropodid species but does not occur in at least one species, the western gray kangaroo. One major difference from delayed implantation occurring in eutherian mammals is the condition of the resting blastocyst. The macropodid blastocyst consists of about 70 to 100 cells of a uniform type termed protoderm. The macropodid blastocyst is surrounded by a shell membrane and an albumen layer. It has not yet differentiated into embryonic (inner cell mass) and extraembryonic (trophoblast) regions like that of the eutherians.

Presence of a joey suckling on a teat presumably evokes release of oxytocin from the pars nervosa. Oxytocin is believed to arrest corpus luteum functions while allowing lactation to occur. Removal of the suckling joey will allow the resting blastocyst to implant. Ovariectomy following ovulation induces diapause, but if ovariectomy is performed during diapause there is no effect on the duration of diapause. Progesterone administered to either intact or ovariectomized females stimulates cessation of diapause and reinstates blastocyst development. Estrogen is also effective, but continued embryonic development is not as successful as following progesterone treatment.

In the red kangaroo, embryonic diapause may be an adaptation to renew pregnancy immediately following the death of the joey living in the pouch. The gestation period for the red kangaroo is 33 days. After birth the newborn must find its way to the pouch virtually unaided. When it reaches the pouch, the joey attaches itself permanently to a teat and continues development as an exteriorized fetus. Soon after parturition, the mother kangaroo enters estrus again and mates. The presence of one joey in the pouch inhibits implantation of the new blastocyst resulting from the second mating. The new blastocyst remains in a suspended state of development for up to 200 days, at which time the first joey normally disengages itself from the teat and ventures into the outside world as a juvenile kangaroo. The newly liberated kangaroo will return at intervals to the teat to which it was formerly attached for nourishment. Meanwhile the detachment of the first joey from the teat either releases an inhibition to implantation or provides an endocrine stimulus for implantation of the waiting blastocyst.

In about 4 weeks, the gestation period terminates in birth of the second joey. The new joey enters the pouch and attaches to a teat. The mother kangaroo again enters estrus and mates, and another blastocyst enters embryonic diapause. Thus a female red kangaroo may have a young juvenile that requires occasional nourishment, a joey attached to a teat, and a blastocyst "waiting in the wings." During extensive periods of drought, the older joey could be denied milk and allowed to die. The implantation of the waiting blastocyst soon provides another joey whose demands upon the mother's nutritional reserves and water supply would be very small in comparison to the demands of the larger joey. Next, the mother would reenter estrus, produce another diapausing blastocyst, and be ready to continue reproducing should conditions improve.

In carnivores, such as the domestic dog, the corpora lutea normally function throughout gestation since the length of the normal luteal phase is equal to the gestation period. In others, the corpora lutea would degenerate much earlier with respect to the time required for gestation if fertilization and implantation were not successful.

A central question puzzled reproductive physiologists for many years: how did mammals "know" they were pregnant and how did they prolong corpora luteal function and prevent premature regression or sloughing of the endometrium? It turns out there are several mechanisms.

The signal for prolongation of corpora luteal function in some species is the synthesis of an LH-like chorionic gonadotropin (CG) by the blastocyst even before implantation. Placental GTHs are structurally very similar to pituitary GTHs and generally produce LH-like effects (see Chapter 4). Their synthesis and release, however, are not influenced in a negative way by steroids in the manner of the steroidal feedback on pituitary GTHs. The trophoblast of the developing human blastocyst begins to secrete hCG prior to implantation. hCG appears in maternal blood within a few days of fertilization and soon after appears in sufficient quantities in urine to be detected with antibody-based pregnancy kits. Later, the trophoblast will contribute to the placenta following implantation and will continue to secrete hCG throughout pregnancy.

In the mare, only fertilized ova ever reach the uterus, implying some sort of early chemical recognition that fertilization has occurred. The equine chorionic gonadotropin is called **pregnant mare serum gonadotropin (PMSG)** and appears in large amounts in the urine of pregnant horses.

LH-like GTHs can prolong the life of the corpus luteum that continues to secrete progesterone and estradiol, thus maintaining the secretory phase of the uterus. Secretion of ovarian steroids by the corpus luteum inhibits hypothalamic centers controlling pituitary GTH release so that follicular development and subsequent ovulation are blocked in pregnant animals. Suppression of subsequent follicular development and ovulation prevents having several embryos in the uterus at different stages of development. This would create the problem of expulsion of the younger embryos and fetuses during parturition of the oldest one(s).

While the HPG system is more or less shut down during pregnancy, the placenta begins to function as a composite HPG axis in the female. Thus, we observe secretion of hypothalamic peptides (e.g., GnRH, TRH, CRH), tropic-like hormones (e.g., ACTH, CG), and gonadal steroids (estrogens, progesterone). Furthermore, during the last third of pregnancy, another pituitary-like hormone, **chorionic somatomammotropin (CS)**, is secreted by the placenta in a number of species (primates, mice, rats, voles, guinea pigs, sheep, chinchillas, and hamsters but not bitches or rabbits). This placental hormone has both growth hormone (GH)-like and PRL-like activities. Antibodies to CS will cross-react with both GH and PRL in at least some of these species. The major roles for CS appear to be effects on metabolism (GH-like) and stimulation of the mammary gland to begin milk synthesis during the later stages of pregnancy. In humans, hCS formerly was called **human placental lactogen (hPL)**. The human placenta also secretes PRL that is identical to pituitary PRL. Placental PRL accumulates in the amniotic fluid during pregnancy where it is thought to regulate volume and ionic composition of amniotic fluid. Levels of amniotic PRL are not affected by drugs that block maternal pituitary PRL release or even by hypophysectomy of the mother.

D. Birth (Parturition)

The birth process requires coordinated hormonal changes that culminate in the expulsion of the fetus and the associated placenta. Birth can be related to levels of estrogens, progesterone, OXY, prostaglandins, relaxin, corticosteroids, and CRH. The pattern varies in different mammals as to what hormones are involved and the patterns of their secretions. For example, the stimulus for birth in humans is not related to a decrease in progesterone levels as shown for sheep (Figure 10-16) but rather to a marked increase in estrogens relative to progesterone (Figure 10-17).

In sheep, there is a marked reduction in circulating progesterone levels just prior to birth that, presumably, sensitizes the uterus to OXY. The contractions of the uterus initiated by OXY result in expulsion of the fetus as well as of the **afterbirth** (the detached placenta). Experimental studies in sheep show that the fetal adrenal axis plays an essential role in the initiation of the birth process. Factors that interfere with adrenal function at any level retards the normal onset of labor, and premature birth can be induced by addition of ACTH or corticosteroids.

In humans, there is no drop in progesterone to trigger birth although there is a relative increase in estradiol production as compared with progesterone (see Figure 10-17). Not only is the fetal adrenal essential for maintaining pregnancy, it also is involved in the events associated with birth (Figure 10-18). Recent studies demonstrate that CRH from the placenta initiates birth by binding to receptors in the uterine myometrium and stimulating the local production of prostaglandins that in turn induce myometrial contractions. Cortisol secreted by the fetal adrenal stimulates increased estradiol secretion by the placenta that changes the

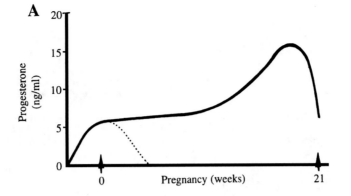

Figure 10-16. **Progesterone levels in pregnant sheep.** Progesterone levels in ewes during the normal cycle (dotted line) and pregnancy. Note the drop in progesterone that occurs prior to birth.

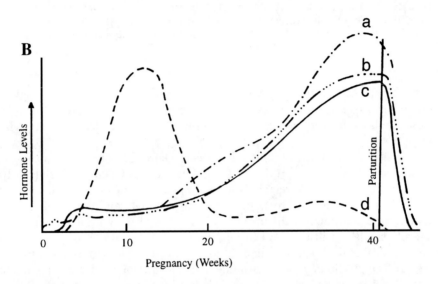

Figure 10-17. **Pattern of hormone secretion during human pregnancy.** Note that maternal progesterone levels do not decrease until detachment of the placenta. (a) hCS, (b) estrogens, (c) progesterone, (d) hCG.

estradiol/progesterone ratio. This change results in increased production of OXY receptors in the uterine myometrium, facilitating contractions. Cortisol also increases CRH production by the placenta at this time, setting up a positive feedback on the fetal adrenal via placental CRH as well as increasing the effects of CRH on the myometrium. Women with higher levels of CRH early in pregnancy are more likely to exhibit higher levels later on and give birth prematurely. Cortisol from the fetus near term also induces the lungs to begin production of surfactants that will be essential for the switch to breathing air that occurs after birth.

Mechanical stimulation of the vagina, cervix, or uterus can release OXY in humans and induce a fetal ejection reflex. Administration of prostaglandins also can induce uterine contractions, and OXY may stimulate prostaglandin synthesis in the uterus. Synthetic OXY is normally used to induce labor in women and frequently is given to reduce postpartum bleeding following detachment of the placenta. OXY is preferred over prostaglandins for clinical uses even though both are involved in normal births because administration of prostaglandins tends to produce strong contractile effects on non-reproductive smooth muscle as well (i.e., gastrointestinal smooth muscle).

Relaxin, an insulin-like peptide unique to pregnancy, was discovered in 1932 to cause relaxation and softening of estrogen-primed pelvic ligaments, allowing the pelvis to stretch and expand (relax) during birth. This expansion allows the relatively large head of the mammalian fetus to pass through the pelvis during parturition. Relaxin reaches peak levels prior to birth and rapidly disappears from the maternal circulation afterward. Spontaneous motility of the uterus may be inhibited by relaxin in some mammals, thereby reducing

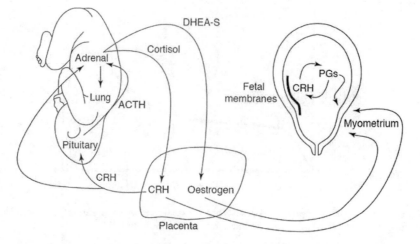

Figure 10-18. **Fetal HPA axis and parturition**. A positive feedback is established between fetal cortisol and placental CRH. Estrogen and CRH cooperate to initiate contractions in the uterine myometrium.[Reprinted with permission from McLean, M., and Smith, R. Corticotropin-releasing hormone in human pregnancy and parturition. *Trends Endocr. Metab.* **10**, 174–178. © 1999, Elsevier Science Inc.]

the risk of premature birth. Relaxin working with estrogens, progesterone, and prostaglandins actually can alter the structural collagen of the uterine cervix, increasing its distensibility at parturition. There are data supporting an action of relaxin in combination with steroids and PRL on the mammary gland and the onset of lactation following birth.

The corpus luteum is the major source of relaxin in species where the corpus luteum is retained throughout gestation (pig, rat, carnivores). Relaxin is produced by the human corpus luteum during early gestation and to some extent by the placenta. Only a little relaxin is found in placentas of sheep, rats, cows, and rabbits, but in horses the placenta is the major source of relaxin. In humans, the ovarian interstitial cells continue to be the major site for relaxin synthesis during pregnancy even after death of the corpus luteum.

Relaxin is chemically similar to insulin and insulin-like growth factors (IGFs) and consists of two short A-chains (22–24 amino acids) and a longer B-chain (26–35 amino acids) joined together by disulfide bonds (see Chapter 3, Figure 3-11). The positioning of the disulfide bonds is the same as for insulin and the IGFs although there are many differences in amino acids sequences. It has been suggested that the relaxin gene arose by duplication from the insulin gene. Subsequent to this duplication, there has been considerable divergence in the relaxin genes among mammals as evidenced by considerable variation in amino acid sequences of mammalian relaxins.

E. Lactation

The development of mammary glands, their synthesis of milk, and the ejection of milk to the suckling offspring are all regulated by hormones. Mammary glands in eutherian mammals usually occur as paired structures, from 2 to 18, and may be located on the thorax (man, elephant, bat), along the entire ventral thorax and abdomen (sow, rabbit), in the inguinal region (horse, ruminants), along the abdomen (whale), or even dorsally (the nutria, a South American rodent). The internal structure is rather uniform and includes supporting stromal cells and a glandular epithelium that is organized into clusters of minute, sac-like structures called **alveoli**. It is this glandular epithelium that is responsible for synthesis of milk. The alveoli are continuous with ducts and various duct-derived enlargements for storing milk. In addition, there are modified epithelial cells that contain muscle-like myofilaments parallel to the long axis of the cells. These cells are termed **myoepithelial cells** and are capable of contracting and causing ejection of milk from the alveoli into the duct system and out of the gland in the region of the nipple.

Information obtained from the mouse and rat indicates that differentiation of mammary glands from ectoderm involves specific induction by a particular underlying mesenchyme. These glands in both mother and fetus normally undergo hyperplasia and hypertrophy with the aid of estrogens during the last third of the gestational period. The placenta is the source of these estrogens. Androgens partially suppress mammary gland development and are presumably responsible for the lack of stimulation seen in the male fetus.

Postnatal mammary development involves hormones from the pituitary, ovaries, and adrenal cortex, at least in mice and rats. Growth of mammary ducts requires estrogens, GH, and corticosterone working in concert. However, expansion of the alveoli (called lobuloalveolar growth) is dependent upon the direct interactions of estrogens, progesterone, PRL, GH, relaxin, and corticosteroids.

Lactation can be separated into two basic processes or phases under separate endocrine control mechanisms. The first phase is milk secretion or **lactogenesis**. This process primarily is controlled by pituitary PRL (or placental CS), growth factors, and glucocorticoids. In primates, lactogenesis also is stimulated by GH. Lactogenesis involves synthesis of milk fat, milk protein, and milk sugar, typically lactose. The synthesis of lactose ultimately depends upon protein synthesis; that is, the enzyme responsible for lactose synthesis, lactose synthetase, must be induced. Lactose synthetase is composed of two protein units, one of which is lactalbumin, which also is found in milk. Lactose, fat, and milk protein (largely casein) are secreted into the lumen of the alveolus. Water and numerous water-soluble substances enter the lumen by osmosis and result in a watery liquid known as milk. Many hormones are present in milk including hypothalamic peptides, pituitary hormones, growth factors, steroids, gastrointestinal peptides, and others (see Table 10-6). In addition, the mammary route may conduct lipid-soluble pollutants such as PCBs and pesticides accumulated by the mother to the offspring especially to the first born.

The composition of milk produced by the mammary gland associated with suckling the young is very different at birth from what it will be shortly thereafter. This first milk, known as **colostrum**, is characterized by having a greater concentration of protein and less carbohydrate than does later milk. Colostrum contains antibodies and other substances that serve to protect the neonate against allergies and diseases while its own immune response system is developing.

The second phase of lactation is **milk ejection**, a simple reflex mechanism controlled by OXY from the pars nervosa. Mechanical stimulation of the nipple (suckling) evokes release of OXY from the pars nervosa via a spinohypothalamic neuronal pathway. Release of PRL also occurs when milk is ejected and stimulates further milk synthesis. OXY stimulates contraction of myoepithelial cells that causes milk to be ejected from the alveoli into the ducts and storage channels of the mammary gland. The suckling by the young animal strips this milk from the gland by expressing it between the tongue and hard palate.

The milk ejection neurohormonal reflex exhibits classical conditioning responses as evidenced by stimulation of milk flow in the cow by sight and sounds of the milking parlor or in women by the cries of their hungry infant. This reflex can be influenced by other neural or chemical inputs to the hypothalamus. For example,

Table 10-6. Some Chemical Regulators Found in Milk[a]

Regulator type	Examples	Regulator type	Examples
Adenohyophysial hormones	PRL	Gastrointestinal peptides	VIP
	GH		CCK
	TSH		Gastrin
	FSH		GIP
	LH		Substance P
	ACTH		Neurotensin
Growth factors	IGF-I	Steroid hormones	Estradiol
	NGF		Progesterone
	EGF		Testosterone
	TGF-α		Corticosterone
	PDGF		Vitamin D
Neurohormones	TRH	Other regulators	Prostaglandins (PGE, PGF$_{2\alpha}$)
	GnRH		cAMP
	SS		Delta sleep-inducing peptide
	GHRH		Relaxin
	Oxytocin		Thyroid hormones (T$_3$, T$_4$, rT$_3$)
			Calcitonin
			Parathyroid hormone

[a] see Appendix A for abbreviations.

stress or physical discomfort can inhibit ejection of milk in the presence of the stimulus that would normally elicit release of OXY.

F. Menopause

In nature, few animals live beyond their peak of reproductive activity due to predation, disease, or other environmentally related phenomenon. In contrast, life after reproductive age is a common occurrence in human females. Whereas men may produce viable sperm most of their lives, the ovary becomes refractory to GTHs, usually during the mid to late 40s. This transitional stage is called **menopause**. Cycles of these women become irregular and eventually they cease to ovulate and menstruate. This is accompanied by a marked depression in circulating levels of gonadal steroids as well as of adrenal androgens and by an elevation in GTH levels. The transition from **premenopausal** (actively reproductive) to **postmenopausal** (non-reproductive) usually is gradual over several years and may be accompanied by additional symptoms including vaginal atrophy, hot flashes or flushes, reduced libido, and accelerated bone resorption leading to calcium deficiency syndromes such as osteopenia and osteoporosis (see Chapter 14). Many studies have shown that heart disease and other cardiovascular disorders increase exponentially in postmenopausal women and deaths due to cardiac disease are several-fold greater than for uterine and breast cancer combined.

Hormone (estrogen or estrogen-progestogen) replacement therapy (HRT) alleviates many of the symptoms for postmenopausal women. When taken with calcium supplements and a regimen of weight-bearing exercise, steroid therapy also can prevent bone resorption that otherwise can lead to decreased bone density associated with osteoporosis (see Chapter 14). However, potential benefits of estrogen therapy need to be considered in the light of recent studies that show prolonged HRT (longer than 5 years) is associated with a small increase in risk for reproductive cancers and cardiovascular disease. Thus, the decision for a postmenopausal woman to elect HRT involves weighing the pros and cons for her specific situation in consultation with a knowledgeable physician.

Exposure to other estrogenic chemicals through food, water, cosmetics, and other sources (i.e., phytoestrogens, bisphenol A, nonylphenols, ethinylestradiol, phthalates, certain pesticides, etc.) should also be considered as they do contribute to the total estrogen exposure. Careful scientific studies have verified that mixtures of estrogenic chemicals at levels unlikely for each to produce estrogenic effects are additive when they all work through the same mechanism (e.g., binding to and activating the estrogen receptor, ERα).

Men also experience reproductive decline with age, although this "male menopause" or **andropause** occurs more gradually and is not so evident as female menopause. Testosterone levels begin to decline after about age 30 and can lead to clinical signs in the 50s and 60s. Symptoms of andropause include reduced libido (sex drive), depression, loss of skeletal muscle mass, increased body fat, declines in cognitive ability, and osteoporosis. Metabolic changes may be responsible for the correlation of low testosterone with increased risk for cardiovascular disease. Although testosterone therapies are appearing on the market, the known relationships between excess androgens and cancer induction should be considered before embarking on either a preventative or restorative course.

VI. Reproductive Cycles in Selected Eutherian Females

In this section, four reproductive cycles are presented as being representative of eutherian mammals: 4-day cycling rats, ewes, women, and elephants. These four examples emphasize both the features described previously that are characteristic of eutherian mammals and some of the differences seen among different species. The cycles of these species are among the best known, but not necessarily representative of all mammals. Ewes and rats are polyestrous species with distinct periods of estrus whereas women have no seasonal estrous behavior and exhibit a menstrual cycle. Both rats and women are continuous breeders, but ewes, like elephants, are distinctly seasonal breeders. Reproductive cycle length varies from 4 or 5 days in rats to 16 days in sheep, 28 days in humans, and 16 weeks in elephants. Cows and pigs have cycles that are essentially like the ewe cycle although they differ somewhat in timing of the various events. Rats have a short gestation period lasting only 22 days whereas elephants at the other extreme have a 22-month gestation period. None of these species exhibits delayed implantation, and all are believed to be spontaneous ovulators except for the rat and possibly the human under special conditions.

A. The Four-Day Cycling Rat

The laboratory rat cycle (Figure 10-19) is separable into **proestrus** (1 day), **estrus** (1 day), and **diestrus** (2 or 3 days) and is cued closely to environmental events. Typically, several follicles develop and ovulate during each cycle resulting in multiple corpora lutea in the postovulatory ovary.

GTHs from the pituitary stimulate ovarian follicle development and steroidogenesis. On the morning of the day prior to estrus (that is, during proestrus), the levels of estrogen in the plasma reaches a peak that stimulates an LH surge accompanied by a small surge in FSH. The GTH surge occurs on the afternoon of proestrus and is followed rapidly by a marked surge of progesterone from several short-lived corpora lutea. Ovulation occurs a few hours after midnight on the day of estrus. Several follicles usually mature simultaneously, and multiple ovulations commonly occur. Estrus lasts about 9 to 15 hours, during which time the female is highly receptive to the male. Ovulation occurs during estrus. Cornified cells, which were produced by the actions of estrogens during proestrus, appear in the superficial layers of the vagina, and their presence in vaginal smears characterizes estrus (Figure 10-20). In fact, this action was used as a bioassay for many years to define whether any compound had estrogenic activity (see Appendix D). Today, we have substituted more molecular techniques to assess estrogen activity (see Chapter 2).

The third and fourth days of the cycle are termed **diestrus I** and **diestrus II**. Vaginal smears prepared during diestrus are characterized by the absence of cornified cells and a pre-dominance of leukocytes in the smear. There is limited secretory function by the corpora lutea, as evidenced by a slight increase in plasma progesterone. Much of this progesterone is produced by ovarian interstitial cells, which constitute what has been called a permanent corpus luteum in the rat ovary. This interstitial tissue responds to LH by secreting both progesterone and 20α-dihydroprogesterone.

Many researchers recognize a short transitional period between estrus and diestrus in rats termed **metestrus**. The female in metestrus is no longer receptive to the male, but some cornified cells still appear in smears prepared from the vaginal mucosa.

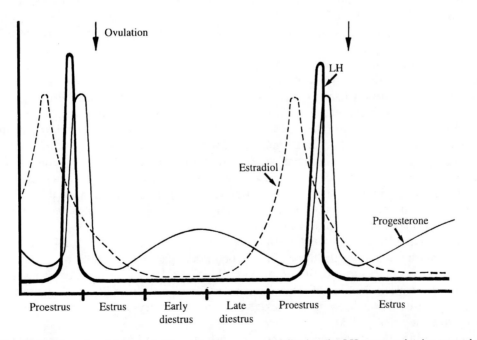

Figure 10-19. Ovulatory cycle of 4-day rat. The progesterone surge following the LH surge and prior to ovulation (arrow) is responsible for increased receptivity in the female for the male. There is a secondary, slow increase and decline in progesterone secretion from the corpus luteum that occurs during diestrous in the unmated female.

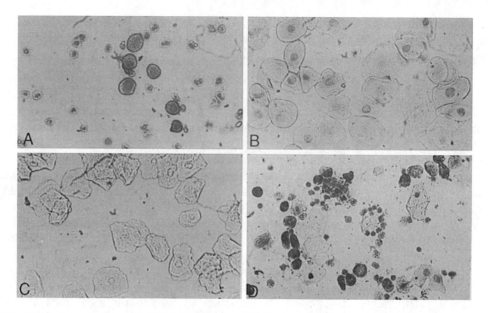

Figure 10-20. **Vaginal smears from rats during estrous cycle.** (A) Diestrus. Absence of cornified (keratinized) cells and presence of small leukocytes. (B) Proestrus. Many live epithelial cells with smooth margins. Leukocytes absent. (C) Estrus. Large cornified cells with irregular margins. (D) Metestrus. Leukocytes have infiltrated among the cornified cells. This stage is transitional between estrus and diestrus.

Mating stimulates the GnRH surge followed by ovulation and consequently the corpora lutea form and begin to secrete significant amounts of progestogens. This increased production of progestogens will inhibit hypothalamus-pituitary function and delay the onset of the next cycle. If fertilization and implantation do not result from mating, the rat will not return immediately to proestrus but will delay resumption of proestrus for a few days. This period of copulation-induced **pseudopregnancy** often occurs in laboratory rodents and sometimes in other domestic mammals. The condition of pseudopregnancy is often accompanied by PRL-like effects on lactation and behavior presumably due to pituitary release of PRL.

If implantation does occur, the corpora lutea continue to secrete progestogens under the influence of placental CG and begin to secrete relaxin. The rat placenta also produces CS, which contributes to stimulation of mammary gland development and lactogenesis prior to birth.

Pheromones have been shown to play central roles in mating and successful pregnancy in rodents. Crowded female mice become anaestrus when no males are present (called the Lee-Boot effect). However, simply the odor from a male mouse can cause them to synchronously ovulate and enter estrus (Whitten effect). The endocrinological basis for these effects is suggested by observations that pheromones from female mice suppress pituitary release of FSH, whereas male pheromone stimulates GTH release that is followed in normal sequence by an LH surge and ovulation. A newly mated female mouse may abort if placed with a "strange" male (not the previous mate), and the likelihood of spontaneous abortion increases with the genetic dissimilarity of the strange male to the male with whom she originally was mated (this is called the Bruce effect). If offspring result, they are always from the "strange" male. This effect also has been observed in wild rodents and may not be peculiar to laboratory mice.

The sexual pheromones involved in the Lee-Boot and Bruce effects are probably modified steroids (steroid metabolites) and are transmitted via the urine of the male to the olfactory apparatus of the female. Male mouse urine induces and accelerates estrous cycles of females (Whitten effect), and the effect is most pronounced on Lee-Boot groups of females. The time of vaginal closing in females is also influenced by male urine. Anosmic females (animals whose nostrils have been blocked or whose olfactory bulbs have been removed surgically) do not respond to male urine.

Pregnant and lactating rats produce pheromones that influence other females. Odors from a lactating female with pups lengthens estrous cycles of non-pregnant females. Thus a socially dominant, lactating female may suppress fertility of other females until she is again in estrus herself.

Males also may be influenced by female pheromones. Pairing of a previously paired male mouse with a strange female results in elevation of plasma testosterone in the male, indicating that endocrine responses of both males and females may be influenced through intersexual encounters.

B. The Ewe

Sheep estrous cycles occur seasonally, and the duration of one complete cycle is 16 days. The ewe may return to proestrus at least once if fertilization does not occur (Figure 10-21). Reproductive cycles can be blocked in ewes by **genistein**, a phytoestrogen found in certain clovers (genistein is also present in some plant products consumed by humans such as soy). The structure of genistein is provided in Chapter 3, Figure 3-28. During the follicular phase (=proestrus), there is a marked increase in estrogen and androgen levels, a peak being reached about 24 hours after the onset of proestrus. About 12 hours later, a surge of plasma LH occurs caused by the action of estradiol on the cyclic hypothalamic neurosecretory center. A high level of circulating androstenedione actually may be responsible for inducing estrous behavior by providing the substrate for estradiol synthesis. Usually, a single ovulation follows the LH surge by about 24 hours, and a corpus luteum forms from the ruptured follicle under the influence of LH. Low levels of LH following ovulation and the estrogen-induced surge of PRL stimulate the corpus luteum to secrete progesterone. Under the influence of progesterone, the uterine endometrium synthesizes a luteolytic prostaglandin ($PGF_{2\alpha}$) that causes degeneration of the corpus luteum and resumption of proestrus unless pregnancy occurs.

It appears that follicle growth, ovulation, and luteinization can be brought about by LH alone, although several studies have shown that FSH can stimulate follicular development, too. However, both postovulatory LH and PRL are necessary to induce progesterone synthesis by the sheep corpus luteum.

Fertilization followed by implantation delays degeneration of the corpus luteum. Although oCG is produced, the conceptus somehow neutralizes the PGFs synthesized under the influence of progesterone so that the corpus luteum may continue to secrete progesterone until the placenta is capable of producing sufficient steroids to maintain gestation. The placenta also secretes oCS throughout gestation. Birth seems to be triggered by a marked reduction in progesterone production near term (birth; see Figure 10-16).

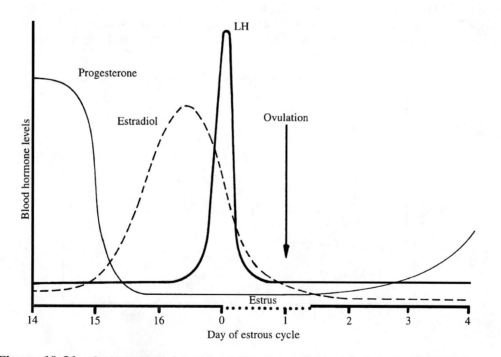

Figure 10-21. Ovulatory cycle of sheep (ewe). Note that ovulation occurs during the later part of estrus.

C. Women

The human female exhibits continuous reproductive cycling with a mean non-pregnancy cycle length of 28 days for most reproductively active women (Figure 10-22). Timing of reproductive events is related to the uterine menstrual cycle. The rhesus monkey also has a menstrual cycle of 28 days, and there are many parallels in the menstrual cycles of these two primates. Thus, studies of the rhesus monkey have provided valuable insight into factors regulating the human menstrual cycle. Although this menstrual cycle is sometimes referred to as a lunar cycle because its periodicity is equivalent to approximately one lunar month, the human menstrual cycle is not correlated with any particular phase of the lunar month and should not be termed lunar. It could be that at one time the menstrual cycle was correlated more closely with moon phases but has become highly modified by numerous environmental and internal factors.

The duration of menstrual cycles of women can vary from as short as 14 days to as long as 360 days, depending upon both endocrine and psychological factors. Furthermore, considerable variation can occur in cycle length in a given woman at different times in her life history. In general, short cycles and irregular cycles are associated with the onset of puberty and with the end of the reproductive life prior to menopause when the ovaries become refractory to pituitary GTHs and both estrogen synthesis and ovulation cease. The absence of circulating estrogens and progesterone releases the hypothalamus from negative feedback, and levels of circulating GTHs are exceptionally high in menopausal and postmenopausal women.

By convention, the menstrual cycle begins at the onset of the menses, which occupies the first five days of the cycle (Figure 10-22). However, as soon as the corpus luteum of a previous cycle begins to regress prior to the onset of menses, there is a depression in plasma gonadal steroids and a resultant moderate elevation in plasma FSH that initiates growth of new follicles. Typically, only one follicle in one of the ovaries will reach maturity in a given cycle, with ovulation often occurring in the alternate ovary during the following cycle. The largest follicle in the other ovary will ovulate the next month (hence the true ovarian cycle is twice as long as the menstrual cycle; i.e., =56 days) with two periods of follicular growth correlated with the proliferative phase of two successive uterine cycles.

The thecal cells of the growing follicles in both ovaries begin to secrete estrogens and progestogens, which peak on about day 14 of the normal menstrual cycle. Steroidogenesis is regulated by LH and FSH operating on the thecal and granulosal cells, respectively. The peak in follicular phase estrogen level stimulates accelerated pulsatile GnRH release from the cyclic center, causing a large surge of LH accompanied by a lesser surge of FSH. Galanin released with GnRH enhances the LH response whereas inhibin secreted by the ovary under the stimulation of FSH actually reduces the release of FSH in response to the GnRH surge. Ovulation of typically only the largest follicle follows the LH surge by about 24 hours, and the LH-stimulated granulosa cells and some thecal cells from the ruptured follicle undergo luteinization to form a corpus luteum. The

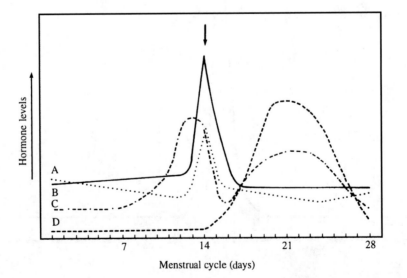

Figure 10-22. Ovulatory cycle of human. (A) FSH. (B) LH. (C) Estradiol. (D) Progesterone. [Reprinted with permission from Bolander, F. F. (1989) "Molecular Endocrinology." Academic Press, San Diego.]

resulting corpus luteum is independent of pituitary hormones and begins production of progesterone and estradiol.

The hypothalamic centers governing LH and FSH release are inhibited by the high levels of these circulating steroids so that neither follicular growth nor ovulation can occur during the early portion of the luteal phase of the cycle. However, the corpus luteum functions for only a few days if the ovum is not fertilized. Unlike the case for sheep, the human uterus plays no active role in causing degeneration of the corpus luteum. Surgical removal of the uterus (hysterectomy) does not affect the duration of the luteal phase. Production of estrone by the corpus luteum of the rhesus monkey increases markedly prior to the onset of luteal degeneration. A similar mechanism employing estrone as a luteolytic factor may be operating in women. As the production of steroids by the corpus luteum decreases, the pituitary is released from steroid-induced inhibition, and a second spurt of follicular growth begins during the latter portion of the luteal phase. The outer portion of the uterine lining begins to slough off following the decline in progesterone levels, and the menses begins.

The limiting factor for follicle growth appears to be the availablility of GTH. Treatment with fertility drugs that enhance GnRH secretion and hence GTH levels often can cause development and ovulation of multiple follicles resulting in multiple births. Hence, women may transition from being non-reproductive to producing litters.

Should fertilization occur at the appropriate time during the menstrual cycle, the trophoblast of the blastocyst begins to secrete hCG prior to implantation, and the production of hCG continues at an accelerated rate during early pregnancy (Figure 10-17). Under the influence of hCG, the corpus luteum continues to secrete both progesterone and relaxin for about 60 days, after which it degenerates even in the presence of exogenous hCG. However, the normal fetal adrenal-placenta unit by this time produces sufficient estrogens and progesterone to continue the inhibition of pituitary GTH release and to maintain the secretory and hyperemic condition of the uterus. The placenta can synthesize progesterone but lacks the necessary enzymes to synthesize androgens. The fetal adrenal provides weak androgens (androstenedione, DHEA, DHEAS) so that the placenta can convert them into estrogens. Failure of the fetal adrenal to produce adequate androgens before the corpus luteum degenerates invariably results in a miscarriage at about 2–3 months following implantation.

At one time, a synthetic estrogen **diethylstilbestrol (DES)**, discovered in 1938, was prescribed for thousands of women who were unable to sustain sufficient estrogen levels to maintain pregnancy. Many women were treated with DES as a precautionary therapy even without a history of miscarriage. Although this treatment was effective in preventing miscarriages, it was found to increase the later incidence of cancer in both the treated women and their offspring, and this practice was discontinued in the early 1970s. Similar observations had been made in animals years before, but the medical community was slow to recognize the danger.

Pheromones have been documented as important agents for coordinating events of sexual reproduction among many mammals, and may even play important roles in human reproduction as inferred from studies of monkeys. Female rhesus monkeys produce a mixture of fatty acids of low molecular weight. The compounds appear in vaginal secretions and stimulate sexual interest of males as well as mounting behavior and ejaculation. The major volatile agents are fatty acids including acetic acid, butanoic acid, propanoic acid, methylbutanoic acid, and methylpropanoic acid. Synthetic mixtures of these fatty acids in appropriate ratios stimulate male interest in females. Estrogens stimulate fatty acid secretions, and progesterone is inhibitory; observations that correlate well with levels of fatty acids observed in vaginal secretions throughout the menstrual cycle.

Human vaginal discharges exhibit a similar cyclical variation in fatty acid composition (Figure 10-23), although human females produce a much greater percentage of acetic acid than do rhesus monkeys. The administration of oral contraceptives to these females effectively obliterates the preovulatory increase in volatile fatty acids suggesting either an inhibition caused by high levels of estrogen or that the specific pheromonal agents are GTH-dependent (recall that negative feedback by the contraceptive steroids blocks GTH release and hence prevents follicle development and ovulation).

Although studies of pheromones in humans are complicated by a number of psychological and social considerations, some evidence exists for production of pheromones and their roles in reproduction. A "dormitory effect" of menstrual synchrony has been described by McClintock for all-female living groups. Even though it is generally accepted that the olfactory sense in humans is limited as compared to most mammals, several studies have shown definite sensitive olfactory discriminations, including sexually based differences in the abilities to perceive certain odors. Trained perfumers can apparently distinguish between different skin and hair types, and some psychiatrists claim to be able to smell schizophrenics because of abnormal production

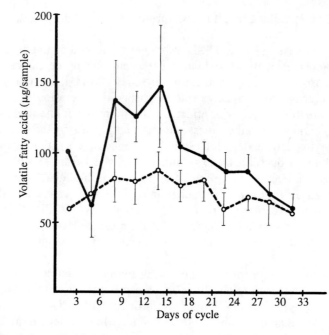

Figure 10-23. **Effect of oral contraceptives on vaginal secretions in humans.** Lipid composition of human vaginal secretions collected at 3-day intervals during the menstrual cycle. Treatment with oral contraceptives (dashed line) reduced the normal midcycle rise observed in the volatile fatty acid content of vaginal secretions in 47 women. [Data originally reported by Michael, R. P., Bonsall, R. W., and Warner, P. (1974). Human vaginal secretion: Volatile fatty acid content. *Science* **186**, 1217–1219.]

and elimination of trans-3-methylhexanoic acid. The ability to detect some odors is sex-dependent, such as the greater sensitivity of women to "boar taint" associated with spoiled pork. Some oders (e.g., licorice, lavender, doughnuts, and pumpkin pie) are claimed to induce sexual arousal. Clearly, controlled experimental studies are needed to establish what roles pheromones have in controlling human behavior and reproductive functions.

D. Elephants

Asian (*Elephas maximus*) and African elephants (*Loxodonta africana*) have similar seasonal reproductive cycles with a 4–5-year birth interval in females due to the relatively long gestation period and extended lactation. The following account merges information from both species. Females are most likely to mate with older males that exhibit **musth**, a period of increased activity, association with females, and aggressiveness toward other males. A female may signal her receptiveness to a male by calling or through pheromones. In the Asian elephant, a forthcoming ovulation is advertised by the excretion of (Z)-7-dodecen-1-yl acetate in urine that arouses interest in males. When a male is in musth, he secretes more fluid from his temporal glands and dribbles strong urine about that is attractive to females during the follicular phase of their ovarian cycles.

The ovarian cycle appears to be 16 weeks in duration with ovulation and a one-week period of estrus occurring near the middle of the cycle (Figure 10-24). There appear to be be two successive LH surges about 2–3 weeks apart, and both are related to elevated estradiol levels. The first surge is believed to stimulate development of accessory corpora lutea and the second LH surge stimulates ovulation. The single follicular that usually ovulates following the second LH surge forms a corpus luteum and together with the other corpora lutea are responsible for the observed rise in circulating progestins that characterize the luteal phase. Typically, only one follicle probably ovulates as twins are rare among elephants and usually only a single offspring is produced following 22 months of gestation. Progestogen levels rise during the luteal phase and remain elevated in the pregnant elephant until about 30 weeks prior to birth, reaching prepregnancy levels about 2–5 days before parturition. Relaxin appears in the blood about 20 weeks after the onset of pregnancy and also shows a decline with the progestogens. However, relaxin rises again during the last 8 weeks of pregnancy. Nothing is known about the factors responsible for initiation of birth in elephants.

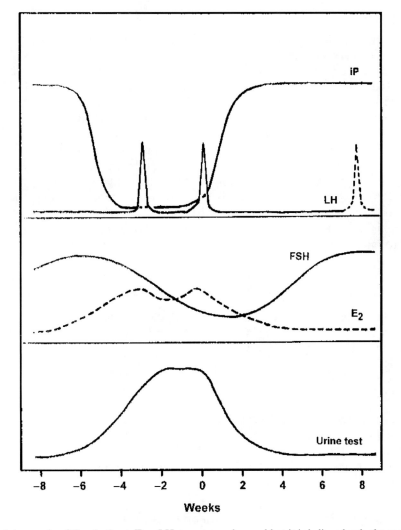

Figure 10-24. **Ovulatory cycle of the elephant.** Two LH surges are observed but it is believed only the second results in ovulation and corpora lutea formation as evidenced by the levels of progestogens (DHP). [Reprinted with permission from Hodges, J. K. Endocrinology of the ovarian cycle and pregnancy in the Asian (*Elephas maximus*) and African (*Loxodonta Africana*) elephant. *Animal Reproduction Science* **53**, 3–18. Copyright 1998 by Elsevier Science Inc.]

Elephants are unique in producing very low amounts of progesterone but instead produce large amounts of the progestogens **5α-dihydroxyprogesterone (DHP)** and **5α-pregnan-3-ol-20-one**. DHP has the strongest affinity for the progesterone receptor and may be the physiologically important progesterone in elephants. Following birth of the offspring, the female elephant enters a prolonged period of lactation during which GTH release is suppressed and the ovary remains quiescent.

VII. Major Human Endocrine Disorders Related to Reproduction

Reproductive disorders have been studied extensively in order to prevent their occurrence as well as to correct defects and increase reproductive capacities of both men and women. Some of the more common reproductive disorders are described here. Additional disorders related to reproduction include congenital adrenal hyperplasia (see Chapter 8) and osteoporosis (see Chapter 14).

The discussion of major endocrine disorders is separated into three major categories. The first two categories consider factors that influence the timing of puberty. The third deals with major genetically based disorders, many of which can result in ambiguous sexual determination.

A. Precocious Puberty

Puberty is a delayed period of development focusing upon activation of the HPG axis and the functional integrity of sex accessory structures that may lead to successful sexual reproduction. **Precocity** is defined as the appearance of any one indicator of puberty at an age earlier than 2.5 to 3 standard deviations below the mean age at which the indicator normally appears in that population (see Table 10-7). The sequence and mean age for appearance of these indicators should be considered only as a guide. Implied precocity may not be evidence of an endocrine disorder, and variations in the sequence of any of these events is normal. Major deviations in a number of indicators may signal precocial endocrine activity of a pathological nature. **Isosexual precocity** involves early appearance of the genetically determined sex. It is termed **heterosexual precocity** if male features develop precocially in a female or if female features appear precocially in a male.

It should be noted that there has been a shortening of the mean prepubertal period in the last several decades resulting in earlier puberty. Evidence from studies of endocrine disruption through accidental exposures to estrogenic compounds such as phthalates suggest environmental causes of this accelerated timing of puberty. Exposure to artificial lighting that extends daylight and perhaps to television and computer monitors also have been hypothesized to influence pineal function (see below) and contribute generally to precocity.

1. Precocity with Normal Endocrinology

Idiopathic (of unknown cause) precocity may be familial. Sexual development and body growth appear normal but are accelerated. Reproduction may be possible at an early age. For example, the youngest mother on record was 5 years 8 months of age at delivery.

2. Precocity and Pineal Tumors

Pineal tumors are not common but occur most frequently in young males. Precocious sexual maturation occurs in about one-third of these cases. Pineal tumors may impair release of melatonin from the pineal and allow sexual maturation to occur prematurely (see Chapter 4). In contrast, some pineal tumors have been related to delayed puberty in a few cases. These tumors possibly secrete more melatonin than does a normal gland and hence delay puberty.

3. Precocity from Ectopic Gonadotropins or Gonadal Steroids

Rarely, pituitary tumors secrete excessive amounts of gonadotropins, and sometimes a non-pituitary tumor secretes chorionic gonadotropin causing premature gonadal maturation. Likewise, certain ovarian or testicular

Table 10-7. Mean Age for Normal Attainment of Certain Indicators of Puberty in Humans

	Mean age (in years ± SD)
Female	
Budding of breasts	11.2 ± 1.1
Sparse public hair	11.7 ± 1.2
Peak vertical growth rate	12.1 ± 1.0
Menarche[a]	
U.K.	13.5 ± 1.0
United States	12.9 ± 1.2
Male	
Enlargement of testes and scrotum	11.6 ± 1.1
Lengthening of penis	12.8 ± 1.0
Sparse pubic hair	13.4 ± 2.2
Peak vertical growth rate	14.1 ± 0.9
Adult genital size and shape	14.9 ± 1.1

[a] Ninety-five percent reach menarche between ages 11 and 15.

tumors can produce sufficient steroids to cause external evidence of puberty although the gonads themselves are still quiescent with respect to gamete production. Heterosexual precocity can occur from feminizing tumors in testes or androgen-secreting tumors of the female adrenals or ovaries. (See also the discussion of congenital adrenal hyperplasia, Chapter 8.)

4. Precocity from Endocrine-Disrupting Chemicals

Exposure of animals to compounds such as phthalates and bisphenol A associated with plastics have been shown to accelerate puberty in laboratory animals. Young girls exposed to phthalates exhibit early and sometimes excessive breast development (thelache).

5. Delayed Puberty

Numerous examples of delayed puberty are known. The causes and characteristics of delayed puberty are unique for males and females. However, mice lacking a G-protein-coupled receptor known as **GPR54** fail to undergo puberty. The natural ligand for GPR54 is **metastin**, a peptide of 54 amino acids that is produced by the *KISS-1* gene. Metastin was named for its ability to suppress the metastatic potential of melanoma and breast carcinoma cells. Knockout mice for GPR54 (so-called Harry Potter strain) failed to undergo puberty. Metastin was later found to stimulate LH and FSH secretion through GPR54 receptors. It also activates GnRH neurons. GPR54 is expressed on GnRH neurons in a cichlid fish, but this has not been shown yet in mammals although GPR54 is expressed in mouse hypothalamus at puberty. Recent clinical studies have observed mutant GPR54 genes in patients with idiopathic hypogonadotropic hypogonadism.

6. Causes of Delayed Puberty in Males

Prevalence of undescended testes or **cryptorchidism** is common at birth (10%) but is reduced to only 1% of males by one year of age. Only about 0.3% of adult males exhibit cryptorchidism, and the case of only one undescended testis is much more common than the bilateral condition. Testicular descent normally is initiated by local effects of DHT. Because of higher temperatures experienced by an undescended testis, the spermatogenetic tissue degenerates at about the time when spermatogenesis would normally begin (at about age 10). Androgen production usually is normal but may be reduced in some cases. The external testis of a unilateral cryptorchid develops normally, and these males usually are fertile.

There are several other causes for **hypogonadism** in males including insufficient levels of LH and FSH due to hypothalamic or pituitary dysfunction. In some very rare cases, the interstitial cells may be unresponsive to GTHs.

7. Causes of Delayed Puberty in Females

Primary amenorrhea is the failure for menarche to occur at the normal time (Table 10-7). This condition can be related to many different causes including disorders of the hypothalamus, pituitary, and ovaries. Poor nutrition, stress, or rigorous athletic training programs can delay puberty through inhibitory actions on the HPG axis. For example, levels of LH and FSH are depressed in women suffering from **anorexia nervosa**, a disorder in which food intake is greatly reduced. Simple weight loss can depress FSH levels for a time but does not inhibit LH secretion.

Secondary amenorrhea occurs after menarche and can result from many endocrine disorders including thyrotoxicosis, drug therapy, and premature menopause as well as from a variety of hypothalamic, pituitary, and gonadal disorders. Two of the more common gonadal disorders associated with secondary amenorrhea are **polycystic ovarian syndrome (PCOS)** and **luteinization of atretic follicles (LAF)**.

The name for PCOS is derived from the general thickening and simultaneous luteinization of several ovarian follicles resulting in formation of numerous cysts in the ovaries. These cysts develop from thecal cells, and there is a corresponding decrease of granulosa cells in these follicles. Progesterone and estrogen production are diminished and gonadotropin secretion consequently is elevated. This resultant elevation of gonadotropins stimulates excessive production of androgenic steroids that cannot be aromatized to estrogens in the absence of granulosa cells. Uterine abnormalities and infertility result as well as obesity, hirsuitism, and occasional balding from the androgens may accompany PCOS. An association has been recognized between diabetes mellitus and the tendency to develop PCOS and it appears to be linked to a persistent metabolic disturbance.

The LAF syndrome results from premature luteinization of ovarian follicles prior to formation of the cumulus oophorus. GTH levels are elevated, but the masculinization described for PCOS usually does not happen. Numerous small ovarian cysts may be present, but these are easily distinguished from the large cysts that characterize PCOS.

B. Hereditary Disorders

Chromosomal rearrangements are common causes for deviations in sexual determination and/or expression. The most common disorders are the consequences of meiotic **nondisjuction** associated with the sex chromosomes; i.e., where the paired sex chromosomes fail to separate during the first meiotic division, resulting in gametes with either 2 or no sex chromosomes. Zygotes produced by such gametes would have only one sex chromosome or would have three sex chromosomes. In addition, numerous disorders have been linked to mutations in single genes.

Occasionally, people are born with a combination of ovarian and testicular tissue and are termed **hermaphrodities**. This term comes from Greek mythology, combining the names of Hermes, a god who sometimes played tricks on lovers, and Aphrodite, the goddess of love. Most hermaphrodites possess an ovotestis on one or both sides of the body. These conditions are also termed intersexes. Rarely, **gynandromorphs** are discovered, individuals with an ovary and attendant mullerian derivatives on one side and a testis with its wolffian duct derivatives on the other. **Pseudohermaphrodites** have gonads of the genetic sex but externally resemble the opposite sex.

1. Klinefelter's Syndrome (XXY)

Person's with **Klinefelter's syndrome** are born with an abnormal number of sex chromosomes: 47,XXY (total number of chromosomes, sex chromosomes). This familial disorder occurs at fertilization and is present in about 0.2 to 0.3% of males. Klinefelter's syndrome can exist without obvious somatic abnormalities, although these persons are infertile and exhibit differing degrees of mental retardation. Similar syndromes have been described with additional sex chromosomes (48,XXYY, 48,XXXY, etc.). Severity of the symptoms increases with the number of X chromosomes present.

2. Turner's Syndrome (XO)

Another disorder arising at fertilization is **Turner's syndrome** in which there is a loss of one sex chromosome so that the resulting genotype is 45,XO (one X chromosome and no Y or no second X chromosome). Sometimes this condition occurs when a twin is found to exhibit Klinefelter's syndrome. Individuals with Turner's syndrome have a female phenotype but are infertile. They also exhibit a number of anatomical defects as well as cardiovascular and kidney disorders. These patients do exhibit H-Y antigen that is characteristic of males but at a lower concentration suggesting some activation of an H-Y antigen gene on the remaining X chromosome. Thus the presence of H-Y antigen in blood cells is not indicative of the presence of a Y chromosome.

3. Galactorrhea

Secretion of a lactescent (milky) fluid from the breasts of either sex is called **galactorrhea**. It is usually caused by excessive secretion of PRL. Breast enlargement is not prerequisite for its appearance. Galactorrhea frequently occurs in severe hypothyroidism characterized by elevated circulating levels of TSH and TRH. Prolactin release may be evoked by the high TRH levels.

4. Testicular Feminization Syndrome

A person with **testicular feminization syndrome** is a genetic male (46,XY). The testes are normal and secrete testosterone. Mullerian duct derivatives are absent because the embryonic testes also secreted MIS. However, the external appearance is that of a woman because of the congenital absence of androgen receptors in the tissues. This is an example of male psuedohermaphroditism.

5. 5α-Reductase Deficiency

A most unusual example of pseudohermaphroditism is the apparent shift of sex at puberty. This condition was first reported from several small villages of the Dominican Republic. This disorder is the result of a genetic deficiency for the ability to synthesize the enzyme 5α-reductase. Males with this defect are born with undescended testes that synthesize testosterone like normal testes. However, these males lacking 5α-reductase cannot convert testosterone to DHT and early development of male external genitalia does not take place. Although testosterone also can bind to the receptors in these tissues, DHT has a much greater affinity for them. Levels of testosterone in normal prepubertal males are too low to activate these receptors sufficiently and hence the need for 5α-reductase to convert testosterone to the more effective androgen, DHT. Apparently, in men with 5α-reductase deficiency, there is sufficient testosterone to stimulate other androgen-dependent structures that develop normally (such as the vasa deferentia, epididymi) but the normally DHT-dependent structures such as the prostate gland, penis, and scrotum do not develop. These males understandably are raised as girls until these latter structures appear at puberty when testicular testosterone levels are elevated suitably to stimulate the appropriate tissues. The marked increase in circulating testosterone at puberty allows the penis and other structures to enlarge and causes facial hair to appear. Although these men usually change gender roles after puberty, they are infertile.

VIII. Summary

The reproductive system includes the HPG axis and sex accessory structures. Primary control resides in pulsatile production of GnRH that controls pituitary production of FSH and LH that in turn cause gamete formation, gonadal steroid secretion, and ultimately the regulation of sexual characters and reproductive behaviors. FSH is involved primarily with gamete production whereas LH is responsible for initiating steroid secretion and release of mature gametes (ovulation and spermiation). FSH and testosterone work cooperatively to produce mature sperm. Androgens, progestogens, and estrogens stimulate other primary reproductive structures and secondary sex characters as well as mating behavior. Numerous paracrine regulators contribute to reproductive events. Pheromones may play important roles in reproductive behavior and in the timing and success of reproduction.

In mammals, the male sex must be determined by the SRY gene that is responsible for production of MIS and androgens by the testis. MIS causes regression of potential female structures, and androgen production allows development of male sex accessory structures and reprograms hypothalamic reproductive centers in the brain to the male secretory pattern. Brain neurosteroids may also play a role in development of male brain differences. The default sex in mammals is female although estrogens are essential for completely normal female development.

Mammalian reproductive cycles show great variations among the major taxonomic groups. Monotremes are egg-laying mammals but nourish their hatchlings with milk from their mammary glands. Marsupials allow their young to develop in a pouch after a short gestation period involving a nonendocrine placenta, relying on the mammary glands to support continued development of an exteriorized fetus. Eutherian mammals have a prolonged period of intrauterine fetal development supported by an endocrine placenta. Mammary glands are still used for extended nutritional support after birth.

Most female mammals exhibit an ovarian-based estrous cycle characterized by a period of enhanced receptivity of the female to the male called estrus. In some species, primates, including humans and the rhesus monkey, a special phase of the uterine cycle occurs, the menses, that involves sloughing and discharge of a portion of the endometrium and trapped blood. Because of this special uterine cycle, their reproductive cycles are typically called menstrual cycles and may (e.g., rhesus monkey) or may not (human) exhibit a distinct period of estrus. The proliferative phase of the uterine cycle corresponds closely to the follicular phase of the ovarian cycle, and the secretory phase of the uterine cycle that follows ovulation coincides exactly with the luteral phase of the ovarian cycle. The uterine secretory phase is followed by a quiescent phase called diestrus in most mammals or by the menses in species having a uterine menstrual cycle. The menses corresponds to the first few days of the next follicular phase in the ovary.

Species may exhibit one (monestrous), two (diestrous), or many reproductive cycles (polyestrous) during the breeding season should fertilization or pregnancy not occur. In eutherians, the cycle can be separated into a follicular phase during which one or more ova develop in follicles and a luteal phase which prepares the uterus for implantation of the blastocyct. The luteal phase is named for one or more corpora lutea that develop from ruptured follicles and possibly from atretic follicles and continue to secrete estrogens and progestogens. These phases are clearly separated by ovulation.

During pregnancy, the eutherian placenta in cooperation with the fetal adrenal functions as an endocrine gland to maintain pregnancy, initiate birth, and prepare the mammary glands for postnatal functions. The corpus luteum performs various roles in pregnancy depending on the species. The placenta also functions in gaseous, nutrient, and metabolic waste exchanges. Numerous modifications of the placenta have evolved in different eutherian groups. OXY, prostaglandins, fetal adrenal steroids, and placental CRH, CG, CS, etc. play important roles in pregnancy and in the birth process. Postnatal functions of the mammary gland are controlled by PRL and oxytocin from the pituitary gland.

Gonadal secretory activites involve two special cell types responsive to FSH and LH, respectively. Ovarian granulosa cells and testicular Leydig cells are responsive primarily to LH and synthesize androgens. Ovarian thecal cells and testicular Sertoli cells as well as Leydig cells respond to FSH with conversion of androgens into estrogens ($P450_{aro}$ activity). FSH also stimulates Sertoli cells to synthesize inhibin, activin, and other local bioregulatory factors. Gonadal cells make many other local regulators (e.g., GnRH, IGFs, OXY,GDF-9, prostaglandins, etc.) in response to GTHs or independently, and these regulators may have autocrine and/or paracrine actions that control local events in the gonads.

Suggested Reading

Books

Adashi, E. Y., and Leung, P. C. K. (1993). "The Ovary." Raven, New York.

Burger, H., and DeKretser, D. (1989). "The Testis," 2nd Ed. Comprehensive Endocrinology Revised Series, Raven, New York.

Campbell, K. L., and Woods, J. W. (1994). "Human Reproductive Ecology: Interactions of Environment, Fertility, and Behavior." *Ann. N.Y. Acad. Sci.* **709**, 1–431.

de Kretser, D. (1993). "Molecular Biology of the Male Reproductive System." Academic Press, San Diego.

Ferin, M., Jewelewicz, R., and Warren, M. (1993). "The Menstrual Cycle: Physiology, Reproductive Disorders, and Infertility." Oxford Univ. Press, New York.

Findlay, J. K. (1994). "Molecular Biology of the Female Reproductive System." Academic Press, New York.

Goodman, H. M. (2003). "Basic Medical Endocrinology." Academic Press, San Diego.

Gruhn, J. G., and Kazer, R. R. (1989). "Hormonal Regulation of the Menstrual Cycle." Plenum, New York.

Henry, H. and Norman, A. (2003). "Encyclopedia of Hormones," Vols. 1–3. Academic Press, San Diego.

Jamieson, B. G. M. (2003). "Reproductive Biology and Phylogeny of Anura." Science Publishers, Inc. Enfield, NH.

Johnson, M., and Everitt, B. (1988). "Essential Reproduction," 3rd Ed. Blackwell, Oxford.

Jones, R. E. and Lopez, K. H. (2006). "Human Reproductive Biology," 3rd Ed. Academic Press, San Diego.

Knobil, E., and Neill, J. D. (1994). "The Physiology of Reproduction," 2nd Ed., Vols. 1 and 2. Raven, New York.

Knobil, E. (1999). "Encyclopedia of Reproduction," Vols. 1–4. Academic Press, San Diego.

Krey, L. C., Gulyas, B. J., and McCracken, J. A. (1989). "Autocrine and Paracrine Mechanisms in Reproductive Endocrinology." Plenum, New York.

Leung, P. C. K., and Adashi, E. Y. (2003). "The Ovary." Academic Press, San Diego.

Neill, J. (2005). "Knobil and Neill's Physiology of Reproduction," Vols. 1–3. Academic Press, San Diego.

Sever, D. M. (2003). "Reproductive Biology and Phylogeny of Urodela." Science Publishers, Inc. Enfield, NH.

Tyndale-Biscoe, H., and Renfree, M. (1987). "Reproductive Physiology of Marsupials." Cambridge Univ. Press, Cambridge.

Wynn, R. M., and Jollie, W. P. (1989). "Biology of the Uterus," 2nd Ed. Plenum, New York.

Yokoyama, A. (1992). "Brain Control of the Reproductive System." Japan Scientific Societies Press, Tokyo, and CRC Press, Boca Raton, FL.

General Articles

Adashi, E. Y., Resnick, C. E., D'Ercole, A. J., Svoboda, M. E., and Van Wyk, J. J. (1985). Insulin-like growth factors as intraovarian regulators of granulosa cell growth and function. *Endocr. Rev.* **6**, 400–420.

Adashi, E. Y. (1990). The potential relevance of cytokines to ovarian physiology: The emerging role of resident ovarian cells of the white blood cell series. *Endocr. Rev.* **11**, 454–464.

Adashi, E. Y., and Rohan, R. M. (1992). Intraovarian regulation: Peptidergic signaling systems. *Trends Endocr. Metab.* **3**, 243–248.

Bilezikjian, L., and Vale, W. W. (1992). Local extragonadal roles of activin. *Trends Endocr. Metab.* **3**, 218–223.

Bourguignon, J.-P. (1995). The neuroendocrinology of puberty. *Growth Gen. Horm.* **11**, 1–6.

Bryant-Greenwood, G. D., and Schwabe, C. (1994). Human relaxins: Chemistry and biology. *Endocr. Rev.* **15**, 5–26.

Burrow, G. N. (1993). Thyroid function and hyperfunction during gestation. *Endocr. Rev.* **14**, 194–202.

Clarke, I. J. (1995). The preovulatory LH surge: A case of a neuroendocrine switch. *Trends Endocr. Metab.* **6**, 241–247.

Crowley, W. R., and Armstrong, W. E. (1992). Neurochemical regulation of oxytocin secretion in lactation. *Endocr. Rev.* **13**, 33–65.

Dey, S. K., Lim, H., Das, S. K., Reese, J., Paria, B. C., Daikoku, T., and Wang, H. (2004). Molecular clues to implantation. *Endocrine Rev.* **25**, 341–373.

Erickson, G. F., and Shimasaki, S. (2000). The role of the oocyte in folliculogenesis. *Trends Endocr. Metab.* **11**, 193–198.

Fitch, R. H., and Deneberg, V. H. (1998). A role for ovarian hormones in sexual differentiation of the brain. *Behav. Brain Sci.* **21**, 311–352.

Fraser, H. M., and Lunn, S. F. (1993). Does inhibin have an endocrine function during the menstrual cycle? *Trends Endocr. Metab.* **4**, 187–194.

Frisch, R. E. (1991). Body weight, fat, and ovulation. *Trends Endocr. Metab.* **2**, 191–197.

Giudice, L. C. (1992). Insulinlike growth factors and ovarian follicular development. *Endocr. Rev.* **13**, 641–649.

Giudice, L. C., and Saleh, W. (1995). Growth factors in reproduction. *Trends Endocr. Metab.* **6**, 60–69.

Griffiths, M. (1984). Mammal: Monotremes. *In* "Marshall's Physiology of Reproduction, Vol. 1, Reproductive Cycles of Vertebrates" (G. E. Lamming, Ed.), pp. 351–385. Churchill Livingston, London.

Grosvenor, C. E., Picciano, M. F., and Baumrucker, C. R. (1993). Hormones and growth factors in milk. *Endocr. Rev.* **14**, 710–728.

Handwerger, S. (1991). The physiology of placental lactogen in human pregnancy. *Endocr. Rev.* **12**, 329–336.

Handwerger, S., Richards, R. G., and Markhoff, E. (1992). The physiology of decidual prolactin and other decidual protein hormones. *Trends Endocr. Metab.* **3**, 91–95.

Hawkins, J. R. (1993). The SRY gene. *Trends Endocr. Metab.* **4**, 328–332.

Hazum, E. (1991). Neuroendocrine peptides in milk. *Trends Endocr. Metab.* **2**, 2528.

Hiller, S. G., Whitelaw, P. F., and Smyth, C. D. (1994). Follicular oestrogen synthesis: The "two cell; two gonadotropin" model revisited. *Mol. Cell. Endocr.* **100**, 51–54.

Hodges, J. K. (1998). Endocrinology of the ovarian cycle and pregnancy in tre Asian (*Elephas maximus*) and African (*Loxodonta africana*) elephant. *Animal Reprod. Sci.* **53**, 3–18.

Hsueh, A. J. W., and LaPolt, P. S. (1992). Molecular basis of gonadotropin receptor regulation. *Trends Endocr. Metab.* **3**, 164–170.

Josso, N., Boussin, L., Knebelmann, B., Nihoul-Fekete, C., and Picard, J.-Y. (1991). Anti-mullerian hormone and intersex states. *Trends Endocr. Metab.* **2**, 227–233.

Kalra, S. (1993). Mandatory neuropeptide-steroid signalling for the preovulatory luteinizing hormone-releasing hormone discharge. *Endocr. Rev.* **14**, 507–538.

Kierszenbaum, A. L. (1994). Mammalian spermatogenesis *in vivo* and *in vitro*: A partnership of spermatogenic and somatic cell lineages. *Endocr. Rev.* **15**, 116–134.

Lee, M. M., and Donahoe, P. K. (1993). Müllerian inhibiting substance: A gonad hormone with multiple functions. *Endocr. Rev.* **14**, 152–164.

Leung, P. C. K., and Steele, G. L. (1992). Intracellular signalling in the gonads. *Endocr. Rev.* **13**, 476–498.

Licht, P., Frasnk, L. G., Pavgi, S., Yalcinkaya, T. M., Siiteri, P. K., and Glickman, S. E. (1992). Hormonal correlates of "masculinization" in female spotted hyaenas (*Crocuta crocuta*). 2. Maternal and fetal steroids. *J. Reprod. Fert.* **95**, 1–12.

Liggins, G. C. (1994). The role of cortisol in preparing the fetus for birth. *Reprod. Fert. Devel.* **6**, 141–150.

Matt, K. (1993). Neuroendocrine mechanisms of environmental integration. *Am. Zool.* **33**, 266–274.

McLachlan, R. I., Wreford, N. G., Robertson, D. M., and de Kretser, D. M. (1995). Hormonal control of spermatogenesis. *Trends Endocr. Metab.* **6**, 95–100.

McLean, M., and Smith, R. (1999). Corticotropin-releasing hormone in human pregnancy and parturition. *Trends Endocr. Metab.* **10**, 174–178.

Mellen, J. D. (1993). A comparative analysis of scent-marking, social and reproductive behavior in 20 species of small cats (*Felis*). *Am. Zool.* **33**, 151–166.

Moore, A., Krummen, L. A., and Mather, J. P. (1994). Inhibins, activins, their binding proteins and receptors: Interactions underlying paracrine activity in the testis. *Mol. Cell. Endocr.* **100**, 81–86.

Newman, J. (1995). How breast milk protects newborns. *Sci. Am.* **273**(6), 76–79.

Nicol, S., Andersen, N. A., and Jones, S. M. (2005). Seasonal variations in reproductive hormones in free-ranging echidnas (*Tachyglossus aculeatus*): Interactions between reproduction and hibernation. *Gen. Comp. Endocr.* **144**, 204–210.

Nicol, S., Anderson, N. A., and Jones, S. M. (2005). Seasonal variations in reproductive hormones in free-ranging echidnas (*Tachyglossus aculeatus*): Interaction between reproduction and hibernation. *Gen. Compa. Endocr.* **144**, 204–210.

Niemuller, C. A., Gray, C., Cummings, E., and Liptrap, R. M. (1998). Plasma concentrations of immunoreactive relaxin activity and progesterone in the pregnant Asian elephant (*Elphas maximus*). *Animal Reprod. Sci.* **53**, 119–131.

O'Dell, W. D., Griffin, J., and Sawitzke, A. (1990). Chorionic gonadotropin secretion in normal nonpregnant humans. *Trends Endocr. Metab.* **1**, 418–421.

Ojeda, S. R., and Dissen, G. A. (1994). Developmental regulation of the ovary via growth factor tyrosine kinase receptors. *Trends Endocr. Metab.* **5**, 317–323.

Pescovitz, O. H., Srivastava, C. H., Breyer, P. R., and Monts, B. A. (1994). Paracrine control of spermatogenesis. *Trends Endocr. Metab.* **5**, 126–131.

Protet, M. (1993). Menstruation as a defense against pathogens transported by sperm. Q. *Rev. Biol.* **68**, 335–386.

Rothschild, I. (2002). The yolkless egg and the evolution of eutherian viviparity. *Biol. Reprod.* **68**, 337–357.

Saez, J. M. (1994). Leydig cells: Endocrine, paracrine, and autocrine regulation. *Endocr. Rev.* **15**, 574–625.

Seron-Fere, M., Ducsay, C. A., and Valenzuela, G. J. (1993). Circadian rhythms during pregnancy. *Endocr. Rev.* **14**, 594–609.

Skinner, M. K. (1991). Cell–cell interactions in the testis. *Endocr. Rev.* **12**, 45–77.

Soares, M. J., Faria, T. N., Roby, K. F., and Deb, S. (1991). Pregnancy and the prolactin family of hormones: Coordination of anterior pituitary, uterine, and placental expression. *Endocr. Rev.* **12**, 402–422.

Tyndale-Briscoe, C. H. (1984). Mammals: Marsupials. *In* "Marshall's Physiology of Reproduction, Vol. 1, Reproductive Cycles of Vertebrates" (G. E. Lamming, Ed.), pp. 386–454. Churchill Livingston, Edinburgh.

Walker, W. H., Fitzpatrick, S. L., Barrera-Saldana, H. A., Resendez-Perez, D., and Saunders, G. F. (1991). The human placental lactogen genes: Structure, function, evolution, and transcriptional regulation. *Endocr. Rev.* **12**, 316–328.

Clinical Articles

Bidart, J.-M., and Bellet, M. (1993). Human chorionic gonadotropin: Molecular forms, detection, and clinical implications. *Trends Endocr. Metab.* **4**, 285–291.

Colledge, W. H. (2004). GPR54 and puberty. *Trends Endocr. Metab.* **15**, 448–453.

Imperato-McGinley, J., and Canovatchel, W. J. (1992). Complete androgen insensitivity: Pathophysiology, diagnosis, and management. *Trend Endocr. Metab.* **3**, 75–81.

Kaltsas, G. A., Isidori, A. M., Besser, G. M., and Grossman, A. B. (2004). Secondary forms of polycystic ovary syndrome. *Trends Endocr. Metab.* **15**, 204–210.

Lufkin, E. G., and Ory, S. J. (1995). Postmenopausal estrogen therapy, 1995. *Trends Endocr. Metab.* **6**, 50–54.

Richardson, M. R. (2003). Current perspectives in polycystic ovary syndrome. *Am. Fam. Physician* **68**, 697–704.

Sam, S., and Dunaif, A. (2003). Polycystic ovary syndrome: Syndrome XX? *Trends Endocr. Metab.* **14**, 365–370.

Sunderland, M. C., and McGuire, W. L. (1991). Hormones and breast cancer. *Trends Endocr. Metab.* **2**, 72–76.

11

Comparative Aspects of Vertebrate Reproduction

An understanding of reproductive patterns and their hormonal control in animals are central to our concerns about environmental quality and the future of aquatic and terrestrial ecosystems that are affected adversely by human activities. Levels of environmental contamination previously considered "safe" because they were not immediately toxic are now being seen to influence reproductive efforts through more subtle mechanisms than the dramatic thinning of bird eggshells by the pesticide DDT described some decades ago. Furthermore, documented declines in reproductive potentials in human males and dramatic increases in reproductive cancers provide even more incentive to examine reproductive mechanisms. It is imperative that biologists learn more about the endocrine-regulated reproductive mechanisms that are most prone to disturbance, how these disturbances occur, and what remedies might be applied. In this respect, we need more information about the roles of natural environmental influences on reproduction as well as the influences of environmental contaminants.

Because of the great diversity among vertebrates and the important role of natural selection on reproductive phenomena, it is even more difficult to generalize about non-mammalian vertebrate reproductive patterns than it was for mammals in Chapter 10. The descriptions provided here are based on the terminology used for mammalian reproduction. In the following accounts, many of the terms employed were introduced in Chapter 10 and will not be redefined here.

I. Some General Features of Vertebrate Reproduction

The hypothalamus-pituitary-gonad (HPG) axis regulates the reproductive success of all vertebrates. It is influenced by a variety of internal (i.e., hormones and other bioregulators) and external cues such as temperature, photoperiod, and pheromones. The HPG axis of non-mammals operates essentially like that of mammals.

Attainment of sexual maturity occurs at a time characteristic for each species and is followed by a series of reproductive cycles closely attuned to certain environmental factors. Bony fishes illustrate the full range of reproductive strategies known for vertebrates. Depending on the species, sexual maturity may be achieved during the first year of life (many teleosts), after more than 15 years of juvenile existence (Atlantic eel, sturgeon) or at some intermediate period. Some animals are semelparous and breed only once after attaining sexual maturity and die soon afterward (for example, Pacific salmon, *Oncorhynchus spp*), whereas most species are iteroparous and exhibit two or more reproductive cycles. Some of these may produce successive broods in a given year or season or may exhibit only one or two cycles per year. A few species may breed as one sex and then change to the opposite sex and breed again. Males may exhibit an associated reproductive pattern in which gonadal steroids are highest during mating or a dissociated reproductive pattern where mating occurs when androgens are reduced (Figure 11-1).

Natural environmental factors, such as temperature and photoperiod and the presence of suitable breeding or nesting sites, influence the central nervous system and the HPG axis and regulate gonadal maturation and secretion of sex hormones. Steroid hormones, pituitary hormones, or both determine development of various sex-dependent characters and influence courtship, breeding, and parental behaviors.

Like mammals, chondrichthyean and bony fishes, amphibians, and reptiles may be either viviparous or oviparous. Females of oviparous species lay eggs whereas viviparous species give birth to live young. Oviparous species all lay eggs with protective coverings from which a larval or juvenile form later will hatch regardless of the state of development at oviposition. Cyclostomes and birds, however, are exclusively oviparous. The term "ovoviviparity" has been applied somewhat inconsistently in vertebrates and will not be used here as suggested by Blackburn (1994; see Table 11-1). For simplicity, use of the term "viviparous" here will indicate live-bearing species regardless of whether there is a placental relationship or not. Hence, "viviparous" will include retention of eggs in the body of the parent prior to hatching so that free-living young are released into the environment.

Internal fertilization, a prerequisite for viviparity, requires evolution of a technique for transferring sperm from the male to the female. Some viviparous anurans (for example, *Nectophrynoides*) and birds transfer sperm through cloacal aposition or what has been termed the cloacal kiss. Aquatic fishes and urodele amphibians, which practice internal fertilization, rely on **spermatophores** for transfer of sperm. The spermatophore consists of a bundle of sperm that are aggregated and enclosed in a gelatinous substance that will not rapidly dissolve in water. This structure allows the male to directly or indirectly transfer sperm to the female without excessive dilution of the "semen." Spermatophore transfer often in facilitated by a sex accessory structure such as a

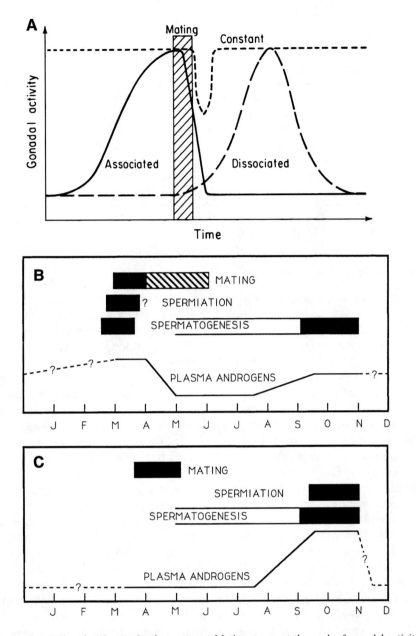

Figure 11-1. **Associated and dissociated reproductive patterns.** Mating occurs at the peak of gonadal activity in species exhibiting the associated pattern whereas mating occurs when gonadal activity is low in the dissociated pattern. [(A) Modified from Whittier, J. M. and Crews, D. (1987). Seasonal reproduction: Patterns and control. In Norris, D. O., and Jones, R. E. (Eds.) "Hormones and Reproduction in Fishes, Amphibians, and Reptiles." Plenum Press, pp. 385–410. (B) and (C) are reprinted with permission from Houck, L. D., and Woodley, S. K., (1995). Field studies of steroid hormones and male reproductive behavior in amphibians. *In* "Amphibian Biology" (H. Heatwole and B. K., Sullivan, Eds.) Vol. 2, Surrey, Beatty & Sons, Chipping Norton, Australia.]

modified fin or a copulatory organ. Elasmobranchs, viviparous teleosts, apodan amphibians, one anuran, and many reptiles possess intromittent organs that allow direct transfer of sperm or spermatophores from male to female. In contrast, an aquatic male urodele typically deposits spermatophores on a substrate and through a complicated behavioral ritual induces the female to pick one up with her cloaca. Frequently the female receiving a spermatophore has a special storage site, the spermatotheca, that is capable in some species of storing viable sperm for months. The spermatotheca has special mechanisms to disperse and nourish sperm so that they can perform their destined functions at a later time.

Table 11-1. Patterns of Reproduction That Have Been Described as Ovoviviparity[a]

Pattern	Description
1	Internal fertilization; partial development of eggs within female reproductive tract; eggs at oviposition contain visible embryos
2	Restricted to anamniotes; site of metamorphosis is central to recognition; young at birth are premetamorphic larvae (amphibians)
3	Nutrients all supplied by yolk and not by placenta; oviductal secretions, or sibling embryos (including yolk)
4	A trace of egg shell appears whereas in viviparous species, no egg shell is shown
5	Includes anurans that brood eggs in vocal sacs, stomachs, dorsal skin pouches, etc.

[a] Based on Blackburn, D. G. (1994). Review: Discrepant usage of the term "ovoviviparity" in the herpetological literature. *Herpetol. J.* **4**, 65–72.

A. Gonad Features in Non-Mammals

Ovarian structures and events occurring in the gonads of non-mammalian vertebrates are similar to those described for mammals. Oocyte development is regulated by pituitary gonadotropins (GTHs). The process of yolk protein formation is called vitellogenesis. Synthesis of these lipoprotein yolk precursors or vitellogenins by the liver is stimulated by estrogens. When released into the blood, these vitellogenins bind calcium ions and result in an elevation of total blood calcium in females undergoing vitellogenesis. Ovarian cells remove vitellogenins from the blood and use them to synthesize yolk proteins. Thus, marked increases in blood calcium can be used as an indicator of vitellogenesis and reflect circulating estrogen levels. Furthermore, vitellogenins are phosphoproteins, and an increase in plasma phosphoproteins can be monitored to provide information on reproductive status. Sensitive immunoassays (e.g., ELISA, see Chapter 2) are available to measure plasma vitellogenin, and measurement of plasma calcium levels or phosphoprotein levels to approximate vitellogenin levels are no longer necessary. Incorporation of vitellogenins by growing oocytes and their conversion to yolk proteins are controlled by GTHs.

There is a major difference in the structure of testes in most anamniotes and amniote vertebrates. Whereas testes of mammals, birds, reptiles, and anurans exhibit a tubular pattern of seminiferous elements with interspersed clumps of interstitial cells, the testes of anamniotes exhibit a cystic organization. In cyclostomes and elasmobranches, the testes consist of isolated cysts whereas the testes of bony fishes and urodele amphibians consist of lobes or lobules, each of which is composed of large cellular cysts. Although the gonads of anurans are described as consisting of seminiferous tubules, they also exhibit a pattern of cystic spermatogenesis even though the lobular organization is absent. Each testicular cyst is derived from a Sertoli (sustentacular or nurse) cell that surrounds a germ cell (Figure 11-2). Mitotic proliferation of the germ cell forms a spermatogonial nest, and all of the cells within a cyst and usually all the cysts within a lobule will be in the same stage of spermatogenesis. The more posterior lobules may be in a more advanced stage of spermatogenesis in repeating breeders than are the more anterior lobules. Spermiation in these anamniotes is usually followed by complete evacuation of sperm from the mature cysts and degeneration of the Sertoli cells. In iteroparous species, differentiation of lobules containing new cell nests occurs anteriorly from connective tissue elements and residual germ cells in the connective tissue covering of the testis, the tunica albuginea. In some fishes, however, all lobules develop and discharge sperm more or less simultaneously, and if breeding recurs there must be extensive regeneration of new cysts and spermatogonial nests prior to the next breeding season. In urodeles, different lobules mature each breeding season and spent lobules do not regenerate.

It was formerly believed on the basis of light microscope observations that interstitial tissues (i.e., Leydig cells) were lacking in many anamniotes, and the synthesis of androgenic hormones occurs in cells lobule boundary cells associated with the lobule walls. The cells formerly identified as lobule boundary cells are actually Sertoli cells. In most cases, Leydig cells are present between cysts in anamniotes, in the periphery of the testes or in a few cases adjacent to the testes.

In the amniote testis Sertoli cells are associated with spermatogonia in seminiferous tubules and the Leydig cells develop between the tubules in the interstitial regions. Furthermore, the amniote Sertoli cell is involved with the entire range of spermatogenetic stages in levels or layers from the spermatogonia at the outside of

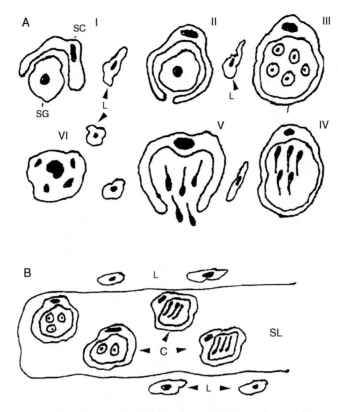

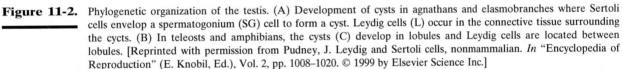

Figure 11-2. Phylogenetic organization of the testis. (A) Development of cysts in agnathans and elasmobranches where Sertoli cells envelop a spermatogonium (SG) cell to form a cyst. Leydig cells (L) occur in the connective tissue surrounding the cycts. (B) In teleosts and amphibians, the cysts (C) develop in lobules and Leydig cells are located between lobules. [Reprinted with permission from Pudney, J. Leydig and Sertoli cells, nonmammalian. *In* "Encyclopedia of Reproduction" (E. Knobil, Ed.), Vol. 2, pp. 1008–1020. © 1999 by Elsevier Science Inc.]

the tubule to spermatids and sperm bordering the tubules lumen (see Chapter 10, Figure 10-6). Furthermore, the amniote Sertoli cell does not degenerate after releasing sperm. However, in birds and reptiles as well as in some mammals, the Sertoli cell regresses considerably after the breeding season.

An additional steroidogenic tissue, the interstitial gland, may develop in the ovaries of non-mammalian gnathostomes similar to that described for mammals in Chapter 10. Interstitial glands develop from thecal cells derived from atretic previtellogenic follicles. It has been suggested that much of the androgen and estrogen synthesized during reproductive cycles in females is from the interstitial gland of the ovary.

B. Reproductive Ducts in Non-Mammals

Permanent reproductive ducts for transporting gametes are absent in the agnathan fishes. In mammals (Chapter 10), sperm are conducted from the epididymis associated with each testis via a vas deferens that is derived from the primitive pronephric (archinephric duct) and embryonically is referred to as the wolffian duct. The paired müllerian ducts develop adjacent to or possibly from the wolffian ducts and give rise to the oviducts, the uterus, and the upper portion of the vagina in females. The upper end of the müllerian duct and hence the oviduct are open to the peritoneal cavity.

Müllerian ducts degenerate in male mammals as do wolffian ducts in females. In elasmobranch fishes, the müllerian ducts definitely develop from the pronephric duct. The müllerian ducts give rise to oviducts in primitive bony fishes but they do not develop in teleosts. Some teleosts have developed a short duct of uncertain homologies, but most teleosts have an oviduct associated with each ovary that develops from a fold of peritoneum. In others, a temporary opening develops in the body wall to allow the extrusions of gametes. The sperm ducts like the oviducts are derived from the coelomic walls and are not homologous to the vasa deferentia of other vertebrates. Amphibians, reptiles, and birds all retain the müllerian duct in females and some male amphibians retain a rudimentary müllerian duct. The wolffian ducts function both as urinary ducts and as sperm ducts in male fishes and amphibians. It is also retained in all females as a urinary duct to drain the mesonephric kidney. In amniotes, the wolffian ducts degenerate in all females since new ducts, the ureters, develop to drain the metanephric kidney. The wolffian ducts are retained as sperm ducts (vasa deferentia) in male amniotes.

C. Endocrine Features in Non-Mammals

The endocrine factors in non-mammalian vertebrates are similar to and in many cases identical to those already described for mammals. The reader is reminded, however, that relatively few vertebrates have been examined with respect to endocrine factors and their involvement in reproduction. For example, about 50 of the 4600 mammals and even fewer of the more than 20,000 teleosts have been studied thoroughly. The same is true of amphibians, reptiles, and birds. So, there is much to be learned before we can be certain these patterns described here will apply to all vertebrates or even within a taxonomic group.

It is clear that the control of reproduction resides in the hypothalamus that controls pituitary and ultimately gonadal functions. One or more gonadotropin-releasing hormones (GnRHs) have been identified in all vertebrate groups (see Chapter 5, Table 5-7) and GnRH-1s are responsible for release of GTHs. A gonadotropin inhibitory hormone (GnIH) has been found in birds and may be a factor affecting GTH secretion in other non-mammals.

There appear to be two distinct GTHs in most non-mammals that are FSH- and LH-like in their actions. Their release generally is under stimulatory hypothalamic control. Follicular development in females and spermatogonial mitoses in males are stimulated by FSH, with meiotic events in males being influenced locally by androgens. Spermiation and ovulation are generally controlled by LH-like GTHs. Teleost fishes exhibit two distinct GTHs (GTH-I and GTH-II) that are now termed FSH and LH, respectively (see Chapter 5). Amphibians, birds, and most reptiles have separate FSHs and LHs. In contrast to fishes and the other tetrapod vertebrates, reproduction in squamate reptiles requires only an FSH-like GTH, and mammalian LH is ineffective in these reptiles (see Chapter 5).

The major circulating estrogen in non-mammals is estradiol, and testosterone or a closely related androgen is characteristic for males. Androgen and estrogen levels are higher than in mammals possibly due to high circulating levels of steroid-binding globulin. Furthermore, relative levels of androgens and estrogens are not correlated with sex. For example, females fishes may exhibit levels of androgens at certain times that exceed estrogen levels. Similarly, males may secrete significant amounts of estrogens. The actions of gonadal steroids, including negative feedback effects on the HPG axis, are similar in non-mammals to those described for mammals. Gonaduct differentiation and function, differentiation and maintenance of sex accessory structures, and induction of certain behaviors are regulated by gonadal steroids.

As in mammals, PRL exhibits in certain species some specialized functions that are closely linked to reproductive events. The specific involvements of PRL will be discussed in some of the accounts that follow.

The relationships between thyroid hormones and reproductive events in non-mammals were discussed in Chapter 7, and actions of corticosteroids on reproduction were described in Chapter 9. Briefly, thyroid hormones appear to enhance the onset of gametogenesis, especially in males. It is only in amphibians and certain avian species that a negative correlation has been reported between thyroid activity and the onset of sexual maturation. Generally, corticosteroids enhance reproduction and typically are elevated during breeding. Stressful stimuli, however, can activate the hypothalamus-pituitary-adrenal (HPA) axis to a level that results in a reduction in or complete cessation of reproductive activities.

D. Sex Determination in Vertebrates

There are several mechanisms of sex determination in vertebrates (Figure 11-3). In mammals, birds, amphibians, and some fishes and reptiles, sex is associated with distinct differences in one pair of chromosomes known as sex chromosomes. The remaining pairs are referred to as autosomes. In the homogametic sex, both sex chromosomes are identical (hence, all gametes produced by members of that sex are the same with respect

Genotypic sex determination

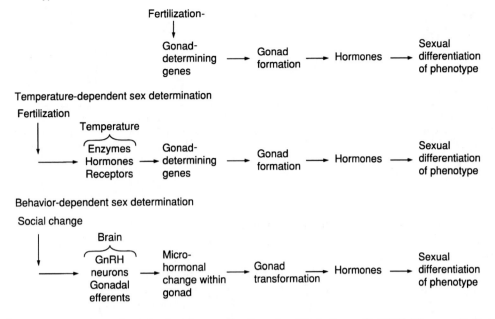

Figure 11-3. **Mechanisms of sex determination**. See text for discussion. [From Crews, D. (1993). The organizational concept and vertebrates without sex chromosomes. *Brain Behav. Evol.* **42**, 202–214.]

to chromosome morphology; i.e., they are homogametic). The opposite sex has unlike sex chromosomes that separate during meiosis, producing two kinds of gametes with respect to the sex chromosomes; hence, the heterogametic sex. When the female is homogametic, as in mammals and most anuran amphibians, the common sex chromosome type is termed an X-chromosome and her sexual genotype is XX. The male is heterogametic with one X-chromosome and one Y-chromosome (genotype = XY). When the male is the homogametic sex, as in birds and most urodele amphibians, the male is designated as ZZ and the heterogametic female is ZW. Typically, the homogametic sex does not require gonadal steroids for early differentiation (i.e., it is the default sex), but gonadal steroids must be present for the heterogametic sex to overcome the default sex. The SRY gene on the Y-chromosome of mammals and SRY-like genes in some other vertebrates are responsible for initiating heterogametic sexual differentiation. When sex is determined by this chromosomally based mechanism, it is called genotypic sex determination (GSD). Sex determination in most non-mammals appears to involve GSD even where chromosomal dimorphism is absent. However, the specific sex-determining genes have not been identified in non-mammals with the exception of two teleost species identified by Yoshi Nagahama and his colleagues (see references at end of chapter).

Many vertebrates do not have distinct sex chromosomes and may exhibit environmentally based mechanisms of sex determination. Although the lack of a morphologically distinct pair of sex chromosomes does not mean there is no genetic basis to sex determination, at least two mechanisms are well-known that depend on environmental temperature or behavior of conspecifics. Temperature-dependent sex determination (TSD) occurs in all crocodilians, many turtles, and some fishes and lizards. TSD is correlated with early nest or water temperatures (Table 11-2). Incubation at a high temperature produces all one sex whereas at a lower temperature all the offspring are the other sex. These temperature effects are "all-or-none" and intermediate temperatures produce equal ratios of males and females (50:50) rather than intersexes. Hormones do not play an initiating role in TSD although the levels of certain enzymes, such as aromatase ($P450_{aro}$) and Δ^5-3β-hydroxysteroid dehydrogenase (3βHSD), are greatest in adrenocortical tissue and mesonephric kidney during sexual differentiation.

A form of TSD has been reported for the Australian brush turkey, *Alectura lathami*, a species that builds mounds in which the eggs are incubated. More females hatch at higher temperature (36°). A 1:1 sex ratio results at 34°C (normal mound temperature), but males predominate at 31°C. Additional observations support a differential mortality as the mechanism of these shifts in the sex ratio at hatching.

Table 11-2. Temperature-Dependent Sex Determination in Vertebrates[a]

Group	Male-producing temperatures (°C)	Female-producing temperatures (°C)
Crocodilians	> 34	< 30
Turtles	23–27	30–33
Lizards	29–33	24–29
Teleosts	17–25	11–19

[a] Crocodilians, most turtles, and some lizards show TSD but snakes apparently do not. TSD also has been confirmed in one teleost (the Atlantic silverside, *Menidia menidia*) and may be a more common occurrence than is now known. Note that only in turtles is the low temperature male-producing. Categories indicate an overwhelming predominance of one sex, if not 100%. Intermediate temperatures produce males and females in more or less equal numbers, but no intersexes are reported.

Social situations (i.e., behavior) can initiate changes in gonadal sex. In sequential hermaphrodites, sex change may be induced by behavioral events and such species are said to exhibit behavioral sex determination (BSD). Most cases of sex change (or sex reversal) occur in adult coral reef fishes as evidenced in the excellent studies by Andrew Bass, Mathew Grober, Charles Kramer, Robert Ross, Robert Warner and their associates. Protogyny (female to male sex change) is the more common and appears to be triggered by environmental cues. Some species are termed diandric in that two types of males are found. One is a genetically determined or primary phase male, and the secondary or terminal phase male is derived through sex change of a female. In many cases, sex change is initiated by loss or removal of a dominant male in the social grouping and the largest ranking female takes his place. Often there are immediate behavioral changes in the dominant female that prevent sex reversal in subordinate females. Gonadal sex change usually follows the behavioral changes.

The bluehead wrasse, *Thalassoma bifasciatum*, is a diandric, sex-changing teleost living in the Carribean. Treatment of females with human chorionic gonadotropin (hCG) induces gonadal sex change within 1 to 6 weeks. Spontaneous reversal is accompanied by a two-fold increase in the number of GnRH-immunoreactive cells in the preoptic area of the brain. A similar increase in GnRH cells can be induced with implants of 11-ketotestosterone into females. How GnRH and GTHs produce a sex change in females previously employing these same hormones for female reproduction is unclear. Possibly the answer lies in changes in brain function that are initiated by environmental cues.

A similar pattern of sex change occurs in a closely related diandric species, the saddleback wrasse (*Thalassoma duperrey*) living on coral reefs in Hawaii. A very different mechanism for triggering sex change operates in *T. duperrey*, a promiscously mating fish that does not live in male-dominated groups. Long-term studies of these fish in underwater cages have determined that the cue for sex change is visual rather than chemical or tactile. The ratio of larger (usually males) to smaller fish (usually females) is perceived visually by the female who undergoes sex reversal if sufficient males are not present. Experimental studies by Earl Larson suggest a role for biogenic amines that in turn influence GnRH and GTH release. Isolation of a female *T. duperrey* results in immediate changes in catecholaminergic neuron activity and sex change that can be duplicated with appropriate pharmacological treatments.

1. Steroid Hormones and Sex Determination

Regardless of the mode of sexual differentiation (GSD, TSD, or BSD), gonadal steroids and neurosteroids appear to have important roles. Androgens and estrogens from the gonads traveling in the blood or locally produced in the brain often determine the pattern of HPG function early in development that persists in adults. Furthermore, exposure to exogenous steroids can interfere with this process and cause reversal of one sex to the other. Typically, there is a window of sensitivity in development for this process (Figure 11-4). When this window occurs, its width varies with the species. Treatment of larval fish, for example with reproductive steroids, during the sensitive window can produce populations of all one sex that may be advantageous in fish farming where one sex may grow more rapidly than the other or where sterile fish spend energy producing muscle and not gametes. Estrogen treatment can reverse the effects of a male-producing temperature in turtles

A   Sex determination window

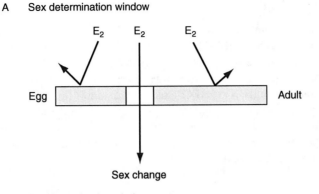

B   Sex determination windows

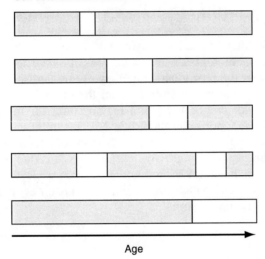

Age

Figure 11-4. **Sex determination windows.** (A) Estrogen (E$_2$) arriving only during the short time (window) when sex determination is occurring in the embryo or larva can alter the genetic sex. This is an example of a trait that is determined by an organizational action of steroids. Exogenous estrogen can alter the genetic sex from male to female if it appears at this time. (B) Illustration that such windows can exist at different times in the life history of animals and can be variable in their duration. Thus, an adult animal can undergo sex reversal even after functioning as a male or as a female.

and augment the actions of a female-producing temperature, but androgens usually cannot override effects of a female-producing temperature. In turtle eggs incubated at a neutral temperature (one that should produce a 50:50 ratio), the sex ratio is sensitive to either androgens or estrogens. However, addition of both androgens and estrogens simultaneously at the neutral temperature will produce intersexes.

One of the major concerns of exposure of developing animals in nature to environmental estrogens relates to the appearance of the disrupting chemical during this window of sensitivity. Depending on dose and time of exposure, we may see complete or partial (intersexes) sex changes. This is also a concern for the human fetus as well where exposure of the mother to estrogenic chemicals from a variety of sources can affect the fetus.

Paradoxical effects of steroid exposure are frequently observed, especially in fishes and amphibians. For example, exposure of a juvenile female catfish to testosterone causes precocial sexual development, while feminization of larval male fish occurs from exposure to a large dose of testosterone.

This early sexual differentiation based on gonadal steroids or temperature resulting in a permanent designation of sex or of a sexual characteristic is known as an organizational effect of steroids. Sexual differentiation of the HPG axis, for example, is an example of an early organizational event in most vertebrates. In the situation described above for the coral reef fishes, sex and related structures and behaviors are not organized at an early age but show that sex determination and differentiation of the gonads is due to an activational effect that occurs later in life.

2. SF-1 and Sex Determination

Considerable evidence has accumulated concerning a role for the orphan nuclear receptor (transcription factor) known as **steroidogenic factor-1 (SF-1)**, also called NR5a1. It was named for its role in stimulating the expression of several steroidogenic enzymes, including aromatase, as well as **steroidogenic acute regulating (StAR) protein**. SF-1 is also associated with GnRH gene regulation and gonadotropin release as well as with formation of the gonads and adrenals. The HPG axis, gonads and adrenals do not develop in SF-1 knockout mice that externally resemble females. Furthermore in mammals and turtles, SF-1 activity is greater during development of the bipotential gonad into a testis and lower during ovarian differentiation, and mutations in the human SF-1 gene have been associated with feminization of genetic males. In contrast, SF-1 levels are elevated in developing bullfrog, American alligator, and chicken.

II. Reproduction in Agnathan Fishes: Cyclostomes

Lampreys (*Petromyzontidae*) are characterized by having no breeding cycle, since all individuals die after a single spawning (i.e., semelparous). In contrast, hagfishes (*Myxinoidea*) apparently breed more than once. However, much less is known about the reproductive biology of the hagfishes than of lampreys.

It appears that the cyclostome gonad arises entirely from the embryonic cortex whether it is destined to be a testis or an ovary. This singular embryonic origin may account for the common observations of what appear to be hermaphroditic gonads among the hagfishes. Males exhibit a single median testis with a cystic pattern of spermatogenesis. Because of fusion of the paired primordia early in development, the adult female lamprey has a single ovary. In contrast, the single ovary of myxinoids is due to the failure of one primordium to develop. Steroid-binding proteins have not been demonstrated in cyclostome blood, and circulating levels of steroids are very low (Table 11-3). Gonaducts are absent in cyclostomes, and the gametes are shed into the coelom from which they exit via abdominal pores.

A. Male Lampreys

The mature lamprey testis consists of lobules with germinal cysts. When the cysts have completed formation of sperm, they simultaneously rupture and release sperm into the body cavity. The testes of parasitic forms, such as *Lampetra fluviatilis*, contain only primary spermatocytes at the time of migration to the breeding grounds. These spermatocytes are transformed rapidly near the time of spawning into sperm masses. Typical interstitial cell masses can be identified cytologically between the lobules in testes of migrating lampreys. These cells accumulate cholesterol-positive lipids and have become densely lipoidal by spawning time. Cytologically, interstitial cells appear to be steroidogenic and exhibit maximal 3β-HSD activity in February and March prior to the time of spawning.

B. Female Lampreys

Oogenesis has been carefully examined in the parasitic sea lamprey *Petromyzon marinus* and in the river lamprey *L. fluviatilis*. In *P. marinus*, oogonia proliferate mitotically in the larvae to form the primary oocytes. By the time of metamorphosis of the larva to the juvenile, there are no oogonia remaining in the ovary. The primary ovarian follicles become more vascularized at this time. During the prolonged parasitic phase of body growth (about 10 to 20 months), the oocytes continue to enlarge slowly. The single follicular cell layer becomes thinner and less vascularized as spawning approaches, and the oocyte enters a period of rapid enlargement to reach the preovulatory condition. The mature follicles rupture immediately before spawning, and the eggs enter the coelom. Follicular atresia occurs throughout the history of ovarian development, and many oocytes undergo atresia, establishing this basic pattern early in the phylogeny of vertebrates. Phagocytes derived from the follicular cells ingest the yolk, and the follicle layers and surrounding stroma collapse into the area formerly occupied by the oocyte.

Table 11-3. Circulating Steroid Levels[a] in Selected Non-Mammalian Vertebrates

Class and species	Testosterone	Estradiol (ng)	Progestogen (ng)
Agnatha			
Petromyzon marinus[b]			
Prespermiating male	275 ng		
Spermiating male	216 ng		
Preovulatory female	156 ng		
Ovulated female	62 ng		
Eptatretus stouti	24 ng		
Myxine glutinosa		1.0	
Chondrichthyes			
Torpedo marmorata (male)	15.6–35 ng		
Raja radiata			
Male	28–102 ng		
Female	0.2–6 ng		
Raja eglanteria			
Male	42.7 ng	0.022	0.150
Female	14 ng	2.48	0.042
Scyliorhinus canicula (male)	2–6 ng		
Osteichthyes			
Oncorhynchus nerka			
Male	17 ng		
Female	78 ng		
Salmo trutta			
Male	2–33 ng		
Female	20–77 ng		
Oncorhynchus mykiss			
Prespawning female	52–235 ng	24–48	8–15
Spawning female	65–84 ng	2–3	354–416
Spent female	2–5 ng	1–2	8–19

[a] Per milliliter of plasma or serum.
[b] 15α-hydroxylated testosterone.
[c] 17β, 20α-dihydroxy-4-pregnen-3-one.

Oocyte growth in parasitic *L. fluviatilis* accelerates markedly just prior to spawning. The granulosa contacts the oocyte only at the vegetal pole and reaches maximal development about one month prior to spawning. The thecal cells are greatly reduced and with the aid of the electron microscope can be seen covering the granulosa layer and the animal pole. The theca interna consists of a single layer of cells in which there is a marked increase in smooth endoplasmic reticulum and mitochondrial differentiation during vitellogenesis. These cells show maximal cytological activity prior to the time of most intensive vitellogenesis, following which they undergo progressive regression until the time of ovulation. The theca externa consists of fibroblasts, collagen fibers, and capillaries. 3β-HSD activity is apparently confined to the thecal cells where peak activity is observed about one month prior to the appearance of secondary sex characters and the acceleration of follicular development.

Vitellogenesis appears to be an estrogen-dependent event in lampreys involving cooperative action of the liver, which produces proteins that are secreted into the blood and are sequestered by the ovary to be incorporated in the developing oocyte. Estrogens stimulate liver hypertrophy and elevate plasma protein-bound calcium, suggesting the presence of a mechanism such as the one that has been documented so carefully in birds and other non-mammals (see below).

In the free-living lampreys that do not feed after metamorphosis, the ovarian events occur over a much shorter time and are consequently more dramatic. In brook lampreys, the immediate post-metamorphic period is marked by the onset of both vitellogenesis and massive atresia. As many as 70% of the follicles present at metamorphosis may become atretic, and phagocytosis of the yolk may provide an essential nutritional source for growth of the remaining oocytes to maturity.

C. Endocrine Function in Lampreys

The importance of gonadal steroids to development of sex accessory structures has been demonstrated through classical experiments involving hypophysectomy, gonadectomy, and appropriate hormone therapy to either hypophysectomized or castrate animals. However, lampreys secrete primarily 15α-hydroxylated steroids that are not secreted by any other vertebrates. Plasma testosterone levels are extremely low. 15α-testosterone levels in sea lampreys do, however, exhibit a dose-response relationship to administered lamprey GnRH, and increases in adults from undetectable levels to more than 200 pg/ml in reproducing males.

Lamprey GnRH or pituitary GTH from various vertebrates stimulate gonadal hormone secretions, which in turn stimulate formation of secondary sex characters. Spermiation also can be induced with lamprey GnRH. The gonads of hypophysectomized *L. fluviatilis* are less developed than those of sham-operated controls, indicating a reliance on the HPG axis.

D. Hagfishes

The reproductive biology of deep-water myxinoids is poorly known. They typically live on muddy ocean bottoms at depths between 100 and 300 meters in northern or arctic waters. Most hagfishes apparently are not seasonal breeders and, unlike the lampreys, exhibit continuous reproduction. *Eptatretus burgeri*, which migrates periodically into the shallow coastal waters of Japan, shows a seasonal cycle of gonadal activity. The brain content of GnRH of the Atlantic hagfish, *Myxine glutinosa*, exhibits a seasonal cycle, and peaks of GnRH activity in females are followed by peaks in plasma estradiol and progesterone (Figure 11-5). There is a single gonad in adult hagfishes similar to that described in lampreys. Hypophysectomy of another Pacific hagfish, *Eptatretus stouti*, results in testicular degeneration in males. However, hypophysectomy of mature females has no effect on either ovarian structure or circulating steroid hormone levels. Vitellogenesis is stimulated by estradiol treatment of *E. stouti*.

Both preovulatory corpora lutea (atretic follicles) and postovulatory corpora lutea have been described and can convert pregnenolone to progesterone in the Atlantic hagfish. Although male hagfishes appear to lack interstitial cells, they do secrete testosterone.

III. Reproduction in Chondrichthyean Fishes

The elasmobranchs have been studied extensively, probably because of the high incidence of viviparity in these species (present in 10 families of sharks and 4 families of rays). Unfortunately, no complete data are available on reproduction in ratfishes. Several different reproductive patterns have been described in elasmobranchs, extending from species that lay a precise number of eggs in a particular sequence, such as the oviparous clearnosed skate *Raja eglanteria*, to the viviparous spotted dogfish, *Scyliorhinus canicula*, that is sexually active throughout the year and may have embryos in different stages of development *in utero* at the same time. Elasmobranchs are characterized by internal fertilization regardless of whether they are viviparous or oviparous. The elasmobranch reproductive system is illustrated in Figure 11-6A, and plasma levels of gonadal steroids are provided in Table 11-3.

A. Male Elasmobranchs

Spermatogenesis in paired testes is of the cystic type. Sertoli cells are present and possess 3β-HSD activity. These cells become densely lipoidal and cholesterol-positive following spermiation and are eventually resorbed. Sertoli cells for the next cycle differentiate from connective tissue cells (fibroblasts) in the walls of the testis. Nests of spermatogonia proliferate from germ cells in the same regions, and they are responsible for producing sperm utilized during the next breeding period. Leydig cells have been described between cysts although they may not be readily discernible throughout the testicular cycle.

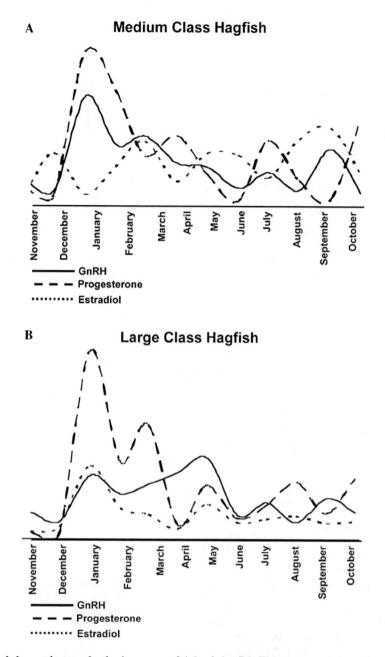

A **Medium Class Hagfish**

GnRH
Progesterone
Estradiol

B **Large Class Hagfish**

GnRH
Progesterone
Estradiol

Figure 11-5. **Seasonal changes in reproductive hormones of Atlantic hagfish.** The patterns are shown for GnRH, progesterone, and estradiol in median-sized and large females of *Myxine glutinosa*. Reprinted with permission from Kavanaugh, S. I., Powell, M. L., and Sower, S. A. (2005). Seasonal changes of gonadotropin-releasing hormone in the Atlantic hagfish *Myxine glutinosa*. *Gen. Comp. Endocr.* **140**, 136–143.

Spermatophores produced by elasmobranchs are the result of secretory activities of male accessory ducts. After spermiation, sperm pass through vasa efferentia and enter the coiled tubules of the Leydig gland, which is derived from the anterior portion of the mesonephric kidney. It is not steroidogenic and should not be confused with the Leydig cells. Sperm and secretions of the Leydig gland pass on to an expanded region of the vas deferens known as the ampulla. Here the sperm are consolidated and receive additional secretory material to form complex spermatophores typical for each species. Fertilization is internal, and spermatophores are transferred to the female by specialized structures termed claspers associated with the paired ventral (pelvic) fins.

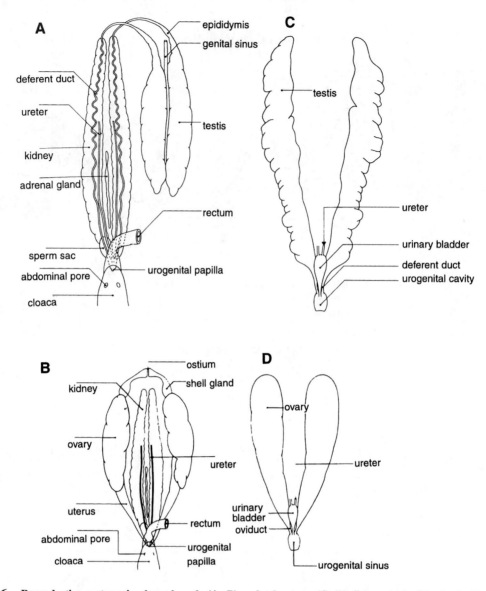

Figure 11-6. **Reproductive systems in elasmobranch (A, B) and teleostean (C, D) fishes.** A dogfish shark, *Mustelus manazo*: (A) Male with testes pushed to the side to reveal kidneys, reproductive ducts, and the interrenal. (B) Female with ovaries obscuring the oviducts running between the shell gland and uterus. A teleost, the carp, *Cyprinus carpio*. (C) Male. (D) Female. [Modified from Matsumoto, A., and Ishii, S. (1987). "Atlas of Endocrine Organs: Vertebrates and Invertebrates." Springer-Verlag, Berlin.]

1. Endocrine Factors in Male Elasmobranchs

The importance of the ventral lobe of the elasmobranch pituitary as the source of GTH controlling spermatogonial proliferation (mitotis) has been demonstrated in the spotted dogfish. Degenerative changes in the testes appear 6 weeks after removal of only the ventral lobe, and 22 months later the testes contain only spermatogonia and mature sperm, indicating that removal of the ventral lobe blocks further differentiation of spermatogonia to spermatocytes, whereas all spermatocytes present at the time of surgery are able to complete meiosis and spermiogenesis. Although testosterone is the principal androgen in elasmobranchs, 11-ketotestosterone has been reported in *R. eglanteria*. Circulating estradiol and progesterone also have been reported in males. Estadiol levels are lower in male *R. eglanteria* than in females, but progesterone levels are greater in males.

B. Female Elasmobranchs

The elasmobranch ovary is covered by germinal epithelium and may contain a cavity derived from large lymph spaces within the stroma. Elasmobranch follicles are similar to those of mammals in possessing several distinct layers of cells. The connective tissue near a nest of oogonia will differentiate into the theca. As each follicle begins to develop, some epithelial cells from the germinal epithelium undergo hypertrophy and hyperplasia to become the granulosa. In some species, the granulosa may consist of only a single layer of cells. These cells are responsible for transfer of vitellogenin during follicle growth as well as for yolk resorption should a given follicle become atretic. Granulosa cells also are thought to be the source of estrogens since they exhibit more 3β-HSD activity than do thecal cells. Most estrogen synthesis occurs in the mature follicle, which has a well-developed granulosa. During follicular development, a theca interna and theca externa can be discerned. However, both layers largely consist of connective tissue elements, and only a small amount of 3β-HSD activity has been observed in the theca interna cells.

The granulosa cells provide the source of both preovulatory (atretic) and postovulatory corpora lutea. The connective tissue layers surrounding these structures are derived from the theca. Corpora lutea of several species possess 3β-HSD activity, and corpora lutea persist during gestation in *Squalus acanthias*, the spiny dogfish. The corpora lutea from pregnant *S. acanthias* produce twice as much progesterone *in vitro* as do those from nonpregnant females, which possess only preovulatory corpora lutea formed from atretic follicles. These observations strongly support an endocrine role for postovulatory corpora lutea in the viviparous elasmobranchs.

Atresia is a common occurrence in elasmobranch ovaries. Depending upon the species being examined, either thecal or granulosa cells may contribute to formation of the preovulatory corpora lutea from atretic follicles.

Elasmobranch females have well-developed müllerian ducts that give rise to the oviducts as well as to the uterus of viviparous species. Oviducts have been examined in oviparous species that secrete horny shells to protect the eggs laid in the ocean as well as in viviparous species, and they possess a number of specialized features. Oviductal or nidamental glands secrete albumin and mucus in oviparious species. Villus-like structures may develop in the uterine portion of the oviducts of certain viviparous females, and they provide nourishment for their young. The oviductal glands of oviparous species are often differentiated into an anterior albumin-secreting area and a posterior shell-secreting region. An intermediate mucus-secreting zone may be found in some species. A spermatotheca (a site for sperm storage in the female genital tract) is present in some species.

1. Endocrine Factors in Female Elasmobranchs

Removal of the ventral lobe of the adenohypophysis blocks oviposition in female *S. canicula*, and all follicles containing oocytes larger than 4 mm in diameter undergo atresia, demonstrating dependence on GTHs. Progesterone can inhibit vitellogenesis in the dogfish, *S. acanthias*, and prevents reinitiation of oocyte growth during early gestation. Estradiol stimulates vitellogenin synthesis in the liver and and growth of the oviduct. The possible role of progesterone from corpora lutea during gestation was suggested earlier.

In the oviparous skate, *Raja erinacea*, estradiol and testosterone levels increase during follicular growth but progesterone shows a peak just prior to ovulation. After ovulation, there is a decline in steroid secretion until oviposition (Figure 11-7). However, estradiol peaks prior to ovulation in the egg-retaining viviparous *S. acanthias* and progesterone remains elevated during the early part of gestation (Figure 11-8). Viviparous rays, *Sypyrna tibuno* and *Dasyatis sabina*, exhibit similar patterns of estradiol and progesterone to *S. acanthias* (Figure 11-9).

The ovaries of viviparous sharks produce a relaxin molecule structurally more similar to mammalian insulins than to mammalian relaxin but with similar biological actions when tested for uterine-relaxing activity in the guinea pig. Mammalian relaxin causes dilation of the uterus of pregnant *S. acanthias* and premature expulsion of embryos. Relaxin appears to have evolved early in vertebrate evolution and performs a similar function in sharks as in mammals. However, this is the only group of non-mammalian vertebrates so far shown to produce a relaxin and to respond to mammalian relaxin.

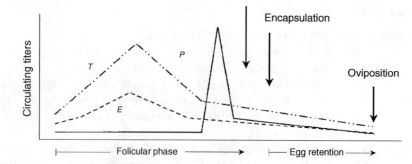
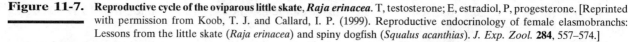

Figure 11-7. **Reproductive cycle of the oviparous little skate,** *Raja erinacea*. T, testosterone; E, estradiol, P, progesterone. [Reprinted with permission from Koob, T. J. and Callard, I. P. (1999). Reproductive endocrinology of female elasmobranchs: Lessons from the little skate (*Raja erinacea*) and spiny dogfish (*Squalus acanthias*). *J. Exp. Zool.* **284**, 557–574.]

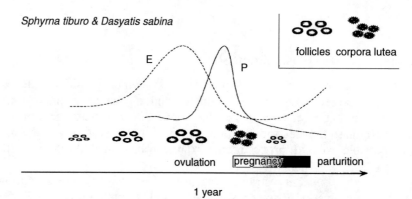

Figure 11-8. **Reproductive cycle of the viviparous shark,** *Squalus acanthias*. E, estradiol; P, progesterone. [Reprinted with permission from Koob, T. J., and Callard, I. P. (1999). Reproductive endocrinology of female elasmobranchs: Lessons from the little skate (*Raja erinacea*) and spiny dogfish (*Squalus acanthias*). *J. Exp. Zool.* **284**, 557–574.]

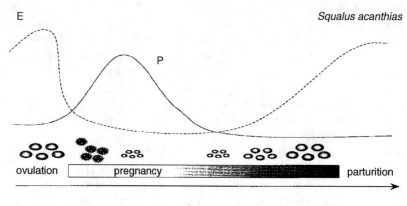

Figure 11-9. **Reproductive cycles of viviparous skates,** *Sphyrna tiburo, Dasyatis sabina*. E, estradiol; P, progesterone. [Reprinted with permission from Koob, T. J., and Callard, I. P. (1999). Reproductive endocrinology of female elasmobranchs: Lessons from the little skate (*Raja erinacea*) and spiny dogfish (*Squalus acanthias*). *J. Exp. Zool.* **284**, 557–574.]

IV. Reproduction in the Bony Fishes

Among the bony fishes, the teleosts exhibit almost every reproductive pattern and strategy known for vertebrates, including some that are unique to these fishes. Most of the account here is based on teleosts, but there are many similarities between teleosts and the other groups of bony fishes. Some features of these other bony fishes will be illustrated, also. But first, some generalizations need to be made.

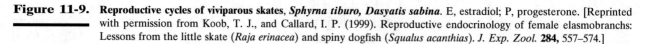

Like that of cyclostomes, the teleost gonad develops only from a cortical primordium. Bony fishes may be gonochoristic (separate sexes), unisexual (all female populations), or ambisexual (simultaneous or sequential hermaphrodites). Hermaphroditism implies that both functional sexes appear in the same body as opposed to intersex that means the present of of features normally characteristic of the opposite sex (i.e., presence of a female character in a male). Among the sequential hermaphrodites, there are numerous examples of **protandry** (*proto*, first; *andro*, male; function first as males and later transform to females) and **protogyny** (*gyno*, female; female first). Most bony fishes are oviparous, but viviparity has arisen in many forms as well.

Fertilization may be external or internal as in the viviparous teleosts and in the viviparous coelacanths, *Latimeria* spp. In some viviparous teleosts, the fertilized egg is known to develop within the ovary. Elaborate patterns of courtship, nest building, parental care, and other specific reproductive behaviors have been reported among diverse groups.

Breeding typically is cyclic but some species are semelparous and only breed once. Each species has a well-defined spawning period regulated by environmental factors (seasonal changes in photoperiod, temperature, etc.). Many iteroparous species spawn several times during a single breeding season (for example, *Reprohanus melanochir*, an Australian garfish of the halfbeak family). In some viviparous species, such as the guppy *Poecilia reticulata*, ovulation is induced by treatment with prostaglandins but is unaffected by steroids or pituitary extracts. Soon after birth of the young, a new batch of oocytes are released and another brood is raised. Other viviparous species require a longer "interbrood period" for oocyte maturation and vitellogenesis (*Mollienesia* and *Gambusia*). However, in *Quintana atrizoma*, oocyte development occurs during gestation so that a new batch of eggs can be fertilized as soon as the young are born.

The endogenous nature of seasonal or annual rhythms has not been demonstrated in fishes although seasonal reproductive cycles clearly are evident (see Figures 11-10 and 11-11) even in tropical species. The effects of

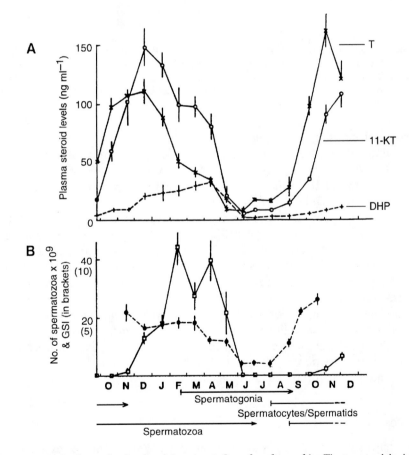

Figure 11-10. **Annual reproductive cycle of male rainbow trout, *Oncorhynchus mykiss*.** The top panel depicts plasma levels of testosterone (T), 11-ketoteosterone (11-KT), and 17,20b-dihydroxy-4-pregnen-3-one (DHP). The lower panel shows the volume of sperm produced (open squares) and the gonadosomatic index (GSI, gonad weight related to body weight). [From Scott, A. P. (1987). Reproductive endocrinology of fish. *In* "Fundamentals of Comparative Endocrinology" (Chester Jones, I., Ingelton, P. M., and Phillips, J. G., Eds.), pp. 223–256. Plenum, New York.]

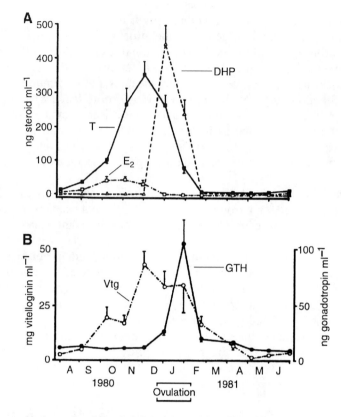

Figure 11-11. **Annual reproductive cycle of female rainbow trout,** *Oncorhynchus mykiss.* The top panel shows plasma levels of testosterone (T), estradiol (E$_2$), and 17,20b-dihydroxy-4-pregnen-3-one (DHP). Plasma levels of vitellogenin (Vtg) and gonadotropin (GTH) appear in the lower panel. [From Scott, A. P., and Sumpter, J. P. (1983). Seasonal variations in sex steroids and gonadotropin in females of autumn and winter spawning strains of rainbow trout (*Salmo gairdneri*). *Gen. Comp. Endocr.* **52,** 79–85.]

artificial lengthening and decreasing of the photophase may accelerate spawning in spring and fall spawners, respectively. A classical demonstration of environmental phasing of reproduction has been demonstrated by transporting a poecilid, *Jenynsia lineata*, from South America, where it normally spawned in January and February, to the northern hemisphere. In the new pond location where photoperiod and seasons were reversed, the fish switched to spawning in July and August. However, the possible importance of the temperature regimen, which was also switched, should not be overlooked. In some species, temperature has been shown to be the critical factor in controlling recrudescence regardless of the light regimen imposed on the fish. Some tropical cichlid fishes that live in permanent bodies of water exhibit successive breeding bouts over most of the year.

In the tropics, where photoperiod and temperature show little or no fluctuations, the reproductive cycles of freshwater and brackish water fishes appear to be tuned to the wet and dry seasons as occurs in many terrestrial vertebrates. Periodic flooding and drying cause marked changes in water availability and also influence salinity and chemical composition of the aquatic environment. During the dry season, the entire habitat of the South American annual killifish, *Austrofundulus limnaeus*, dries up and all adults die. However, the last eggs produced by these fish enter a state of diapause and survive in a desiccated state until the next rainy season. When the temporary ponds fill with water, the eggs hatch and the young grow rapidly, mature, reproduce repeatedly, and die when the ponds dry again.

A. Male Bony Fishes

Spermatogenesis in bony fishes is of the cystic tubular type, that is, the testes have a tubular organization but cystic spermatogenesis. Nests of spermatogonia proliferate from germ cells in the tunica albuginea and are surrounded by sertoli cells. The major circulating androgens in teleosts are 11-ketotestosterone and testosterone by interstitial or heydig cells. Many species show marked seasonal development in gonaducts,

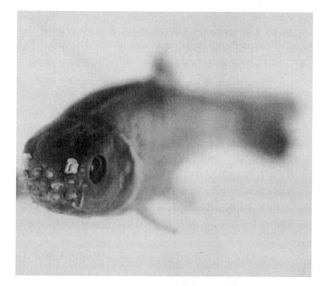

Figure 11-12. **Nuptial tubercles on the snout of a minnow.** These androgen-dependent secondary sexual characters are found on a number of cyprinid teleosts.

accessory glands, and secondary sexual characters that are presumed to be under androgenic control. For example, testosterone induces formation of nuptial tubercles on the head of fathead minnows (Figure 11-12), a distinctive male sexual characteristic in several cyprinid species. Viviparous teleosts, like their distant elasmobranch relatives, produce spermatophores, employing secretions by the male gonaducts. The gonaducts and the endocrine control of their secretory activities have not been examined sufficiently in teleosts.

B. Female Bony Fishes

The teleost ovary has been studied in considerable detail with respect to gonadal differentiation, oogenesis, vitellogenesis, and ovulation, in both oviparous and viviparous species. The ovary of most teleosts is hollow, whereas solid ovaries have been reported in most lungfishes and chondrostean fishes. A few teleosts also have solid ovaries. Unlike the hollow ovary of elasmobranchs and amphibians, in the ovary of teleosts the cavity as well as the outer surface are lined with germinal epithelium. Each hollow ovary is continuous with an oviduct that is not homologous to the mullerian duct-derived oviducts of other vertebrates. Eggs are discharged from the ovary directly into the oviduct. In species with solid ovaries, the eggs are discharged into the body cavity from which they pass to the exterior via oviducts or directly through temporary openings in the body wall. Teleost GnRH-1 or LH induces ovulation in teleosts *in vivo* or *in vitro*.

Basically, the teleost ovary consists of masses of follicles embedded in a rather sparse stroma. Each follicle begins as a single-layered epithelium derived from the germinal epithelium and surrounding an oocyte. As the follicle grows, these epithelial cells undergo hyperplasia and hypertrophy to form the granulosa. Connective elements in the stroma near the follicular nest will differentiate into a theca, which may further differentiate into a theca externa and a theca interna. The granulosa cells are responsible for yolk deposition in the oocyte during follicular growth and resorption of yolk during atresia. In salmonids, receptors that will bind FSH are found on both thecal and granulosa cells, and FSH is responsible for synthesis of estrogens during follicular growth. The LH receptors occur only on granulosa cells where they are associated with synthesis of the steroid $17,20\beta$-dihydroxy-4-pregnen-3-one (DHP) that is responsible for final oocyte maturation and ovulation in many species. The discovery and subsequent identification of DHP was accomplished by Yoshi Nagahama and his colleagues in Japan. A related derivative of progesterone, $17,20\beta,21$-trihydroxy-4-pregnen-3-one ($17,20\beta,21$-P), has been found to be responsible for these events in some species. A corticosteroid, deoxycorticosterone (DOC), is responsible for ovulation and final oocyte maturation in an Indian catfish, *Heteropneustes fossilis*.

Three developmental patterns for ovaries can be identified in teleosts. In the synchronous ovary, all oocytes are in the same stage of development. Species with a synchronous ovary are semelparous (for example, *Anguilla* spp. and most members of the genus *Oncorhynchus*). Species such as rainbow trout, white sucker, and flounder have a group-synchronous ovary with at least two populations of oocytes. These iteroparous species generally spawn once each year during a short breeding season. The last type is the asynchronous ovary that has oocytes in all stages of development at all times during the breeding season. These species spawn frequently each year during a prolonged breeding season.

Teleost ovarian tissue synthesizes estrogens *in vitro* from radioactive precursors and also synthesizes testosterone and DOC. These steroids have been identified in the peripheral plasma of females from several teleost species. The levels of testosterone often are greater in prespawning females than they are in males (Figure 11-10, 11-11), suggesting a behavioral role for androgens in females as reported for some female mammals.

All groups of bony fishes develop preovulatory, secretory corpora atretica as a result of atresia of developing follicles and develop short-lived corpora lutea following ovulation. However, a convincing endocrine function for corpora lutea is not yet established.

Vitellogenesis by the liver is stimulated by estradiol, and consequently total plasma calcium and phosphoprotein levels usually are elevated during oogenesis (Table 11-4). Calcium and vitellogenins are sequestered by the granulosa cells and are transferred to growing oocytes where they are transformed into yolk proteins (Figure 11-13).

C. Reproductive Behavior in Bony Fishes

Many aspects of reproductive behavior have been studied in teleosts, including migration, courtship, nest building, spawning, copulation, and parental care. Most of this work has concentrated on roles of testis, testosterone, and synthetic androgens in males. Male behaviors are regulated by 11-ketotestosterone and hence do not appear in females, which rarely produce 11-ketotestosterone. Castration of males blocks breeding behavior and causes reversal to non-breeding condition of androgen-dependent characters. Exposure to environmental estrogens has similar effects in males. Some variations have been reported for agonistic (territorial) behavior, which often accompanies breeding, depending upon the time of castration. In *Gasterosteus aculeatus*, form *trachurus*, castration more than a week before building of the first nest abolishes all related behaviors. If castration is performed within the week prior to building of the first nest, however, agonistic behavior remains at a high level for 3 to 4 weeks. In some species, castration does not result in a decrease in agonistic behavior, and androgens may not be required to maintain the behavior once it has been induced in these fishes.

The roles of estrogens and androgens in relation to the breeding behaviors of females have been studied less than the roles of androgens in males. Castration of females may result in complete abolition of all reproductive behavior, loss of only some or only a decrease in intensity. In one case, ovariectomized *G. aculeatus*, form *leiurus*, show more aggressive behavior than intact females, implying that ovarian steroids normally depress aggressive behavior in females. Estrogens have proven ineffective in inducing female behavior in females. Possible roles for androgens have not been studied, but the relatively high level of plasma androgens in prespawning females is suggestive of a behavioral role.

Table 11-4. Reproductive State and Serum Calcium Levels during the Spring in Steelhead Trout (*Oncorhynchus mykiss*) from a Natural Population

Sexual state	N	Mean body weight (g)	Mean serum calcium (mg/dl ± SE)
Immature males and females	12	38.4	11.6 ± 0.43
Sexually mature male prior to spawning	11	213.6	11.5 ± 0.74
Sexually mature females[a] after ovulation but prior to spawning	9	204.9	15.5 ± 1.44

[a] Sexually mature female trout differ significantly ($p < 0.01$) from sexually mature males and immature trout.

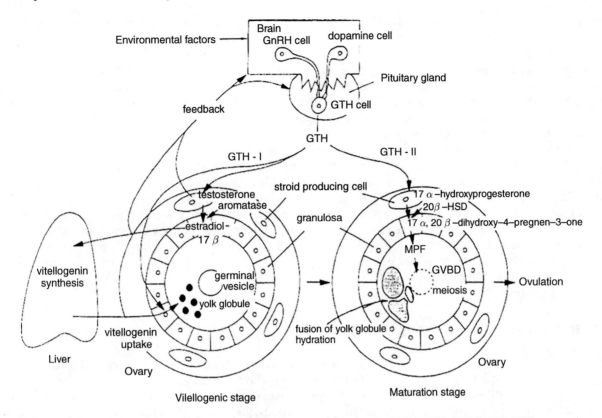

Figure 11-13. **Vitellogenein synthesis and incorporation into oocyes in teleosts.** GTH-I, FSH; GTH-II, LH; MPF, maturation promoting factor; GVBD, germinal vesicle breakdown; HSD, hydroxysteroid dehydrogenase. [Reprinted with permission from Connaughton. M. A., and Aida, K. (1999). Female reproductive system, fish. *In* E. Knobil, Eds. "Encyclopedia of Reproduction," Vol. 2, pp. 193–204, Academic Press, San Diego.]

Spawning behavior in females appears to be under control of GnRH and GTHs, although in *Fundulus heteroclitus*, neurohypophysial preparations or synthetic oxytocin induces reflexive spawning movements in hypophysectomized or castrated females (see Chapter 5). This spawning reflex is a behavior not dependent upon shedding of ova. Similar observations have been reported for a few additional species. Spawning behavior in female goldfish is stimulated by ovarian prostaglandins.

Communication by pheromones is important in the reproduction of teleosts. Following ovulation, females of numerous oviparous species emit pheromones that attract and arouse sexual activity in males. For example, female *Bathygobia soporator* secrete a pheromone from the ovary that elicits courtship behavior by intact males but not by anosmic males (treated to prevent olfactory detection). A priming pheromone released in the urine of female salmonids increases production of DHP in recipient males that in turn causes spermiation. The chemical nature of this pheromone is not known. Parental behavior is stimulated in *Heterochromis bimaculatus* by chemicals secreted by the young. Several species recognize their own young by using olfactory cues, and the offspring of some species use chemical recognition to identify their parents.

The goldfish has become a model system for investigations of pheromonal communication in teleost reproduction primarily due to the pioneering discoveries by Norman Stacey at the University of Alberta and his collaborators. During the final stages of oocyte development, the ovaries synthesize a mixture of C21-steroids including DHP and 17,20β,21-P. These steroids not only induce final oocyte maturation but also act as a pheromone in males to induce LH secretion, gamete release, and competence for spawning behavior. In addition, sulfated forms (DHP-S, 17,20β,21-P-S) are produced by goldfish ovaries and these too are potent stimulators of males. Recent evidence indicates that different regions of the male olfactory epithelium can detect 17,20β,21-P and distinguish selectively between DHP and 17,20β,-P-S. The physiological correlates of this ability have not been demonstrated, but should be forthcoming as this research continues.

In addition to releasing free and conjugated progestogens, goldfish ovaries also release considerable quantities of the androgen androstenedione that also plays a pheromonal role. Androstenedione release precedes release of DHP and inhibits the responsiveness of males to DHP. This mechanism may prevent premature gamete release in males. The presence of steroids and steroid mimics in wastewater effluents could alter reproduction in sensitive fish species.

Mammalian PRL has been shown to influence certain aspects of parental behavior in fishes. Fanning behavior associated with aeration of the eggs can be stimulated in *Symphysodon aequifasciata* and *Pterophyllum scalars* by PRL treatment. However, similar treatment inhibits fanning behavior in sticklebacks. PRL stimulates secretion of mucus that is fed to young *S. aequifasciata*, but it is not clear if the behavior of feeding the young also is PRL-dependent in these parent fish.

The implication of hormones in migratory behavior is largely circumstantial. The gonads and their secretions probably do not play a causative role since gonadal maturation usually occurs during migration. Thyroid hormones have been claimed to be causative factors of migratory behavior, and increased thyroid activity coincides with migratory behavior as does increased corticosteroid secretion. It is possible that the increased activity of the thyroid and adrenal glands are correlated to "permissive" effects of these hormones related to metabolism and osmoregulation. These hormones may only enhance the physiological states favorable to migration, whereas the behavioral changes are neurally controlled through actions of environmental factors such as photoperiod and temperature or possibly by endogenous rhythmic neural cycles that are regulated by these environmental factors.

V. Reproduction in Amphibians

Many amphibians are characterized as terrestrial or semi-terrestrial adults with an aquatic larval form. The importance of the aquatic intermediate larval stage is that it allows for an aquatic feeding stage where growth can be optimized without using energy stores or food resources of the terrestrial parents. During metamorphosis of these fish-like amphibian larvae to terrestrial-type tetrapods, the same problems are encountered and solved that confronted the evolution of terrestrial vertebrates from aquatic animals.

Although only a few of the almost 6000 known species of amphibians have been studied thoroughly, it is clear that there is a great diversity of reproductive patterns within this group of animals, and several trends in reproductive patterns are evident (Figure 11-14). All three extant orders (anurans, urodeles, and apodans) show a reduction in the use of the aquatic habitat with a tendency toward terrestrial development. This trend is accompanied by greater reliance on internal fertilization, a reduction in clutch size (number of eggs produced per breeding), and development of simple parental care of eggs and young. Mate selection and courtship patterns have become very elaborate in some species, often related to these complex patterns. Finally, oviparity apparently has given rise to viviparity independently on several occasions in each group: anurans, urodeles, and apodans.

The male gonaducts function as both urinary ducts and as sperm ducts or vasa deferentia. Enlargement and differentiation of the wolffian ducts to the functional male condition is caused by either testosterone or dihydrotestosterone (DHT) but is antagonized by estrogens. In marked contrast, although normal ovarian differentiation of müllerian ducts can be stimulated by estrogens, both DHT and testosterone are effective at stimulating müllerian duct enlargement in tiger salamanders although only testosterone is effective in frogs.

A. Oviparity in Amphibians

Most anuran amphibians studied are oviparous with external fertilization, although internal fertilization occurs in several species. Breeding in oviparous species is tied closely to a seasonal cycle involving photoperiod, temperature, availability of moisture, or a combination of these, although a few species are continuous breeders (e.g., the Indian frogs *Rana tigrina* and *R. erytrea* and the South American toads *Bufo arenarum* and *B. paracmenis*).

One predominant reproductive pattern is found in temperate oviparous anurans. Spermatogenesis and ovarian follicular development are completed in the fall, and the animals simply "hibernate" until suitable breeding conditions occur in the spring. Many oviparous species lay their eggs in temporary or permanent ponds with the eggs developing into free-swimming larvae. Tadpole larvae are the characteristic limbless, fish-like larval forms of anurans and differ markedly from the larvae of urodeles that possess external gills and four

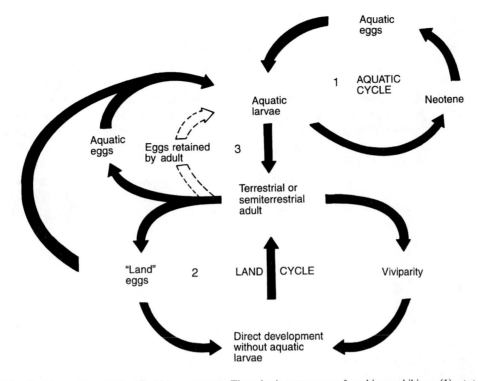

Figure 11-14. **Summary of amphibian life history patterns.** Three basic patterns are found in amphibians: (1) a totally aquatic cycle with sexually mature larvae (e.g., neotenes, see page 575); (2) a totally terrestrial or land cycle; (3) an aquatic-land pattern with terrestrial or semi-terrestrial adults and aquatic larval stages. Within these patterns are some distinct variations such as viviparity vs. laying an egg on land within the land cycle.

limbs at hatching. Anurans have internal gills like fishes and obtain their limbs later during metamorphosis. One anuran (*Ascaphus*) is known to lay its eggs in streams, and the tadpole larvae that result have special modifications to keep from being swept downstream. Some anuran and urodele species lay their eggs on land, usually in moist places such as under logs, in the axil of tree branches, or in temporary ponds held within the leaves of certain tropical plants. Terrestrial eggs require considerable parental care. For example, the male midwife toad, *Alytes obstetricans*, periodically carries the eggs, that are wrapped around his legs, to water to remoisten them. Larvae developing from terrestrial eggs either drop into the water after hatching or are carried to water by the watchful parents. Terrestrial eggs that are heavily yolked often develop directly into miniature adults, and no aquatic larval stage exists except as a transitional state within the egg.

Oviparous urodeles exhibit several reproductive patterns. In some species (e.g., *Triturus cristatus, Notophthalmus viridescens*), the pattern is similar to that of oviparous anurans. In the hellbender *Cryptobranchus alleganiensis*, spermatogenesis occurs in July shortly before breeding in August and September. Other species such as the mudpuppy, *Necturus* spp., transfer sperm to the females in the fall, and oviposition and fertilization occur the next spring when males are not present.

A number of oviparous apodans have been described, all of which lay terrestrial eggs. In *Ichthyophis*, the eggs are laid in a burrow near a stream, and each newly hatched larva must emerge from the burrow and find its way to the stream. Apodans generally produce larger eggs than do the other amphibian groups, and clutch sizes are proportionally small.

B. Viviparity in Amphibians

Two European land salamanders, *Salamandra salamandra* and *S. atra*, give birth to live offspring that develop in the posterior portion of the oviducts. In *S. atra*, one young develops and undergoes metamorphosis in each oviduct during a 4-year gestation period. Gestation is shorter in *S. salamandra* that gives birth to larval salamanders. The large size of these offspring indicates considerable nutrient contributions are made by the mother during these prolonged gestation periods. Details of these contributions and the mechanisms for their transfer have not been reported.

Viviparity in anurans typically involves a modification of a pouch that allows the eggs to develop into tadpoles on the body of the maternal animal. The South American tree frogs carry their eggs in a single mass on their back. A fold of skin may develop that completely covers the eggs in a pouch such as that found in the so-called marsupial frogs, *Gastrotheca* spp., of South America. In others, such as the African frog *Pipa pipa*, each egg develops in its own dermal chamber that forms on the back of the parent. Oviductal incubation of eggs occurs in *Nectophrynoides* and *Elutherodactylus*. One anuran incubates its young in its vocal sacs and at least one Australian species broods its young in its gut. Although this latter species was discovered very recently, it is now believed to be extinct.

It is estimated that viviparity occurs in the majority of apodan species. The contribution of maternal energy through oviductal secretion to support the developing young also is considerable. In *Typhlonectes*, one female may give birth to as many as nine larvae, each of which weighs about 40% of the mother's body weight at birth.

C. Reproduction in Male Amphibians

Male anurans and urodeles secrete both testosterone and dihydrotestosterone (DHT) in response to LH. Additionally, urodeles may produce some 11-ketotestosterone. Circulating androgens, FSH, and LH vary seasonally, but estradiol levels are very low. Highest values for reproductive hormones occur during mating in some species (e.g., *Rana catesbeiana*) but not in others (*Rana esculenta*, *A. tigrinum*) where gametogenesis is dissociated from time of spawning and development of accessory structures is dependent on steroids.

1. Male Urodeles

Spermatogenesis is of the cystic type in urodeles. The urodele testis (Figure 11-15) consists of one or more lobes, each containing several ampullae, which in turn are comprised of several germinal cysts (Figure 11-16). Germ cells associated with a germinal cyst divide mitotically to produce a cluster of secondary spermatogonia. These cells undergo synchronous differentiation to primary spermatocytes and enter meiosis. All of the cysts within an ampulla develop synchronously although it is typically only the more posterior ampullae that exhibit spermatogenesis prior to a given breeding season. The other ampullae represent the source of sperm for future breeding seasons. Sertoli cells develop from fibroblasts in the cyst walls while the spermatogonial divisions are taking place. As the ampullae mature, the posterior portion of the testis becomes swollen with sperm, whereas ampullae of the anteriormost portion consist primarily of spermatogonia. The posterior portion of the testis becomes dense and whitish because of masses of sperm. After spermiation occurs, the collapsed ampullae that have discharged their sperm into the male ducts are resorbed, and after breeding, spermatogenesis is initiated in the anterior portion of the testis. If spermiation occurs in the fall, spermatogenesis will not be resumed until the next summer. New ampullae differentiate from connective tissue elements and germ cells in the tunica albuginea.

Androgen levels exhibit distinct seasonal cycles in urodeles and anurans (Figure 11-17, Table 11-5). Seasonal patterns of androgen secretion have been reported for *Taricha granulosa*, *Cynops pyrrhogaster*, and *Ambystoma tigrinum*. Androgen levels appear to be low during breeding and high levels are more closely associated with development and maintenance of the vas deferentia that store sperm until breeding. Androgens also stimulate development of cloacal glands in males that are associated with spermatophore production and possibly with production of pheromones used in breeding. Contraction of the vasa deferentia and discharge of sperm during mating and spermatophore production are caused by AVT.

Androgens also stimulate development of sex accessory structures called nuptial pads in the newt *N. viridescens*, but maximal development is obtained by simultaneous treatment with PRL and androgen. Development of skin glands also are influenced by androgens. In urodeles such as *N. viridescens*, *T. cristatus*, and *A. tigrinum*, PRL is known to influence the movement of land-phase animals to water for

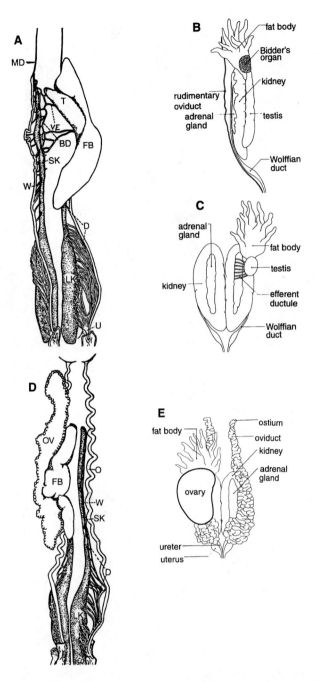

Figure 11-15.   **Amphibian gonads**. (A) Reproductive system of male salamander, *Ambystoma tigrinum*. Note the vasa efferentia (VE) that carry sperm from the testis to the wolffian duct (W) that doubles as both vas deferens and ureter. Many urinary-collecting ducts (D) connect the lumbar portion of the kidney (LK) to the wolffian duct. One testis and its corresponding fat body (FB) have been removed. Even in the adult, a remnant of the mullerian duct persists (MD). (B) The male toad *Bufo japonicus* with Bidder's organ anterior to the testis and a rudimentary oviduct, a remnant of the mullerian duct that persists in adults. This condition is common in all species of *Bufo* but is not found in other genera of anurans. Only one side of the reproductive system is shown. (C) In the male bullfrog, *Rana catesbeiana*, as in most anurans, there are no remnant female structures. One testis and its fat body have been removed. (D) In female tiger salamanders, the wolffian duct is reduced. The oviduct typically is much longer and folded in mature animals than is shown here. (E) Female bullfrog, *R. catesbeiana*. One ovary and its fat body have been removed to reveal the convoluted oviducts. [(A) and (D) from Rodgers, L. T., and Risley, P.L. (1938). Sexual differentiation of urogenital ducts of *Ambystoma tigrinum*. *J. Morphol.* **63**, 119–139. © 1938 John Wiley & Sons. Reprinted by permission of John Wiley & Sons, Inc. (B), (C), and (E) are from Matsumoto, A., and Ishii, S. (1992). "Atlas of Endocrine Organs: Vertebrates and Invertebrates." Japanese Society for Comparative Endocrinology and Springer-Verlag, Berlin.]

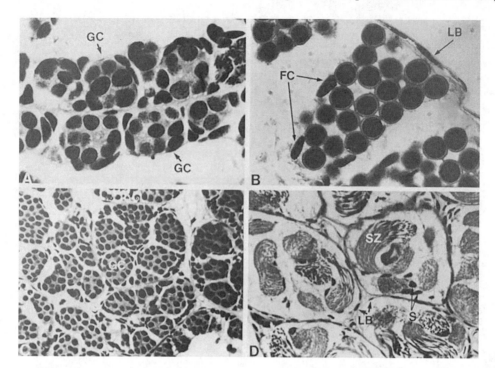

Figure 11-16. **Testis of the newt, *Taricha granulosa*.** (A) Early germinal cysts (GC). (B) Older cyst containing secondary spermatogonia. Follicle cells (FC) have flattened nuclei. LB, lobule boundry cell. (C) Lower magnification showing several ampullae each containing 6 to 8 cysts. (D) Enlargement of cysts from another region of the testis containing mature sperm (Sz) and prominent Sertoli cells (S) derived from follicle cells. (Courtesy of Frank L. Moore, Oregon State University, Corvallis.)

breeding and also induces heightening of the tail fin, which is a male secondary sex character in some species.

Internal fertilization in both aquatic and terrestrial urodeles occurs through transfer of a spermatophore from the male to the female. The spermatophore is produced through the actions of an array of specialized cloacal glands. The spermatophore consists of a glycoprotein matrix to which a packet of coagulated sperm is attached. The glycoprotein matrix acts as a base upon which the sperm packet rests. Following a complex courtship procedure, the female is induced to pick off the sperm packet using her cloacal lips. The sperm packet may then be stored in a specialized portion of the female's cloaca (spermatotheca) until ovulation and fertilization occur.

2. Male Anurans

The anuran testis is structurally unlike that of urodeles and is more similar to that of amniotes, consisting of a homogeneous mass of seminiferous tubules with a permanent germinal epithelium and conspicuous Leydig cells (Figure 11-18). The Leydig cells resemble mammalian Leydig cells ultrastructurally and possess 3β-HSD activity. The lipid cycle within the Leydig cells and the degree of 3β-HSD activity closely parallel the development of androgen-dependent sex accessory structures such as the enlarged thumb pads of ranid frogs. Leydig cells of post-spawning anurans exhibit considerable lipoidal accumulation but very low 3β-HSD activity, and thumb pads regress in ranids at this time.

During winter months, Sertoli cells of ranid testes lack lipid, but these cells elongate and exhibit small lipoidal granules as the breeding season approaches. Sertoli cells of breeding animals have a well-developed smooth endoplasmic reticulum, and 3β-HSD activity is detectable. After spermiation the Sertoli cells detach from the tubule wall and degenerate. New cells for the next reproductive period differentiate from fibroblasts in the tubule walls.

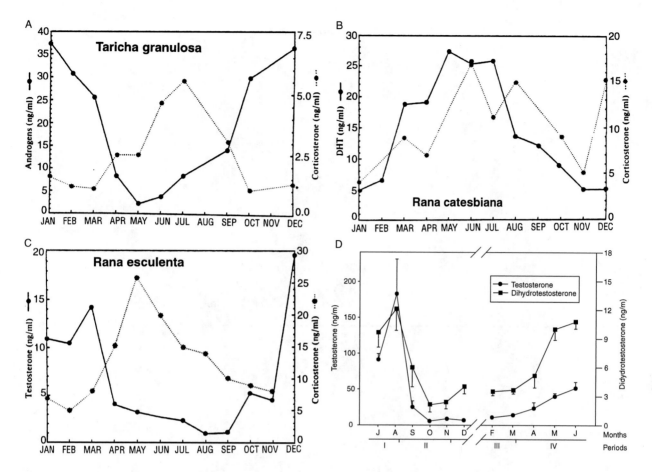

Figure 11-17. **Comparision of androgen and corticosterone levels during the reproductive cycles of amphibians.** Androgen levels appear to be negatively correlated to corticosterone levels in the newt *Taricha granulosa* (A) and the frog *Rana esculenta* (C) but dihydrotestosterone (DHT) is positively correlated with corticosterone in bullfrogs, *Rana catesbeiana* (B). The toad, *Bufo arenarum* (D), showns a similar pattern of androgen secretion to *R. esculenta*. [(A–C) From Moore F. L., and Deviche, P. (1988). Neuroendocrine processing of environmental information in amphibians. *In* "Processing of Environmental Information in Vertebrates" (M. Stetson, Ed.), pp. 19–45. Springer-Verlag, Berlin. (D) from Medina, M. F., Ramos, I., Crespo, C. A., Gonzalez-Calvar, S.I., Fernandez, S. N. (2004). Changes in serum sex steroid levels throughout the reproductive cycle of *Bufo arenarum* females. *Gen. Comp. Endocr.* **136**, 143–151.]

Table 11-5. Seasonal Extremes in Androgen Levels[a] in Selected Male Amphibians[b]

Species	Testosterone		5α-Dihydrotestosterone		Total androgens	
	High	Low	High	Low	High	Low
Urodeles						
Ambystoma tigrinum	32	0.4	7	0.3	39	0.7
Taricha granulosa					37	3
Triturus carnifex					28	2
Anurans						
Bufo japonicus	203	47	115	27	318	74
Bufo mauritanicus[c]	183		52			
Rana blythi[d]	4		1		5	
Rana catesbeiana					35	3
Xenopus laevis	39	19				
Xenopus laevis females	20	16				

[a] In nanograms per milliliter of plasma.
[b] Note the much higher levels reported for *Bufo* as compared to other anurans and urodeles.
[c] For breeding animals only.
[d] Continuously breeding tropical frog.

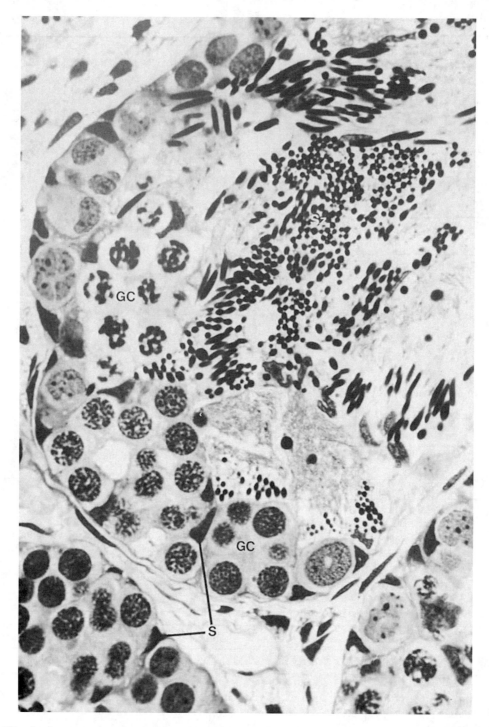

Figure 11-18. Section through testis of bullfrog, *Rana catesbeiana*. Note how all cells in a germinal cyst (GC) are in the same stage of development. Compare to urodele testis in Figure 11-10. (Courtesy of Charles H. Muller, University of Washington.)

3. Male Apodans

Male caecilians differ from urodeles and almost all anurans by possessing an elaborate intromittent organ, the phallodeum, associated with the posterior part of the cloaca. The pallodeum is employed for transferring sperm to the female reproductive tract. Consequently, fertilization is internal in all apodans. Another unique feature is the retention of only the most posterior portion of the müllerian ducts in males as the müllerian glands. These tubular apocrine glands are believed to produce seminal fluid and hence would be analogous to the prostate of mammals. The structure of the lobed apodan testes is similar to that of urodeles, but the cell nests within an ampulla are not synchronized and do not exhibit the same stage of spermatogenesis.

D. Reproduction in Female Amphibians

1. Female Anurans and Urodeles

Amphibian ovaries are hollow, sac-like structures derived from the embryonic cortex and covered by germinal epithelium (Figure 11-19). A derivative of embryonic medullary tissues forms the inner lining of the ovary. Oogonia are present in the germinal epithelium, and they give rise to nests of oocytes. The follicular epithelium is derived from the germinal epithelium and consists of a single layer of granulosa cells throughout the maturation period. A very thin thecal layer does form around the follicle, but it is only obvious when viewed with the aid of the electron microscope (compare Figures 11-19 and 11-20).

Granulosa cells and thecal cells contain 3β-HSD activity, but there is no steroidogenic activity in the ovarian interstitial cells of the ovary. Both thecal and granulosa cells may be sources of circulating ovarian steroids, but cytological evidence favors the granulosa as the major source. GTHs stimulate these cells to synthesize estrogens.

At the end of a breeding season, the ovary typically contains young follicles that will become the next crop of mature oocytes, numerous cell nests that will become the young follicles of the next vitellogenic period, and primary germ cells that will give rise to new cell nests for future generations of oocytes. Progression from primary germ cells to mature oocytes may require three breeding seasons or more for completion.

Ovarian estrogens control development of sex accessory structures such as the hypertrophy of oviducts prior to sexual maturation and during each season prior to ovulation. The oviducts regress when estrogen synthesis declines after breeding. In the marsupial frog *Gastrotheca riobambae*, the development of the brood pouch that will be used to incubate the eggs is dependent upon estrogens secreted from preovulatory follicles.

Postnuptial ovaries frequently contain postovulatory corpora lutea, which are short-lived in oviparous species. Granulosa cells hypertrophy after ovulation and accumulate cholesterol-positive lipids. The follicle collapses and becomes a central mass of lipoidal cells surrounded by a fibrous capsule derived from the thecal layer. Postovulatory corpora lutea of *T. cristatus* and *R. esculenta* possess 3β-HSD activity and are sources for steroids. However, no functional endocrine role for postovulatory corpora lutea has been demonstrated in these oviparous species.

In viviparous amphibians such as the anuran *Nectophrynoides occidentalis*, postovulatory corpora lutea are capable of converting pregnenolone to progesterone and persist throughout gestation. Corpora lutea are required for about the first 25 to 30 days of the 100- to 125-day gestational period in the pouch of the marsupial frog, *G. riobambae*, and ovariectomy after day 40 has no effect on gestation. The granulosa-lutein cells of the postovulatory corpora lutea in viviparous *S. salamandra* possess 3β-HSD activity and appear cytologically to be steroidogenic. Thirty or more corpora lutea persist in each ovary during the first two years of gestation and gradually decrease in both size and number over the next two years until the young larvae are born.

Development of new oocytes may be arrested by the presence of corpora lutea. In *N. occidentalis* as well as in oviparous *Taricha torosa*, the succeeding crop of follicles begins development only after degeneration of the postovulatory corpora lutea. These latter data suggest an inhibitory action of progesterone produced in the postovulatory corpora lutea on release of GTHs from the adenohypophysis.

Atresia occurs frequently during follicular development in amphibians. Granulosa cells are responsible for phagocytosis of yolk and formation of the preovulatory corpora lutea (corpora atretica) as they were in fishes. Since no 3β-HSD activity has been identified in these structures, they probably should be termed corpora atretica.

The process of vitellogenesis in the liver and yolk deposition in oocytes of oviparous amphibians has been examined extensively. In *X. laevis*, GTH stimulates micropinocytosis of vitellogenin by oocytes. Micropinocytotic vesicles of vitellogenin are hydrolyzed enzymatically in the yolk platelets to produce the yolk proteins **phosvitin** and **lipovitellin**. The yolk platelets containing these yolk proteins are utilized as an energy source during early embryogenesis. Estrogens will induce vitellogenin synthesis in both female and male livers when

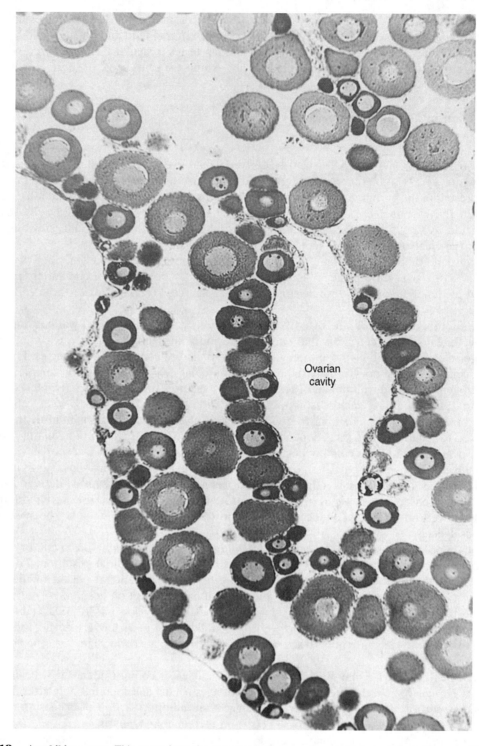

Figure 11-19. **Amphibian ovary.** This ovary from the cane toad, *Bufo marinus*, is typical of the hollow amphibian ovary with follicles attached to the germinal epithelium. (Courtesy of Charles H. Muller, University of Washington.)

administered *in vivo*. Circulating vitellogenin binds free calcium ions, resulting in elevated total plasma calcium levels through release of calcium from storage sites.

Hypophysectomy results in atresia of all vitellogenic follicles in excess of about 0.4-mm diameter, indicating the importance of endogenous pituitary GTHs in the process of vitellogenesis and maintenance of follicular

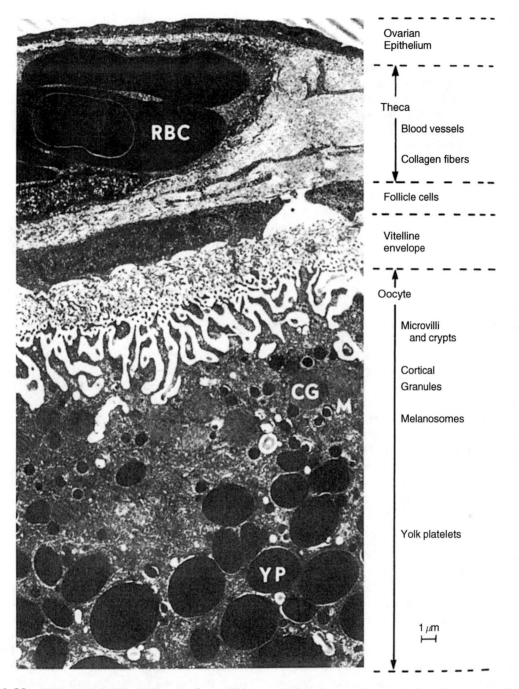

Ovarian
Epithelium

Theca

Blood vessels

Collagen fibers

Follicle cells

Vitelline
envelope

Oocyte

Microvilli
and crypts

Cortical
Granules

Melanosomes

Yolk platelets

1 μm

Figure 11-20. **Vitellogenic follicle of** *Xenopus laevis*. This transmission electron micrograph shows the vascular theca and its relationship to microvillous processes projecting from the surface of the developing oocyte. YP, yolk platelets. [From Dumont, J. N., and Brummett, A. R. (1978). Oogenesis in *Xenopus laevis* (Daudin). V. Relationships between developing oocytes and their investing follicular tissues. *J. Morphol.* **155**, 73–97. Reprinted with permission of the authors, publisher, and the Oak Ridge National Laboratory operated by Union Carbide Corporation for the Department of Energy.]

growth. Mammalian FSH will augment the growth of vitellogenic follicles and prevent atresia following hypophysectomy. The failure of GTHs to stimulate formation and growth of previtellogenic follicles (i.e., follicles of less than 0.4-mm diameter) coupled with their apparent insensitivity to hypophysectomy has led to the suggestion that these processes are completely independent of pituitary control. However, experimental studies have not ruled out completely a role for GTHs in the development of previtellogenic follicles, and it is possible that low endogenous levels of amphibian GTHs are necessary for even the earliest events in gametogenesis.

Amphibian ovaries *in vitro* produce progesterone, estradiol, estrone, testosterone, DOC (like teleosts), and DHT. The high levels of circulating testosterone reported for some female anurans may be related to a precursor role for peripheral aromatization to estrogens or to a behavioral role of their own.

Ovulation is under control of an LH-like GTH and progesterone. *In-vitro* studies of the ovary, initiated by Paul Wright about 60 years ago and subsequently elaborated by others, indicate that LH as well as a wide variety of steroids can induce oocyte maturation (completion of meiosis and breakdown of the germinal vesicle) and ovulation *in-vitro*. Progesterone is the most potent maturational steroid, and it is reasonable to presume that progesterone or a closely related steroid plays a key role in normal ovulatory events. The synthesis of progesterone is under control of LH, and the action of progesterone is believed to be indirect, operating through stimulation of a "maturation-promoting factor." Recent studies with *X. laevis* have shown that it may be the enzymatic conversion of progesterone into testosterone in the follicle that actually triggers final oocyte maturation and ovulation. PRL enhances the sensitivity of oocytes to GTH or progesterone (or testosterone?) both *in vivo* and *in vitro*. This enhancement can be blocked by simultaneous *in-vivo* treatment with thyroxine (T_4).

Ovarian maturation typically is completed in autumn, and ovulation is delayed over winter until favorable conditions occur in the spring. The endocrine basis for this diapause is not clear but may involve direct inhibition of ovulation by one or more pituitary hormones. Hypophysectomy of gravid anurans and at least one urodele result in ovulation and oviposition. Furthermore, hypophysectomy of gravid neotenic tiger salamanders increases their sensitivity to induced ovulation in response to a single injection of hCG. This "reflexive" ovulation could be due to inadvertent release of GTHs by the operation itself or to removal of an active inhibitory substance of pituitary origin or to both.

Growth of amphibian oviducts is stimulated by either estrogens or androgens. The feminizing action of androgens is another example of a paradoxical effect. In mature females, contraction of oviducts is caused by AVT, which presumably is the hormonal stimulus in oviposition. Oviducts of breeding animals are more sensitive to AVT than are those of non-breeding adults. Progesterone induces responsiveness to AVT in immature oviducts of salamanders, but estrogens are not effective. Possibly the pre- or postovulatory follicle releases sufficient progesterone in response to LH to alter receptor levels for AVT in the muscles of the oviducts. Androgens and estrogens do not affect the sensitivity of oviducts to AVT. The adrenocortical cells have been implicated as an additional progesterone source and may influence the response of oviducts.

2. Bidder's Organ

Among both sexes of bufonid toads are found rudimentary ovaries or Bidder's organs (Figure 11-15) that develop from cortical remnants of the embryonic genital ridge prior to normal gonadal differentiation. Histologically, Bidder's organ consists of a compact mass of small oocytes. In males, the bidderian oocytes undergo a limited seasonal growth and degeneration cycle correlated with the testicular cycle (Figure 11-21). These bidderian oocytes never reach the vitellogenic stage in males, however. The presence of 3β-HSD activity suggests they are steroidogenic during this time. After castration of male bufonids, Bidder's organ hypertrophies, presumably under the influence of increased GTHs, and forms a functional ovary. In castrated males, the rudimentary müllerian ducts may develop into functional oviducts and such sex-reversed animals may breed as females. The presence of isolated oocytes in the testes of bufonids is a common condition in at least one species, *Bufo woodhousei*.

3. Fat Bodies

Conspicuous masses of adipose tissue called fat bodies are located adjacent to the gonads of amphibians (Figure 11-15). In female anurans and urodeles, the size of the fat body is correlated inversely with gonadal weight, and it has been proposed that the lipoidal substances stored in the fat bodies are utilized for oocyte growth. The size of the fat bodies also is correlated with food availability. Fat bodies of both male and female European newts (*T. cristatus*) can synthesize steroids and therefore may influence gonadal function, accessory

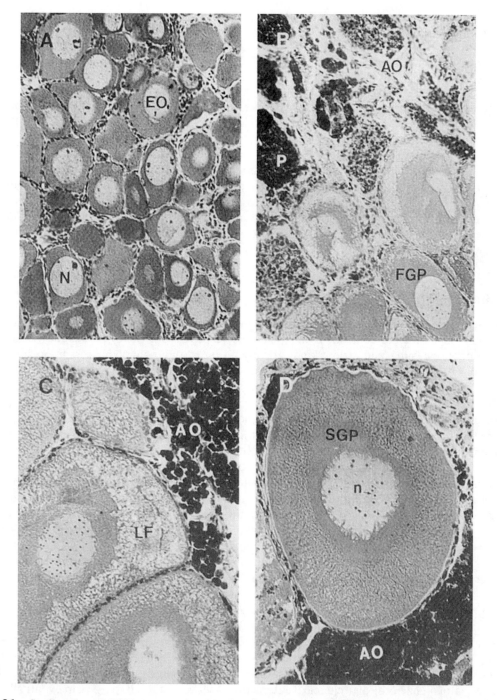

Figure 11-21. **Sections through Bidder's organ from male *Bufo woodhousii*.** These figures at the same magnification show the effects of castration and gonadotropin treatment on oocytes of Bidder's organ. (A) Sham-operated toad treated with saline injections for 26 days shows unstimulated follicles. EO, early previtellogenic follicle; N, nucleus. (B) Sham-operated toad treated with mammalian gonadotropins for 26 days shows moderately enlarged follicles. AO, atretic follicle; P, pigment granules; FGP, first growth phase follicle (previtellogenic). (C) Castrated toad treated with saline for 26 days shows oocyte and follicle growth into the late previtellogenic stage (LF). (D) Castrated toad treated with gonadotropins showing vitellogenic or second growth phase oocyte (SGP). [From Pancak-Roessler, M. K., and Norris, D.O. (1991). The effects of orchidectomy and gonadotropins on steroidogenesis and oogenesis in Bidder's organ of the toad *Bufo woodhousii. J. Exper. Zool.* **260**, 323–336. © 1991 John Wiley & Sons, Inc. Reprinted by permission of John Wiley & Sons, Inc.]

sex structures, or both. In the European frog, *R. esculenta*, the steroidogenic function of fat bodies appears to be regulated by pituitary GTHs.

4. Female Apodans

Fertilization in apodans normally occurs in the upper portion of the oviduct following intromission by the male, and the fertilized eggs either are laid in burrows or are retained in the oviducts until the developing larvae have completed metamorphosis. Ovarian development is very similar to that described for anurans and urodeles, but in apodans the eggs tend to be larger and fewer. Postovulatory corpora lutea develop in the ovaries, and they appear to be important for maintaining oviductal secretion (even in oviparous species) and pregnancy. Oviductal secretions in viviparous species provide nutrition for the developing young, and these secretions may be controlled by hormones released from the corpora lutea.

Relatively few apodans have been examined and it is not possible to describe the seasonality of breeding and ovarian cycles in caecilians. Even the endocrine factors involved in reproductive events can only be inferred from studies on anurans and urodeles.

E. Reproductive Behavior in Amphibians

Numerous aspects of reproductive behavior have been described for amphibians, but little is known about the mechanisms of endocrine control for most species. Reproductive behavior includes migration, calling, courtship, clasping, spawning, and various kinds of parental care. Studies involving castration, hypophysectomy, and/or injections of pituitary hormones support the conclusion that testicular hormones are involved in calling, courtship, and clasping. In neotenic *A. tigrinum*, a species with dissociated mating, androgens are not high at the time of mating. Although most species examined exhibit associated mating, attempts to stimulate reproductive behavior with androgens alone often have not been successful.

Even knowing plasma androgen levels may not tell the entire story. In the European crested newt, *Triturus carnifex*, inactive males have higher testosterone levels than courting males. Clasping of the female does not occur in these newts and courtship involves progressive stages: approaching, fanning, tail lashing, and spermatophore deposition. $P450_{aro}$ activity increases in the brain and gonad during courtship, and courting males have significantly higher levels of estrogen in brain and plasma during the approach stage of courtship.

Neural peptides (AVT, GnRH, ACTH) trigger mating behavior in androgen-primed animals. For example, when a female frog that is not ready to spawn is clasped by a courting male, she croaks to signal her non-receptivity. A receptive female will not emit this release call. This receptive female has accumulated water that will be used in ovulation and oviposition. Water retention is caused by AVT (see Chapter 5), and administration of AVT inhibits the release call, possibly through effects on the brain.

According to extensive studies by Frank Moore and associates at Oregon State University, reproductive behavior by male rough-skinned newts (*T. granulosa*) also is stimulated by AVT although androgens and other factors are involved (Figure 11-22). During courtship, males in the breeding pond will attempt to clasp a female along the back. Attempts by several males to clasp the same female result in the formation of mating balls that persist for a time, but the unsuccessful males soon drop off, leaving only one clasping the female. A series of behavioral and chemical interactions between the clasping pair eventually will lead to spermatophore transfer. Androgens play a priming role than enhances the sensitivity of the newts to AVT. Stress or injection of corticosterone can rapidly repress clasping behavior within minutes. Clasping can be activated by cloacal stimulation and is controlled by neurons located in the rostral portion of the medulla. Furthermore, activity of these neurons is increased by AVT treatment but decreased by administration of corticosterone.

Pheromones are used in courtship by many urodeles that possess hedonic glands or cloacal glands. These glands are known to be sources of potent pheromones. Male plethodontid and desmognathid salamanders employ a tubular mental (chin) gland for stimulating courtship behavior in females. Ambystomatids and salamandrid salamanders rely on pheromonal secretions from one of their cloacal glands, the abdominal gland, to stimulate females. Female attractants released into a stream readily attract reproductively active male *T. granulosa*. Furthermore, males of this species are attracted to females by airborne cues as well (see

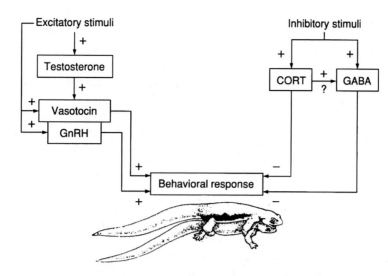

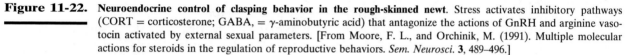

Figure 11-22. **Neuroendocrine control of clasping behavior in the rough-skinned newt.** Stress activates inhibitory pathways (CORT = corticosterone; GABA, = γ-aminobutyric acid) that antagonize the actions of GnRH and arginine vasotocin activated by external sexual parameters. [From Moore, F. L., and Orchinik, M. (1991). Multiple molecular actions for steroids in the regulation of reproductive behaviors. *Sem. Neurosci.* **3**, 489–496.]

Table 11-6. Sex-Dependent Conspecific Odor Preferences in *Taricha granulosa*: Directed Locomotor Response of Newts to Newt and Non-Newt Odors[a,b]

No. of tests	Sex of test newt	Sex of stimulus newt	Ratio of S[c]/NS[d]	Probability that choices were random
10	Male	Male	7/3	0.0570
10	Male	Female	10/0	0.0003
20	Male	Male/female	17/3	0.0004
10	Female	Male	4/6	0.625
10	Female	Female	6/4	0.625
20	Female	Male/female	10/10	0.987

[a] Unpublished data of M. Schwartz, D. Duvall, and D. O. Norris (1978).
[b] Examined in a simple olfactometer.
[c] Subject chose air from stimulus animal.
[d] Subject chose air from nonstimulus source (no newt).

Table 11-6). Two peptide pheromones have been isolated from the abdominal cloacal glands of newts (*Cynops pyrrhogaster, Cynops ensicauda*) and a 22-kD protein was found in the mental gland of the salamander, *Plethodon jordani*. These secretions are used to attract the female to a spermatophore. The pheromone from *C. pyrrhogaster*, **sodefrin**, is released by the action of AVT on the abdominal gland, and it binds to receptors in the female's vomeronasal organ. The number of receptor cells for sodefrin in the female increases during the breeding season. The responsiveness of the vomeronasal epithelium to sodefrin is enhanced by exposure of the animals to PRL and estrogens.

In contrast, there is little evidence for chemical communication among anuran species, and mating is accomplished presumably by using auditory, tactile, and visual cues. For example, estrogen levels are enhanced in female Túngara frogs, *Physalaemus pustulosus*, by listening to calling males. However, another peptide with female attractant properties has been isolated from the skin glands of a male anuran, *Litoria splendida*.

Nest-building is a complex form of parental care that is exemplified by the terrestrial foam nest frog, *Chiromantis xerampilina*. As many as 40 females may contribute to production of a huge, communal foam nest in which fertilized eggs are deposited. The females produce the foam by beating water with their hind limbs. Males are much smaller than females and they attract females by making soft clicking sounds. When a female arrives at a calling site, males drop from above onto her back. One male occupies the central position with up to seven peripheral males hanging on. This central position is considered to be the most advantageous postion for fertilizing eggs emanating from the female's cloaca. In experiments where the cloacae of males were sheathed to prevent sperm release, no eggs were fertilized. When only the central male was sheathed, about half of the eggs were still fertilized, but they were fertilized by the unsheathed peripheral males. In another study, 10 of 15 naturally breeding females were shown to produce clutches having 2 or more feathers. Thus, cooperation not only occurs in nest-building behaviors in this species but also in mating, which ensures a good mixing of genetic material in the following generation.

VI. Reproduction in Reptiles

Living reptiles are members of diverse orders, and it is not surprising that considerable differences occur, making it difficult to generalize about reptilian reproduction. In many respects, the squamate reptiles possess features unique to their order, whereas the other orders may be more typical of reptiles as a group with respect to exhibition of primitive features. Most reptilian species are oviparous and exhibit well-defined annual reproductive cycles and breeding seasons. In addition, many examples of viviparity are known among snakes and lizards, and viviparity has been hypothesized to have evolved many times in these groups. Only a few, heavily yolked eggs are produced by most reptilian species although clutch sizes may be relatively large in some turtles, crocodilians, and snakes. Fertilization is internal in all reptiles, and males have intromittent organs for placing sperm into the cloaca of a female. Mating frequently follows complicated behaviors including male–male territorial and aggressive interactions. Following mating, females of many species can store sperm in the cloaca for months.

In males, the vas deferens develops from the wolffian ducts as described for amphibians (Figure 11-23). The vas deferens conducts no urine in reptiles, however, as the mesonephric kidney is completely replaced in reptiles by the evolution of the metanephric kidney with its own ureter connecting to the urinary bladder. As elegantly demonstrated in the American alligator, müllerian ducts degenerate in males prior to hatching as a consequence of a müllerian-inhibiting substance (MIS) secreted by the testes as in mammals (Figures 11-24 and 11-25).

Crocodilians and turtles produce two distinct GTHs, but squamate reptiles rely on a single FSH-like hormone. The hypothalamus produces GnRH-1 that regulates GTH release in response to environmental stimuli such as photoperiod and temperature (see Chapter 5).

Reptiles classically have been characterized by a lack of parental behavior and, in some cases, even lack of recognition of their offspring. In recent years, however, studies have demonstrated that there is considerable investment in parental care even among oviparous species. Although members of the oldest extant group, the chelonians, typically abandon their nests once the eggs are laid, many squamates exhibit parental behavior. Crocodilian parents participate in the hatching process and in protecting the young. Evidence of nest-building and parental care has been unearthed for some extinct dinosaurs as well. Thus, complex parental care did not appear *de novo* in birds and mammals but already had evolved in early reptiles.

A. Male Reptiles

The male reproductive system (Figure 11-26) is typical of amniotes, and the testes consist of convoluted seminiferous tubules (Figure 11-27), each surrounded by a connective tissue sheath, the tunica propria. The entire testis is enclosed by a tunica albuginea. Spermatogenesis recurs soon after the breeding season and is completed in most species prior to the onset of winter. Pituitary GTHs stimulate spermatogenesis in a variety of reptilian species. Sperm may be stored in the vas deferens for up to several months prior to mating. Sertoli cells are common, and they are steroidogenic. After spermiation and testicular collapse, the Sertoli cells fill with cholesterol-positive lipid that is depleted under the influence of FSH at the time mitosis resumes

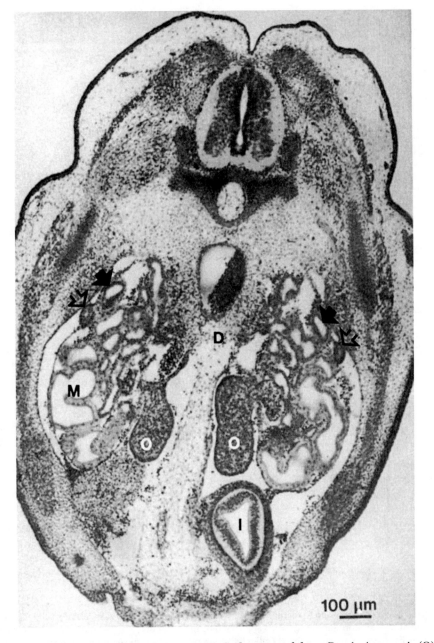

Figure 11-23. **Cross-section through an embryo of the lizard,** *Sceloporus undulatus*. Developing gonads (O), mesonephros (M), mullerian ducts (open arrows), wolffian ducts (solid arrows), intestine (I), dorsal mesentary (D). [From Austin, H. (1988). Differentiation and development of the reproductive system in the iguanid lizard, *Sceloporus undulatus*. *Gen. Comp. Endocr.* **72**, 351–363.]

in the spermatogonia. Typical interstitial cells have been described in the reptilian testis (Figure 11-27), and they undergo cyclical changes associated with androgen secretion and sexual changes in androgen-dependent sex accessory structures (Figure 11-28). Representative plasma androgen levels are provided in Table 11-7.

In sexually active squamates, a portion of the kidney tubules, known as the sexual segment of the kidney, undergoes hypertrophy under the influence of androgens. The sexual segment appears to secrete materials that help maintain sperm that are stored in this region prior to ejaculation, and it may be homologous to the seminal vesicles of male mammals.

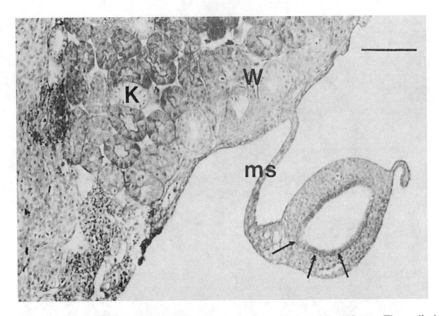

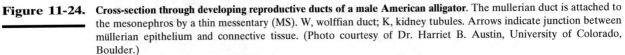

Figure 11-24.   **Cross-section through developing reproductive ducts of a male American alligator.** The mullerian duct is attached to the mesonephros by a thin messentary (MS). W, wolffian duct; K, kidney tubules. Arrows indicate junction between müllerian epithelium and connective tissue. (Photo courtesy of Dr. Harriet B. Austin, University of Colorado, Boulder.)

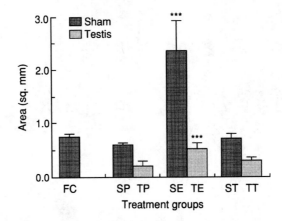

Figure 11-25.   **Effects of testis grafts and hormone treatment on mullerian ducts of female American alligator embryos.** The source of mullerian inhibitory substance (MIS) appears to be the testis, and MIS is antagonized by the presence of estradiol (E). This figure shows mean epithelial cell height of mullerian ducts in sham-operated (S) and testis-grafted (T) animals. Estradiol (E) treatment stimulated mullerian ducts (SE) and reduced the degree of regression (TE) caused by the presence of a testis (TP). Testosterone had no effect in either group (ST, TT). [From Austin, H. B. (1990). The effects of estradiol and testosterone on Mullerian-duct regression in the American alligator (*Alligator mississippiensis*). *Gen. Comp. Endocr.* **76**, 461–472.]

B. Female Reptiles

Reptiles have paired hollow ovaries with little stromal tissue. Oogonia are present in the mature ovary as described for anamniotes and give rise to primary oocytes throughout reproductive life. The developing oocyte (Figure 11-29) becomes invested with granulosa cells derived from the germinal epithelium. The granulosa cells are separated from the surrounding thecal cells by a connective tissue layer, the membrana propria. In reptiles, the theca is differentiated into an inner, glandular theca interna surrounded by a fibrous theca externa. The cells of the granulosa in most species are considered the primary source of follicular estrogen during ovarian recrudescence, although histochemical evidence in skinks (genus *Lamproholis*)

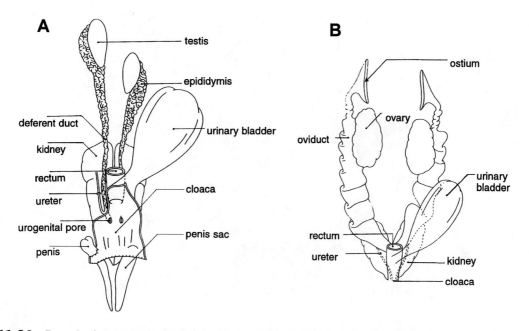

Figure 11-26. **Reproductive system of a lizard.** (A) Male. The top wall of the cloaca has been removed to show the duct openings and the penis. (B) Female. [Modified from Matsumoto, A., and Ishii, S. (1987). "Atlas of Endocrine Organs: Vertebrates and Invertebrates." Springer-Verlag, Berlin.]

implies that thecal cells rather than the granulosa cells are steroidogenic. Histochemical changes in ovarian cholesterol-positive lipid inclusions and 3β-HSD activity parallel estrogen-dependent oviductal growth and changes in other sex accessory structures as well as changes in the gonadotropes in the adenohypophysis. As the oocyte enlarges, it begins to project into the ovarian cavity and out from the surface of the ovary.

The squamate granulosa contains a unique flask-shaped cell type, the pyriform cell (Figure 11-29), that is in direct contact with the developing oocyte. These cells apparently are involved with early steps in oocyte development as they either degenerate or transform into typical granulosa cells soon after the onset of vitellogenesis.

As ovulation approaches, the granulosa cells as well as some thecal cells accumulate cholesterol-positive lipids, and, following ovulation, proliferate and luteinize to form corpora lutea. These corpora lutea are well vascularized, exhibit 3β-HSD activity, and synthesize progesterone. They persist throughout egg laying in oviparous species or during gestation in most viviparous forms. Corpora lutea of viviparous species synthesize greater amounts of progesterone than do those of oviparous species. Plasma progesterone levels are greatest following ovulation and are maintained at elevated levels throughout gestation in most viviparous lizards and snakes. Preovulatory peaks of progesterone are found in oviparous turtles, crocodilians, and lizards (Table 11-8).

Only a few of the follicles that begin development reach maturity at a given time; the majority undergo atresia. Follicular atresia and formation of corpora atretica is a common occurrence in reptilian ovaries as in other vertebrates. The importance of corpora atretica is unknown, but the absence of 3β-HSD activity in corpora atretica makes it unlikely they would have an endocrine function. However, steroidogenic cells from atretic follicles may give rise to an "interstitial gland" that is believed to be a major source of ovarian estrogens.

Ovaries of reptiles show different patterns of follicular maturation and ovulation. Some produce several eggs simultaneously from each ovary (most reptiles). Others may alternate production of a single egg from each ovary (anoline lizards). Differences in follicular atresia rather than in the number of oocytes beginning development may be responsible for these patterns. Still others (e.g., certain turtles) may produce most of their eggs in one ovary during one season and most from the other ovary the next season.

Exogenous GnRH produces direct actions on ovarian follicles that may reflect a paracrine role for ovarian GnRH. Treatment of lizards (*Podacris sicula sicula*) with salmon GnRH (sGnRH) increases secretion of

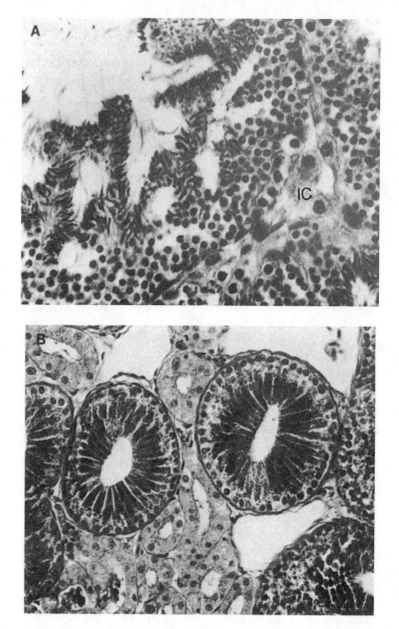

Figure 11-27. **Spermatogenesis and the sexual segment in sceloporine lizards.** (A) Spermatogenesis in the testis of *Sceloporus jarrovi*. Portions of three seminiferous tubules can be seen, separated by several large Leydig (interstitial, IC) cells. Note the dense, elongated sperm heads. (B) Section through kidney of *Sceloporus undulatus* showing small, lightly stained renal tubules and large, darkly stained sexual segments of renal tubules modified for sperm storage. This enlargement is due to the action of testosterone. (Courtesy of Dr. John Matter, Juniata College.)

prostaglandin ($PGF_{2\alpha}$) from mid- to late follicles and early corpora lutea and increases secretion of progesterone from follicles. Antagonists of GnRH produce opposite results. The physiological relevance of these observations is open to interpretation, but it does suggest paracrine effects of GnRH are not limited to mammals.

Alternation of ovulation in the ovaries of the anoline lizard *A. carolinensis* has been investigated extensively by Richard Jones. There is a definite alteration in catecholamine activity in the hypothalamus that mirrors ovarian alternation. These observations may be explained by sensory neural connections between the ovaries and the hypothalamus that are transmitting information responsible for regulating the alternating pattern of ovulation.

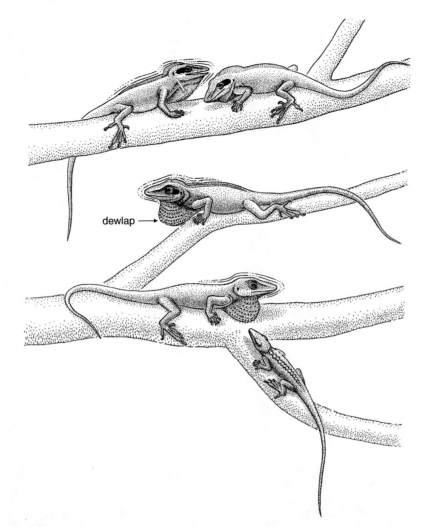

Figure 11-28. **Displays exhibited by male *Anolis carolinensis*.** The dewlap is an androgen-dependent structure that may be extended from the throat region. On the top limb, two males are performing an aggressive bout. Head-bobbing and dewlap extension are common components of displays. Note the postorbital black pigment spot that appears in response to elevated epinephrine. The lone male on the middle limb is exhibiting an assertion-challenge display normally performed by the dominant animal following an aggressive bout. Note the postorbital spot is less intensely blackened. The male on the bottom main limb is making a courtship display to the smaller female on the branch below. This display includes dewlap extension and head-bobbing, but there is no evidence of the postorbital pigment spot. [Reprinted with permission from Crews, D. (1978). Integration of internal and external stimuli in the regulation of lizard reproduction. *In* "The Behavior and Neurology of Lizards" (N. Greenberg and P. D. McLean, Eds.), pp. 149–171. NIMH, Rockville, Maryland.]

Oviductal development apparently is under the influence of ovarian estrogens, and progesterone is without effect. In oviparous species, estrogens probably influence the secretion around the egg of albumin and shell from the anterior end of each oviduct. Estrogens also stimulate synthesis of vitellogenic proteins by the liver and cause increases in serum calcium of snakes, lizards, and turtles (Table 11-9). This increased availability of calcium is important for secretion of the shell by specialized cells in the lining of the oviduct. Undoubtedly the details of this process are very similar to those described for amphibians, although vitellogenesis has not been investigated as extensively in reptiles as in anamniotes. It is known that crocodiles produce yolk proteins that are biochemically similar to those of birds.

Oviposition or birth of live young is controlled by AVT, prostaglandins, and β-adrenergic innervation in turtles, lizards, and snakes. In the American chameleon, *A. carolinensis*, the sensitivity of the uterus to AVT is determined by presence or absence of a corpus luteum in the adjacent ovary.

Table 11-7. Plasma Steroid Levels[a] in Reptiles

Species	Testosterone	Estradiol	Progesterone
Turtles			
Chrysemys picta			
Male	15–40 ng		
Preovulatory female	3.2–5.7 ng	0.79–1.37 ng	1.2–1.5 ng
Postovulatory female	0.2 ng	UND[b]	0.3–0.5 ng
Stenotherus ordonatus			
Female	250–1500 pg	500–5000 pg	700–4000 pg
Male	10–75 ng		
Lizards			
Lacerta vivipara	27–390 ng		
Uromastix hardwicki			
Preovulatory female	0.37 ng	0.18 ng	1.6 ng
Gravid female	1.57 ng	0.46 ng	13.41 ng
Iguana iguana			
Male	100 pg	79 pg	
Female	3 pg	270 pg	
Snakes			
Natrix fasciata (female)	50–1065 pg	10–540 pg	90–1445 pg
Naja naja			
Male	60–2300 pg		
Female	30–700 pg	10–310 pg	1.4–25 ng
Nerodia sipedon (male)	2–21 ng		

[a] Per milliliter.
[b] UND, undetectable.

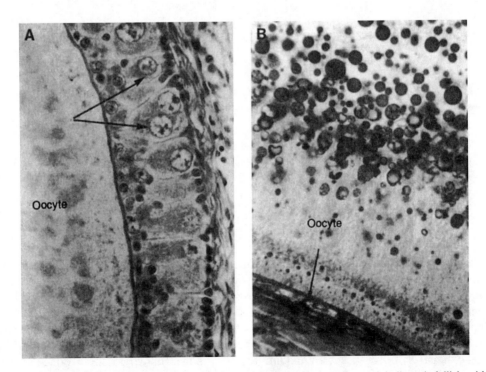

Figure 11-29. **Ovary of the iguanid lizard, *Ctenosaura pectinata*.** (A) Section through a perivitellogenic follicle with large pyriform cells (arrow) in the granulosa layer. (B) Lower magnification of a vitellogenic follicle. Note the granulosa (arrow) is flattened. (Courtesy of Dr. Mari Carmen Uribe, Facultad de Ciencias, UNAM, Mexico.)

Table 11-8. Circulating Progesterone Levels[a,b] during Reproductive Cycles of Turtles, Lizards, and Snakes

Species	Period of early follicle growth	Preovulatory stage	Early postovulatory	Mid-pregnancy	Late pregnancy
Turtles					
Chrysemys picta (oviparous)	0.2±0.06	5.0±1.02	0.5±0.01	—	—
Chelonia mydas (oviparous)	0.2±0.08	1.8±0.13	0.7±0.88	—	—
Lizards					
Sceloporus cyanogenys	0.7±0.15	0.9±0.38	3.3±0.48	—	3.5±0.34
Chamaelo pumilis	0.9	1.0±0.71	5.0±3.90	2.3±0.34	—
Snakes					
Natrix taxispilota	0.4±0.04	0.9±0.08	1.9±0.24	—	—
Nerodia sipedon	1.3±0.19	3.9±0.83	5.0±1.41	6.9±0.78	2.8±0.44
Thamnophis elegans	—	—	1.7±0.30	6.2±1.00	—

[a] Modified from Lance, V., and Callard, I. P. (1978). *In vivo* responses of female snakes (*Natrix fasciata*) and female turtles (*Chrysemys picta*) to ovine gonadotropins (FSH and LH) as measured by plasma progesterone, testosterone, and estradiol levels. *Gen. Comp. Endocrinol.* **35**, 295–301.

[b] In nanograms per milliliter of plasma.

Table 11-9. Effect of Estradiol on Serum Calcium Levels of Ovariectomized Female Lizards (*Anolis carolinensis*)[a]

Treatment	N	Serum calcium (mg/dl ± SE)
Ovariectomized saline-injected females	5	14.8±1.05
Reproductively active, sham-operated females	4	21.2±3.47
Ovariectomized females injected with 1.0 μg of estradiol per day for 7 days	5	213.2±9.88
Ovariectomized females injected with 10 μg of estradiol per day for 7 days	7	256.0±22.13

[a] Unpublished data of K. Faber and D. Norris (1975).

C. Environment, Behavior, and Reproduction in Reptiles

The role that physical and biological components of the environment play in sexual behavior and reproduction has been extensively studied in reptiles. Species living in temperate climates exhibit distinct seasonal patterns of hormonal secretion and reproductive events. Reproduction in tropical reptilian species varies from cyclic patterns to continuous breeding. There is a strong tendency for an observed increase in the incidence of viviparity among species inhabiting colder climates (altitude or latitude), but it is not clear which is cause or consequence.

Among temperate lizards, temperature is the dominant environmental factor influencing reproduction. Photoperiod, humidity, and nutritional status play decisive roles in some species. Other groups of reptiles have not been studied as extensively as lizards.

Although visual cues are the primary mechanism employed in reptilian courtship, evidence for pheromonal communication can be inferred from some experimental studies in all major reptilian groups. Male lizards of several families (Scincidae, Lacertidae, Teidae, Gekkonidae) have androgen-dependent femoral glands located on the inner thighs as well as special cloacal glands that seem to play important roles in courtship and territorial behavior in association with breeding. Inguinal and axillary glands of chelonians have been implicated in reproductive behavior, too. Crocodilians appear to use chemical communication in courtship, but little detail is available.

When a female red-sided garter snake, *Thamnophis sirtalis*, emerges from its winter hibernaculum, she is immediately courted by a large number of males who had emerged previously. This behavior produces a mating ball of males, all attempting to copulate with a single female. The skin of the reproductive female produces methyl ketone that apparently in the presence of estrogens attracts the males and signals them that she is ready to mate. As soon as one male successfully copulates with the female, she secretes another semiochemical that immediately turns off male mating behavior. Although injection of estrogens into adult males does not make them attractive to other males, some males with high testosterone and aromatase levels also are attractive to normal males, presumably because of the conversion of testosterone to estrogens. These "she-males" are more successful in achieving copulation with females than are normal males, presumably because the "she-males" confuse normal males who attempt to mate with them rather than with the true female, thus reducing their competition.

One model for studying reptilian behavioral studies is exemplified by the work of David Crews and his collaborators at the University of Texas. In general, estrogen and progesterone are responsible in reptiles as in most vertebrates for stimulating female receptive and mating behaviors whereas androgens, typically testosterone, control male behaviors. As previously mentioned, in a number of cases, androgens may be converted to estrogens by aromatase in order to produce behavioral effects. Among the species of whiptail lizards in the genus *Cnemidophorus*, about one-third are unisexual. These species consist only of females, which are further unusual in that these females are all triploid (3n). Studies by Crews have employed one 3n species, the desert-grasslands whiptail *C. uniparens*, which apparently evolved from hybridization of two 2n species, the rusty rump whiptail *C. burti* and the little striped whiptail *C. inornatus*. Since *C. uniparens* has two sets of chromosomes derived from *C. inornatus* and only one from *C. burti*, Crews focused his behavioral studies on *C. uniparens* and *C. inornatus* (that exhibits normal sexual reproduction). A similar system occurs among the salamanders of the *Ambystoma jeffersonianum* complex except that there the 3n females must mate with a male from a 2n species to activate cleavage in the egg although no genetic material is contributed. In *C. uniparens*, mating does not occur with males of diploid species but rather the 3n females alternate between expressing female (receptive) and male (mounting) mating behaviors (Figure 11-30). Although estradiol levels in the 3n females is 5X less than in 2n females, this results in higher hypothalamic levels of estrogen receptor mRNA in the 3n brains and hence greater sensitivity to low plasma levels of estradiol. The postovulatory decrease in estrogen allows

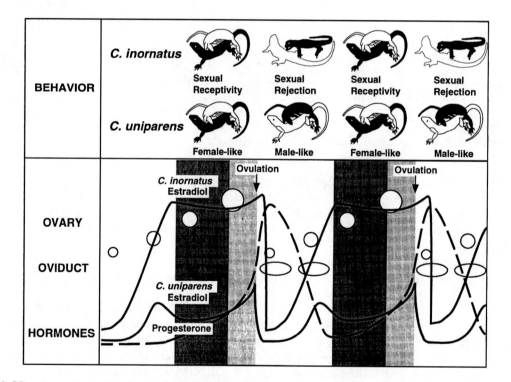

Figure 11-30. **Comparison of mating behavior in unisexual and bisexual lizards.** Female-like and male-like behavior in the all female desert-grasslands whiptail lizard (*C. uniparens*) is compared with female receptive behavior in a bisexual lizard, the little striped whiptail (*C. inornatus*). The differences in estradiol levels for the two species are illustrated. Female-like behavior in *C. uniparens* is elicited by a lower estrogen level and is followed by male-like copulatory behavior. The circles represent size of the ovarian follicles and the ovals indicate presence of eggs in the oviduct. [Reprinted with permission of the publisher from Young, L. J., and Crews, D. Comparative neuroendocrinology of steroid receptor gene expression and regulation: Relationship to physiology and behavior. *Trends Endocr. Metab.* **6**, 317–323. Copyright 1995 Elsevier Science Inc.]

for appearance of male-like mounting behavior or pseudocopulation although the exact chemical stimulus is not clear.

VII. Reproduction in Birds

The HPG axis of birds appears to be controlled by both the production of GnRH-1 in the PVN but also by a GnIH neuropeptide from the same nucleus in the hypothalamus (see Chapter 5). Secretion of this GnIH appears to be regulated by melatonin from the pineal gland. These dual factors regulating reproduction in birds may be related to the importance of photoperiodic information for reproduction.

Avian reproductive organs (Figure 11-31) reflect the reductional anatomical adaptations to flight that characterize most bird systems. In females of most species, only the left ovary and its attendant oviduct develop, whereas the right-hand components remain in a rudimentary state. Should the left ovary be removed surgically or destroyed by disease, the right rudiment may develop, but it will usually form an ovotestis or a testis rather than another ovary. This left-right asymmetry is reflected in the male where the left testis usually is larger than the right although both are functional.

Avian gonads develop from a pair of undifferentiated primordia associated with the embryonic nephrotome. These primordia are invaded by primordial germ cells that migrate through the blood from the splanchnopleure and develop into the germinal epithelium. The embryonic gonad goes through a bipotential state in which both cortical and medullary components are present. Differentiation of cortical tissue is necessary for ovarian development and the medullary portion is suppressed. The reverse condition prevails in male birds. In contrast to mammals, it is the male bird that is the homogametic sex (similar sex chromosomes, ZZ), and it is the female that has unlike sex chromosomes (ZW). Developing a female phenotype requires estrogens, and castration of a young female may cause development of male plumage.

Development or suppression of the müllerian and wolffian ducts eventually depends on the direction of gonadal development as it does in other vertebrates. In females in which only the left half of the reproductive system usually develops, the left ovary receives the larger proportion of germ cells that migrate to the gonads. The mechanism behind this disproportionate distribution of germ cells is not known. Degeneration of the müllerian duct occurs only on the side of the smaller ovary and is induced by MIS produced in ovarian cells.

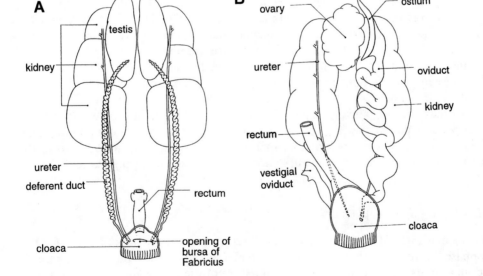

Figure 11-31. **Reproductive organs of the pigeon.** The top of the cloaca has been removed in both sexes to illustrate connection of the gonaducts. (A) The male. (B) The female. Note that the right ovary is absent in most birds (the left in others) as well as the corresponding oviduct. This regression is due to production of MIS in the embryo by the remaining ovary, which secretes estradiol locally and protects the mullerian duct on that side from MIS. [From Matsumoto, A., and Ishii, S. (1992). "Atlas of Endocrine Organs: Vertebrates and Invertebrates." Japanese Society for Comparative Endocrinology and Springer-Verlag, Berlin.]

Local secretion of estrogens by the larger ovary is believed responsible for preventing oviduct degeneration on that side.

All birds are oviparous but display significantly more parental behavior than any non-mammalian group of vertebrates. Birds are endothermic like mammals and use their body heat to support development of the embryo within the egg much as the mammal does *in utero*. Consequently, birds can breed successfully under conditions that are too cold for their reptilian relatives. The adaptation of long-distance flight coupled with high body temperatures allows utilization of polar and subpolar regions where winter conditions are too severe for survival but where the summer months provide adequate warmth and food to breed and rear young birds to a size sufficient for successful fall migration to warmer latitudes for winter.

Reproduction is decisively cyclic in adult birds and is closely attuned to environmental factors (Figures 11-32 and 11-33). Migratory and non-migratory high-latitude and temperate species typically exhibit seasonal cycles with breeding occurring in the spring and sometimes continuing through much of the summer. On the other hand, species occupying arid regions may show irregular cycles cued to the availability of water, which may not occur with any seasonal regularity. One tropical species, *Zonotrichia capensis*, has been reported to breed every 6 months regardless of rainfall as long as food is available.

Generally, ovaries and testes remain small in non-breeding birds and undergo tremendous hypertrophy in a very short time at the onset of the breeding season. This is especially advantageous for migratory species or species relying on particular stimuli for breeding where gonadal recrudescence can await arrival on the breeding grounds or appearance of suitable conditions such as abundant food.

A. Male Birds

Unlike the case for many mammalian species, bird testes are permanently located in the body cavity, and each testis consists of a mass of convoluted seminiferous tubules lined with a germinal epithelium and surrounded by connective tissue. Both developing germ cells and steroidogenic Sertoli cells as well as numerous fibroblasts can be seen in the germinal epithelium. As in mammals and other vertebrates, the cytoplasm of the Sertoli cells completely envelops the germ cells. Typical steroidogenic interstitial cells occur between the seminiferous tubules as seen in reptiles and mammals.

In non-breeding birds, testes are very small, and histologically these quiescent testes appear to be composed largely of interstitial cells. However, this is only an artifact produced by a marked post-breeding regression of spermatogenetic tissue. The onset of spermatogenesis (recrudescence) results in a rapid and marked increase in testicular size. Such rapid and extreme growth (to as much as 500 times the resting gonad weight) results in considerable strain and damage to the tunica albuginea surrounding the testis, and it must be replaced each year during the postnuptial phase of the testicular cycle. Replacement is accomplished through differentiation of fibroblasts and formation of a new tunica directly beneath the damaged one. It is often possible to distinguish histologically between juvenile birds and postnuptial birds by the presence of two connective tissue capsules around the testis in the latter.

Testicular recrudescence may involve a single synchronous spermatogenetic event or separate spermatogenetic waves, depending on whether a given species produces successive clutches during a particular breeding season. In either event, following spermiation, sperm migrate to expanded distal ends of the vasa deferentia known as seminal sacs from which sperm will be ejaculated forcefully during mating.

1. The Avian Testicular Cycle

The annual testicular cycle of temperate birds has three more or less distinct phases: (1) the regeneration or preparatory phase; (2) the acceleration or progressive phase; and (3) the culmination phase. Similar phases can be identified in all birds regardless of the seasonal nature of their reproductive cycles or what environmental factors control testicular events.

The most common environmental factor influencing development of the avian testis is photoperiod. Placing quiescent, temperate birds, such as ostriches (Figure 11-32) on long-day photoperiods will typically stimulate testicular recrudescence, whereas maintenance of these birds on short-day photoperiods even into the normal breeding season represses anticipated testicular events. In contrast, some birds such as the emu (*Dromaius*

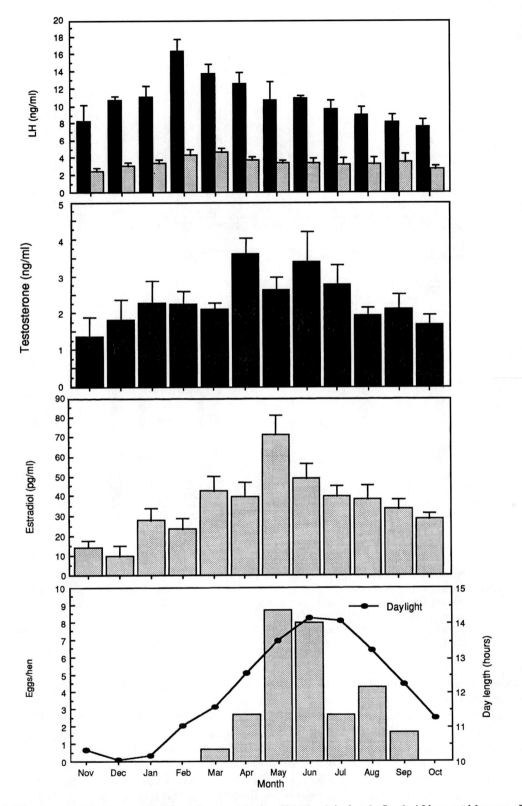

Figure 11-32. **Plasma LH, plasma estradiol, and egg production (light bars) in female South African ostriches are affected by photoperiod**. Plasma LH and testosterone levels in males are indicated by the black bars. [From Degen, A. A., Weil, S., Rosenstrauch, A., Kam, M., and Dawson, A. (1994). Seasonal plasma levels of luteinizing and steroid hormones in male and female domestic ostriches (*Struthio camelus*). *Gen. Comp. Endocr.* **93,** 21–27.]

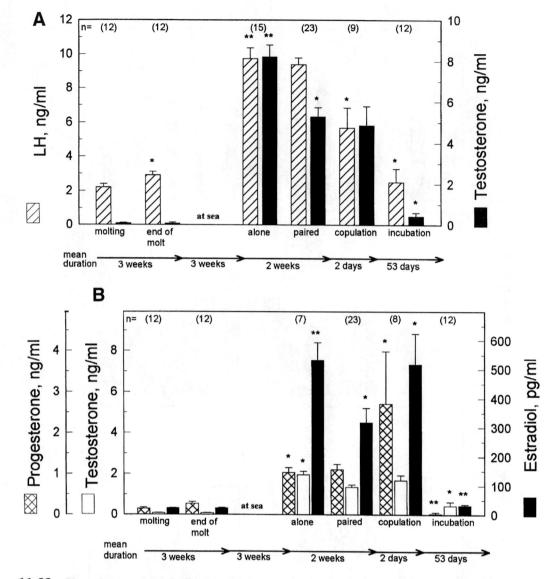

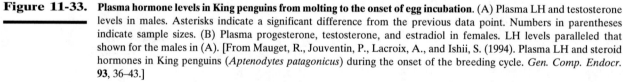

Figure 11-33. **Plasma hormone levels in King penguins from molting to the onset of egg incubation**. (A) Plasma LH and testosterone levels in males. Asterisks indicate a significant difference from the previous data point. Numbers in parentheses indicate sample sizes. (B) Plasma progesterone, testosterone, and estradiol in females. LH levels paralleled that shown for the males in (A). [From Mauget, R., Jouventin, P., Lacroix, A., and Ishii, S. (1994). Plasma LH and steroid hormones in King penguins (*Aptenodytes patagonicus*) during the onset of the breeding cycle. *Gen. Comp. Endocr.* **93**, 36–43.]

novaehollandiae) are short-day breeders with peak testicular function occurring during the winter months and quiescence is maintained under long-day photoperiods.

The preparatory phase of testicular development begins immediately after the reproductive period and is characterized by marked collapse of the testis. Animals in the preparatory phase are insensitive to effects of long photoperiod and are termed "photorefractory." The end of the preparatory phase is heralded by restoration of photosensitivity. The endocrine basis for the photorefractory period in birds is not clear, and more than one mechanism may be involved in different species. Some studies suggest that feedback of testosterone on the hypothalamus is responsible for induction of the photorefractory period and for lower levels of LH during the photorefractory period (Figures 11-32 and 11-33). Other investigations point to changes in hypothalamic sensitivity and/or steroid metabolism and not testosterone feedback. An intriguing hypothesis proposed by Peter Sharp involves the inhibitory role of PRL that determines GnRH secretion in both long-day and short-day breeders.

Photosensitivity is separable into two phases, although there may be a continuum of the events associated usually with one phase. During the progressive phase, there is an increase in GTH secretion brought about by actions of lengthening photoperiod on the HPG axis. Increased circulating GTHs stimulate both spermatogenesis and androgen secretion by the interstitial cells. An increasingly intensive period of sexual activity and song occurs, and males of some species may begin exhibiting territorial behavior and mate selection. This effect of long photoperiod can be blocked by low temperatures and may involve elevated glucocorticoids (see Chapter 9).

The culmination phase coincides with the time of ovulation in females and includes the time of insemination. The male typically is ready for breeding before the female, and his testes will be bulging with sperm. Successful breeding involves a complex, hormonally dependent series of events involving precise male-female behavioral interactions.

2. Leydig Cells in Birds

A characteristic lipid cycle occurs in avian Leydig cells similar to that described for other vertebrates. There is accumulation of lipid in young birds followed by rapid depletion coincident with onset of the first breeding season and spermatogenesis. The Leydig cells of adult birds are small and sparsely lipoidal in winter although they occupy a large proportion of the testis because of the regressed nature of the seminiferous tubules. There is gradual accumulation of lipids, including cholesterol, throughout the progressive phase as well as an increase in 3β-HSD activity. At the time of maximal sexual display, there is rapid depletion of Leydig cell lipid. Cholesterol disappears completely, but 3β-HSD activity remains strong, indicating lipid depletion is a consequence of rapid synthesis and secretion of androgens. The activity of 17α-hydroxylase is also high at this time (see Chapter 3 for its specific role in androgen synthesis). A massive disintegration of interstitial cells occurs during the preparatory phase, and new Leydig cells differentiate from fibroblasts.

3. Sertoli Cells in Birds

Cyclical changes in lipid content are characteristic of avian Sertoli cells that ultrastructurally resemble steroidogenic cells. Both 3β-HSD and 17β-HSD activities have been reported for these cells. They become densely lipoidal following the breeding season, and no detectable 3β-HSD activity remains. The stored lipid is depleted with the onset of the next period of spermatogenesis.

4. Endocrine Control of Testicular Function

The hypothalamus contains two gonadotropic centers that separately control release of LH and FSH from the adenohypophysis. Hyperplasia of Leydig cells is caused by LH, and they become lipoidal and exhibit increased 3β-HSD activity. Avian testes are much more sensitive to avian LH than to mammalian LH. Androgens secreted by these cells stimulate sex accessory structures and secondary sexual characters. Similarly, purified mammalian FSH is less effective than avian FSH in stimulating spermatogenesis. Local effects of androgens from Sertoli cells are responsible for stimulating meiosis. Androgens are known to maintain spermatogenesis even in hypophysectomized birds.

Prolactin is present in the male pituitary and has been reported to inhibit FSH release and block spermatogenesis in some species. The formation of incubation patches on males of certain species is induced in part by PRL working cooperatively with testicular steroids.

5. Sex Accessory Structures in Male Birds

Wolffian ducts give rise to paired vasa deferentia, vasa efferentia, and the epididymides and their associated testes, all of which exhibit hypertrophy with the onset of sexual activity. These events are all prevented by castration. A testis is connected to the vasa efferentia by small rete tubules in the tunica albuginea that become enlarged during the breeding season. The vasa efferentia show increased secretory activity during the breeding season and coalesce to form a long, coiled tube, the epididymis. Hypertrophy of the epididymis is accompanied by secretion of seminal fluid. Mature sperm leave the epididymis and enter the enlarged vas deferens for storage. The distal end of each vas deferens (seminal sac) fills with sperm. The posterior walls of the seminal sacs protrude into the cloaca as erectile papillae that facilitate transfer of sperm to the female. During copulation, the male's cloaca is everted and these erectile papillae are brought into contact with the vagina of the female. In some species, the cloaca actually is modified into a penis-like intromittent organ.

B. Female Birds

In spite of the extensive literature available on domestic fowl, few studies of avian reproduction have employed wild species. However, assessment of ovarian function in domestic species is relatively complete and provides a basis for comparison with wild species. In many respects, ovarian function in birds is like that of their oviparous ancestors, the chelonians, squamates, and especially the crocodilians.

The domestic hen differs most importantly from wild birds by being selected for continuous breeding. Prior to hatching there is a proliferation of oogonia to produce thousands of primary oocytes that will serve the hen throughout her long and busy reproductive life. As in mammals, few if any oocytes will be formed after hatching, unlike the situation for many anamniotes and reptiles. However, most of these oocytes will undergo atresia during early maturational stages. The primary follicle consists of an oocyte surrounded by a layer of granulosa cells. As the follicles grow, thecal layers are added, and the follicles become highly vascularized. Both granulosa and thecal cells are steroidogenic, possess 3β-HSD activity, and produce steroids as described for mammals. However, in birds, the steroidogenic process may involve three cells rather than two. In the domestic turkey, progesterone is synthesized by the granulosa cell while androgens are made in cells of the theca interna and converted to estrogens in the theca externa. This pattern has yet to be confirmed in wild species.

Estrogens secreted from the follicular cells cause the liver to produce large quantities of calcium-binding vitellogenin for the growing oocytes. This mechanism brings calcium to the oviducts, where it is used to construct the shell. Vitellogenin is enzymatically hydrolyzed to produce phosvitin and lipovitellin, which are stored in the yolk of the egg. The liver also synthesizes large quantities of triglycerides that are transported in the blood as β-lipoproteins and also are incorporated into growing oocytes. Micropinocytosis of these phosphoproteins and triglycerides by the oocytes is stimulated by FSH. Antrum formation as described for mammalian follicles does not occur in birds.

The large developing follicles of birds bulge conspicuously from the surface of the ovary, giving it the appearance of a bunch of grapes. The largest follicles are highly vascularized except for a rough, avascular spot, the stigma, where the follicle will rupture at ovulation.

Atresia of developing follicles may occur at any time during follicular development. These atretic follicles can be easily recognized by an influx of fibroblasts that phagocytize the yolk materials. Granulosa and thecal cells are lipoidal and contain cholesterol. There are many corpora atretica at all times in the ovary, but their importance, if any, is not recognized. As they disintegrate, some of the cells of the corpora atretica may become stromal interstitial cells and secrete estrogens.

Birds are characterized by the absence of persistent corpora lutea following ovulation. This feature is correlated with the absence of viviparity among the more than 8000 known species of birds. Following ovulation, collapsed follicles consist largely of granulosa cells containing progesterone, abundant smooth endoplasmic reticulum, and considerable 3β-HSD activity. The only evidence for a functional role, however, is the observation that surgical removal of these ruptured follicles increases the time that the ovulated egg is retained in the oviduct.

1. Endocrine Control of Ovarian Function in Birds

There is a close correlation between pituitary GTH content and ovarian function in both domestic and wild birds (Figure 11-32). Hypophysectomy causes ovarian regression and extensive follicular atresia, which can be prevented by GTH replacement therapy. Follicular development is stimulated by FSH, and FSH will maintain oviducts in hypophysectomized but not in ovariectomized birds. Estrogen secretion is controlled by both LH and FSH. Mammalian GTHs, however, are not always as effective in birds as are avian pituitary extracts or avian GTH preparations. Furthermore, avian FSH is very effective at stimulating follicle development in lizards, emphasizing the close similarity between reptilian and avian pituitary hormones and the cautions necessary when interpreting the effects of mammalian hormones.

As is the case for certain reptiles, growth of follicles and ovulation is a continual process throughout the breeding season. Studies on the ovary of laying chickens have demonstrated an oocyte-derived growth differentiation factor (GDF9) that appears to exert a paracrine regulation of surrounding granulosa cells similar to that reported for the mammal (see Chapter 10). As in mammals, GFD9 appears to play a role in follicle development and can suppress progesterone synthesis by granulosa cells. Ovarian function is regulated so that typically only one egg is discharged at a time. This condition is reminiscent of the human and the lizard *A. carolinensis*, in which only one ovum is discharged, and the ovaries alternate in providing the ovum. However, birds have only one functional ovary with a hierarchy of graded follicle size. The endocrinological basis for establishment and maintenance of this hierarchy is not known for reptiles, birds, or mammals, and it represents one of the major unanswered questions in reproductive biology.

The synthesis of vitellogenin by the avian liver is induced by estrogens as was described for other oviparous vertebrates. Total serum calcium concomitantly increases, which is related to the binding of calcium by vitellogenin (Table 11-10). In addition to incorporation of vitellogenic proteins into the oocyte, circulating calcium is sequestered by the shell glands of the "uterus" (an expanded region of the oviduct) for construction of the eggshell.

Pituitary LH is responsible for triggering ovulation of the fully mature follicle. Plasma LH peaks about six to eight hours before ovulation in domestic hens as well as in Japanese quail, but the magnitude of the avian LH surge is considerably smaller than that observed in mammals. This lower surge of LH might be an adaptation to ensure only sufficient LH for ovulating the largest follicle.

Calcium availability may be a potent factor regulating reproduction in female birds. Production of shelled eggs in domestic species directs as much as 10% of the body calcium stores per day into eggs. If large amounts of calcium are not available in the diet, the reproductive axis of the egg factory is shut down before damage to the skeleton occurs. When sufficient calcium becomes available, the birds resume laying. Although continuous egg laying does not occur in wild birds as it does in domestic fowl, it is possible that calcium depletion in wild birds contributes to cessation of breeding and induction of the refractory period.

Another pituitary hormone, PRL, plays essential roles in reproduction including the development of a specialized, defeathered region in some species known as an incubation patch, which aids in incubating eggs. Secretion of crop milk by the pigeon crop sac for use in feeding young birds also is induced by PRL and has resulted in development of a most useful biological assay for PRL activity in all tetrapod pituitaries (see Appendix D). Prolactin does not affect steroidogenesis in cultured chick granulosa cells and probably has no effect on progesterone synthesis.

2. The Avian Oviduct

Estrogens secreted by the growing follicle stimulate hypertrophy of the oviduct and differentiation of secretory regions. Five differentiated regions can be identified in the mature avian oviduct which are like those of crocodilians: infundibulum, magnum, isthmus, shell gland, and vagina. After ovulation, the ovum moves through the body cavity, enters the open end of the **infundibulum**, and is fertilized in the upper portion of the oviduct before the egg white protein albumen is added. The middle portion of the oviduct or **magnum** becomes highly glandular under the influence of estrogens, forming tubular glands and goblet cells. Estrogens

Table 11-10. Effect of Mammalian Parathyroid Extract and the Influence of the Egg-Laying Cycle on Total Serum Calcium of Chicken[a]

Subject	Control (mg/dl $\pm$ SE)	Treated with parathyroid extract (mg/dl $\pm$ SE)
Rooster	10.1 ± 0.2	19.5 ± 3
Nonlaying hen	13.4 ± 2	19.5 ± 4
Laying hen	29.8 ± 11	47.7 ± 9

[a] Assenmacher, I. (1973). The peripheral endocrine glands. *In* "Avian Biology" (D. S. Farner and J. R. King, Eds.), Vol. 3, pp. 183–286. Academic Press, New York.

stimulate synthesis of **ovalbumen** protein by these tubular glands, whereas progesterone stimulates the goblet cells to secrete the other major egg white protein, **avidin**. After accumulation of several coatings of ovalbumen, the egg passes from the magnum to the muscular **isthmus** where two shell membranes are applied. These membranes are composed of fibrous proteins cemented together with albumin. The shell consists largely of calcium salts supported by a fibrous protein matrix deposited on the outermost shell membrane by the **shell gland** or "uterus." After the shell has been applied, contraction of a powerful sphincter muscle causes the egg to rotate in the muscular **vagina** and enter the cloaca pointed-end first. Movement of the egg into the cloaca as well as its extrusion into the nest (oviposition) is controlled by AVT and prostaglandins. An increase in plasma AVT together with a concomitant decrease in neurohypophysial AVT coincides with oviposition. Treatment with AVT can cause premature oviposition.

3. Incubation Patches

In many avian species, a ventral region of skin called the **apterium** becomes defeathered, highly vascularized, and edematous just prior to or during egg laying. In addition, the epidermis of this region may exhibit hyperplasia. This specialized region is the **incubation** or **brood patch**, and when in contact with the eggs provides an efficient transfer of warmth from the parent bird to the eggs. Incubation patches may form in females, males, or both, depending upon the species and which sex is responsible for incubating eggs. However, mere possession of an incubation patch is not proof of incubating behavior. Male house sparrows, *Passer domesticus*, have no incubation patch, yet exhibit incubating behavior. Conversely, male flycatchers (genus *Empidonax*) develop an incubation patch but do not show incubating behavior.

Formation of incubation patches involves cooperative actions of both estrogens and PRL. Estrogens seem to stimulate vascularization of the patch region, and PRL stimulates defeathering and epidermal hyperplasia. There typically is a concomitant transformation of pituitary lactotropes to a stimulated morphology known as "broody cells." Both PRL and estrogens are necessary for normal patch development. Furthermore, the response of epidermis in forming a patch is both site-specific and tissue-specific. After transplant to the dorsal surface ventral skin will still respond to PRL but not to estrogen. Vascularization of the ventral skin occurs only when it is in its normal location. Dorsal skin transplanted to the normal patch site will not respond to either estrogens or PRL.

C. Androgen-Dependent Secondary Sex Characters in Male and Females Birds

Androgens play important roles in both male and female birds. In a number of species, a change in bill color is associated with breeding. Such changes are induced in both sexes by androgens but not by estrogens or progesterone. However, there is at least one case in which bill color change occurs only in the female, and, in that case, the color change is induced by estrogens.

Plumage color changes also may be controlled by androgens. This can occur even in the case of phalarope birds where the females possess the more colorful or nuptial plumage. One cannot presume androgens are responsible unless specific studies have been performed to verify this fact, because androgens are not always responsible for nuptial plumage. For example, development of nuptial plumage in castrated male weaver finches, *Euplectes orix*, has been used as the classical bioassay for LH (see Appendix D). In some instances, estrogens actively inhibit formation of nuptial dress, and castration of females will cause development of male plumage. Assumption of nuptial dress in males also can be blocked with estrogens, verifying that it is the absence of estrogens that allows male plumage to develop and not the presence of androgens.

In some strains of chicken, both sexes have female-type plumage and castration causes development of male plumage. Treatment of castrated males with testosterone causes a return to female-type plumage, but growth of the comb and wattle are stimulated (a normal male trait). If castrated males are treated with DHT, the growth of the comb and wattle are stimulated, but there is no reversion to female plumage. In these strains of chicken, the skin aromatizes testosterone to estrogens and stimulates female plumage. In the comb and wattle, 5α-reductase converts testosterone to DHT. Since DHT is not readily aromatizable, the plumage of DHT-treated, castrated males does not revert to the female type.

D. Reproductive Behavior in Birds

Each avian species exhibits a precise sequence of endocrine-dependent behaviors such as migration, acquisition of territory, advertisement by song, attraction of mate, pairing, nest-building, egg laying, incubating eggs, and rearing young birds. The actual sequence of events and their endocrinological bases are species-specific and cannot easily be generalized. Successful breeding involves a complex interaction of male and female behaviors in precise sequences (that is, if male does A, then female does B, which stimulates male to do C, and so forth) as well as the presence of suitable environmental cues such as proper nesting material, availability of water, etc. Little experimental work has been done with wild birds since it is difficult to get them to perform under laboratory conditions although several descriptive studies on hormone levels and behavior are available. Much of our knowledge of wild birds comes from the work of John Wingfield at the University of Washington and his many associates.

Androgens appear to be responsible for territorial display and aggression in wild birds as it is in domesticated species. Aggressive behavior also can be stimulated by FSH but not by LH in males. Courtship appears to involve negative feedback of testosterone on FSH levels, which results in reduction in circulating androgens and allows for subsequent, less aggressive behaviors. In domestic ring doves, the initial aggressive behavior involves testosterone, and copulatory behavior coincides with reduced androgens and increased P450$_{aro}$ activity. Androgens antagonize incubation patch development, and a reduction in circulating testosterone may be necessary for patch development in males of certain species.

Bowing behavior in feral pigeons coincides with maximal androgen synthesis but decreases prior to egg laying, coincident with an increase in progesterone levels. Progesterone is a well-known stimulus for incubation behavior in laying pigeons, and removal of the postovulatory follicle from chickens blocks nesting behavior.

Mate choice is a complicated pattern of male-female interactions with clear hormonal overtones. These behaviors appear to have activational and organizational components involving steroids and possible nonapeptides as shown in mammals.

VIII. Summary

Reproduction involves a precise integration of environmental factors (photoperiod, temperature, availability of nesting sites, etc.), physiological factors (nutritional state, general endocrine state with respect to thyroid hormones, adrenocortical functions, etc.), and specific endocrine secretions (FSH, LH, androgens, estrogens, progestogens, PRL, etc.). Reproductive patterns are finely tuned to environmental conditions in order to maximize evolutionary success, and this results in frequent observations of greater similarities in reproductive patterns between phylogenetically divergent species facing similar environmental problems than between closely related species living in diverse environments.

Environmental factors operate through the nervous system and specifically the hypothalamus to control release of GTHs and in certain cases PRL. Prolactin molecules or PRL activity as well as FSH and LH molecules have been identified in all tetrapods. Fishes have a unique PRL-like hormone. In both fishes and tetrapods, FSH initiates spermatogenesis in males and follicular development in females. Local androgens secreted from testicular cells under the influence of FSH appear to be necessary for initiating reductional division (meiosis) of primary spermatocytes. Luteinizing hormone induces androgen synthesis by interstitial (Leydig) or lobule-boundary cells in males and estrogen synthesis and ovulation in females. Androgen synthesis in female mammals also may be stimulated in thecal cells or ovarian interstitial cells by LH. It is thought that thecal androgens are converted to estrogens by granulosa cells.

Follicular atresia associated with formation of corpora atretica is a common occurrence in female vertebrates. Atresia appears to be a mechanism for effectively reducing the biotic potential and placing reliance in production of a smaller number of offspring with better individual survival for evolutionary success. Corpora lutea form in many vertebrates primarily from granulosa cells of ruptured follicles, and corpora lutea usually synthesize progesterone, which is related to gestation or behavior in many viviparous species. Many examples of autocrine and paracrine regulation in the gonads are known.

Courtship and breeding behavior appear to be controlled primarily by gonadal steroids although evidence is accumulating for participation of peptides. In addition, estrogens produce dramatic effects on vitellogenesis in non-mammalian liver and bring about a consequent disturbance in calcium metabolism. The basic oviparous mode of reproduction has become modified with respect to the development of viviparity in all non-mammalian groups except birds and agnathan fishes.

Suggested Reading

Books

Balthazart, J. (1990). Hormones, brains and behavior in vertebrates. 1. Sexual differentiation, neuroanatomical aspects, neurotransmitters and neuropeptides. *In* "Comparative Physiology" (A. K. H. Kinne, E. Kinne-Saffran, and K. W. Beyenbach, series eds.), Vol. 8. Karger, Basel.

Balthazart, J. (1990). Hormones, brains and behavior in vertebrates. 2. Behavioral activation in males and females—social interactions and reproductive endocrinology. *In* "Comparative Physiology" (A. K. H. Kinne, E. Kinne-Saffran, and K. W. Beyenbach, series eds.), Vol. 9. Karger, Basel.

Becker, J. B., Breedlove, S. M., and Crews, D. (1992). "Behavioral Endocrinology." MIT Press, Cambridge, MA.

Duellman, W. E., and Trueb, L. (1986). "Biology of Amphibians." McGraw-Hill, New York.

Halliday, T. (1980). "Survival in the Wild—Sexual Strategy." Univ. of Chicago Press, Chicago.

Hoar, W. S., Randall, D. G., and Donaldson, E. M. (1983). "Fish Physiology, Volume IX. Reproduction, Part A. Endocrine Tissues and Hormones. Part B. Behavior and Fertility Control." Academic Press, New York.

Jamieson, B. G. M. (2003). "Reproductive Biology and Phylogeny of Anura". Science Publishers, Inc. Enfield, NH.

Jones, R. E. (1978). "The Vertebrate Ovary." Plenum, New York.

Lamming, G. E. (1984). "Marshall's Physiology of Reproduction. Volume 1: Reproductive Cycles in Vertebrates." Churchill Livingston, Edinburgh.

Nelson, R. J. (1995). "An Introduction to Behavioral Endocrinology." Sinauer, Sunderland, MA.

Norris, D. O., and Jones, R. E. (1987). "Hormones and Reproduction in Fishes, Amphibians, and Reptiles." Plenum, New York.

Schreibman, M. P., and Jones, R. E. (1991). Reproduction. *In* "Vertebrate Endocrinology: Fundamentals and Biomedical Implications" (P. K. T. Pang and M. P. Schreibman, Eds.), Vol. 4, Parts A and B. Academic Press, San Diego.

Sever, D. M. (2003). "Reproductive Biology and Phylogeny of Urodela". Science Publishers, Inc. Enfield, NH.

Sharp, P. J. (1993). "Avian Endocrinology." The Society for Endocrinology, Bristol, UK.

Taylor, D. H., and Guttman, S. I. (1977). "The Reproductive Biology of Amphibians." Plenum, New York.

Van Tienhoven, A. (1983). "Reproductive Physiology of Vertebrates," 2nd Ed. Cornell Univ. Press, Ithaca, NY.

Articles

General

Blackburn, D. G. (1991). Evolutionary origins of the mammary gland. *Mammal Rev.* **21**, 81–96.

Blackburn, D. G. (1994). Review: Discrepant usage of the term "ovoviviparity" in the herpetological literature. *Herpetol. J.* **4**, 65–72.

Callard, I. P., Fileti, L. A., Perez, L. E., Sorbera, L. A., Giannoukos, G., Klosterman, L. L., Tsang, P., and McCracken, J. A. (1992). Role of the corpus luteum and progesterone in the evolution of vertebrate viviparity. *Am. Zool.* **32**, 264–275.

Crews, D. (1993). The organizational concept and vertebrates without sex chromosomes. *Brain Behav. Evol.* **42**, 202–214.

Jones, R. E., and Baxter, D. C. (1991). Gestation, with emphasis on corpus luteum biology, placentation, and parturition. *In* "Vertebrate Endocrinology: Fundamentals and Biomedical Implications" (P. K. T. Pang and M. Schreibman, Eds.), Vol. 4, Part A, pp. 205–302. Academic Press, San Diego.

Lange, I. G., Hartel, A., and Meyer, H. H. D. (2003). Evolution of estrogen functions in vertebrates. *J. Stero. Biochem. Mol. Biol.* **1773**, 1–8.

Polzonetti-Magni, A. M., Mosconi, G., Soverchia, L., Kikuyama, S., and Carnevali, O. (2004). Multihormonal control of vitellogenesis in lower vertebrates. *Intl. Rev. Cytol.* **239**, 1–46.

Pudney, J. (1999). Leydig and Sertoli cells, nonmammalian. In E. Knobil, Ed., "Encyclopedia of Reproduction," Vol. 2, pp. 1008–1020.

Wourms, J. P., and Callard, I. P. (1992). Evolution of viviparity in vertebrates. *Am. Zool.* **32**, 251–354.

Young, L. J., and Crews, D. (1995). Comparative neuroendocrinology of steroid receptor gene expression and regulation: Relationship to physiology and behavior. *Trends Endocr. Metab.* **6**, 317–323.

Fishes

Bryan, M. B., Young, B. A., Dlose, D. A., Semeyn, J., Robinson, T. C., Bayer, J., and Li., W. (2006). Comparison of synthesis of 15α-hydroxylated steroids in males of four North American lamprey species. *Gen. Comp. Endocr.* **146**, 149–156.

Callard, G. V. (1988). Reproductive physiology. Part B. The male. *In* "Physiology of Elasmobranch Fishes" (T. J. Shuttleworth, Ed.), pp. 292–317. Springer-Verlag, Berlin.

Callard, I. P., and Klosterman, L. (1988). Reproductive physiology. Part A. The female. *In* "Physiology of Elasmobranch Fishes" (T. J. Shuttleworth, Ed.), pp. 277–291. Springer-Verlag, Berlin.

Connaughton. M. A., and Aida, K. (1999). Female reproductive system, fish. *In* "Encyclopedia of Reproduction," Vol. 2 (E. Knobil Eds.), pp. 193–204.

Cottone, E., Camantico, E., Gustalla, A., Aramu, S., Polzonetti-Magni, A. M., and Franzoni, M. (2005). Are the Cannabinoids involved in bony fish reproduction? *An. NY Acad. Sci.* **1040**, 273–276.

Davis, K. B., Goudie, C. A., Simco, B. A., Mac Gregor, R., and Parker, N. C. (1986). Environmental regulation and influence of the eyes and pineal gland on the gonadal cycle and spawning in channel catfish (*Ictalurus punctatus*). *Physiol. Zool.* **59**, 717–724.

Devlin, R. H., and Nagahama, Y. (2002). Sex determination and sex differentiation in fish: An overview of genetic, physiological, and environmental influences. *Aquaculture* **208**, 191–364.

Dickoff, W. W., Yan, L., Plisetskaya, E. M., Sullivan, C. V., Swanson, P., Hara A., and Berrard, M. G. (1989). Relationship between metabolic and reproductive hormones in salmonid fish. *Fish Physiol. Biochem.* **7**, 147–155.

Larson, E. T., Norris, D. O., Grau, E. G., and Summers, C. H. (2003). Monoamines stimulate sex reversal in the saddleback wrasse. *Gen. Comp. Endocr.* **130**, 289-298.

Grober, M. S., Jackson, I. M. D., and Bass, A. H. (1991). Gonadal steroids affect LHRH preoptic cell number in a sex/role changing fish. *J. Neurobiol.* **22**, 734–741.

Kavanaugh, S. I., Powell, M. L., and Sower, S. A. (2005). Seasonal changes of gonadotropin-releasing hormone in the Atlantic hagfish *Myxine glutinosa. Gen. Comp. Endocri.* **140**, 136–143.

Koob, T. J., and Callard, I. P. (1999). Reproductive endocrinology of female elasmobranches: Lessons from the little skate (*Raja erinacea*) and spiny dogfish (*Squalus acanthias*). *J. Exp. Zool.* **284**, 557–574.

Mommsen, T. P., and Walsh, P. J. (1988). Vitellogenesis and oocyte assembly. *In* "Fish Physiology, Volume XI, The Physiology of Developing Fish. Part A. Eggs and Larvae" (W. S. Hoar and D. J. Randall, Eds.), pp. 348–407. Academic Press, San Diego.

Nagahama, Y., Yoshikuni, M., Yamashita, M., and Tanaka, M. (1994). Regulation of oocyte maturation in fish. *In* "Fish Physiology. Molecular Endocrinology of Fish" (N. M. Sherwood and C. L. Hew, Eds.), Vol. XIII, pp. 393–439. Academic Press, San Diego.

Parenti, L. R., and Grier, H. J. (2004). Evolution and phylogeny of gonad morphology in bony fishes. *Integ. Comp. Biol.* **44**, 333–348.

Parsons, G. R., and Grier, H. J. (1992). Seasonal changes in shark testicular structure and spermatogenesis. *J. Exp. Zool.* **261**, 173–184.

Reinboth, R. (1999). Fish, mode of reproduction. *In* "Encyclopedia of Reproduction," Vol. 2 (Knobil, E., Ed.), pp. 365–372.

Ross, R. M., Hourigan, T. F., Lutnesky, M. M. F., and Singh, I. (1990). Multiple spontaneous sex changes in social groups of a coral-reef fish. *Copeia* **1990**, 427–433.

Sorenson, P. W., Scott, A. P., Stacey, N. E., and Bowdin, L. (1995). Sulfated 17,20β-dihydroxy-4-pregnen-3-one functions as a potent and specific olfactory stimulant with pheromonal actions in the goldfish. *Gen. Comp. Endocr.*. **100**, 128–142.

Stacey, N., Chojnacki, A., Narayanan, A., Cole, T., and Murphy, C. (2003). Hormonally derived sex pheromones in fish: Exogenous cues and signals from gonad to brain. *Can. J. Phys. Pharm.* **81**, 329–341.

Stacey, N. E., Sorenson, P. W., Van Der Kraak, G. J., and Dulka, J. G. (1989). Direct evidence that 17α, 20β-dihydroxy-4-pregnen-3-one functions as a goldfish primer pheromone: Preovulatory release is closely associated with male endocrine responses. *Gen. Comp. Endocr.* **75**, 62–70.

Warner, R. R., and Swearer, S. E. (1991). Social control of sex change in the bluehead wrasse, *Thalassoma bifasciatum* (Pices: Labridae). *Biol. Bull.* **181**, 199–204.

Wourms, J. P., and Lombardi, J. (1992). Reflections on the evolution of piscine viviparity. *Am. Zool.* **32**, 276–293.

Amphibians

Del Pino, E. M., and Sanchez, G. (1977). Ovarian structure of the marsupial frog *Gastrotheca riobambae* (Fowler). *J. Morphol.* **153**, 153–162.

Houck, L. D., and Woodley, S. K. (1994). Field studies of steroid hormones and male reproductive behaviour in amphibians. *In* "Amphibian Biology" (H. Heatwole, Ed.), Vol. 2. Social Behaviour. Surrey Beatty and Sons, Chipping Norton, Australia.

Jorgensen, C. B. (1992). Growth and reproduction. *In* "Environmental Physiology of the Amphibians" (M. Feder and W. W. Burggren, eds.), pp. 439–466. Univ. of Chicago Press, Chicago.

Kikuyama, S., Nakada, T., Toyoda, F., Iwata, T., Yamaoto, K., and Conlon, J. M. (2005). Amphibian pheromones and endocrine control of their secretion. *Ann. NY Acad. Sci.* **1040**, 123–130.

Lofts, B. (1984). Amphibians. *In* "Marshall's Physiology of Reproduction. Volume 1: Reproductive Cycles in Vertebrates" (G. E. Lamming, Ed.), pp. 127–205. Churchill Livingston, Edinburgh.

Lutz, L. B., Cole, L. M., Gupta, M. K., Kwist, K. W., Auchus, R. J., and Hammes, S. R. (2001). Evidence that androgens are the primary steroids produced by Xenopus laevis ovaries and may signal through the classical androgen receptor to promote oocyte maturation. *Proc. Nat. Acad. Sci.* **98**, 13728–13733.

Lynch, K. S. and Wilczynski, W. (2006). Social regulation of plasma estradiol concentration in a female anuran. *Hormones and Behavior* **50**, 101–106.

Moore, F. L. (1987). Reproductive biology of amphibians. *In* "Fundamentals of Comparative Endocrinology" (I. Chester-Jones, P. M. Ingleton, and J. G. Phillips, Eds.), pp. 207–221. Plenum, New York.

Moore, F. L., and Orchinik, M. (1991). Multiple molecular actions for steroids in the regulation of reproductive behaviors. *Semin. Neurosci.* **3**, 489–496.

Polzonetti-Magni, A. M. (1999). Amphibian ovarian cycles. *In* "Encyclopedia of Reproduction," Vol. 1 (E. Knobil, Ed.). Academic Press, San Diego, pp. 154–160.

Rastogi, R. K. and Iela, L. (1999). Female reproductive system, amphibians. *In* "Encyclopedia of Reproduction," Vol. 2 (E. Knobil, Ed.). Academic Press, San Diego, pp. 183–189.

Rose, J. D., Kinnaird, J. R., and Moore, F. L. (1995). Neurophysiological effects of vasotocin and corticosterone on medullary neurons: Implications for hormonal control of amphibian courtship behavior. *Neuroendocr.* **62**, 406–417.

Wake, M. H. (1985). Oviduct structure and function in nonmammalian vertebrates. *In* "Functional Morphology in Vertebrates" (H.-R. Duncker and G. Fleischer, Eds.), pp. 427–435. Gustav Fischer Verlag, Stuttgart.

Reptiles

Blackburn, D. G. (1992). Convergent evolution of viviparity, matrotrophy, and specializations for fetal nutrition in reptiles and other vertebrates. *Am. Zool.* **32**, 313–321.

Cree, A., Guillette, L. J., Jr., Cockrem, J. F., Brown, M. A., and Chambers, G. K. (1990). Absence of daily cycles in plasma sex steroids in male and female tuatara (*Sphenodon punctatus*), and the effects of acute capture stress on females. *Gen. Comp. Endocr.* **79**, pp. 103–113.

Crews, D. (1983). Alternative reproductive tactics in reptiles. *Bioscience* **33**, 562–566.

Duvall, D., Guillette, L. J., Jr., and Jones, R. E. (1982). Environmental control of reptilian reproductive cycles. *In* "Biology of the Reptilia" (C. Gans and H. Pough, Eds.), Vol. 13, Academic Press, New York, pp. 201–231.

Guillette, L. J., Jr. (1990). Prostaglandins and reproduction in reptiles. *In* "Progress in Comparative Endocrinology." Wiley-Liss, New York, pp. 603–607.

Guillette, L. J., Jr. (1993). The evolution of viviparity in lizards. *Biosci.* **43**, 742–751.

Jones, R. E., Propper, C. R., Rand, M. S., and Austin, H. B. (1991). Loss of nesting behavior and the evolution of viviparity in reptiles. *Ethology* **88**, 331–341.

Licht, P. (1984). Reptiles. *In* "Marshall's Physiology of Reproduction. Volume 1: Reproductive Cycles in Vertebrates" (G. E. Lamming, Ed.), Churchill Livingston, Edinburgh, pp. 206–282.

Mason, R. T. (1993). Chemical ecology of the red-sided garter snake, *Thamnophis sirtalis parietalis. Brain Behav. Evol.* **41**, 261–268.

Owens, D. W., and Morris, Y. A. (1985). The comparative endocrinology of sea turtles. *Copeia* **1985**, 723–735.

Stewart, J. R. (1992). Placental structure and nutritional provisions to embryos in predominantly lecithotrophic viviparous reptiles. *Am. Zool.* **32**, 303–312.

Birds

Adkins-Regan, E. (2005). Female mate choice. *In* " Functional Avian Endocrinology," (A. Dawson and P. J. Sharp, Eds.). Narosa Publishing House, New Dehli, pp. 341–350.

Ball, G. F. (1993). The neural integration of environmental information by seasonally breeding birds. *Am. Zool.* **33**, 185–199.

Balthazart, J., and Ball, G. F. (1995). Sexual differentiation of brain and behavior in birds. *Trends Endocr. Metab.* **6**, 21–29.

Deviche, P. (1995). Androgen regulation of avian premigratory hyperphagia and fattening: From ecophysiology to neuroendocrinology. *Am. Zool.* **35**, 234–245.

Fivizzani, A. J., Colwell, M. A., and Oring, L. W. (1986). Plasma steroid hormone levels in free living Wilson's phalaropes, *Phalaropus tricolor. Gen. Comp. Endocr.*. **62**, 137–144.

Follett, B. K. (1984). Birds. *In* "Marshall's Physiology of Reproduction. Volume 1: Reproductive Cycles in Vertebrates" (G. E. Lamming, Ed.). Churchill Livingston, Edinburgh, pp. 283–350.

Göth, A. and Booth, D. T. (2004). Temperature-dependent sex ratio in a bird. *Biology Letters* **1**, 31–33.

Lofts, B., and Murton, R. K. (1973). Reproduction in birds. *In* "Avian Biology" (D. S. Farner and J. R. King, Eds.), Vol. 3. Academic Press, San Diego, pp. 1–107.

Sharp. P. J. (2005). Photoperiodic regulation of seasonal breeding in birds. *Ann. NY Acad. Sci.* **1040**, 189–199.

Staub, N., and De Beer, M. (1997). The role of androgens in female vertebrates. *Gen. Comp. Endocr.* **108**, 1–24.

Strüssmann, C. A., and Nakamura, M. (2002). Morphology, endocrinology, and environmental modulation of gondal sex differentiation in teleost fishes. *Fish Physiol. Biochem.* **26**, 13–29.

Wingfield, J. C., Ball, G. F., Dufty, A. M., Hegner, R. E., and Ramenofsky, M. (1987). Testosterone and aggression in birds. *Am. Sci.* **75**, 602–608.

Wingfield, J. C., O'Reilly, K. M., and Astheimer, L. B. (1995). Modulation of the adrenocortical response to acute stress in arctic birds: A possible ecological basis. *Am. Zool.* **35**, 285–294.

Yoshida, N., Mita, K., and Yamashita, M. (2000). Comparative study of the molecular mechanisms of oocyte maturation in amphibians. *Comp. Biochem. Physiol. B* **126**, 189–197.

12

Bioregulation of Feeding, Digestion, and Metabolism

Survival of any vertebrate requires ingestion of a nutrient source, enzymatic digestion of its macromolecules, and absorption of the end products of digestion. Once absorbed, these substrates may be used as energy sources, for synthesis of various molecules, or stored for later utilization. The processes responsible for these events are closely regulated by the nervous system and by hormones arising from the gastrointestinal (GI) tract, the endocrine pancreas, and the hypothalamus-pituitary system. In this chapter, we will first examine hormones that influence feeding behavior, hormones that regulate the processes involved in digestion of food as well as the biochemical pathways involved in metabolism of ingested nutrients in mammals. These processes for non-mammals are discussed in Chapter 13.

I. Bioregulation of Feeding

Ingestion of food is regulated by a complex system of peptide hormones and neural factors that is incompletely understood at this time. Numerous bioregulators have been described that stimulate or inhibit appetite and feeding behavior. Most of these factors are known as well for other roles related to metabolism or other events. Some of these bioregulators are produced in the hypothalamus whereas others come from the gastrointestinal tract or adipose tissue. A brief account of some of the better-known factors is provided here. Other peptides, such as apelin, resistin, and Acrp30 from adipose cells, that appear to be involved may soon be established as important regulators of feeding and obesity, possibly the major clinical concern of the 21st century (see ahead).

Early brain lesion studies identified the ventromedial region of the hypothalamus as the "satiety center" and the lateral hypothalamus as the "feeding center." Subsequent studies on the neural circuits involved and the location of receptors for regulatory factors that influence feeding have implicated a number of hypothalamic centers including the arcuate nucleus (ARC), the ventromedial nucleus (VMN), the dorsomedial nucleus (DMN), the lateral hypothalamus (LatH), and the paraventricular nucleus (PVN). Bioregulators that stimulate appetite and feeding are termed **orexic agents** (*orexin*, appetite) whereas those that suppress appetite and feeding are termed **anorexic agents**.

A. Stimulation of Feeding

An important hypothalamic orexic agent in mammals is **neuropeptide Y (NPY)**. Repeated or continuous administration of NPY produces hyperphagia (excessive eating), weight gain, and obesity. Blocking NPY neuronal activity reduces hyperphagia. The **agouti-related protein (AgRP)** is co-localized in NPY neurons, and overexpression of AgRP also can lead to obesity. Overexpression of the hypothalamic peptide called **melanin-concentrating hormone, MCH** (see Chapter 4), in the LatH or administration of MCH also elevates feeding. Furthermore, MCH knockout mice are hypophagic (reduced feeding) and are excessively lean. Studies of the **endogenous endocanabinoids**, such as **anandamide**, suggest a central role for these compounds and their receptors, especially the **CB$_1$ receptor**. Discovery of these bioregulators was a result of investigations of the mechanisms of action for the active ingredient of marijuana, **9-tetrahydrocannabinol (THC)**. Endogenous endocanabinoids are potent stimulators of food intake and appear to be important in the development of obesity. They also have stimulatory peripheral effects on lipogenesis in liver and adipose cells. Knockout mice for the CB$_1$ receptor (CB$_1^{-/-}$) are very lean and are resistant to dietary-induced obesity.

Orexins are peptides that stimulate feeding. There are two forms of orexin that are derived from the same prohormone. Human orexin A consists of 33 amino acids and orexin B is a peptide of 28 amino acids (Figure 12-1). Orexins A and B were also named **hypocretin-1** and **hypocretin-2** by another laboratory that isolated them at about the same time. In addition to stimulation of appetite, orexins have been found to have multiple actions on hormone release, gastric secretion, metabolic rate, and some behaviors (Figure 12-2).

Ghrelin, a 28-amino acid peptide (Figure 12-3), was first discovered as an endogenous ligand for the **growth hormone (GH) secretogogue receptor (GHS-1a)** in the ARC that can result in release of GH from the pituitary. Ghrelin is secreted by cells in the stomach epithelium and stimulates feeding. Plasma levels of ghrelin increase prior to mealtimes as well as at night (Figure 12-4) and may be a hunger signal for the brain. Ghrelin-secreting neurons also are present within the brain and appear to be involved in control of feeding. It has been associated with reduced gastric emptying that probably contributes to a sense of satiety.

Reports claim that **galanin**, the same peptide that stimulates LH release from the pituitary (Chapter 4), triggers a craving for fatty foods. Levels of galanin rise in the general circulation prior to lunch and dinner. Galanin is also thought to cause a weight increase in adolescent girls at puberty. This action fits with its known role in reproduction.

B. Inhibition of Feeding

Numerous peptides have been demonstrated to inhibit feeding behavior and induce satiety. In the brain, a short version of the intestinal **cholecytokinin** (CCK$_8$) may play a role in regulating food intake. CCK produced in the intestinal epithelium plays an important role in the regulation of digestion (see ahead). CCK$_8$ secreted

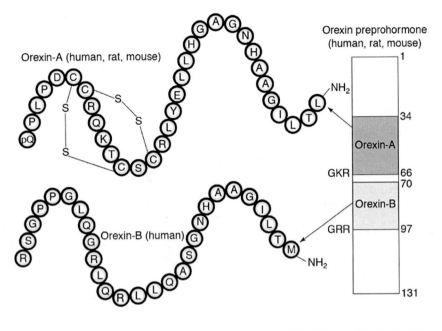

Figure 12-1. **Structure of orexins**. Orexin A (= hypocretin-1) and Orexin B (= hypocretin-2) are derived from the same prohormone. See Appendix C for explanation of amino acid abbreviations. [Reprinted with permission of the publisher from Samson, W. K., and Resch, Z. T. The hypocretin/Orexin story. *Trends Endocr. Metab.* **11**, 257–262. Copyright 2000 Elsevier Science Inc.]

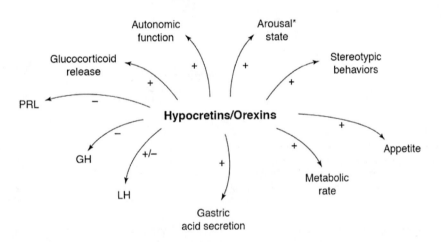

Figure 12-2. **Orexin actions**. [Reprinted with permission of the publisher from Samson, W. K., and Resch, Z. T. The hypocretin/Orexin story. *Trends Endocr. Metab.* **11**, 257–262. Copyright 2000 Elsevier Science Inc.]

by hypothalamic neurons decreases food intake (appetite suppression) in rats. Furthermore, rats of an obese strain exhibit lower than normal brain levels of CCK_8. The use of CCK antagonists decreases satiety in humans, suggesting a similar mechanism is operational. Investigators also have reported increased food intake and accelerated weight gain in pigs treated with antibodies against CCK_8. The physiological stimulus for CCK_8 effects is not known, and it is not clear that CCK_8 is a regulator of appetite.

A large peptide (167 amino acids) called **leptin** (*leptos*, thin) that curbs appetite and increases metabolic rate was first isolated from adipose tissue. Leptin was discovered in mice as a result of studies of a mutant gene called the obese gene (*ob*). Mice homozygous for this mutant (*ob/ob*) are obese, are deficient in leptin, and have higher levels of endogenous canabinoids. Leptin is secreted in greater amounts when an animal puts

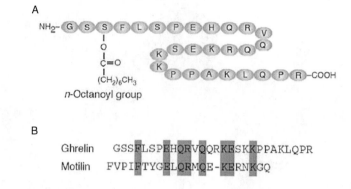

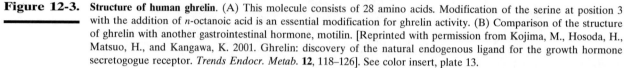

Figure 12-3.   **Structure of human ghrelin.** (A) This molecule consists of 28 amino acids. Modification of the serine at position 3 with the addition of *n*-octanoic acid is an essential modification for ghrelin activity. (B) Comparison of the structure of ghrelin with another gastrointestinal hormone, motilin. [Reprinted with permission from Kojima, M., Hosoda, H., Matsuo, H., and Kangawa, K. 2001. Ghrelin: discovery of the natural endogenous ligand for the growth hormone secretogogue receptor. *Trends Endocr. Metab.* **12**, 118–126]. See color insert, plate 13.

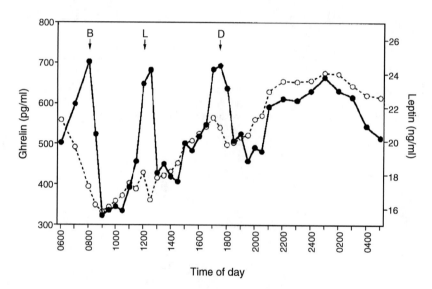

Figure 12-4.   **Daily pattern for Ghrelin and leptin levels in blood.** Note the rise in Ghrelin occurs prior to each meal (B, breakfast; L, lunch; D, diner) whereas there is a steady rise in appetite suppressing leptin during the day. [Reprinted with permission from Cummings, D. E., Purnell, J. Q., Frayo, R. S., Schmidova, K., Wisse, B. E., and Weigle, D. S.(2001). A preprandial rise in plasma ghrelin levels suggests a role in meal initiation in humans. *Diabetes* **50**, 1714-1719.]

on fat; it then reduces appetite and causes the animal to lose weight (Figure 12-5). Leptin binds to receptors in the hypothalamus that operate through a JAK-STAT (Janus Kinase—Signal Transducer and Activator of Transcription) pathway. It may operate in part by blocking the orexic action of the peptide ghrelin in the brain. In obese humans, leptin levels are about 5X those of lean people, suggesting that either this protein is not regulating fat levels in humans or that obese people do not respond to this signal in the same manner as do leaner people. Leptin also has been claimed to have affects on reproduction, and its anorexic action may delay puberty.

POMC neurons (see Chapter 4) in the brain are associated with anorexia and have receptors for leptin. These neurons secrete α-MSH as a neuromodulator/neurotransmitter that binds to MC3 and MC4 receptors in the hypothalamus. Knockout mice lacking MC4 receptors (MC4$^{-/-}$) or mice possessing a mutant MC4 receptor gene exhibit obesity. POMC neurons that co-express **cocaine-amphetamine-regulated transcript (CART)**, a potent inhibitor of food intake, exhibit leptin receptors and may be mediators of leptin action. **Neurotensin (NT)** neurons also appear to be leptin targets and can stimulate neurons that release **corticotropin-releasing hormone (CRH)**, a potent anorexic agent that also functions as a mediator for leptin.

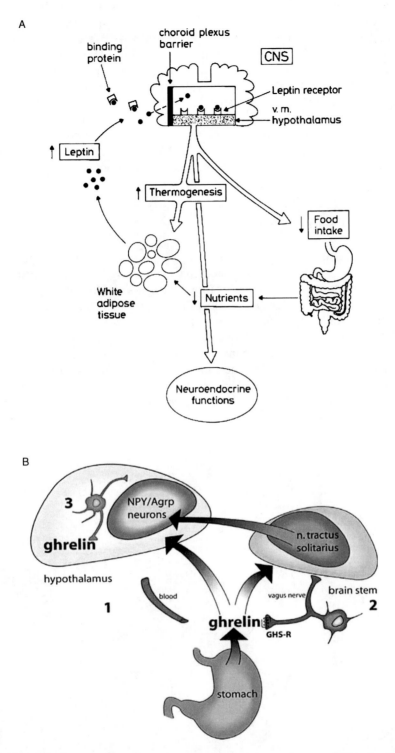

Figure 12-5. **Actions of leptin and grehlin on food intake**. (A) Leptin from adipocytes inhibits food intake through actions at the hypothalamus. [Reprinted with permission of the publisher from Sahu, A. Leptin signaling in the hypothalamus: Emphasis on energy homeostasis and leptin resistance. *Frontiers in Neuroendocr.* **24**, 225–253. Copyright 2003 Elsevier Science Inc.] (B) Ghrelin produced in the stomach also operates at the hypothalamus to alter food intake. See text for details. [Reprinted with permission of the publisher from Korbonits, M., Goldstone, A. P., Gueorguiev, M., and Grossman, A. B. Ghrelin—a hormone with multiple functions. *Frontiers Neuroendocr.* **25**, 27–68. Copyright 2004 Elsevier Science Inc.] See color insert, plate 11.

Several other gastrointestinal peptides have been shown to suppress appetite. **Intestinal peptide YY (PYY)** is a gut peptide that also suppresses appetite. PYY inhibits release of NPY and stimulates α-MSH release through actions at the ARC. Furthermore, **pancreatic polypepetide (PP)** from the endocrine pancreas appears to reduce appetite, but its physiological role in not yet confirmed. **Oxyntomodulin**, a byproduct of post-translational processing of the glucagon preprohormone in intestinal and brain tissue, also suppresses appetite. One of the more interesting peptides in this grouping is **glucagon-like peptide 1 (GLP-1)**, an intestinal hormone that reduces appetite and food intake. GLP-1 also enhances pancreatic secretion of insulin (see below).

Some additional peptides have been found to have anorexic actions. A peptide originally named **prolactin-releasing peptide (PrRP)** has been reported to be a more affective appetite suppressant especially in fishes where it also has prolactin-releasing action. Urocortin-II (Ucn-II), a hypothalamic peptide that binds to the CRH_2 receptor (see Chapter 4), has been shown to be a powerful appetite suppressant.

II. Bioregulation of Digestion

The GI tract secretes a variety of peptides that control digestion. Many of these peptides also have important roles in the nervous system as well as in the HP-system; e.g., **vasoactive intestinal peptide, VIP**. You may recall that the study of endocrinology began with identification by Bayliss and Starling of the first hormone, **secretin**, produced by the duodenal mucosa. A few years later, Edkins proposed that **gastrin** from the antral stomach controlled secretion of acid. Cholecystokinin (CCK) was soon proposed to stimulate gallbladder contraction and release of bile into the gut. And this was followed by evidence of **pancreozymin** that stimulates enzyme secretion by the pancreas. However, it was many years before these gastrointestinal hormones were finally isolated and characterized chemically due to the diffuse nature of the secretory cells responsible for their production. These endocrine cells do not form distinct glands but occur as isolated cells or small groups of cells distributed along the GI epithelium (Figure 12-6). A summary of these GI regulators is provided in Table 12-1.

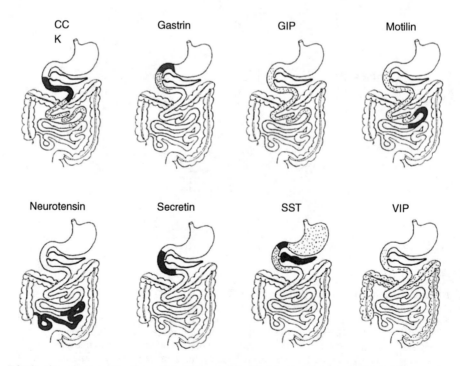

Figure 12-6. **Distribution of some endocrine cells in the gastrointestinal tract and pancreas.** High density regions are in black. Dots indicate lower density. See text for explanation of abbreviations. Based on numerous sources.

Table 12-1. Mammalian Regulators of Feeding and Digestion

Hormone	Number of amino acids	Cellular source	Primary function
Gastrin	17, 34	Antral G cell	Stimulates gastric acid secretion
Somatostatin (SST)	14, 28	Gastric D cell	Inhibits gastric acid secretion
Cholecystokinin (CCK)	8, 33, 39, 58	Intestinal I cell	Stimulates pancreatic enzyme secretion, gallbladder contraction, and bile release
CCK$_8$		Brain neuron	Anorexic
Secretin	27	Intestinal S cell	Stimulates pancreatic HCO_3^- secretion
Vasoactive intestinal peptide (VIP)	28	Neurons	Relaxes arteriole smooth muscle and increases blood flow to intestines
Glucose-dependent insulinotropic peptide (GIP)	43	Intestinal K cells	Stimulates insulin release in presence of glucose
Motilin	22	Intestinal M cells	Stimulates migrating motor complex; causes intestinal contractions
Enteroglucagons: GLP-I	36	Intestinal L cells (EG cells)	Stimulates insulin release and inhibits glucagon release; anorexic
Neurotensin (NT)	13	Intestinal N cells and neurons	May inhibit gastric acid secretion and motility
		Brain neurons	Anorexic
Gastrin-releasing peptide (GRP)	27	Gastric and intestinal neurons	Stimulates gastrin release
Calcitonin gene-related peptide (CGRP)	37	Gastric and intestinal neurons	May inhibit gastric secretion
Galanin	29/30	Intestinal neurons	May inhibit gastric acid secretion
		Brain neurons	May stimulate appetite for fats (orexic)
Peptide YY	36	Intestinal L cell	Inhibits pancreatic secretion; anorexic
Peptide histidine isoleucine (PHI)	27	Intestinal neurons	Released with VIP and may have same actions
Melanin-concentrating hormone (MCH)	33	Brain neurons	Orexic
Neuropeptide Y (NPY)	36	Brain neurons	Orexic
Orexin A (Hypocretin-1)	33	Brain neurons	Orexic
Orexin B (Hypocretin-2)	28	Brain neurons	Orexic
Ghrelin	28	Brain neurons, stomach cells	Orexic
Prolactin-releasing peptide (PrRP)	31	Brain neurons	Anorexic
Leptin	167	Brain neurons, adipose cells	Anorexic
Melanocortin (α-MSH)	13	Brain neurons	Anorexic

A. The Human Digestive System

In addition to the secretions of the GI epithelium, digestion is aided by three essential exocrine glands: (1) the salivary glands; (2) the liver; and (3) the exocrine pancreas. Several pairs of salivary glands secrete a solution called saliva containing salts and a starch-digesting enzyme, salivary amylase. The liver and pancreas have exocrine functions, too, and they secrete enzymes and other substances directly into the small intestine via ducts.

The first detailed and systematic knowledge of human digestive processes came in the early 1800s from observations of Dr. William Beaumont on his patient Alexis St. Martin, a French Canadian who, while visiting Fort Mackinac, Michigan, was accidentally shot in the chest from close range with a shotgun. St. Martin had two fractured ribs, his lungs were lacerated, and his stomach was perforated. Beaumont assumed that St. Martin would not live the night, but he miraculously survived. The wound in St. Martin's stomach, however, never healed completely, resulting in a permanent opening to the outside (what we now call a **gastric fistula**) through which Beaumont was not only able to observe the progression of gastric digestion under varying conditions over a period of years, but through which he could remove samples of gastric contents for closer analysis. The accidental production of a gastric fistula in St. Martin provided the inspiration for a variety of surgical techniques in other animals, including production of gastric fistulas and gastric or intestinal pouches (isolated pouches no longer connected with the lumen of the gut). Transplantation of denervated pouches or pieces of digestive tract or pancreas to sites under the skin where revascularization can occur has enabled subsequent investigators to separate endocrine and extrinsic nervous regulatory mechanisms. Such isolated organs still contain functional elements of the enteric division of the autonomic nervous system, however, and may exhibit endogenous nervous regulation. Development of crossed circulatory systems between experimental animals confirmed the transfer of chemical factors (later to be called hormones) through the blood to target tissues. *In-vitro* studies of pancreatic slices or mucosal tissues from various regions of the gut were used to identify the various GI regulatory peptides as well as the factors regulating their release. Table 12-1 summarizes the actions of some GI peptides in mammals as well as their cellular sources.

B. Embryonic Origin of Gastrointestinal Endocrine Cells

Although the use of immunological and fluorescent techniques has enabled investigators to identify the actual cellular sources for many of the GI peptides, there is still considerable controversy with respect to the embryonic origin or origins of these cells in mammals. Pearse proposed that all of these GI cellular types as well as calcitonin-secreting C-cells of the thyroid gland, parathyroid chief cells, endocrine cells of the pancreas, melanin-containing cells, adenohypophysial cells, and the chromaffin cells of the adrenal medulla belong to the APUD cellular series (APUD = amine content and amine precursor uptake and decarboxylation; see Chapter 4). These APUD cells are derivatives of neural crest or other neural ectoderm cells, suggesting that GI endocrine cells are of neural ectodermal rather than of endodermal origin in the mucosa and that they have migrated into the gastric or intestinal mucosa during early development. The neural origin for many of these endocrine cells has been confirmed, although the majority of these GI endocrine cells do not come from neural crest cells *per se* as originally postulated by Pearse. The occurrence of many of the GI peptides in brain tissue and peripheral neurons argues strongly for the neural origin for these GI hormone-secreting cells. A single evolutionary origin for GI endocrine cells is supported further by observations that immunoreactive gastrin, CCK, and glucagon appear to be co-localized in a single intestinal cellular type in an invertebrate chordate (amphioxus) and in the cyclostome fishes.

C. Hormonal and Neural Regulation of Gastric Digestion

Neural control of gastric secretion occurs at two levels. The **cephalic phase** involves stimulation of secretion via parasympathetic discharges elicited by the same stimuli that cause salivation; that is, sight, smell, taste, thought, or presence of food. In the **gastric phase** of secretory control, the presence of food in the stomach elicits secretion through vago-vagal reflexes and/or through the gastrin mechanism. In addition, neural factors can stimulate secretion of a hormone produced in the gastric epithelium that stimulates certain aspects of gastric secretion. It has not been possible to determine which of these mechanisms is more important in controlling gastric secretion; probably all of these mechanisms operate in the normal digestive process.

1. The Gastrin Theory and Acid Secretion

Edkins in 1905 showed that extracts prepared from the most posterior portion of the stomach, the antrum, stimulated acid secretion by the gastric glands, and he suggested the name "gastrin" for the active substance in these extracts. He found no gastrin activity in extracts prepared from the other portions of the stomach. Edkin's **gastrin hypothesis** temporarily lost credibility with the discovery of **histamine**, a potent stimulator of gastric acid secretion, and the demonstration of histamine in extracts of the gastric mucosa. It was almost 30 years before it was shown that histamine-free extracts from the mucosa of the antral portion of the stomach possessed the ability to stimulate the acid-secreting **parietal cells** of the gastric glands. Nevertheless, it was not until gastrin was finally isolated almost 60 years later and characterized chemically by Gregory and Tracey that the term "gastrin theory" finally was discarded, and the hormone gastrin was confirmed.

There are two peptide forms of gastrin, each composed of 17 amino acids: **gastrin I**, and a sulfated form, **gastrin II**, which has a sulfate group attached at position 6 near the C-terminal end. A larger form of gastrin called **big gastrin** also has been found in the circulation. Big gastrin consists of gastrin I or II plus a different 17-amino acid peptide component. Only about 5% of the circulating gastrin occurs as big gastrin, however.

The preprohormone for gastrin is composed of 104 amino acids and is cleaved several times to release big and little gastrins. Most of the biological activity of these gastrins resides in the four carboxy-terminal amino acids consisting of Trp-Met-Asp-Phe-NH$_2$. Several peptides that possess this terminal sequence (see Figure 12-7) have been shown to stimulate acid secretion. A synthetic pentapeptide (**pentagastrin**) incorporating the terminal tetrapeptide sequence is frequently used for experimental studies.

The control mechanism for acid secretion combines the observations that parasympathetic stimulation, acetylcholine (ACh), histamine, gastrin, and some other peptides all cause acid secretion (see Figure 12-8). In contrast, atropine (an anticholinergic drug acting on muscarinic cholinergic receptors), procaine (an anesthetic), sympathetic stimulation, and certain antihistamines tend to reduce acid secretion under some experimental conditions. Cephalic stimulation through the parasympathetic system (ACh) can release gastrin from the **G-cell** in the mucosa of the antral portion of the stomach. Gastrin travels via the blood through the systemic circulation to the body of the stomach where it stimulates the release of histamine from **tissue mast cells** situated in the mucosa. Gastrin also activates the synthesis of **histidine decarboxylase**, the enzyme responsible for histamine synthesis. Histamine in turn stimulates release of HCl from the parietal cells. Gastrin may stimulate parietal cells directly without employing histamine as an intermediate, and some investigators conclude that histamine is not involved in endogenous acid secretion. Vagal stimulation or application of ACh may stimulate the parietal cells directly to secrete HCl.

The gastrin receptor is a G-protein-linked molecule that works through inositol trisphosphate (IP$_3$) and phosphokinase C (see Chapter 3), to activate H$^+$-ATPase and cause secretion of H$^+$ resulting in decreased pH of the stomach contents. Although the mechanism activating H$^+$ secretion is not fully understood, an increase in cytosolic Ca^{2+} follows the binding of gastrin by the parietal cell.

During active digestion, the pH of the human stomach may be between 1 and 2. Low pH in the antral portion of the stomach (especially near the pyloric sphincter) reduces gastrin release (feedback), probably acting through local release of somatostatin (SST) by **D-cells** in the antral stomach.

In the 1930s, the term **enterogastrone** was coined to designate humoral inhibitors of intestinal origin that reduced gastric secretion and/or motility. Several peptides secreted by the small intestine may be candidates as enterogastrones either by evoking SST release or through more direct inhibitory actions (Figure 12-9).

2. Gastrin-Releasing Peptide

A novel peptide isolated from the mammalian stomach and intestine stimulates gastrin release and hence was named **gastrin-releasing peptide (GRP)**. This peptide of 27 amino acids bears a remarkable structural similarity to the 14-amino acid peptide **bombesin** that previously was isolated from the skin of frogs in the genus *Bombina*. In the stomach, immunoreactive GRP appears exclusively in neurons, but the axonal tips of these neurons do not contact the G-cells directly, implying that this neurocrine behaves in a paracrine fashion whereas intestinal GRP acts in the manner of a true hormone.

In addition to its action on gastrin release, GRP stimulates secretion of pancreatic enzymes, contraction of gastric, intestinal, and gallbladder smooth muscle, and release of several gastrointestinal and pancreatic hormones. GRP also produces mitogenic effects resulting in hyperplasia of pancreatic, intestinal, and other tissues. Thus, GRP may play multiple roles in modulating GI physiology.

Administration of GRP or bombesin into the ventricles of the brain causes a dramatic cessation of gastric acid secretion regardless of the stimulus used to evoke gastric secretion. This effect appears to be mediated via sympathetic nerves and suggests another level for the involvement of this peptide in gastric function.

Peptide	Residues				
Human gastrin II	17	EEPWL	EEEEE	A Y*	G W M D F-NH$_2$
Caerulein	10		QQD	Y* T	G W M D F-NH$_2$
CCK$_8$	8		D	Y* M	G W M D F-NH$_2$

Figure 12-7. **Peptides that stimulate gastric acid secretion.** Caerulein is a peptide isolated from frog skin that has the common amino-terminal pentapeptide and hence similar activity to gastrin II. The same sequence occurs in all CCKs although only CCK$_8$ is shown. Y* indicates a sulfate group is attached to that tyrosine in each of these peptides. See Appendix C for explanation of the letters coding for individual amino acids. [From Walsh, J. H., and Dockray, G. J. (1994). "Gut Peptides." Raven, New York.]

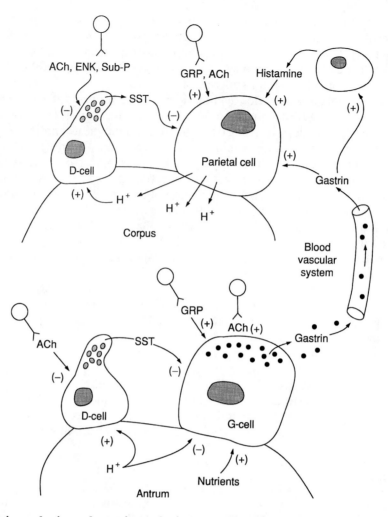

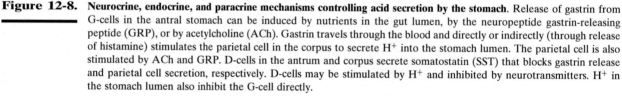

Figure 12-8. **Neurocrine, endocrine, and paracrine mechanisms controlling acid secretion by the stomach.** Release of gastrin from G-cells in the antral stomach can be induced by nutrients in the gut lumen, by the neuropeptide gastrin-releasing peptide (GRP), or by acetylcholine (ACh). Gastrin travels through the blood and directly or indirectly (through release of histamine) stimulates the parietal cell in the corpus to secrete H+ into the stomach lumen. The parietal cell is also stimulated by ACh and GRP. D-cells in the antrum and corpus secrete somatostatin (SST) that blocks gastrin release and parietal cell secretion, respectively. D-cells may be stimulated by H+ and inhibited by neurotransmitters. H+ in the stomach lumen also inhibit the G-cell directly.

3. Secretion of Pepsinogen

The major gastric enzyme in adult humans and carnivorous vertebrates is the protease **pepsin** that is secreted by the **chief cells** of the gastric mucosa in an inactive form called **pepsinogen**. Conversion of inactive pepsinogen to pepsin is accomplished by the presence of an excess of H+ supplied by the parietal cells. The optimum pH for vertebrate pepsins lies between 1 and 2, the normal pH range observed in the stomach following stimulation of acid secretion. Pepsin is inactive above a pH of about 4.5. The presence of acid on the surface of the gastric mucosa may activate a cholinergic reflex that evokes pepsinogen release. Parasympathetic stimulation via the vagus nerve causes release of pepsinogen, and hormonal control of pepsinogen secretion may be absent. Gastrin causes release of pepsinogen only when applied in doses large enough to inhibit acid secretion by the parietal cells, implying that gastrin is not the normal factor causing pepsinogen release from the chief cells.

Several other GI peptides can invoke pepsinogen release but do so only when applied in pharmacological doses. However, one duodenal peptide (motilin, see ahead) has been implicated in regulating pepsinogen secretion at physiological levels. Inhibition of pepsinogen release is caused by SST or by sympathetic stimulation.

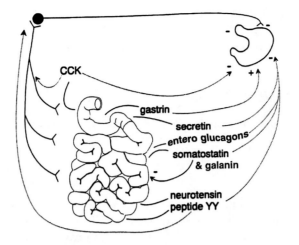

Figure 12-9. **Enterogastrones.** Several peptides released from the small intestine inhibit acid secretion and slow processing of food in the stomach. [Modified from Lloyd, K. C. K., and Walsh, J. H. (1994) Gastric secretion. *In* "Gut Peptides" (J. H. Walsh, and G. J. Dockray, Eds.), pp. 147–173. Raven, New York.]

D. Regulation of Intestinal Digestion

The duodenal mucosa contains many secretory cells, including cells responsible for secretion of several digestive enzymes as well as a variety of hormone-secreting and mucus-secreting cells. The intestinal mucosa is organized into thousands of tiny finger-like projections called "villi." The presence of villi greatly increases the total surface area of the small intestine for releasing digestive secretions and for absorption of digestive products. The number of villi and secreting cells in the mucosa of the small intestine decreases progressively from the duodenum to the jejunum and ileum.

Three stages or phases of intestinal regulation can be identified involving neural and endocrine mechanisms. There appears to be a distinct **cephalic phase of intestinal regulation** mediated via vagal stimulation that influences pancreatic secretion. A **gastric phase of intestinal regulation** involves vagal and vago-vagal stimulation of gastrin release that appears to influence pancreatic secretion. Finally, the **intestinal phase** relies primarily on release of peptides stimulated directly by the composition of the intestinal contents.

1. Secretin

The presence of acidic chyme (pH less than 4.5) from the stomach directly stimulates the **S-cell** in the duodenal mucosa to release the peptide secretin into the blood. Although H[+] are the primary stimulus, secretin release also is stimulated by bile salts, fatty acids, sodium oleate, and several herbal extracts. Secretin stimulates the pancreas to secrete basic juice (rich in HCO_3^-) and helps to neutralize the acidity of the chyme that has entered the small intestine. Although secretin levels in the blood do not increase following ingestion of a meal, the action of secretin on the exocrine pancreas is potentiated by another intestinal peptide hormone, CCK, that also increases in the blood following ingestion of a meal (see below).

Originally, it was believed that secretin also was responsible for stimulating secretion of the digestive enzymes normally present in the pancreatic juice, including the proteases chymotrypsin and trypsin, pancreatic lipase, pancreatic amylase, and nucleases for DNA and RNA. After 40 years of controversy following the demonstration of secretin, it was confirmed finally by Harper and Raper (1943) that purified secretin stimulates secretion of pancreatic fluid that is rich in sodium bicarbonate but poor in digestive enzymes. Secretion of the digestive enzymes was attributable to a second duodenal peptide that was found to contaminate some secretin preparations. Since zymogen granules represent vesicles of stored enzyme within the acinar (exocrine) pancreatic cell, the peptide that caused extrusion of zymogen granules from pancreatic acinar cells initially was called **pancreozymin** (pancreas-zymogen). It was postulated that the release of pancreozymin into the blood in response to the presence of peptides and amino acids in the chyme is due to direct actions of these molecules on pancreozymin-producing cells, similar to the action of H[+] on the S-cell. Sometimes the term **secretagogue** is applied to substances present in food, substances secreted from the mucosa into the gut lumen, or products

	1	11	21
Pig, cow	H S D G T F T S E L	S R L R D S A R L Q	R L L Q G L V
Dog	H S D G T F T S E L	S R L R E S A R L Q	R L L Q G L V
Rat	H S D G T F T S E L	S R L Q D S A R L Q	R L L Q G L V
Human	H S D G T F T S E L	S R L R E G A R L Q	R L L Q G L V
Chicken	H S D G L F T S E Y	S K M R G N A Q V Q	K F I Q N L M

Figure 12-10. **Comparision of secretins from mammals and the chicken.** Mammalian secretins are very conservative whereas more than half of the amino acids are different in the bird. See Appendix C for explanation of the letters coding for individual amino acids. [Based on Leiter, A. B., Chey, W. Y., and Kopin, A. S. (1994) Secretin. In "Gut Peptides." (J. H. Walsh, and G. J. Dockray, Eds.), pp. 147–173. Raven, New York.]

of digestion that induce gastric or intestinal secretions. Pancreozymin later turned out to be another intestinal peptide hormone previously named for a different function (CCK, see below).

Secretin consists of 27 amino acids and chemically is related to several other peptides of the PACAP family (see Chapter 4), several of which are involved in digestion. Secretin has been isolated from several mammalian species and evolutionarily appears to be very conservative (Figure 12-10) although mammalian secretins differ markedly from avian secretin. Receptors for secretin are G-protein-linked, and secretin apparently operates through production of a cAMP second messenger to stimulate pancreatic HCO_3^- secretion (see Chapter 3).

2. Cholecystokinin (CCK)

In 1928, Ivy and Goldberg proposed that fat in the chyme or some of the products from fat digestion was a secretogogue for release of an intestinal peptide hormone that they named CCK (*chole* bile + *kystis* bladder + *kinein* move). CCK travels via the blood to the gallbladder, where it stimulates contraction of smooth muscles comprising the walls of the gallbladder. At the same time, it causes relaxation of the sphincter of Oddi, a muscle that controls exit of bile from the gallbladder. As a result, bile is expelled from the gallbladder, enters the bile duct, and is transported to the duodenum. Bile is a viscous, complex mixture consisting largely of bile salts (derived from excess cholesterol; see Chapter 3) and bile pigments. Bile salts are powerful emulsifiers (i.e., surfactants). Bile pigments are breakdown products of hemoglobins, and they give bile and feces their characteristic colorations. Many other substances produced by the liver are present in bile, including metabolites of steroid hormones, thyroid hormone metabolites, and inorganic iodide from deiodination of thyroid hormones. When bile enters the duodenum, the bile salts emulsify globules of fat, causing them to be dispersed as small fat droplets within the aqueous digestive fluids. The emulsification of fats or **triacylglycerides (TAGs)** allows for a marked reduction in the volume-to-surface ratio of the fat droplets, facilitating hydrolytic attack by pancreatic lipase to release **monoacylglycerides (MAGs)** and **nonesterified fatty acids** (NEFAs; also called free fatty acids, FFA) for absorption by intestinal mucosal cells.

Isolation and purification of the first GI peptides were accomplished by Mutt and Jorpes in Sweden more than half a century after the discovery of secretin by Bayliss and Starling. Mutt and Jorpes discovered that the biological functions previously ascribed to pancreozymin and CCK resided in the same peptide consisting of 33 amino acids. Consequently, the rather cumbersome name **pancreozymin-cholecystokinin (PZCCK)** was proposed to designate the single peptide that for many years had been described in the literature under separate names. Because CCK was described first, Grossman (1970) proposed that we continue to use CCK for both actions and that we drop the PZ. In general, this proposal has been adopted. The **I-cell** in the intestinal mucosa has been identified as the synthetic source for CCK.

Several CCK peptides have been identified, including molecules composed of 8 amino acids (CCK_8), 33 (CCK_{33}), 39 (CCK_{39}), and 58 (CCK_{58}). Recent studies indicate that the larger forms predominate and all forms are cleaved from the same gene product. In the central nervous system, CCK_8 is the common form present. CCK activity is very low in the general circulation and it is difficult to obtain quantitative information on its various potential forms. However, CCK_8, CCK_{39}, and CCK_{58} are measureable in blood plasma of the dog, but it is not known if they are secreted in these forms or whether the shorter forms are produced by peptidase activity in the blood following secretion of the larger form(s).

The separate functional roles of secretin and CCK have been demonstrated elegantly *in vitro* using slices of exocrine pancreas. Physiological levels of CCK do not evoke release of basic pancreatic juice except in the presence of secretin, implying a permissive role for CCK, enhancing the action of secretin. As mentioned above, purified CCK, but not secretin, causes extrusion of zymogen granules from the acinar cells of the exocrine pancreas. Acetylcholine also causes extrusion of zymogen granules, suggesting direct parasympathetic (cephalic) control of enzyme release from the exocrine pancreas. Parasympathetic influence via the vagus nerve and CCK probably operate via separate mechanisms since atropine blocks the effects of ACh but not of CCK on enzyme release. Furthermore, CCK does not require neural factors for its action.

Two G-protein-linked receptors have been characterized for CCK. One type predominates in target cells of the digestive or alimentary tract (CCK-A receptor) and preferentially binds larger or sulfated forms of CCK. The second receptor type (CCK-B) occurs in the brain and has highest affinity for CCK_8. Once occupied, CCK receptors stimulate production of second messengers, IP_3 and DAG. The former causes an increase in cytosolic Ca^{2+} and the latter activates phosphokinase C. There also is evidence suggesting CCK may work through a cAMP mechanism to produce some of its effects.

Fats, proteins, and amino acids in the gastric effluent entering the duodenum are the most potent, direct secretagogues for CCK release. Conversely, active proteases such as trypsin in the duodenum inhibit CCK secretion (negative feedback). The presence of bile elements also may reduce CCK release. Basal levels of CCK are very low (about 1 pM/L of plasma) but increase following eating to between 5 and 8 pM in about 10–45 minutes followed by a slow decline until the stomach is empty.

In addition to releasing enzymes in response to CCK, the rat exocrine pancreas also secretes a **monitor peptide** (61 amino acids) that stimulates CCK release that in turn increases pancreatic secretion (positive feedback). The intestine also secretes a similar peptide that causes CCK release during early phases of digestion. During periods of fasting, this peptide is rapidly destroyed by the low levels of trypsin present in the duodenal lumen. However, when food enters from the stomach, the trypsin is further diluted so that the intestinal peptide is not degraded so rapidly, which in turn elevates CCK release.

In rats and dogs, bombesin and GRP are also potent releasers of CCK and hence pancreatic enzyme secretion. However, direct actions of bombesin and GRP have been demonstrated on pancreatic acinar cells as well. Furthermore, acinar cells are innervated by GRP-secreting neurons providing another possible mechanism for enzyme release.

In several species, CCK slows the rate of gastric evacuation (emptying) through relaxation of gastric smooth muscle and contraction of the pyloric sphincter, thus slowing peristalsis and preventing passage of material from the stomach. These contradictory actions of CCK on gastric smooth muscle and the pyloric sphincter are similar to the effects observed on gallbladder smooth muscle (contraction) and the sphincter of Oddi (relaxation). CCK receptor antagonists accelerate gastric emptying in some human studies, suggesting a similar enterogastrone-like role for CCK. Intestinal blood flow also may be altered by CCK. Certain neurons supplying blood vessels in the gut can release CCK, which causes relaxation of smooth muscle in arterioles and increases intestinal blood flow.

E. Intestinal Regulation of Gastric Secretion

In 1930, Kosaka and Lim proposed the existence of an intestinal peptide that they called enterogastrone. This hypothetical hormone was released in response to arrival of fat from the stomach and was believed to inhibit gastric motility (peristalsis) as well as reduce acid secretion by the gastric parietal cells. These actions would slow the entrance of fat into the small intestine and allow more time for proper processing of fat already present in the duodenum. There may be numerous enterogastrones, and several peptides with entrogastrone-like activity have been isolated from the small intestine (Figure 12-9). The possible action of CCK on gastric secretion and peristalsis was discussed earlier. Three additional intestinal peptides with enterogastrone-like actions are described below.

1. Gastric Inhibitory Peptide or Glucose-Dependent Insulinotropic Peptide

A peptide first called **gastric-inhibitory peptide (GIP)** was isolated from the intestine and shown to inhibit gastric function. GIP is produced by the **K-cell** in the duodenal mucosa. Chemically, GIP is similar in amino

	1	11	21	31	41

Porcine
GIP   Y A E G T F I S D Y   S I A M D K I R Q Q   D F V N W L L A Q K   G K K S D W K H N I   T Q

Human
GIP   Y A E G T F I S D Y   S I A M D K I H̄ Q Q   D F V N W L L A Q K   G K K N̄ D W K H N I   T Q

Bovine
GIP   Y A E G T F I S D Y   S I A M D K I R Q Q   D F V N W L L A Q K   G K K S D W Ī H N I   T Q

Rodent
GIP   Y A E G T F I S D Y   S I A M D K I R Q Q   D F V N W L L A Q K   G K K N̄ D W K H N L̄   T Q

Figure 12-11. **Comparison of mammalian GIP structures.** These peptides are highly conservative and there have been few substitutions. See Appendix C for explanation of the letters coding for individual amino acids. [Modified from Pederson, R. A. (1994). Gastric inhibitory peptide. *In* "Gut Peptides" (J. H. Walsh, and G. J. Dockray, Eds.), pp. 217–259. Raven, New York.]

acid sequence to secretin but is considerably larger (42 amino acids). Introduction of fat or glucose into the duodenum evokes GIP release. Ingestion of a meal results in a five- to six-fold elevation in plasma GIP that remains elevated for about six hours.

GIP has been extracted from several mammals, and its structure is rather conservative (Figure 12-11). GIP blocks both gastrin-stimulated secretion of acid and enzyme by the stomach but is effective only in the experimentally denervated stomach, suggesting this may not be a physiological role for GIP. It may produce its inhibitory effects by stimulating release of SST that in turn directly inhibits acid secretion by the parietal cell. In humans, large (pharmacological) doses of GIP are required to obtain even a weak effect on gastric acid secretion, implying that this is not a major role for GIP.

Other studies suggest the physiological role for GIP is to stimulate insulin release from the endocrine pancreas to facilitate absorption and distribution of glucose and amino acids. A dose-dependent release of insulin is caused by physiologically relevant amounts of GIP both *in vivo* and *in vitro*. Since it is believed this action represents the true role for GIP, the peptide has been renamed **glucose-dependent insulinotropic peptide**, providing a more descriptive name while retaining the original acronym, GIP.

2. Peptide YY

Another potential enterogastrone may be PYY that was first isolated from the pig intestine. It also is called peptide tyrosine-tyrosine and has both a C-terminal and an N-terminal tyrosine for which the abbreviation is "Y." The peptide consists of 36 amino acids and is chemically very similar to neuropeptide Y (NPY) and pancreatic polypeptide (see ahead). PYY inhibits secretion by the exocrine pancreas and reduces gastric acid secretion. Release of PYY into the circulation occurs following the introduction of fat into the duodenum, and physiologically relevant levels of PYY produce a dose-dependent inhibition of gastric acid secretion.

3. Calcitonin Gene-Related Peptide

Calcitonin is a calcium-regulating hormone produced in mammals by the thyroid C-cells (see Chapters 6 and 14). **Calcitonin gene-related peptide (CGRP)** is formed in neurons by an alternative post-translational processing of the calcitonin gene product resulting in this peptide of 37 amino acids. CGRP, which inhibits gastric acid secretion, has been isolated from human, rat, rabbit, bovine, and porcine sources (Figure 12-12). Two forms have been isolated from humans and rats, each produced by a separate gene. A related peptide is **amylin** (also consisting of 37 amino acids) that has about 40–50% homology to CGRP (Figure 12-12). Amylin, however, is co-secreted with insulin when pancreatic B-cells are exposed to glucose.

Unlike most of the GI regulators, the distribution of CGRP-immunoreactive axons differs greatly among the species examined to date. For example, CGRP is virtually absent from gastric neurons in humans and pigs but is abundant in the stomachs of the rat, hamster, mouse, mole, and ferret. Intermediate amounts of CGRP occur in stomachs of cats, dogs, and guinea pigs.

Most of the gastric CGRP-containing neurons are primary (sensory) afferent neurons. The cell bodies of these sensory neurons often are present in the dorsal root ganglia. CGRP neurons occur throughout the

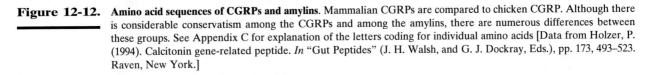

CGRPS	1										11										21										31						37
Human CGRP-I	A	C	D	T	A	T	C	V	T	H	R	L	A	G	L	L	S	R	S	G	G	V	V	K	N	N	F	V	P	T	N	V	G	S	K	A	F-NH₂
Human CGRP-II	A	C	N	T	A	T	C	V	T	H	R	L	A	G	L	L	S	R	S	G	G	M	V	K	S	N	F	V	P	T	N	V	G	S	K	A	F-NH₂
Rat CGRP-I	S	C	N	T	A	T	C	V	T	H	R	L	A	G	L	L	S	R	S	G	G	V	V	K	D	N	F	V	P	T	N	V	G	S	E	A	F-NH₂
Rat CGRP-II	S	C	N	T	A	T	C	V	T	H	R	L	A	G	L	L	S	R	S	G	G	V	V	K	D	N	F	V	P	T	N	V	G	S	K	A	F-NH₂
Rabbit CGRP	G	C	N	T	A	T	C	V	T	H	R	L	A	G	L	L	S	R	S	G	G	M	V	K	S	N	F	V	P	T	N	V	G	S	E	A	F-NH₂
Bovine CGRP	S	C	N	T	A	T	C	V	T	H	R	L	A	G	L	L	S	R	S	G	G	V	V	K	S	N	F	V	P	T	N	V	G	S	E	A	F-NH₂
Porcine CGRP	S	C	N	T	A	T	C	V	T	H	R	L	A	G	L	L	S	R	S	G	G	M	V	K	S	N	F	V	P	T	D	V	G	S	E	A	F-NH₂
Chicken CGRP	A	C	N	T	A	T	C	V	T	H	R	L	A	D	F	L	S	R	S	G	G	V	G	K	N	N	F	V	P	T	N	V	G	S	K	A	F-NH₂
Amylins																																					
Human amylin	K	C	N	T	A	T	C	A	T	Q	R	L	A	N	F	L	V	H	S	S	N	N	F	G	A	I	L	S	S	T	N	V	G	S	N	T	Y-NH₂
Rat, mouse, amylin	K	C	N	T	A	T	C	A	T	Q	R	L	A	N	F	L	V	D	S	S	N	N	F	G	P	V	L	P	P	T	N	V	G	S	N	T	Y-NH₂
Guinea-pig amylin	K	C	N	T	A	T	C	A	T	Q	R	L	T	N	F	L	V	D	S	S	H	N	F	G	A	A	L	L	P	T	D	V	G	S	N	T	Y-NH₂
Cat amylin	K	C	N	T	A	T	C	A	T	Q	R	L	A	N	F	L	I	D	S	S	N	N	F	G	A	I	L	S	P	T	N	V	G	S	N	T	Y-NH₂

Figure 12-12. **Amino acid sequences of CGRPs and amylins.** Mammalian CGRPs are compared to chicken CGRP. Although there is considerable conservatism among the CGRPs and among the amylins, there are numerous differences between these groups. See Appendix C for explanation of the letters coding for individual amino acids [Data from Holzer, P. (1994). Calcitonin gene-related peptide. *In* "Gut Peptides" (J. H. Walsh, and G. J. Dockray, Eds.), pp. 173, 493–523. Raven, New York.]

mammalian digestive tract, but endocrine cells secreting CGRP have been found only in the human small intestine and the rat pancreas. CGRP-containing motor neurons from the brain stem have been described in the esophagus of monkeys and cats, and some CGRP-containing motor neurons as well as some CGRP-enteric neurons are seen in the stomach and intestine.

CGRP is released from the gastric mucosa of rats by the neurotoxin **capsaicin** (the active component in hot peppers) or by an increase in acidity of the duodenal contents to pH 6. CGRP probably stimulates SST release within the gastric mucosa that in turn inhibits gastric acid secretion.

4. Motilin

A small peptide (22 amino acids) that stimulates motility in the gastrointestinal tract and possibly the secretion of pepsinogen by the stomach has been isolated from the duodenum. This peptide is called **motilin** for its stimulatory action on smooth muscle that hastens the passage of material through the small intestine. Motilin is structurally unlike the other GI peptides (Figure 12-13). In most mammals, alkaline conditions in the duodenum cause release of motilin from the **M-cells** of the small intestine. However, in humans, motilin apparently is released by acidic solutions.

In the fasting human, an endogenous rhythmic secretion of motilin activates a wave of muscular contraction called the **migrating motor complex (MMC)**. This MMC begins at the antral end of the stomach every 75 to 90 minutes and moves along the intestine to sweep materials into the colon. This mechanism also prevents movement of bacteria from the large intestine into the small intestine, especially when food is absent.

5. Vasoactive Intestinal Peptide (VIP)

Relaxation of vascular smooth muscle increases blood flow to the viscera. This relaxation is caused by another peptide first isolated from the intestinal mucosa, **vasoactive intestinal polypeptide (VIP)**. Increased blood flow into the small intestine may enhance absorption of digestion products into the blood. In addition, VIP relaxes gastric smooth muscle and slows gastric processing.

	1					11					21	
Canine	F	V	P	I	F	T H S E L	Q K I R E	K E R N K	G Q				
Porcine	F	V	P	I	F	T Y G E L	Q R M Q E	K E R N K	G Q				

Figure 12-13. **Amino acid sequences of canine and porcine motilins.** See Appendix C for explanation of the letters coding for individual amino acids. [Data from Poitras, P. (1994). Motilin. *In* "Gut Peptides" (J. H. Walsh, and G. J. Dockray, Eds.), pp. 261–304. Raven, New York.]

Pig	HSDDAV	FTDNY	[T]RLRL	QMAVK	KLYNS	[I]L N-NH2
Guinea pig	HSDDA[L]	FTDTY	[T]RLRL	QMAMK	KLYNS	VLN-NH2
Chicken	HSDDAV	FTDNY	SRFRL	QMAVK	KLYNS	VL T-NH2
Alligator	HSDDAV	FTDNY	SRFRL	QMAVK	KLYNS	VL T-NH2
Frog	HSDDAV	FTDNY	SRFRL	QMAVK	KLYNS	VL T-NH2
Rainbow trout	HSDDA[I]	FTDNY	SRFRL	QMAVK	KLYNS	VL T-NH2
Cod fish	HSDDAV	FTDNY	SRFRL	QMAAK	KLYNS	VL A-NH2
Bowfin	HSDDA[I]	FTDNY	SRFRL	QMAVK	KLYNS	VL T-NH2
Dogfish shark	HSDDAV	FTDNY	SRIRL	QMAVK	KLYNS	[L]L A-NH2

Figure 12-14. **Comparison of vertebrate VIPs.** This neuropeptide shows few substitutions have been made in the molecule through its long evolutionary history from fishes to mammals. See Appendix C for explanation of the letters coding for individual amino acids. [Modified from Wang, Y., and Conlon, J. M. (1995). Purification and structural characteristics of vasoactive intestinal polypeptide from trout and bowfin. *Gen. Comp. Endocr.* **98**, 94–101.]

VIP consists of 28 amino acids and is structurally similar to both secretin and GIP (Figure 12-14). The immunoreactive VIP found in the brain is structurally identical to intestinal VIP. In the intestine, VIP is produced typically in neurons, but a pyramidal-shaped **H-cell** found in the small intestine and in the colon of some species also may secrete VIP. Post-translational processing of the preprohormone produces not only VIP but another similar peptide consisting of 27 amino acids with an N-terminal histidine and a C-terminal isoleucine reflected in its name: **peptide histidine isoleucine**, or **PHI**. In humans, this VIP-like peptide exhibits methionine in place of isoleucine and is termed **PHM**. Some of the actions previously attributed to VIP may be due to an interaction of PHI and VIP on the target cells. Sufficiently high doses of VIP have been shown to produce weak secretin-like effects on the pancreas as well as to induce a hyperglycemic response. These actions of VIP on the exocrine pancreas and blood sugar levels may be pharmacologic as a consequence of the similarity of amino acid sequence when applied at pharmacological doses.

A major role for VIP is that of an inhibitory neurotransmitter produced by intestinal nerves. It inhibits vascular smooth muscle but stimulates glandular epithelia. It is the inhibitory action on vascular smooth muscle that increases blood flow into intestinal tissues.

Another proposed action for VIP is on the secretion of Brunner's glands in the duodenal mucosa. In response to the entrance of acidic chyme into the duodenum, Brunner's glands secrete a viscous, alkaline mucus that is believed to help in neutralizing gastric acid and protecting the duodenal mucosa.

6. Enteroglucagons

The **L-cells** (also called EG-cells) in the small intestinal mucosa produce several peptides that collectively can be called the **enteroglucagons**. These peptides are structurally and functionally like pancreatic glucagons (see below). Enteroglucagons are extractable in a large form named **glicentin** (69 amino acids). Two other glucagon-like peptides (GLP-I and GLP-II) are also cleaved from the same preprohormone as glicentin (Figure 12-15). A truncated (shortened) form of GLP-1 (**tGLP-I**) has been reported as well. In addition to their possible role in feeding, enteroglucagons may stimulate insulin secretion while inhibiting pancreatic secretion of glucagon following ingestion of a meal. Furthermore, enteroglucagons may inhibit gastric acid secretion and delay gastric emptying. The physiological role for enteroglucagons and their relationship to pancreatic glucagon and glucose metabolism are considered below.

7. Other Gastrointestinal Peptides

Somatostatin (SST), a paracrine inhibitor produced by **D-cells** in the stomach, also is produced by neurons and D-cells located throughout the small intestine. Here, it seems to function in paracrine fashion by inhibiting release of virtually all other GI peptides. SST has been demonstrated in the arterial circulation of dogs following a meal and may act as a hormone to inhibit release of gastrin, insulin, glucagon, and pancreatic polypeptide, PP (see below). Two forms of SST have been isolated. The first is identical to the hypothalamic tetradecapeptide neurohormone (SST_{14}). The second consists of SST_{14} plus an additional 14 amino acids (SST_{28}).

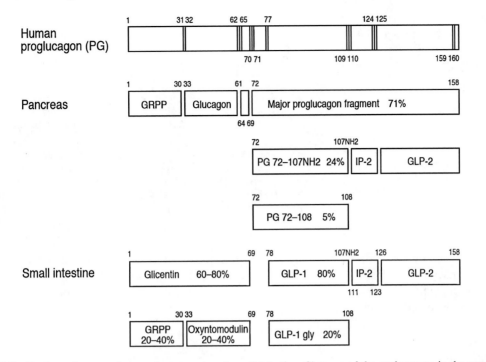

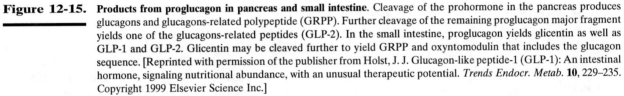

Figure 12-15. **Products from proglucagon in pancreas and small intestine.** Cleavage of the prohormone in the pancreas produces glucagons and glucagons-related polypeptide (GRPP). Further cleavage of the remaining proglucagon major fragment yields one of the glucagons-related peptides (GLP-2). In the small intestine, proglucagon yields glicentin as well as GLP-1 and GLP-2. Glicentin may be cleaved further to yield GRPP and oxyntomodulin that includes the glucagon sequence. [Reprinted with permission of the publisher from Holst, J. J. Glucagon-like peptide-1 (GLP-1): An intestinal hormone, signaling nutritional abundance, with an unusual therapeutic potential. *Trends Endocr. Metab.* **10**, 229–235. Copyright 1999 Elsevier Science Inc.]

Neurotensin (NT), a tridecapeptide, is another neurotransmitter first identified in the central nervous system that is found in the intestine. In addition to localization in neurons, NT also is found in epithelial **N-cells** that directly contact the lumen of the small intestine. Although it has been shown to produce many effects, including acting as an enterogastrone, no clear role has been established for intestinal NT.

Substance P (onadecapeptide) was the first peptide to be identified in both the intestine and the brain (in 1931). It is not clear whether substance P and NT function only as neurotransmitters or if they have paracrine functions in the intestine. Some of the substance P-containing neurons may be primary afferent (sensory) and nociceptive (pain) neurons.

Dynorphin, a heptadecapeptide opioid discussed earlier in the central nervous system (Chapter 4), is also present in the intestine. It is produced by neurons and probably acts as a local inhibitor of the neurotransmitter substance P.

Galanin consists of 29 or 30 amino acids (Figure 12-16) and is concentrated in the duodenum. It is capable of inhibiting gastric acid secretion and can block secretion of several other GI regulators including NT, enteroglucagons, SST, PYY, and pancreatic hormones. Galanin may be a modulator of GI functions including motility, secretion, and blood flow. Hypothalamic galanin also is a releaser of luteinizing hormone (LH) from the pituitary (see Chapter 4). It also functions as a hypothalamic orexic factor (see above).

F. Complex Interactions of Gastrointestinal Peptides

Many studies have been published in the past few years that involve observation of the effects of administering combinations of GI peptides as well as the influences of one peptide on the release of another. Studies of this type indicate considerable overlap in the actions of the various peptides (for example, glucagon-like activity in secretin) although pharmacological doses usually are necessary to produce these effects. The observation

	1	6	11
Common sequence (1–15)	G W T L N	S A G Y L	L G P H A -
Variable sequence (16–30)	16	21	26
Pig (29)	I D N H D	S F H D K	Y G L A -NH₂
Sheep (29)	I D N H D	S F H D K	H G L A -NH₂
Cow (29)	L D S H D	S F Q D K	H G L A -NH₂
Rat (29)	I D N H D	S F S D K	H G L T -NH₂
Chicken (29)	V D N H D	S F N D K	H G L T -NH₂
Human (30)	V G N H D	S F S D K	N G L T S -NH₂

Figure 12-16. **Comparison of mammalian galanins with chicken galanin.** All have the same 15 C-terminal amino acids with only moderate differences among the N-terminal sequence. See Appendix C for explanation of the letters coding for individual amino acids. [Data from Rokaeus, A. (1994). Galanin. *In* "Gut Peptides" (Walsh, J. H., and Dockray, G. J., Eds.), pp. 425–552. Raven, New York.]

that many of these peptides double as neurotransmitters makes it even more difficult to interpret studies employing pharmacological doses. At the present time, it is difficult to sort out interactions due to structural similarities, pharmacological doses, or both from those interactions that might represent true synergisms, functional overlaps, or inhibitions.

III. Bioregulation of Metabolism

The term **metabolism** represents the total of all enzymatic processes occurring within the cells of the body. Metabolism frequently is subdivided into specific pathways. One such subdivision is **intermediary metabolism** that involves the metabolism of carbohydrates for energy and serves as the linkage between **protein metabolism** and **lipid metabolism**. Intermediary metabolism is especially important in the liver, which has the major responsibility for converting amino acids and fatty acids into carbohydrates for energy, especially during periods of fasting, and providing glucose to the circulatory system.

A. Major Elements of Metabolism in Vertebrates

This section provides an overview of the major features of carbohydrate, lipid, and protein metabolism and their interrelationships. In addition, differences among tissues in their metabolic capabilities will be illustrated. This discussion will set the foundation for understanding how hormones regulate certain aspects of metabolism. Although the same metabolic enzymes and pathways are present in most vertebrates, the specific forms of these enzymes and their characteristics differ from group to group and from tissue to tissue within a group. The following account will address a generalized pattern of metabolism for all vertebrates.

1. Intermediary Metabolism

The major pathway in intermediary metabolism involves the oxidation of glucose to produce ATP to drive energy-requiring reactions in cells. This oxidative process is known as **cellular respiration**. About 70% of the glucose used in cellular respiration is oxidized through **glycolysis** (Figure 12-17) with the remainder being oxidized via the pentose phosphate pathway or **pentose shunt** (Figure 12-18). These two pathways operate under both anaerobic and aerobic conditions. The pentose shunt produces reduced **nicotinamide adenine dinucleotide phosphate (NADPH)** that is necessary for the synthesis of fatty acids, for inactivation of steroids, and for detoxification of many drugs. Some intermediates produced in the pentose shunt can feed into the glycolytic pathway (e.g., glyceraldehyde 3-P). Furthermore, some of the five-carbon sugars for which the pathway is named may be utilized for synthesis of ribose and deoxyribose used for making the nucleotides found in RNA and DNA, respectively.

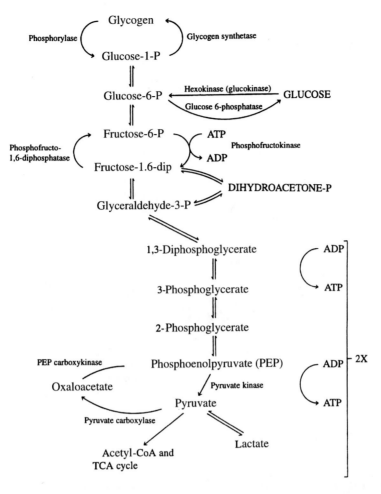

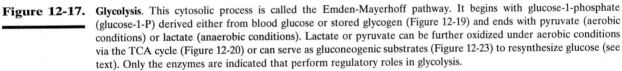

Figure 12-17. **Glycolysis**. This cytosolic process is called the Emden-Mayerhoff pathway. It begins with glucose-1-phosphate (glucose-1-P) derived either from blood glucose or stored glycogen (Figure 12-19) and ends with pyruvate (aerobic conditions) or lactate (anaerobic conditions). Lactate or pyruvate can be further oxidized under aerobic conditions via the TCA cycle (Figure 12-20) or can serve as gluconeogenic substrates (Figure 12-23) to resynthesize glucose (see text). Only the enzymes are indicated that perform regulatory roles in glycolysis.

2. Glycolysis

The initial steps of glucose oxidation all occur in the cytosol. There are three limiting steps in glycolysis, each of which is catalyzed by a unidirectional enzyme (i.e., the reaction is irreversible because of thermodynamic considerations). Free glucose enters a cell by a protein carrier-mediated mechanism or **glucose transporter (GLUT)** that is responsible for carrier-mediated facilitated diffusion of glucose into or from cells depending on the concentration gradient of glucose. Once glucose enters a cell, it is immediately phosphorylated to glucose-6-phosphate in most tissues by a unidirectional enzyme called **hexokinase** (recall that a kinase is a phosphorylating enzyme). In liver, this enzyme often is called **glucokinase**. Once glucose has been phosphorylated, it can no longer be transported across the cell membrane and, in most tissues, is committed either to storage or to use for energy. However, in liver tissue (and in the kidney to a limited extent), the enzyme **glucose-6-phosphatase**, can remove the phosphate from glucose-6-phosphate, creating free glucose that can leave the liver cell. Glucose-6-phosphatase hydrolytic activity is lacking in almost all other tissues, so the liver is the only tissue that can readily supply glucose to the rest of the body. In general, virtually all glucose in the blood is either absorbed following digestion of food or is contributed by the metabolic activities of the liver.

Glucose-6-phosphate can be metabolized through glycolysis or the pentose shunt, or it can be converted to glucose-1-phosphate and polymerized with the aid of the enzyme **glycogen synthetase** (glycogen syntase) to a storage form of polysaccharide called **glycogen**. This process is called **glycogenesis**.

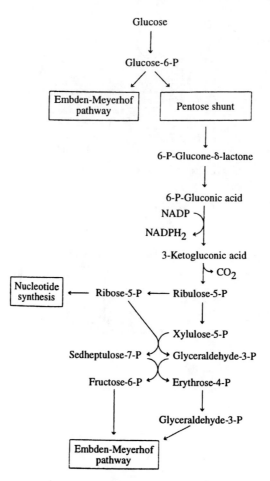

Glucose
↓
Glucose-6-P

Embden-Meyerhof pathway | Pentose shunt

↓

6-P-Glucone-δ-lactone
↓
6-P-Gluconic acid

NADP
NADPH$_2$

3-Ketogluconic acid
→ CO$_2$

Nucleotide synthesis ← Ribose-5-P ← Ribulose-5-P

Xylulose-5-P

Sedheptulose-7-P ⇄ Glyceraldehyde-3-P

Fructose-6-P ⇄ Erythrose-4-P

Glyceraldehyde-3-P

Embden-Meyerhof pathway

Figure 12-18. **The pentose shunt**. This alternate pathway within glycolysis (Figure 12-17) generates substrates for fatty acid and nucleotide synthesis. See text for details.

The enzyme **phosphorylase-a** is responsible for hydrolyzing glycogen back to glucose as needed (see Figure 12-19).

Following complete assimilation of a meal or during fasting, plasma glucose levels are maintained by the liver initially through hydrolysis of glycogen to glucose-6-phosphate (a process called **glycogenolysis**). Glucose-6-phosphate can be dephosphorylated to glucose and exit the liver cell. The liver also produces glucose from amino acids, lactate, fatty acids, and glycerol (see ahead).

The second one-way conversion occurs early in glycolysis by the action of **phosphofructose kinase (PFK)** with ATP and fructose-6-phosphate to form fructose-1,6-diphosphate. This commits the cell to further oxidation by splitting that 6-C sugar to two phosphorylated trioses through the glycolytic pathway that yields a small amount of ATP.

In the third irreversible step, **pyruvate kinase (PK)** converts **phosphoenolpyruvate (PEP)** to pyruvate. In the presence of oxygen, PEP can be further oxidized to produce additional ATP or, in the absence of sufficient oxygen, converted to lactate (Figure 12-17).

3. The Tricarboxylic Acid (TCA) Cycle and the Electron Transport Chain

In the presence of oxygen and coenzyme A, pyruvate leaves the cytosol and enters a mitochondrion where it interacts with coenzyme A and is coverted to **acetyl-coenzyme A (acetyl-CoA)** plus CO$_2$. Acetyl-CoA combines with the 4-carbon compound called "oxaloacetate" to produce citric acid or citrate (Figure 12-20). Through a series of reactions that generates two additional CO$_2$ molecules and a number of important reduced

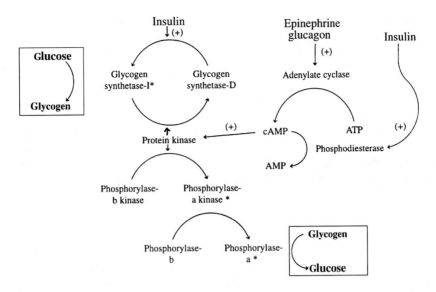

Figure 12-19. Glycogenesis and glycogenolysis. Enzymes are converted from inactive to active forms by various hormones that alter the availability of glucose for metabolism. Insulin favors glucose storage as glycogen whereas epinephrine and glucagon favor glucose oxidation or release into the blood. The asterisk (*) denotes the active form.

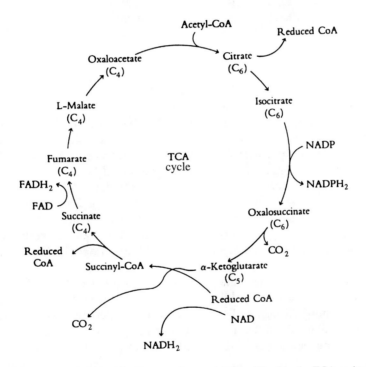

Figure 12-20. The tricarboxylic acid (TCA) cycle. Pyruvate is completely oxidized in the TCA cycle to CO_2 that is released from the cell. Electrons (plus associated hydrogen ions) are transferred to electron-acceptors (FAD, NAD, NADP) that will be used by the electron-transport chain (cytochromes) to synthesize ATP and water. The TCA cycle and the cytochromes are confined within the mitochondria.

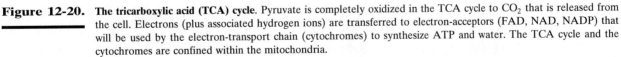

compounds (NADPH, NADH, FADH), the citrate is oxidized back to oxaloacetate that can combine with another acetyl-CoA generated from glucose. This series of cyclic events constitutes the **tricarboxylic acid** or **TCA cycle**, so named because citrate has three carboxyl groups in its structure. It also is known as the "citric acid cycle," since it begins with the combination of acetyl-coA and succinate to form citric acid, as well as the "Krebs cycle," after the man who discovered it.

The reduced compounds generated by the TCA cycle are used to transfer electrons to a series or chain of electron-transfer molecules called cytochromes. This **electron transport chain** also is located in the mitochondrion. A final electron transfer is made to oxygen that results in the generation of water. The energy released by the sequential transfers of electrons from higher to lower energy levels along the electron-transport chain is used to generate ATP. Thus, the complete oxidation of glucose to CO_2 and water requires glycolysis, the TCA cycle, the electron transport chain, and oxygen as the final electron acceptor in order to produce a large number of ATPs. This process is referred to as **aerobic cellular respiration**, or simply as **aerobic respiration**. In the absence of oxygen, the oxidative pathway stops in the cytosol at pyruvate with only a small amount of ATP produced. The excess pyruvate is converted by the enzyme **lactate dehydrogenase** to lactate. This process is called **anaerobic respiration**. When oxygen is available, lactate can be converted back to pyruvate by the same enzyme. In some animals, a portion of the pyruvate is converted irreversibly to ethanol and CO_2.

B. Protein Metabolism

Proteins are composed of more than 20 different amino acids. In animals that have a protein-rich diet, including most predators, ingested proteins are hydrolyzed to amino acids and absorbed through the intestine. These amino acids can be used to synthesize proteins and the excess can be converted to carbohydrate for energy use or to lipids for storage. Under conditions of starvation, hydrolysis of proteins located primarily in muscle cells provides amino acids for energy production in the muscle cells and amino acids for conversion to glucose by the liver (see below).

Some organisms can synthesize all the amino acids required for protein synthesis, but many vertebrates cannot. Humans and some other vertebrates must rely on a dietary source of what have been called **essential amino acids**. In humans, nine amino acids are considered to be essential and must be obtained through the diet.

C. Lipid Metabolism

Lipogenesis is the synthesis of lipids. The most important lipids are the triacylglycerols or TAGs (oils, fats), fatty acids, and steroids. TAGs are also known as triglycerides. Synthesis of a TAG begins with glycerol and one fatty acid and progresses stepwise to the TAG by the actions of a series of acylglycerol enzymes. This synthetic process is usually called **esterification**. The first step in esterification is formation of a monoacylglycerol (MAG) consisting of a molecule of glycerol esterified to a fatty acid (Figure 12-21). This step is catalyzed by a **monoacylglycerol synthetase** and occurs more commonly in the liver. Addition of a second esterified fatty acid produces a **diacylglycerol (DAG)**, and a third addition produces a TAG. If the attached fatty acids have many double bonds or are unsaturated, the TAG is likely to appear as an oil at room temperatures. If there are few double bonds in the esterified fatty acids, the compound is a solid at room temperature and we call it a fat. We will not distinguish between these saturated and unsaturated TAGs in the following discussions, although most of the natural compounds are saturated.

The liver sends TAGs to other tissues (mainly muscle and adipose tissues) for storage or utilization. Hydrolysis of TAGs in storage tissues is called **lipolysis** and occurs through the actions of **triacylglycerol lipase** and **diacylglycerol lipase**. Although lipolysis of stored TAGs is initiated primarily in muscle and adipose tissue, **monoacylglycerol lipase** is active only in the liver. Fatty acids are freed through lipolysis and become NEFAs. They can be released into the blood where they bind reversibly to serum proteins and are transported to the liver.

NEFAs can be synthesized in the liver and other tissues from acetyl-CoA. However, acetyl-CoA generated within the mitochondrion cannot cross the mitochondrial membrane and enter the cytosol where fatty acid synthesis occurs. Instead, citrate is transported into the cytosol and used to regenerate acetyl-CoA. The rate-limiting enzyme **acetyl-CoA carboxylase** initiates fatty acid synthesis from cytoplasmic acetyl-CoA. Glucose metabolism provides glycerol that is enzymatically coupled to a fatty acyl-CoA complex to form an MAG.

The steroid cholesterol may be absorbed following a meal or may be synthesized from cytoplasmic acetyl-CoA (see Chapter 3). This synthetic process involves activation of the rate-limiting enzyme **hydroxymethylglutaryl-CoA (HMG-CoA) reductase** and ends with the synthesis of cholesterol in the cytosol. Cholesterol and cholesterol esters (cholesterol linked by an ester bond to a fatty acid) may be extruded in

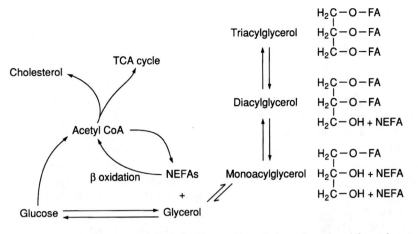

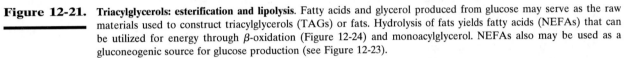

Figure 12-21. **Triacylglycerols: esterification and lipolysis.** Fatty acids and glycerol produced from glucose may serve as the raw materials used to construct triacylglycerols (TAGs) or fats. Hydrolysis of fats yields fatty acids (NEFAs) that can be utilized for energy through β-oxidation (Figure 12-24) and monoacylglycerol. NEFAs also may be used as a gluconeogenic source for glucose production (see Figure 12-23).

lipoprotein droplets and transported through the blood to sites of cholesterol utilization or may be converted to bile salts and transported to the gallbladder for use in digestion (see above). Cholesterol synthesis may be in direct competition with fatty acid synthesis for the cytoplasmic substrate acetyl-CoA, and the regulation of the rate-limiting enzymes for these pathways is critical. Cholesterol is necessary for building cell membranes (especially in dividing cells) and is the precursor for the synthesis of all of the steroid hormones as described in Chapter 3.

Following absorption of a meal, excess carbohydrates and amino acids are converted into TAGs by the liver. These TAGs plus cholesterol are surrounded by a phospholipid membrane in which are embedded special proteins called **apoproteins**. These lipoprotein droplets are extruded into the blood as **very-low-density lipoprotein droplets (VLDLs)**. The apoproteins apparently act as "docking proteins" for attachment to receptors on the endothelial cell membranes of capillaries. These receptors are called **LDL-receptors** and have a high affinity for apoprotein-e. The endothelial cells express a TAG-digesting enzyme called **lipoprotein lipase**. This enzyme is most prevalent in the endothelial cells of capillaries in adipose tissue and to some extent in capillaries of skeletal muscle. Lipoprotein lipase converts TAGs to MAGs and NEFAs that diffuse into the adipose or muscle cell where they are reconstituted to TAGs. The lipoprotein droplet that has lost some of its TAGs has a relatively higher concentration protein, and therefore is now more dense. After the VLDLs have lost about 50% of their TAG content, they are classified as **intermediate-density lipoproteins (IDLs)**. When IDLs again reach the liver, they bind to LDL-receptors and may be refilled with TAGs prior to making another journey to the storage sites as VLDLs. If the IDLs by chance remain in the circulation longer, they continue to lose TAGs to tissues. After they lose about 90% of their TAG content, they begin to lose the special protein **apoprotein-e** and are renamed the **low-density lipoproteins (LDLs)**. Furthermore, without apoprotein-e, they bind poorly to the LDL-receptors and remain longer in the circulation, meanwhile transferring their load of cholesterol to other cells, especially endothelial cells of arteries. However, **apoprotein-B100** is still present on the surface of the LDL and can bind to the LDL-receptor but not as strongly as apoprotein-e. This causes LDLs to be bound in the liver at a much slower rate than IDLs. Hence, they have a much longer biological half-life in blood than do IDLs. Thus, LDLs tend to accumulate in the blood and continue to deliver cholesterol to arterial sites for deposition.

Another group of lipoprotein droplets called **high-density lipoprotein droplets (HDLs)** represent a special group of droplets that are high in cholesterol as well as apoproteins. A special role for HDLs is to remove cholesterol from tissues. In addition, HDLs can transfer excess apoprotein-e to LDLs, allowing them to be removed more rapidly from the blood and recycled by the liver, thereby reducing their opportunity to interact with other cells. It is presumed that a higher ratio of HDLs to LDLs represents a shorter turnover time for LDLs and thus less opportunity for them to transfer cholesterol to arterial cells.

D. Gluconeogenesis

The synthesis of glucose from non-carbohydrate sources is termed **gluconeogenesis**, and this term is used today to encompass the conversion of amino acids, lactate, glycerol, or lipids into glucose. Because glucose and its hydrolysis products are used for ATP synthesis by all cells, gluconeogenesis is essential when the diet consists largely of protein and/or TAGs. Amino acids may simply be transaminated (deaminated) to produce intermediates of glycolysis or the TCA cycle (Figure 12-22). For example, transamination of the amino acids alanine, serine, and glycine results in formation of pyruvate. Pyruvate also can be produced by conversion of lactate by mitochondria in liver or muscle cells in the presence of oxygen. It then can be a source for production of the TCA cycle intermediate oxaloacetate. Transamination of aspartate also yields oxaloacetate. These transaminations require α-ketoglutarate as a recipient for the amino group of the amino acid. Regeneration of α-ketoglutarate from glutamate can be accomplished by urea cycle enzymes or by direct deamination of the amino acids arginine, lysine, or histidine. Of the amino acids mentioned above, only lysine cannot be resynthesized in humans.

The rate-limiting enzyme for gluconeogenesis is **phosphoenolpyruvate carboxykinase (PEPCK)** that converts oxaloacetate to PEP that in turn can be used to synthesize glucose (see Figure 12-23). The ratio of PK to PEPCK can be used as an index to assess the gluconeogenic activity of a tissue under differing conditions.

TAGs contribute to energy metabolism and glucose synthesis in two ways. Hydrolysis of monoacylglycerol in the liver frees glycerol that can be used to resynthesize glucose. NEFAs released from hydrolysis of TAGs are metabolized through special pathways (see below) to cytoplasmic acetyl-CoA and other metabolites that can be used for energy. Acetyl-CoA also can be used to synthesize cholesterol and bile salts.

E. Fatty Acid Metabolism and Ketogenesis

NEFAs can be hydrolyzed through a pathway known as **β-oxidation** in liver cells (Figure 12-24). This process results in formation of cytoplasmic acetyl-CoA that can be transported into the mitochondria for ATP synthesis or to form glucose through gluconeogenesis. However, certain byproducts of β-oxidation known as **ketone bodies** are produced whenever NEFAs are broken down. These ketone bodies are not metabolized in the liver but are released into the blood. The most common ketone bodies are **acetone, acetoacetate**, and **β-hydroxybutyrate**. Under certain circumstances (e.g., during starvation), other tissues may utilize ketone bodies directly as energy sources (see below). If the body is using a great deal of lipid for energy production, excessive liver ketogenesis results that can alter blood pH significantly. Ketone bodies are weakly acidic and their excessive production (**ketogenesis**) and subsequent elevation in the blood (**ketonemia**) lead to a lowering of blood pH or **ketosis** (acidosis). Thus, ketosis can reduce the ability of hemoglobin to deliver oxygen to the brain, leading to coma and eventually to death. Increased appearance of ketone bodies in the urine is termed **ketonuria**.

IV. The Mammalian Pancreas

The mammalian pancreas is a mixed gland of exocrine and endocrine components that play essential roles in digestion and metabolism, respectively. The digestive role of the pancreas is accomplished by the exocrine

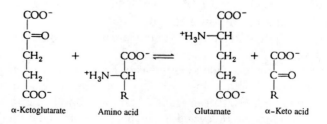

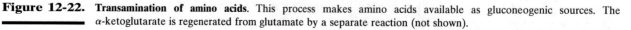

Figure 12-22. Transamination of amino acids. This process makes amino acids available as gluconeogenic sources. The α-ketoglutarate is regenerated from glutamate by a separate reaction (not shown).

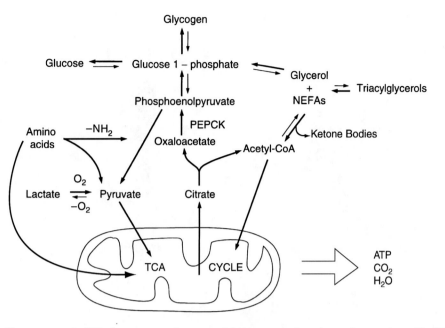

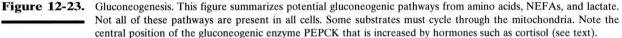

Figure 12-23. Gluconeogenesis. This figure summarizes potential gluconeogenic pathways from amino acids, NEFAs, and lactate. Not all of these pathways are present in all cells. Some substrates must cycle through the mitochondria. Note the central position of the gluconeogenic enzyme PEPCK that is increased by hormones such as cortisol (see text).

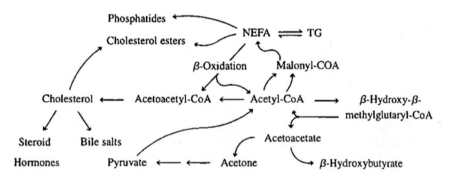

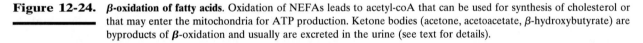

Figure 12-24. *β-oxidation of fatty acids.* Oxidation of NEFAs leads to acetyl-coA that can be used for synthesis of cholesterol or that may enter the mitochondria for ATP production. Ketone bodies (acetone, acetoacetate, β-hydroxybutyrate) are byproducts of β-oxidation and usually are excreted in the urine (see text for details).

portion that produces digestive enzymes and secretes an alkaline pancreatic fluid. The endocrine portion of the pancreas secretes hormones that regulate carbohydrate, lipid, and protein metabolism.

The exocrine or acinar pancreas secretes critical digestive enzymes into the pancreatic duct whereby they reach the lumen of the small intestine. (An acinus is similar in structure to an endocrine follicle except that the lumen of the acinus makes contact with a duct through which the secretory products of the epithelium [acinar cells] are transported.) This pancreatic juice also contains bicarbonate ions that buffer the acidic material entering the small intestine from the stomach. As described above, these pancreatic activities are regulated by the hormones secretin and CCK from the intestines.

The endocrine pancreas or the **islets of Langerhans** consists of small masses or islands of endocrine cells scattered among the acinar tissue (Figure 12-25). The pancreatic islets secrete at least four regulators: **insulin, glucagon**, SST, and an additional peptide known as **pancreatic polypeptide (PP)**. Insulin is primarily a hypoglycemic agent that lowers blood glucose, whereas glucagon is a hyperglycemic hormone. Glucagon and insulin may produce opposing effects on lipid metabolism as well, with glucagon promoting lipolysis. The major role of pancreatic SST may be as a paracrine agent released by neural stimulation that inhibits local release of the

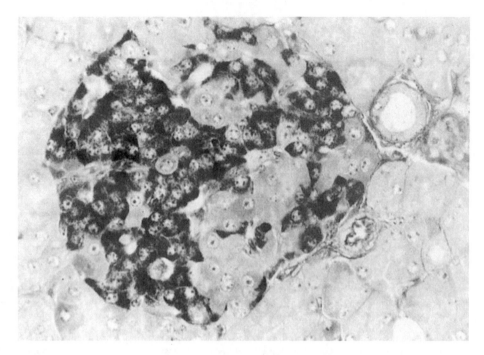

Figure 12-25. **Pancreatic islet of Langerhans.** This islet from guinea pig pancreas contains mostly darkly stained B cells and lightly stained A cells. D cells are rare in this islet and indistinguishable here from A cells. [From Matsumoto, A., and Ishii, S. (1992). "An Atlas of Endocrine Organs." Japanese Society for Comparative Endocrinology and Springer-Verlag, Berlin.]

other pancreatic peptides. The role for PP is not well established, but its increase in the circulation following ingestion of a meal suggests a role in postabsorptive metabolism.

The endocrine pancreas has been linked with blood glucose regulation since the first observations of the clinical syndrome **diabetes mellitus**. This disease was first described by the Greek physician Aretaeus in about 1500 B.C. as a condition where "flesh and bones run together" and are siphoned into the urine. The term "diabetes" comes from the Greek word "diabainein" (*dia* through + *bainein* to go). Indian physicians reported the sweet taste of the diabetic's urine in the 6th century, but it was not until the 18th century that the word "mellitus" referring to the presence of glucose in the urine was added to the name. Diabetes mellitus was always fatal and even today shortens the lives and decreases the quality of life for afflicted people. It is rapidly increasing in developed countries and as a consequence is a leading cause of death in the US. We now recognize two major forms of diabetes mellitus; one is related to insufficient production of insulin, and the second involves an unresponsiveness of target cells to insulin (i.e., insulin resistance; see ahead).

Diabetes mellitus generally is characterized by the production of large quantities of glucose-containing urine. Normally little or no glucose should appear in the urine, and its presence contributes osmotically to the larger urine volume produced by the untreated diabetic. It was the presence of glucose in the urine (**glucosuria**) of pancreatectomized dogs demonstrated by von Mering and Minkowski in 1889 that first linked diabetes mellitus to a possible disorder of the pancreas.

The occurrence of glucose in the urine results from excessively high circulating levels of glucose as a result of the failure by the endocrine pancreas to secrete adequate amounts of insulin and/or the inability of cells to react to insulin. There follows excessive lipolysis and gluconeogenesis of NEFAs. Consequently, blood levels of glucose become elevated resulting in more glucose in the glomerular filtrate produced in the kidney. The oxidation of NEFAs for gluconeogenesis increases production of ketone bodies by the liver yielding ketonemia. Under normal conditions, the proximal convoluted portion of each nephron transports all glucose that appears in the glomerular filtrate back into the blood. However, should blood sugar levels be sufficiently high, so much glucose enters the glomerular filtrate that the carrier-mediated transport mechanism in the nephron is saturated, and all of the glucose cannot be returned to the blood. The glucose remaining in the lumen of the nephron upsets the osmotic balance and less water can be reabsorbed from the filtrate, resulting in production of a greater volume of urine. Ketonuria also contributes to osmotic water losses. Because of the increased water loss associated with glucosuria and ketonuria, this syndrome achieved the descriptive title of "the pissing evil" during the Middle Ages. Several endocrine and metabolic alterations occur in an attempt to compensate for these nutrient losses.

Other consequences of the inadequacy of insulin production contribute to metabolic disturbances and additional water losses. Low insulin levels not only allow increased utilization of fats but also amino acids through gluconeogenesis to replace the lost glucose. Proteins are hydrolyzed to amino acids that are in turn transaminated or deaminated to produce carbohydrates plus ammonia. Most of the highly toxic ammonia is converted to less toxic urea in the liver and excreted through the urine. Elevated urea in the urine also contributes to increased urine production and additional water losses. The loss of glucose into the urine and increased production of nitrogenous wastes and ketone bodies all contribute to a process of desiccation or dehydration. Should the diabetic person enter a coma due to ketonemia-caused acidosis, he or she would be unable to compensate for water losses through drinking. Resultant dehydration may cause a marked decrease in blood volume and blood pressure that can lead to cardiac failure and death if proper treatment does not occur.

A. Development of the Mammalian Pancreas

The mammalian pancreas, like that of other vertebrates, develops from the endodermal lining of the primitive or embryonic gut. A dorsal bud from the embryonic intestine fuses with one or two ventral buds to form the definitive pancreas. Usually only the dorsal connection to the intestine is retained as the exocrine pancreatic duct. The exocrine tissue in the developing pancreas can be identified by the formation of small ductules. These ductules coalesce into larger ducts until they form a large pancreatic duct connecting the exocrine pancreas with the lumen of the small intestine. Small buds develop from the ductules and become the islets of Langerhans. In addition, some of the endocrine cells may be scattered singly or in groups of only a few cells throughout various regions of the pancreas. Immunoreactivity of the various peptides occurs in humans at about 8 to 10 weeks of development, marking the first synthesis of pancreatic hormones (Table 12-2).

Although the islets originate as outgrowths from the pancreatic ductules, the actual embryonic origin for the endocrine cells is not clear. It has been suggested that they arise from mesoderm or from neural crest cells of neuroectodermal origin or from endoderm of the gastrointestinal tract. However, experiments have shown that the islet cells are not derived from neural crest (see discussion of APUD cells in Chapter 4), at least in birds, and it is probable that mammalian islet cells are not derived from either neural crest or other neuroectoderm. Transplantation of quail neural crest cells containing a unique cytological marker into chick embryos confirms their incorporation into the avian pancreas, but they do not give rise to the pancreatic endocrine cells. Instead they differentiate into parasympathetic ganglia that, as we shall see, are important for regulating islet cell activity. Until the origin of its secretory cells is confirmed, the endocrine pancreas can be considered to be of endodermal origin.

Several functional schemes have been proposed for the origins of the endocrine pancreatic cells that are divorced from their possible germ-layer origins. These endocrine cells may represent modified gastrointestinal mucosal cells that initially synthesized "inducers." Exocrine cells in teleosts that are considered to be homologous to avian and mammalian islet cells often possess a concentration of protein granules (zymogen mantle), presumably induced by secretions of the adjacent pancreatic endocrine cells. Another suggestion is that these

Table 12-2. Appearance of Pancreatic Cell Types in Mammalian Fetuses[a]

Cell type	Human	Rat
A cells (glucagon)	8 weeks	12 days
B cells (insulin)	8 weeks	17 days
D cells (SS)	8 weeks	15 days
PP cells	10 weeks	—

[a] As determined by the presence of immunoreactive material (humans) and cell ultrastructure (rat).

cells originally secreted hydrolytic enzymes related to digestion but that these "enzymes" lost their catalytic properties and acquired hormonal functions. In the fetal guinea pig pancreas, immunoreactive glucagon, PP, insulin, and SST can be demonstrated in cells of the pancreatic tubules about 10 to 15 days before they appear in the islets, supporting the notion that they are derived from exocrine enzyme-secreting cells. These modified mucosal cells presumably lost their contact with the gut mucosa and specialized as centers for internal secretion. The similarity of peptides produced in the islet cells and those of the gastrointestinal tract described earlier supports a common origin for these pancreatic and intestinal cells.

B. Cellular Types in Pancreatic Islets

At least five different cellular types have been identified in the mammalian endocrine pancreas: B, A, D, PP, and amphophils. Although first identified by their staining characteristics, they now are identified by their immunoreactivity to antibodies prepared against the specific pancreatic peptides. Immunocytochemistry reveals that several peptides may be localized in one cell type, and the pattern of co-localization may differ markedly in different animals (Figure 12-26).

1. B-Cells

The first cellular type identified in the pancreatic islets was the **B-cell** (= β-cell in an alternative scheme for naming pancreatic cellular types) that stains with aldehyde fuchsin (AF+) and pseudoisocyanin (PIC+). The latter staining procedure applied following an oxidation step has been claimed to be specific for insulin granules, but it stains other intracellular structures in non-pancreatic tissues that do not contain insulin (for example, neurosecretory granules). Immunocytochemical techniques have verified that insulin is produced and stored in the B-cell as granules of about 300 nm in diameter.

Several drugs, such as **alloxan** and **streptozotocin**, selectively destroy the B-cells and impair the ability of the pancreas to secrete insulin. The affected B-cells undergo a process of **hydropic degeneration** that is characterized by clumping of nuclear chromosomal material (formation of pyknotic nuclei) and eventual cell death. This technique of chemically induced degeneration is often used in experimental animals to selectively remove the insulin-secreting cells without altering the ability of the islets to secrete other pancreatic peptides.

2. A-Cells

Cells of the pancreatic islets that are acidophilic and argyrophilic (affinity for silver-staining techniques) are called **A-cells** (= α- or α_2-cells). They do not stain with AF or PIC procedures. The A-cell is the source of the second major pancreatic hormone, glucagon, that is shown by immunocytochemistry to be stored in secretory granules of about 235-nm diameter. In some species, the secretory granules of A-cells may contain other peptides in addition to glucagon (see Table 12-3). The round secretory granules in the cytoplasm of the A-cells are morphologically distinct from the angular insulin granules of the B-cells, making these cells easy to distinguish with the aid of the transmission electron microscope. This difference in granule shape is not found in all mammals, however. Treatment with cobalt selectively impairs the ability of A-cells to secrete glucagon, but such treatment does not lead to destructive degeneration such as alloxan produces in the B-cells.

3. PP-Cells

Pancreatic polypeptide (PP) has been localized by immunocytochemical techniques in 125-nm granules of cells found at the periphery of the endocrine islets as well as in cells scattered throughout the exocrine pancreas. These **PP-cells** are distinct cytologically and immunologically from other cell types. The distribution of these PP-secreting cells (= F-cells) on the periphery of the islets varies greatly among different species, and it is difficult to generalize for all mammals.

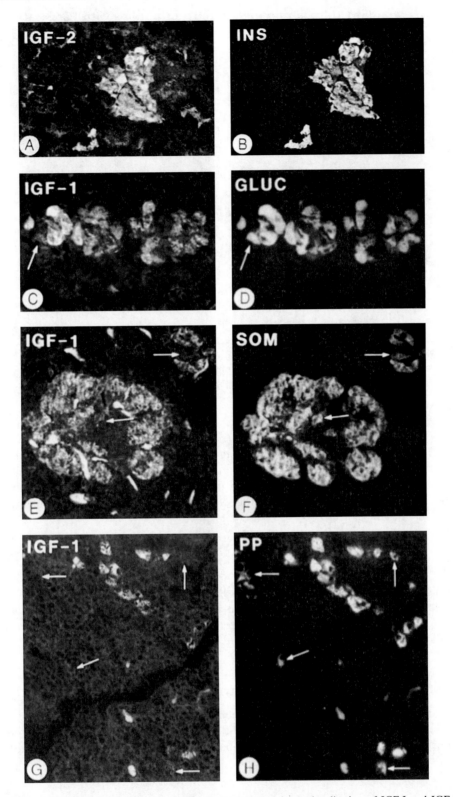

Figure 12-26. **Pancreatic cell types.** The four pancreatic cell types showing co-localization of IGF-I and IGF-2. Although these are from different vertebrates, the patterns are similar for mammals. (A–B) IGF-II and insulin in the B-cells of *Scincus officinalis* (bird). (C–D) IGF-I and glucagon in A-cells of *Psamorphis leniolatum* (snake). (E–F) IGF-I and somatostatin in the D-cells of *Coluber ravergieri* (snake). (G–H) IGF-I and pancreatic polypeptide in PP-cells of *Lacerta viridis* (lizard). [From Reinecke, M. *et al.* (1995). Immunohistochemical localization of insulin-like growth factor I and II in the endocrine pancreas of birds, reptiles, and Amphibia. *Gen. Comp. Endocr.* **100**, 385–396].

Table 12-3. Some Peptides Co-Localized in Selected Vertebrates with Pancreatic Hormones[a]

Cell type and hormone	IGF-I[b]	IGF-II	Gastrin	CRH[b]	GIP[b]	PP[b]	Endorphin	CCK[b]
A-cell (glucagon)	Frog			Catfish	Human	Frog	Rat	Rat
				Toad	Rat	Rat		Human
				Lizard	Pig	Human		
				Chicken	Dog			
				Cat	Cat			
				Mouse	Guinea pig			
				Monkey				
				Rat				
				Human				
B-cell (insulin)		Fish						
		Frog						
		Lizard						
		Snake						
		Bird						
		Mammal						
D-cell (somatostatin)	Lizard		Human	Human				
	Snake			Rat				
	Bird			Guinea pig				
PP cell	Frog							
(pancreatic	Lizard							
polypeptide)	Bird							

[a] Co-localization was determined by immunocytochemistry.
[b] IGF, insulin-like growth factor; CRH, corticotropin-releasing hormone; GIP, glucose-dependent insulinotropic peptide; PP, pancreatic polypeptide; CCK, cholecystokinin.

4. D-Cell

Immunoreactive SST is localized in the cytoplasmic granules of **D-cells** (also called α_1-cells or δ-cells). Although D-cells contain cytoplasmic granules similar in size to those of A-cells, they are cytochemically distinguished from A-cells by applying the toluidine blue staining procedure and from both A-cells and B-cells by their staining with PIC following methylation but not following oxidation. Granule size (230 nm) is very similar to that of A-cells.

5. Amphophils

Amphophilic cells have been demonstrated in the islets of many mammalian species as well as in sharks, teleosts, amphibians, and reptiles, but no conclusions have been generated regarding their functional roles. They may represent either ungranulated and/or differentiating or granule-depleted degenerating forms of any of the four cellular types described above.

C. Hormones of the Mammalian Endocrine Pancreas

The two major pancreatic hormones are the hypoglycemic, antilipolytic, lipogenic hormone called insulin, and the hyperglycemic, lipolytic hormone glucagon. In addition, the pancreatic endocrine cells produce somatostatin and PP, but their roles in the bioregulation of metabolism are not as dramatic as are those for insulin and glucagon.

1. Insulin: The Hypoglycemic Hormone

Von Mering and Minkowski in 1889 first observed the correlation between the pancreas and blood sugar regulation when they induced diabetes mellitus in dogs following pancreatectomy. The suspected hypoglycemic factor of the pancreas was later named "insuline" (from L., *insula*, island) to emphasize its origin from the islets of Langerhans previously identified from histological observations. Purified insulin, however, was not isolated until a physician, Frederick Banting, and a graduate student in physiology and biochemistry, Charles Best, teamed up at the University of Toronto in the summer of 1921. Much of their success was due to the collaborative efforts of the biochemist J. B. Collip, who purified insulin, and the project's director, J. J. R. Macleod.

The presence of proteolytic enzymes in the exocrine pancreas had thwarted earlier attempts to extract insulin from a whole pancreas. Since it had been shown that tying off the pancreatic duct caused degeneration of the acinar pancreatic tissue but did not affect the islet tissue, Banting suggested they employ this technique to avoid contamination of their extracts with digestive enzymes. The hypoglycemic factor they isolated was first named isletin, but they later changed its name to conform to the name proposed earlier by von Mering and Minkowski. The importance of the successful isolation of insulin and its use to alleviate the fatal symptoms of diabetes mellitus led to the awarding of the Nobel Prize in Physiology and Medicine for 1923 to Banting and Macleod. Best and Collip were not officially recognized in the award, although the recipients acknowledged them for their contributions. This pioneering research with experimental animals also is recognized for having saved millions of human lives.

a. Measurement of Insulin and Insulin-Secreting Capacity

Insulin may be bioassayed *in vitro* for its ability to stimulate uptake of glucose from the medium into cells. Muscle cells from the rat diaphragm are often employed in this bioassay.

Radioimmunoassay (RIA), however, is routinely employed to measure circulating insulin levels, and many commercial RIA kits are available for performing these analyses. Insulin RIAs are highly specific, and some can detect the difference between porcine and human insulins that vary in only one amino acid substitution.

The standard measure of the ability of the pancreas to secrete insulin is the **glucose tolerance test**. Following a period of fasting, a glucose load (excessive amount of glucose) is administered orally or intravenously, and its rate of disappearance (clearance) from the blood is measured. The clearance rate for a given glucose load is directly proportional to the secretion of insulin and hence reflects the ability of the pancreas to respond to hyperglycemia with elevated insulin secretion (Table 12-4). Another common indicator of normal insulin secretion is to measure plasma glucose following a 12-hour fast.

b. Chemistry and Synthesis of Mammalian Insulins

Insulin is a very conservative and phylogenetically old molecule, occurring throughout the animal kingdom (Table 12-5) and even among unicellular organisms. The insulin molecule is a small protein composed of two different polypeptide chains linked together by disulfide bridges. It is structurally very similar to the insulin-like growth factors (IGFs) and relaxin described earlier although each has its own receptor type (see Chapter 3). The insulin prohormone is a single-polypeptide chain that can be designated into three regions, A, B, and C. The C-peptide is cleaved post-translationally. Secretion granules of B-cells contain crystals of insulin and C-peptide fragments as well as some uncleaved proinsulin. The insulin fragment forms a complex with available zinc ions to produce a crystalline hexamer within the secretory granule. It is this crystalline structure that imparts the unique, angular structure to insulin secretion granules in the B-cell.

Table 12-4. Comparison of Human Responses to a Standard Glucose Tolerance Test[a]

Subject status	Venous glucose level (mg/dl)			
	Fasting	30 min	60 min	120 min
Normal person	<100	<160	<160	<100
Probable diabetic	<100 or 100–120	130–159	160–180	110–120
Diabetic	<100 or >100	>150	>160	>120

[a] An abnormal glucose tolerance test can also occur as a result of factors other than diabetes mellitus, including improper feeding prior to test, malnutrition, obesity, infection, fever, hyperthyroidism or hypothyroidism, acromegaly, kidney disease, and islet cell tumors.

Table 12-5. Occurrence of Some Pancreatic Peptides in Invertebrate Animals

Group	Insulin	Glucagon	PP	SS
Mollusk hepatopancreas	+	+		
Starfish	+			
Tunicate (urochordate)	+		+	+
Amphioxus (cephalochordate)	+	+		

c. Regulation of Insulin Release

Hyperglycemia can stimulate release of insulin through a direct action of glucose on the B-cell. It is apparently not the presence of glucose but events associated with its uptake and metabolism by the B-cell that stimulate insulin secretion. Decreases in circulating glucose cause a reduction in the secretion of insulin, and it appears that the basic regulatory control mechanism is directed through changes in blood levels of glucose. Any agent capable of elevating circulating glucose levels also will evoke insulin release. Amino acids, especially arginine, also can stimulate insulin release although the mechanism is not well-understood.

The discovery that GIP released from cells of the small intestine after ingestion of a meal was a potent releaser of insulin was the basis for the alternative name for this peptide: glucose-dependent insulinotropic polypeptide. Elevated glucose appears in human hepatic portal blood in 2 minutes after ingesting 75 g of glucose, and elevated GIP and insulin follow within 5 minutes. Insulin, GIP, and glucose all reach maximal levels within 30 minutes and then decline to normal within 3 hr. Following ingestion of a "standard" mixed meal, maximal levels of circulating GIP are achieved within 45 minutes and remain elevated for 6 hr. A similar elevation of circulating glucose induced through direct intravenous injection of glucose evokes a smaller insulin response than did the meal. Although GIP release has been demonstrated following ingestion of long-chain but not short-chain fatty acids, the augmentation of insulin release by GIP apparently requires a simultaneous increase in glucose levels. Release of insulin by GIP only occurs when accompanied by hyperglycemia. This seems to relegate the insulinotropic role of GIP to that of a permissive effect, but a physiologically important action nevertheless.

In recent years, the importance of inhibitory nervous regulation of insulin secretion has been demonstrated. Non-myelinated autonomic axonal fibers are present in the islets. Similarly, acetylcholine or activation of parasympathetic nerves stimulates insulin release, whereas the anti-cholinergic drug atropine blocks insulin release. Norepinephrine from sympathetic neurons blocks insulin release. Epinephrine, which is a hyper-glycemic agent affecting liver, muscle, and adipose tissue, also directly blocks the release of insulin. Thus, circulating epinephrine can potentiate its own hyperglycemic action by blocking the normal response of the B-cell to increased blood glucose resulting from epinephrine's action on adipose and liver cells.

SST inhibits release of insulin by a direct action on the B-cell, and it may play a paracrine role in regulating insulin release locally in the pancreas. It is not known what regulates SST release from the pancreatic D-cells, but studies show that both acetylcholine (parasympathetic) and α-adrenergic (sympathetic) agents can block SST release whereas VIP and β-adrenergic agents stimulate its release.

The neuropeptide galanin has been identified in pancreatic islet neurons of dogs and humans, sometimes co-localized with other peptides such as NPY. Release of insulin from the B-cell by glucose or amino acids is blocked directly by galanin. Various stimulators of insulin release operate via different cellular mechanisms (e.g., blocking K^+ channels, activating IP_3/DAG-mediated Ca^{2+} influx, inhibition of adenylyl cyclase), all of which can be blocked by galanin. The physiological importance of this inhibitory mechanism and its relation to inhibition of insulin release by SST are not clear.

A peptide of 49 amino acids was isolated first from the porcine pancreas and named **pancreostatin (Pst)** for its ability to block glucose-induced release of insulin. Pst may be a product of a large acidic protein, **chromogranin A**, a member of a family of similar proteins that also is associated with the secretory granules of catecholamine-secreting cells of the adrenal medulla (see Chapter 8), some gastrointestinal endocrine cells, and both catecholaminergic and peptidergic neurons. Although its physiological role is uncertain, a phylogenetic survey reveals Pst-immunoreactivity in the gastric mucosa and pancreatic islets of all vertebrates examined including pig, human, chicken, Japanese quail, lizard, frog, shark, ratfish, and hagfish. No Pst-immunoreactivity was observed in either the rat or in cephalochordates or urochordates.

d. Actions of Insulin on Target Tissues

After insulin binds to its membrane receptor, there is an increase in the transport of glucose, amino acids, fatty acids, nucleotides, and various ions into the target cell. Within a few minutes, enhancement of anabolic pathways and a decrease in catabolic pathways occur. Through delayed effects on nuclear transcription and protein synthesis, some cellular growth is stimulated. This growth-promoting action is due to an interaction between insulin and growth hormone (GH)-dependent, circulating IGFs that operate through separate receptors but through similar intracellular pathways.

Insulin appears to bring about hypoglycemia through stimulating increased uptake of glucose through activation of GLUT 4 protein that is responsible for facilitated diffusion of glucose from the blood. Insulin facilitates transport of glucose into muscle and fat cells as well as transport of amino acids into muscle cells. Activity of hexokinase also is enhanced by insulin, which stimulates glucose oxidation and favors lipogenesis (adipose tissue) and protein synthesis (muscle). Insulin also prevents glycogen breakdown (glycogenolysis) and enhances glycogen synthesis following uptake of glucose in muscle and liver. This is accomplished through simultaneous inhibition of the cAMP-dependent enzyme phosphorylase-a and stimulation of the enzyme glycogen synthetase (Figure 12-19).

Glucose oxidation increases the intracellular pools of precursors for fat synthesis, that is, glycerol, acetyl-CoA, and fatty acids. In addition to indirectly enhancing esterification by stimulating acylglycerol synthetases, insulin inhibits triacylglycerol lipase and prevents lipolysis in adipose tissue. This reduces release of NEFAs and monoacylglycerol into the blood and hence reduces hepatic fatty acid oxidation and ketogenesis. These actions of insulin on adipose tissue and lipid metabolism are marked in carnivores, but there is little effect of insulin on either glucose metabolism or lipogenesis in herbivorous mammals. Consequently, carnivorous mammals are more sensitive to pancreatectomy than are herbivores.

The increase in intracellular glucose-6-phosphate and amino acids in both liver and muscle cells promotes protein, lipid, and glycogen synthesis. These are important actions of insulin immediately following ingestion of a meal and the entry of large quantities of digestive products such as glucose and amino acids into the blood.

e. Mechanism of Action for Insulin

The many actions of insulin on its target cells have prompted many different schemes to explain these diverse actions. At last, a unified picture is beginning to emerge that eventually may explain all of insulin's actions. Insulin binds to a tyrosine kinase transmembrane receptor that occurs as a dimer in the cell membrane (see Chapter 3). The occupied receptor undergoes autophosphorylation and then acts as a tyrosine kinase to phosphorylate various substrates including **insulin response (IRS) proteins**. One of these substrates is involved in a chain of phosphokinase events called the kinase cascade (see Chapter 3). This mechanism activates glycogen synthetase (causing storage of glucose as glycogen) and alters levels of certain transcription factors responsible for the delayed actions of insulin on protein synthesis.

f. "Oral Insulins"

The term "oral insulin" refers to the synthetic hypoglycemic drugs known as sulfonylureas and related compounds (Figure 12-27). Because they are not proteins and thereby not subject to enzymatic degradation in the gut, the sulfonylureas may be taken orally and can relieve some of the symptoms of diabetes mellitus. Oral insulins thus have considerable therapeutic value in certain types of insulin-deficiency disorders. The effectiveness of these drugs may be related to their abilities in displacing insulin from nonspecific binding sites and non-effective linkages in plasma, connective tissues, and islet cells to provide marginally effective quantities of insulin for binding to effective (target) sites. If too high a dose is employed, the oral insulin also may block the effective sites as well, and no hypoglycemic effect is observed. The oral insulins are useful only in disorders related to insulin insufficiency and would not be useful in totally pancreatectomized animals or in humans who can not produce insulin. Furthermore, oral insulins are effective only if diet is carefully controlled.

2. Glucagon: The Hyperglycemic Hormone

The discovery of glucagon was not marked by great publicity or special prizes, as was that of insulin, and this second pancreatic hormone has always been overshadowed by the clinical importance of insulin. Glucagon is only one of several hyperglycemic factors, and more attention has been given to growth hormone (GH) and

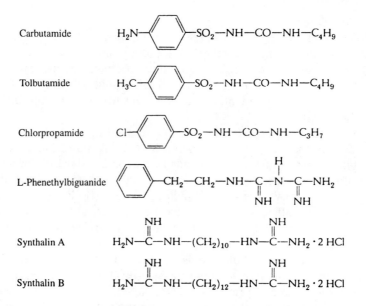

Carbutamide H_2N—〈 〉—SO_2—NH—CO—NH—C_4H_9

Tolbutamide H_3C—〈 〉—SO_2—NH—CO—NH—C_4H_9

Chlorpropamide Cl—〈 〉—SO_2—NH—CO—NH—C_3H_7

L-Phenethylbiguanide 〈 〉—CH_2—CH_2—NH—C—N—C—NH_2

Synthalin A H_2N—C—NH—$(CH_2)_{10}$—HN—C—$NH_2 \cdot 2\ HCl$

Synthalin B H_2N—C—NH—$(CH_2)_{12}$—HN—C—$NH_2 \cdot 2\ HCl$

Figure 12-27. **Oral insulins.** These synthetic molecules cannot substitute for insulin but enhance the activity of insulin already present. These drugs are useful only in the treatment of type 2 diabetes.

epinephrine as hyperglycemic hormones. Glucagon is more important in fasting carnivores and in herbivores than it appears to be in fed humans or carnivores. It also is more important than insulin in birds and lizards for regulating metabolism.

a. Chemistry of Glucagon

Glucagon is a straight-chain polypeptide hormone consisting of 29 amino acid residues and with a molecular weight of 3485 daltons. It is a member of the PACAP family of peptides (see Chapter 4). Thus, glucagon is chemically similar to secretin and CCK. In addition to the peptide glucagon, proglucagon also contains the two glucagon-like peptides GLP-1 and GLP-2 discussed above. Glucagon is a conservative peptide among mammals and has been identified immunocytochemically in all vertebrates as well as in a number of invertebrates. Non-mammalian glucagons are structurally conservative, too.

Another extrapancreatic glucagon-like hyperglycemic factor has been characterized in extracts of submaxillary salivary glands obtained from rats, mice, rabbits, and humans. Release of this salivary glucagon is influenced *in vitro* in the same manner as pancreatic glucagon. SST, however, does not block release of salivary glucagon.

b. Actions of Glucagon on Target Tissues

Glucagon promotes glycogenolysis in liver cells, its primary target with respect to raising circulating glucose levels. This effect appears to be mediated through stimulation of adenylyl cyclase and production of intracellular cAMP and activation of phosphorylase-a. Increased glycogenolysis accompanied by decreased intracellular oxidation of glucose directs the movement of glucose from liver cells into the blood. Lipolysis is stimulated by glucagon in fasting animals through activation of hormone-dependent lipase (triacylglycerol lipase) in adipose tissues. The release of NEFAs into the blood further increases β-oxidation followed by ketogenesis and gluconeogenesis in liver. Glucagon also increases levels of PEPCK, the critical enzyme in gluconeogenesis, in liver cells.

3. Pancreatic Polypeptide: A Third Pancreatic Hormone

Pancreatic polypeptide (PP) was discovered in the chicken pancreas and since has been purified from the usual mammalian sources (ovine, bovine, canine, porcine, rat, and human pancreatic tissue) as well as from wild equines (Przewalski's horse, zebra), rhino, tapir, several birds, and the alligator. The average molecular weight for PP is 4200, and all peptides isolated consist of 36 amino acid residues (see Chapter 13, Figure 13-7). Structurally, PP is similar to NPY and peptide YY (PYY). The physiological role of PP is unknown, although there are several reasons for giving PP hormonal status. In humans, ingestion of a protein meal such as ground beef causes an increase in plasma levels of PP from pre-ingestion levels of 57 pg/ml, plasma to 229 pg/ml, 400 pg/ml, and 580 pg/ml, respectively, in 5, 10, and 240 minutes. Infusion or ingestion of glucose does not evoke this sort of increase in hPP, and it appears that the rapid increase in plasma hPP following ingestion of protein is at least in part a neural response mediated via the vagus nerve. This release of hPP can be blocked by SST, although it is not known whether SST is involved in the normal regulation of PP release. A second phase of elevated PP occurs later and may last for several hours. The initial phase of PP secretion can be induced with experimental gastric distention, but the later response occurs only following protein- or fat-rich meals. Bovine PP is reported to be a potent inhibitor of pancreatic exocrine secretion, but it does not seem to influence carbohydrate (glucose) metabolism. Resting levels of plasma PP in humans increase with age from about 50 pg/ml in 25-year-olds to more than 200 pg/ml at age 70. This increase is paralleled by a progressive increase in the number of PP-cells in the islets.

4. Somatostatin: Paracrine Regulator of Pancreatic Secretion

The D-cell is believed to be the source of pancreatic SST that is chemically identical with hypothalamic SST. In mammals, both SST_{14} and SST_{28} have been identified in the pancreas. Levels of SST in pancreatic extracts of rats are equivalent to those of hypothalamic extracts. Pancreatic SST is believed to locally inhibit the release of insulin, glucagon, and PP in a paracrine fashion.

Regulation of pancreatic SST release is not understood. The observed inhibitory actions of acetylcholine and norepinephrine mentioned earlier possibly mimic parasympathetic and sympathetic innervation, respectively.

V. Hormones Regulating Mammalian Metabolism

Metabolism is affected by many hormones that directly or indirectly affect key enzymes in glycolysis, gluconeogenesis, glycogen synthesis or degradation, lipogenesis, lipolysis, and in the synthesis and utilization of proteins (Table 12-6). These hormones include insulin and glucagon from the endocrine pancreas as well as epinephrine from the adrenal medulla (Chapter 8), glucocorticoids from the adrenal cortex (Chapter 8), GH from the adenohypophysis and the IGFs from liver (Chapter 4), thyroid hormones (Chapter 6), and gonadal steroids (Chapter 10). A hormone may be classified according to its general actions as being **glycolytic** (favoring glycolysis), **glycogenolytic** (favoring glycogen hydrolysis to glucose-phosphate), **gluconeogenic** (favoring conversion of lipids and/or proteins or their intermediates into glucose production), **lipogenic** (favoring synthesis of TAGs or steroids), **lipolytic** (favoring hydrolysis of TAGs to NEFAs and MAGs), protein anabolic (favoring protein synthesis), or **protein catabolic** (favoring breakdown of proteins to amino acids). A hormone may affect directly or indirectly many metabolic processes, and several of the above descriptors may be applied to the same hormone (see glucocorticoid effects, Table 12-7). These metabolic actions may be due to effects

Table 12-6. Generalized Actions of Hormones with Respect to Protein, Carbohydrate, and Lipid Metabolism

Hormone	Protein metabolism	Carbohydrate metabolism	Lipid metabolism
Insulin	Anabolic	Hypoglycemic, glycogenic, antiglycogenolytic	Lipogenic, antilipolytic
Epinephrine		Glycogenolytic, hyperglycemic, gluconeogenic	Lipolytic
Glucagon		Hyperglycemic, glycogenolytic	
Growth hormone	Anabolic	Hyperglycemic, gluconeogenic	Lipolytic
Glucocorticoids	Antianabolic	Hyperglycemic, gluconeogenic, inhibits peripheral utilization	
Thyroxine	Anabolic or catabolic	Hyperglycemic, glycogenolytic	Lipolytic
Androgens	Anabolic		

Table 12-7. Metabolic Actions of Glucocorticoids in Different Mammalian Tissues[a]

Process	Liver	Adipose	Heart, diaphragm	Skeletal muscle
Glucose uptake		−	−	
Glycogenesis	+		+	−
Amino acid uptake	+		+	−
Gluconeogensis	+		+	
Protein synthesis			−	
Protein catabolism				+
Lipogenesis	+			
Lipolysis		+P		

[a] Note that the responses of each tissue to the same hormone are specific to the tissue. +, stimulatory; −, inhibitory; P, permissive effect.

on enzyme activity or effects on transport at the cell membrane and hence affect the availability of substrates for various pathways. Although a detailed analysis of this topic is beyond our scope, we will briefly describe some hormonal interactions in the following sections that occur under some common conditions in mammals.

A. Endocrine Regulation of Metabolism Following Feeding

In carnivores and omnivores, the most important hormones following ingestion of a meal and following its absorption into blood are insulin and GH as well as GIP. This time period is termed **postprandial** and is characterized by elevated blood levels of glucose, amino acids, and lipids in proportion to the composition of the meal. Release of insulin is evoked directly by an increase in circulating glucose in the blood supplying the pancreatic islets. In addition, there is evidence of early enhancement of the glucose-stimulated release of insulin caused by release of GIP from the small intestine in response to the presence of glucose in the small intestine (feed forward). It is not clear what the role of circulating PP is in humans and dogs after a meal. No convincing evidence for a direct metabolic action of PP has been demonstrated, and this peptide may be limited to regulating digestive functions. Direct neural stimulation of insulin release also may occur following or during ingestion, but this does not appear to be a major regulatory pathway.

Insulin stimulates the uptake of glucose by muscle cells, liver cells, and adipocytes. In the liver, insulin promotes glycogenesis and formation of VLDLs from glucose whereas in muscle cells it favors glycogenesis and glycolysis. These effects are mediated largely through reduction in the enzyme phosphorylase-a (which normally would cause hydrolysis of glycogen) and an increase in the enzyme glycogen synthetase. In the liver, there also is a reduction in glucose-6-phosphatase and glucokinase that also favors glycogenesis. In adipose cells, synthesis and storage of triacylglycerols as well as inhibition of lipolytic pathways are favored by the intracellular actions of insulin. Increased lipoprotein lipase activity also is favored in adipose tissue by insulin which enhances incorporation of NEFAs and MAG from VLDLs and LDLs. In addition, insulin enhances transport of amino acids into muscle cells, thereby enhancing protein synthesis. In liver cells, insulin favors protein synthesis and reduces both deamination (transanimation) of amino acids and gluconeogenesis.

Release of GH may occur much later after a meal and together with insulin causes stimulation of protein synthesis in muscle cells. During sleep, insulin levels typically are low and GH release is maximal. GH stimulates additional protein synthesis as well as glycogenolysis and lipolysis.

B. Effects of Acute and Chronic Stress on Metabolism

The details of the stress response are described in Chapter 8. Acute stress, such as the "flight-or-fight" response and exercise, causes release of epinephrine from the adrenal medulla. Epinephrine brings about important changes in energy metabolism resulting in increased glycogenolysis and hyperglycemia. Glucagon levels also may increase, contributing to hyperglycemia. Chronic stress involves the gluconeogenic and hence hyperglycemic actions of the glucocorticoids (see Table 12-7). In cases of fasting or starvation, GH and glucagon as well as glucocorticoids play important metabolic roles.

1. Acute Stress and Metabolism

An early response to stress is the elevation in epinephrine release from the adrenal medulla. Epinephrine activates adenylyl cyclase in muscle cells, resulting in increased glycogenolysis even in the face of elevated insulin. Because glucose-6-phosphate resulting from glycogenolysis cannot be converted into free glucose and leave the muscle cell, it is used directly in glycolysis. This reduces the need for muscle cells to remove glucose from the blood and spares blood glucose for use by the nervous system during stressful times. Another cAMP pathway is stimulated by epinephrine in adipose cells and enhances the activity of triacylglycerol lipase. This in turn increases the availability of NEFAs and glycerol for gluconeogenesis and a trend toward ketogenesis during stress. However, the lipolytic actions of epinephrine result primarily from sympathetic innervation of adipose tissue and circulating epinephrine from the adrenal medulla does not play a major role.

2. Chronic Stress and Metabolism

If stressful conditions persist beyond the acute phase, the HPA axis is stimulated such that additional glucocorticoid is released. The most important role for glucocorticoids is to prevent utilization of amino acids for protein synthesis and favor conversion of amino acids to carbohydrate via gluconeogenesis. In the liver, gluconeogenesis from amino acids provides glucose that can be added to the circulation, producing a subsequent hyperglycemia. This action also protects circulating glucose as an energy source for the nervous system by forcing muscle cells to employ amino acids for energy production and prevent use of circulating glucose by these cells.

During starvation, GH and glucagon have important roles in metabolism. Although glucagon normally stimulates glycogenolysis in the liver, the absence of significant glycogen stores means that glucagon can have little direct effect on circulating glucose levels. However, GH and glucagon both stimulate lipolysis in adipose tissue and increase the levels of NEFAs for energy production as well as ketogenesis. Meanwhile, glucocorticoids continue to encourage muscle cells to catabolize protein stores and to use the resulting amino acids as a major gluconeogenic source. Protein catabolism in muscle cells also provides amino acids for liver gluconeogenesis and thereby can contribute indirectly to blood glucose. Gluconeogenesis from amino acids produces toxic nitrogenous wastes (ammonia, urea, uric acid) that must be eliminated by the kidney with attendant loss of water. In turn, muscle cells will utilize some of the circulating ketone bodies produced during the metabolism of NEFAs as an energy source. The rest of the ketone bodies are excreted in the urine along with the nitrogenous wastes from protein catabolism. As described earlier, addition of ketone bodies to the urine contributes to water loss and dehydration.

Chronic starvation can result in severe protein deficiencies as a consequence of the emphasis on gluconeogenesis from proteins to meet the glucose demands of the nervous system. Accompanying ketogenesis from use of NEFAs can produce disturbances in acid-base balance as well. Calculations based on analyses of energy metabolism associated with acute starvation indicate that most humans could only survive about 21 days of total starvation before they would die of protein deficiencies. However, as early as 3 days after the onset of total starvation, the brain undergoes a remarkable decrease in its metabolic requirement for glucose and begins to utilize ketone bodies produced from lipid metabolism to provide the bulk of its energy needs. This change not only enhances lipolysis as a source of ketone bodies for brain metabolism and for gluconeogenesis in the liver but also spares the need for amino acids as an energy source and reduces the rate at which proteins are catabolized. Consequently, the anticipated protein deficiencies do not occur until much later. However, once the body's lipid stores are exhausted, protein remains as the only source to sustain life.

What causes this shift in brain metabolism during total starvation is unknown at this time, but we do know it only occurs under conditions of total starvation. If there is any caloric intake, the switch to ketone utilization is prevented. Consequently, people experiencing semi-starvation (where caloric intake is less than required to balance energy expenditures) commonly suffer from protein deficiencies because they employ protein stores to make up the energy deficit in preference to lipid stores. Humans who undertake self-regulated semi-starvation (commonly called "dieting") run the risk of developing protein deficiencies and reducing body weight more in terms of lean muscle mass than of fat. The losses of water involved with additional excretion of nitrogenous wastes accounts for most of the initial weight losses associated with "dieting" unless balanced carefully by increased water intake. Furthermore, it appears that protein stores can only be protected by simultaneously stimulating protein synthesis. Periodic bouts of strenuous exercise result in enhanced protein synthesis during non-exercise periods that is directed in part by episodes of GH release.

C. Protein Anabolic Hormones

Alterations in nitrogen retention and excretion reflect episodes of protein synthesis and protein catabolism for gluconeogenesis, respectively. Many hormones have been shown to enhance nitrogen retention through actions on protein synthesis. These **protein anabolic** agents include GH, androgens, estrogens, thyroid hormones, and insulin. We have already considered the actions of GH and insulin above. Since thyroid hormones are protein anabolic in thyroidectomized animals but not in hypophysectomized animals (lacking GH as well as the other tropic hormones), it is safe to conclude that the thyroid effect on protein synthesis is brought about by its interactions with GH (see Chapters 4 and 6).

The earliest suggestion of a protein anabolic role for androgens was the claim for their rejuvenating power by Brown-Sequard in 1889 that he reportedly discovered after treating himself with extracts prepared from animal testes. In the 1930s, Charles D. Kochakian and his coworkers began 40 years of research that clearly established the unique role of androgens as **protein anabolic steroids**. Although estrogens were shown to stimulate protein synthesis in a few tissues (e.g., uterus, mammary gland, skin, skeleton), only the **androgenic-anabolic steroids** had such a profound effect on skeletal muscles that they determined an overall nitrogen retention by the body. Progesterone is protein anabolic on uterus but overall causes increased nitrogen excretion.

The greater muscle masses of male mammals as compared to female mammals long has been recognized and is attributed to the actions of androgens. In non-mammalian vertebrates, androgens have been shown to have sex-specific effects on certain muscles in males. Many analogues of the naturally occurring androgens have been prepared, but it has not been possible to separate their androgenic action from their protein anabolic effect. Androgenic-anabolic steroids do not influence transport of amino acids into muscles cells but apparently affect the levels of amino acid-activating enzymes employed in protein synthesis.

The potential effect of anabolic-androgenic steroids on muscle strength and endurance resulted inevitably in their use by humans for athletic training programs. Although their effect on muscle mass is easily demonstrated, the improvement of athletic performance is mostly anecdotal and is not well-supported by controlled studies. Regardless, the established effects of anabolic-androgenic steroids on reduced reproductive performance (through negative feedback on the HPG axis), increased liver dysfunction (80% of subjects in one study), and correlations with hepatitis, liver failure, and fatal liver cancer should serve to warn people to avoid their use for unsubstantiated, short-term benefits on athletic performance.

VI. Clinical Aspects of Pancreatic Function

A. Diabetes Mellitus

Diabetes mellitus is a complex, heterogeneous assemblage of disorders having the common feature of the appearance of glucose in the urine. Diabetes mellitus is always fatal if not treated, and even if treated, serious complications may develop including blindness, kidney disease, and circulatory or circulation-based problems.

Obesity is one of the major risk factors for development of diabetes mellitus. People with a body mass index [BMI = weight(lb.)/height(inches^2) × 703] greater than 25 are considered to be overweight. Obesity is defined as having a BMI > 30. The average female in the USA is 5′4″ tall and should weigh less than 134 lbs to achieve BMI < 25. For the average 5′9″ US male, an appropriate weight would be 125-168 lbs. Approximately 62% of US females and 68% of US males are overweight. This translates into 127 million adults in the USA are overweight and 60 million are obese. In addition, another 9 million can be categorized as extremely obese (BMI > 40). The US Centers for Disease Control and Prevention estimates that 47 million Americans exhibit a metabolic syndrome or "Syndrome X" that is characterized by insulin resistance, obesity, hypertension, and elevated indicators of cardiovascular disease (high blood levels of triglycerides and cholestrol).

In the early 1990s, obesity levels exceeded 15% in populations of only 4 states. By 2003, only 15 states exhibited rates as low as 15–19% obesity whereas 31 states had obesity rates of 20–24%, and the populations of 4 states exceeded 25% percent obesity (Figure 12-28). Of increasing concern is the rapid increase in obesity among children and adolescents. The effects of obesity are especially reflected in the incidence of

Obesity Trends* Among U.S. Adults
BRFSS, 1991, 1996, 2003
(*BMI ≥30, or about 30 lbs overweight for 5'4" person)

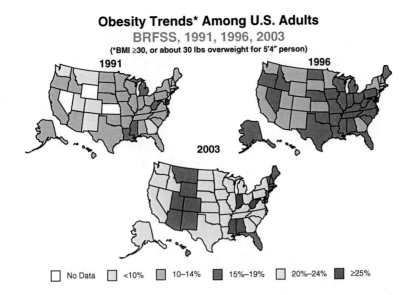

1991   1996

2003

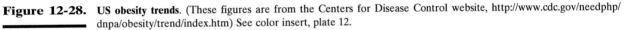

☐ No Data   ☐ <10%   ☐ 10–14%   ■ 15%–19%   ☐ 20%–24%   ■ ≥25%

Figure 12-28. **US obesity trends.** (These figures are from the Centers for Disease Control website, http://www.cdc.gov/needphp/dnpa/obesity/trend/index.htm) See color insert, plate 12.

diabetes mellitus. Current figures indicate that approximately 6% of the US population exhibits diabetes mellitus with another 14% exhibiting pre-diabetes (dangerously elevated blood glucose levels). Moreover, cardio-renal-vascular complications resulting from diabetes mellitus are responsible for an additional 300,000 deaths annually, making diabetes a leading contributor to death in the United States.

Most cases of diabetes mellitus have been characterized as either **maturity onset diabetes** (ketosis-resistant; insulin-independent) or as **juvenile onset diabetes** (ketosis-prone; insulin-dependent). "Maturity" and "juvenile" are not entirely appropriate terms since the former can occur occasionally in children and adolescents, whereas the latter can occur with low frequency in middle-aged or older adults. Consequently, these disorders were renamed first as **Type-1 diabetes** and **Type-2 diabetes** and sometimes are called **insulin-dependent diabetes mellitus (IDDM)** and **noninsulin-dependent diabetes mellitus (NIDDM)**, respectively. Several features of these two types of diabetes are compared in Table 12-8. There are some additional forms of diabetes now recognized, but they are rare.

Type 2 diabetes, accounting for approximately 90–95% of the reported cases, typically occurs in overweight people (80% of cases) who are over 40 years of age. Much of the increase in diabetes observed in the US in recent years is due to an increasing proportion of elderly people in the population coupled with an increasing tendency toward obesity. Type 2 diabetes has a slow onset with no obvious symptoms. Insulin levels

Table 12-8. Comparison of Symptoms for Two Forms of Diabetes Mellitus

Features	Type1 (IDDM)	Type2 (NIDDM)
Age at onset	Usually during childhood or puberty	Frequently over 45 years
Type of onset	Abrupt onset of overt symptoms	Usually gradual
Genetic basis	Frequently positive relationship	Commonly positive relationship
Nutritional status	Usually undernourished	Usually obesity present to some degree (about 80% of cases)
Symptoms	1. Polydipsia, polyphagia, polyuria 2. Ketosis frequently present 3. Hepatomegaly rather common 4. Blood glucose fluctuates widely in response to small changes in insulin dose, exercise, and infection	1. May be none 2. Ketosis uncommon except under stress 3. Hepatomegaly uncommon 4. Blood sugar fluctuations less marked than for juvenile onset
Fasting blood sugar levels	Elevated	Often normal
Requirement for insulin	Necessary for all patients	Necessary for 20–30% of patients
Effectiveness of oral agents	Rarely effective	Effective when diet is controlled

in type 2 diabetes are usually normal or in excess of normal. Apparently, the target cells become insensitive to insulin, possibly due to a decrease in receptor populations or to a deficiency in the mechanism of action of insulin after it is bound to the cell. Another possible cause might be an increase in non-specific binding of insulin to non-target cells that reduces insulin availability for specific receptors. Whatever the defect, dietary regulation and the removal of excess weight will bring these patients back into normal carbohydrate balance, and the regulation of carbohydrate metabolism will return to normal. In more severe cases, oral agents (e.g., sulfonylureas, thiazolidinediones, biguanides) are used to reduce blood glucose levels in these patients along with rigid control of dietary intake.

There is evidence to support a familial or genetic component in type 2 diabetes. A series of studies on twins indicates that if one twin develops type 2 diabetes after age 50, the other twin develops type 2 diabetes in almost every case.

Type 1 diabetes usually develops in persons under 20 years of age and is characterized by an abrupt onset of symptoms. A small percentage of people over 40 who contract diabetes mellitus also exhibit this form of the disease. Typically, the pancreatic B-cells are reduced markedly (usually to less than 10% of normal), and insulin levels are very low or absent. Glycogen stores are depleted readily and fatty acid metabolism is accelerated, resulting in accumulation of ketone bodies in the blood which in about 48 hours will produce ketoacidosis and eventually lead to coma and death unless insulin is administered. Patients with type 1 diabetes have an absolute requirement for exogenous insulin for the rest of their lives. Because of this reliance on exogenous insulin and difficulties in administering the appropriate dose when needed, the diabetic must always be prepared for the onset of hypoglycemia following excessive insulin. Hypoglycemia can also induce coma and usually can be counteracted by consuming a high glucose source.

There is some evidence to suggest a role of infection as a cause of type 1 diabetes. The symptoms of type 1 diabetes appear abruptly, and there is a higher incidence of onset during the fall and winter months when the incidences of infectious diseases also increase. In certain genetic strains of mice, type 1 diabetes has been linked to a specific virus. There also appears to be a correlation between the occurrence of certain viral diseases (e.g., mumps, rubella *in utero*) and the later appearance of type 1 diabetes.

The major cause of type 1 diabetes, however, seems to be an autoimmune reaction that destroys the B-cells. Although characterized by an abrupt onset of severe symptoms soon leading to death if untreated, type 1 diabetes actually has a long incubation period (sometimes years). Only after about 80% of the insulin-secreting capacity of the pancreas is destroyed do the classic symptoms appear. The presence of lymphocytes and monocytes (white blood cells) in the islets at first seem to support the infection hypothesis. However, antibodies to components of B-cells have been found in the blood of patients with type 1 diabetes and in people believed to be at risk. One of these antibodies reacts against a ganglioside found within all B-cells, and a second antibody reacts to a 64-kD protein known only from the cell membranes of B-cells. A third antibody reacts with insulin itself. The antibody against the 64-kD protein is probably the one that initially damages the B-cells. Apparently, these antibodies are present in the blood long before diabetes presents clinically, and administration of anti-immune system drugs to date have prevented the onset of type 1 diabetes in experimental subjects who would have developed the disease eventually. Although the circulating antibodies have been demonstrated, many scientists still believe that cell-mediated immunity is the cause of type 1 diabetes. Nevertheless, the ability to identify these circulating antibodies may prove to be an important diagnostic tool allowing early detection and possible prevention of irreversible damage to the B-cells.

Dietary restrictions are similar for treating both type 1 diabetes and type 2 diabetes patients although a reduction in total caloric intake also is necessary for overweight type 2 diabetes patients. Specific diets must be determined individually for every patient. Carbohydrates are still essential to the diabetic diet but need to be in the form of polysaccharides (e.g., starch). Mono- and disaccharides are usually avoided because of rapid uptake and resultant hyperglycemia soon after ingestion. The ingestion of simple sugars is less a problem for the type 2 diabetes patient as the pancreas can respond with some insulin release.

B. Extrapancreatic Tumor Hypoglycemia

This disorder sometimes appears in patients with cancer. Patients with **extrapancreatic tumor hypoglycemia (EPTH)** exhibit normal to low levels of insulin and normal IGF levels, but have high levels of circulating proIGF-II. This proIGF-II is of tumor origin and can bind to the insulin receptor and produce insulin-like hypoglycemia.

VII. Summary

Feeding is regulated by peptides secreted by the hypothalamus, the gastrointestinal tract, and adipose cells. Orexic factors that stimulate feeding include orexin A and B, NPY, AgRP, ghrelin, galanin, and endocanabinoids, Anorexic factors that suppress appetite and feeding include CCK_8, leptin, α-MSH, CART, CRH, Ucn-II, PYY, and PP.

The existence of three major GI hormones (gastrin, secretin, and CCK) postulated to be present in mammals at the beginning of this century has been established, and their chemical structures have been elucidated. Gastrin is produced by the G-cell of the antral gastric mucosa in response to the presence of food. The parietal cell of the fundic and corpus portions of the stomach secretes HCl in response to gastrin or direct neural (vagal) stimulation. Histamine may play a role as an intermediate in the action of gastrin on the parietal cell. Parasympathetic stimulation stimulates acid secretion and also evokes secretion of pepsinogen from the chief cell in the gastric mucosa. SST produced in gastric D-cells blocks gastric secretion. Release of gastrin also can be elicited by GRP.

Neural stimulation may be involved to a limited degree in the intestinal phases, but the endocrine factors predominate. Secretin is produced by the S-cell of the duodenal mucosa in response to the presence of acidic chyme entering the small intestine from the stomach. The major hormonal action of secretin is to cause release of basic juices from the exocrine pancreas. The presence of peptides, amino acids, or fats in the chyme causes release of CCK from the I-cell of the intestinal mucosa, which in turn stimulates secretion of pancreatic enzymes and release of bile from the gallbladder. This pancreatic action of CCK originally was postulated to be due to a hormone called pancreozymin that later was shown to be identical to CCK.

Four additional peptides have been isolated from the mucosa of the small intestine and established as GI hormones. GIP from the K-cell stimulates release of insulin from the pancreas and may inhibit gastric activity under certain circumstances. Motilin from the M-cell stimulates gastric motility and possibly secretion of pepsinogen but does not influence acid secretion. VIP is a neurotransmitter that stimulates blood flow to the viscera. It is secreted along with PHI which both are derived from the same preprohormone. Enteroglucagons (glicentin, GLP-I, GLP-II, tGLP-I) produced by the L-cells have been identified in the intestinal mucosa and appear to stimulate insulin release but inhibit pancreatic glucagon secretion. Additional GI peptides that appear to have regulatory roles include NT, PYY, dynorphin, CRGP, and galanin. Several peptides have been shown to have enterogastrone action (they inhibit gastric function), including enteroglucagons, NT, CGRP, galanin, and GIP.

Overall metabolism is the sum of all anabolic and catabolic reactions occuring in the body. Intermediary metabolism consists of pathways involved in energy production from carbohydrates which are connected to pathways for protein and lipid metabolism such that excess carbohydrates can be converted to protein or lipid for storage or the latter can be used to supply carbohydrates for energy production via gluconeogenesis. The carbohydrate pathways include glycolyosis and the pentose shunt (anaerobic), the tricarboxcylic acid cycle, and the cytochrome system (which together with glycolysis and the pentose shunt constitute aerobic metabolism). Lipids (fatty acids, TAGs, cholesterol, phospholipids) are synthesized from carbohydrates and can be converted to carbohydrate via gluconeogenesis from glycerol and NEFAs (β-oxidation). Ketone bodies (ketogenesis) are formed during the β-oxidation of NEFAs. Amino acids derived from protein catabolism can be converted (by transamination) to carbohydrates and participate in gluconeogenesis. However, in many animals it is not possible to resynthesize all of the necessary amino acids from carbohydrate and some must be obtained through the diet (the essential amino acids).

The endocrine pancreas secretes hormones that are directly involved in the regulation of metaboism. The predominant cellular types in the vertebrate endocrine pancreas are the A-cell, B-cell, and D-cell. The A-cell and B-cell have been identified as the sources for glucagon and insulin, respectively. The D-cell produces somatostatin. A fourth cellular type located at the periphery of the mammalian pancreatic islet produces PP. It is not certain what the germ-layer origins are for the pancreatic endocrine cells. They do not come from the neural crest in spite of their APUD characteristics, and it is not clear whether they are of endodermal or ectodermal origin.

Glucagon is one of several hyperglycemic regulatory factors in vertebrates, and it stimulates glycogenolysis and lipolysis in liver and adipose cells while inhibiting glucose oxidation. These actions of glucagon appear to be mediated through activation of adenylyl cyclase and formation of cAMP. Low blood sugar levels stimulate glucagon release, and somatostatin blocks glucagon release. High levels of circulating fatty acids (NEFAs) stimulate glucagon release in birds and herbivorous mammals.

Insulin is the only naturally occurring hypoglycemic factor in vertebrates. It is present in many invertebrate species as well and may even function there as a hypoglycemic factor. The many actions of insulin include permeability effects on the plasmalemma, resulting in the increased uptake of glucose and amino acids into muscle cells and the uptake of glucose by adipose cells. Insulin inhibits phosphorylase a activation and stimulates glycogen synthetase to favor glucose storage. Lipogenesis increases after binding of insulin to the plasmalemma of adipose cells because of the increased availability of substrates as a consequence of glucose uptake and oxidation as well as effects on enzymes that increase lipogenesis and inhibit lipolysis. Growth effects occur in cooperation with IGFs produced under the influence of GH.

High circulating glucose levels stimulate release of insulin from the B-cells of the pancreatic islets. It is both the uptake and the metabolism of glucose that actually are responsible for causing insulin release. Neural factors (parasympathetic) and other hormones (for example, GIP, GLP-I) also may stimulate insulin release. SST, epinephrine, and gastrin, as well as low blood glucose levels, all inhibit insulin release.

Metabolism is controlled by the actions and interactions of many hormones under different nutritional conditions, which maintain a healthy organism with energy reserves necessary for maintenance and for reproduction. The major metabolic hormone is insulin, which is protein anabolic, lipogeneic, antilipolytic, glycogenic, antiglycogenolytic, and hypoglycemic. These actions are most important following ingestion of a meal and show lesser importance under postprandial conditions and during starvation. Insulin's actions are opposed primarily by six other hormones including GH (protein anabolic, lipolytic, gluconeogenic, hyperglycemic), glucagon (lipolytic, glycogenolytic, hyperglycemic), epinephrine (lipolytic, glycogenolytic, gluconeogenic, hyperglycemic), glucocorticoids (protein catabolic, gluconeogenic, hyperglycemic), thyroid hormones (lipolytic, glycogenolytic, hyperglycemic), and anabolic-androgenic steroids (protein anabolic). Epinephrine directly inhibits insulin release. Glucocorticoids also prevent peripheral use of glucose especially by muscle.

Suggested Reading

Books

Bliss, M. (1982). "The Discovery of Insulin." The University of Chicago Press, Chicago.

Campaigne, B. N., and Lampman, R. M. (1994). "Exercise in the Clinical Management of Diabetes." Human Kinetics, Champaign, IL.

Chivers, D. J., and Langer, P. (1994). "The Digestive System in Mammals: Food, Form and Function." Cambridge Univ. Press, Cambridge.

Epple, A., and Brinn, J. E. (1987). "The Comparative Physiology of the Pancreatic Islets." Springer-Verlag, Berlin.

Holmgren, S. (1989). "The Comparative Physiology of Regulatory Peptides." Chapman & Hall, New York.

Kochakian, C. D. (1984). "How It Was: Anabolic Action of Steroids and Remembrances." Univ. Alabama School of Medicine, Birmingham, AL.

LeRoith, D., Olefsky, J. M., and Taylor, S. I. (1996). "Diabetes Mellitus: A Fundamental and Clinical Text." Lippincott-Raven, Harestown, MD.

Samols, E. (1991). "The Endocrine Pancreas." Raven, New York.

Schultz, G. M. (1989). "Handbook of Physiology, Section 6, The Gastrointestinal System." American Physiological Society, Bethesda, MD.

Stevens, C. E. (1988). "Comparative Physiology of the Vertebrate Digestive System." Cambridge Univ. Press, Cambridge.

Thompson, J. C. (1990). "Gastrointestinal Endocrinology." Academic Press, San Diego.

Walsh, J. H., and Dockray, G. J. (1994). "Gut Peptides." Raven, New York.

Articles

Bates, S. H. Y., and Myers, M. G. Jr. (2003). The role of leptin receptor signaling in feeding and neuroendocrine function. 2003. *Trends Endocr. Metab.* **14**, 447–452.

Casanueva, F. F., and Dieguez, C. (1999). Neuroendocrine regulation and actions of leptin. *Frontiers Neuroendocr.* **20**, 317–363.

Conlon, J. M. (1995). Peptide tyrosine-tyrosine (PYY)—an evolutionary perspective. *Am. Zool.* **35**, 466–473.

Cooper, G. J. S. (1994). Amylin compared with calcitonin gene-related peptide: Structure, biology, and relevance to metabolic disease. *Endocr. Rev.* **15**, 163–201.

Fehmann, H.-C., Goke, R., and Goke, B. (1995). Cell and molecular biology of the incretin hormones glucagon-like peptide-I and glucose-dependent insulin releasing polypeptide. *Endocr. Rev.* **16**, 390–408.

Ferguson, A. V., and Samson, W. K. (2003). The orexin/hypocretin system: A critical regulator of neuroendocrine and autonomic function. *Frontiers Neuroendocr.* **24**, 141–150.

Johnsen, A. H. (1998). Phylogeny of the cholecystokinin/gastrin family. *Frontiers Neuroendocr.* **19**, 73–99.

Korbonits, M., Goldstone, A. P., Gueorguiev, M., and Grossman, A. B. (2004). Ghrelin—a hormone with multiple functions. *Frontiers Neuroendocr.* **25**, 27–68.

McIntosh, C. H. S. (1995). Control of gastric acid secretion and the endocrine pancreas by gastrointestinal regulatory peptides. *Am. Zool.* **35**, 455–465.

Morely, J. E. (1995). The role of peptides in appetite regulation across species. *Am. Zool.* **35**, 437–445.

Sahu, A. (2003). Leptin signaling in the hypothalamus: emphasis on energy homeostasis and leptin resistance. *Frontiers Neuroendocr.* **24**, 225–253.

Samson, W. K., and Resch, Z. T. (2000). The hypocretin/orexin story. *Trends Endocr. Metab.* **11**, 257–262.

Small, C. J., and Bloom, S. R. (2004). Gut hormones and the control of appetite. *Trends Endocr. Metab.* **15**, 259–263.

General Articles

Baskin, D. G., Figlewicz, D. P., Woods, S. C., Porte, D., Jr., and Dorsa, D. M. (1987). Insulin in the brain. *Ann. Rev. Physiol.* **49**, 335–347.

Bliss, M. (1989). Special lecture: J. J. R. Macleod and the discovery of insulin. *Q. J. Exp. Physiol.* **74**, 79–96.

Fehmann, H.-C., and Habener, J. F. (1992). Insulinotropic glucagonlike peptide-I(7-37)/(7-36) amide: A new incretin hormone. *Trends Endocr. Metab.* **3**, 158–163.

Geary, N. (1990). Pancreatic glucagon signals postprandial satiety. *Neurosci. Biobehav. Rev.* **14**, 323–338.

Hazelwood, R. L. (1993). The pancreatic polypeptide (PP-fold) family: Gastrointestinal, vascular, and feeding behavioral implications. *Proc. Soc. Exp. Biol. Med.* **202**, 44–63.

Heidenreich, K. A. (1991). Insulin in the brain: What is its role? *Trends Endocr. Metab.* **2**, 9–12.

Larner, J. (1988). Insulin signaling mechanisms. Lessons from the Old Testament of glycogen metabolism and the New Testament of molecular biology. *Diabetes* **37**, 262–275.

McDermott, A. M., and Sharp, G. W. G. (1993). Mini review: Inhibition of insulin secretion: A fail-safe system. *Cell. Signal.* **5**, 229–234.

Quon, M. J. (1994). Insulin signal transduction pathways. *Trends Endocr. Metab.* **5**, 369–376.

Sargeant, R., Mitsumoto, Y., Saraba, V., Shillabeer, G., and Klip, A. (1993). Hormonal regulation of glucose transporters in muscle cells in culture. *J. Endocr. Invest.* **16**, 147–162.

Thissen, J.-P., Ketelslegers, J.-M., and Underwood, L. E. (1994). Nutritional regulation of the insulin-like growth factors. *Endocr. Rev.* **15**, 80–101.

Clinical Articles

Atkinson, M. A., and Maclaren, N. K. (1990). What causes diabetes. *Sci. Am.* **263(1)**, 62–71.

Bach, J.-F. (1994). Insulin-dependent diabetes as an autoimmune disease. *Endocr. Rev.* **15**, 516–542.

Bretherton-Watt, D., and Bloom, S. R. (1991). Islet amyloid polypeptide: The cause of type-2 diabetes? *Trends Endocr. Metab.* **2**, 203–206.

Eisenbarth, G. S., and Ziegler, A. (1995). Type I diabetes mellitus. *In* "Molecular Endocrinology: Basic Concepts and Clinical Implications" (B. D. Weintraub, Ed.), pp. 269–282. Raven, New York.

Holst, J. J. (1999). Glucagon-like peptide-1 (GLP-1): An intestinal hormone, signaling nutritional abundance, with an unusual therapeutic potential. *Trends Endocr. Metab.* **10**, 229–235.

Macintyre, J. G. (1987). Growth hormone and athletes. *Sports Med.* **4**, 129–142.

Sima, A. A. F., and Kamiya, H. (2004). Insulin, C-peptide, and diabetic neuropathy. *Sci. Med.* **9**, 308–319.

Van der Lely, A., Tschop, M., Heiman, M. L., and Ghigo, E. (2004). Biological, physiological, pathophysiological, and pharmacological aspects of ghrelin. *Endocrine Rev.* **25**, 426–457.

Weindruch, R. (1996). Caloric restriction and aging. *Sci. Am.* **Jan. 1996**, 46–52.

13

Comparative Aspects of Feeding, Digestion, and Metabolism

The endocrine regulation of feeding, digestion, and metabolism in non-mammals has been poorly studied when compared to mammals. Most of the factors were only discovered in mammals within the last decade, so it is not surprising that little is known for non-mammals with respect to feeding regulation. Most of the published research has been conducted with fishes, and relatively little is known about these processes in non-mammalian tetrapods. Chapter 12 provides a general description of these processes in mammals, and definitions provided there will not be repeated here.

I. Hormones and Feeding in Non-Mammals

Studies in fish have shown that several but not all mammalian orexigenic and anorexic factors are effective in fishes. A summary of known actions in fishes is provided in Figure 13-1. A few studies in amphibians and birds also have been done

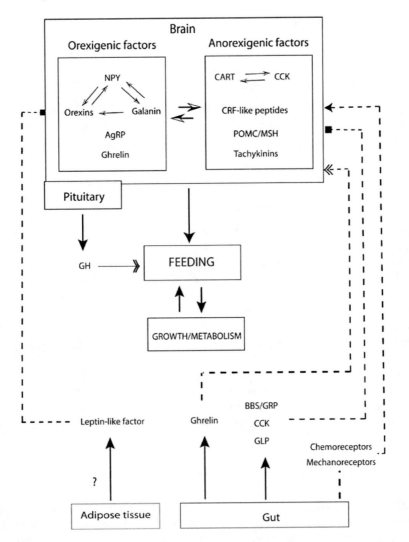

Figure 13-1. **Bioregulation of feeding in fishes.** BBS, bomesin; see text for explanation of other abbreviations. [From Volkoff, H., Canosa, L. F., Unniappan, S., Cerda-Reverter, J. M., Bernier, N. J., Kelly, S. P., and Peter, R. E. (2005). Neuropeptides and the control of food intake in fish. *Gen. Comp. Endocr.* **142**, 3–19.]

A. Orexigenic Factors in Teleost Fishes

Ghrelin has been identified in the stomach and brain of several teleosts. Both human and goldfish ghrelin stimulate feeding behavior in goldfish. Starvation increases production of mRNA for preproghrelin in goldfish. It is not known if any other peptides like ghrelin that are related to growth hormone (GH) secretion are involved in appetite regulation (e.g., somatostatin, growth hormone-releasing hormone) but they are located in brain regions known to influence feeding. Neuropeptide Y also is a potent stimulator of appetite as are pharmacological NPY agonists in teleosts. NPY increases in the brain prior to feeding and decreases after feeding. As in mammals, NPY appears to interact with a number of other factors, including corticotropin-releasing hormone (CRH), cocaine and amphetamine regulated transcript (CART), leptin, orexins, and galanin. Galanin is distributed throughout several brain regions in goldfish and have been shown to stimulate food intake. Orexins synergize with galanin and also enhance NPY effects on feeding. Although changes have been observed in levels of agouti-related peptide (AgRP), it is not clear if it has any regulatory role such as described for the related agouti-signaling protein (ASP) in mammals. Anorexic actions have been reported for CRH, CCK, Bombesin (BBS), GLP-1, and CART. Although melanin-concentrating hormone (MCH) has been characterized as an orexigen in mammals, it appears to be primarily a bioregulator of body color and an antagonist of α-MSH. There is some evidence for an effect of MCH on appetite in teleosts, but no direct support as yet.

B. Anorexogenic Factors in Teleost Fishes

Cholecystokinin (CCK$_8$), CRH and the related Urotensin-I, and CART all decrease feeding in goldfish although CCK$_8$ stimulated feeding in rainbow trout. Prolactin-releasing peptide (PrRP) is an appetite suppressant in fishes in addition to its role in prolactin release (see Chapter 5). Data for roles by leptin, α-MSH, and tachykinins are rather sketchy at this time.

C. Bioregulation of Feeding in Other Non-Mammals

Orexin A and B have been identified in *Xenopus laevis*. Orexin immunoreactive neurons were present only in the suprachiasmatic nucleus (SCN) of the tree frog, *Hyla cinera*, but immunoreactive (ir) Orexin B was found in the SCN as well as in the anterior preoptic area and the magnocellular and ventral hypothalamus of *Rana ridibunda*. Leptin and leptin receptors have been characterized in the newt *Triturus cristatus carnifex* and in the stomach of a frog. In addition, a version of a 26RFamide peptide was isolated from the frog brain that can stimulate feeding in mice. Immunoreactive ghrelin is present in bullfrog stomachs and increases in both mucosa of the stomach and in the blood following a short period of starvation. Urocortins are anorexic in *X. laevis*. Leptin was also reported from the stomachs of a lizard and a snake and ghrelin is present in the gastric mucosa of a turtle.

Leptin has been isolated from chickens and was shown to reduce food intake in chickens and great tits (*Parus major*), and circulating leptin is reduced by starvation in chicks. Administration of orexin to chicks did not stimulate feeding nor did fasting affect levels of orexin in either the lateral hypothalamus or the periventricular nucleus (PVN) although there was a 2X increase in AgRP in the infundibular (arcuate) nucleus.

II. Hormones and Digestion in Non-Mammals

The investigation into comparative regulation is hampered by the lack of basic understanding of the general physiology of digestion in non-mammalian species. For example, although extensive research in teleost fishes of commercial importance has been accomplished with respect to diets, growth, and feeding ecology, few experiments have been concerned with physiological control mechanisms. There are many unique situations with respect to digestive processes of non-mammals. For example, many fishes lack stomachs and may have other specialized structures (e.g., pyloric caeca) that imply major differences in control mechanisms. Also, digestion in fishes, amphibians, and reptiles may require days to accomplish what birds and mammals do in a few hours with elevated body temperatures.

Data on gastrointestinal peptides in non-mammals indicate that many of the peptides described in mammals also are present in non-mammals. However, functional studies are considerably behind the assessments available for mammals, and we are aware of their functions in relatively few species.

Using immunocytochemical techniques, a number of mammalian peptides have been demonstrated in invertebrate species. There appears to be a broad phylogenetic distribution for these peptides among invertebrate animals (see Chapter 12, Table 12-5). Many of these peptides are similar to or identical with peptides located in vertebrate guts and vertebrate nervous systems as well. For example, immunoreactive gastrin/CCK-like peptides have been extracted from the GI tract of a tunicate, two molluscan species, and several insects. However, only the octapeptide cionin extracted from the tunicate *Ciona intestinalis* appears to be a true gastrin/CCK peptide, establishing the origin of this peptide family at about 500 million years ago.

A. Agnathan Fishes: Cyclostomes

Cyclostomes are stomachless fishes and therefore studies have emphasized the intestinal and pancreatic tissues. Cytological studies by Ostberg and coworkers on the intestine of the Atlantic hagfish *Myxine glutinosa* have revealed the presence of primitive open-type endocrine cells. These cells extend from the basal portion of the intestinal epithelium to border on the lumen of the gut. Hagfish intestinal endocrine cells do not possess APUD characteristics, although APUD-type cells have been reported in the pancreatic islets that differentiate into insulin-producing B-cells. These intestinal endocrine cells in the Atlantic hagfish do not resemble zymogen cells either, suggesting a separate origin for the endocrine and enzyme-secreting cells. Immunoreactive CCK, gastrin, glucagon-like peptides, somatostatin (SST), substance P, glucose-insulinotropic peptide (GIP = gastric inhibitory peptide), and vasoactive intestinal peptide (VIP) have all been reported in the hagfish intestine. Gallbladder strips prepared from a Pacific hagfish, *Eptatretus stouti*, however, did not respond *in vitro* with contractions to porcine CCK although ACh caused contractions. Secretion of intestinal lipase in this same species is stimulated by porcine CCK.

In contrast to the hagfishes, the intestinal epithelium of larval and adult lampreys (*Lampetra* spp.) contains APUD-type cells. Immunoreactive glucagon-like peptides, neuropeptide Y (NPY), peptide YY (PYY), SST_{14}, SST_{34}, and pancreatic polypeptide (PP) have been reported in the intestines of several lamprey species. Secretin-like and CCK-like activities are present in extracts prepared from intestines of river lampreys, *Lampetra fluviatilis*, and sea lampreys, *Petromyzon marinus*. Both secretin and CCK activities in these extracts were assayed by monitoring pancreatic secretions in the anesthetized cat.

B. Chondrichthyean Fishes

In their classical studies, Bayliss and Starling reported the presence of secretin-like activity in extracts prepared from dogfish shark and skate intestines and bioassayed in mammals. Intestinal extracts prepared from the holocephalan *Chimaera monstrosa* exhibited CCK activity. Likewise, porcine CCK stimulates contractions in strips of gallbladder prepared from dogfish sharks, and the intensity of the response is proportional to the dose of CCK. Immunoreactive SST and glucagon-like peptides (GLPs) have been reported in the gastric glands of five elasmobranch species, and VIP has been isolated from the dogfish, *Scyliorhinus canalicula* (for structures, see Chapter 12, Figure 12-14).

C. Bony Fishes: Teleosts

Only a few of the more than 20,000 species of teleosts have been investigated. The first observations were those of Bayliss and Starling, who reported that intestinal extracts prepared from salmon possessed secretin-like and possibly CCK-like activities. Similar activities were reported for pike, *Esox lucius*, and cod, *Gadus morhua*, using either avian or mammalian bioassays. CCK activity is present in the intestine of the Atlantic eel, *Anguilla anguilla*, and the pike. Isolated strips of gallbladder from Pacific salmon (*Oncorhynchus*) contract in the presence of porcine CCK, indicating sensitivity of the salmon gallbladder to the mammalian peptide. Intestinal strips from codfish contract in response to either gastrin or CCK_8.

A gastrin-histamine type of mechanism is present in the stomach of the majority of teleosts (cyprinid and labrid fishes lack stomachs). Extracts from the gastric mucosa of sunfish (*Lepomis macrochirus*) stimulate acid secretion in bullfrogs, and large doses of histamine (1015 mg/kg weight) induce acid secretion in the European catfish *Silurus glanis*. Histamine-induced acid secretion in cod (15 mg/kg) is blocked by certain antihistamines, supporting the existence of a mammalian-like regulatory system. Fish stomachs contain one cell type that secretes both pepsinogen and H^+ and probably secrete both products simultaneously in response to gastrin or histamine. Administration of CCK_8 slows gastric emptying in salmoinids.

Ten immunoreactive cell types were identified in *Sparus auratus* including stomach cells reacting to neurotensin (NT), secretin, serotonin, substance P, and SST. Intestinal cells reacted to antibodies for gastrin, CCK, glucagon-like peptides, PP, substance P, and the opioid met-enkephalin. Similar examination of the intestine of a stomachless fish, *Barbus conchonius*, exhibited all but the substance P immunoreactive cell types. SST_{14} is present in the cod stomach where it inhibits acid secretion. Both SST_{14} and SST_{28} have been found in the intestines of several teleosts but not in the mudsucker, *Gillichthyes mirabilis*. VIP has been isolated and characterized chemically from the bowfin (a non-teleost, bony fish) and two teleosts (see Chapter 12, Figure 12-14), but its physiological role is not understood.

D. Amphibians

Regulation of gastric mechanisms in amphibians has been studied almost exclusively in frogs. It appears that amphibians possess mechanisms very much like those of mammals, involving both neural and endocrine mechanisms. Stomachs of intact frogs or isolated gastric mucosa prepared from frogs (including *Rana pipiens*, *R. catesbeiana*, *R. temporaria*, and *R. esculenta*) respond with acid secretion when subjected to ACh, histamine, synthetic pentagastrin, or crude gastrin preparations from non-mammals or mammals. Similarly, gastric mucosa isolated from a urodele, *Necturus*, secretes acid in response to pentagastrin. Treatment with atropine or surgical vagotomy reduces acid secretion in frogs as it does in mammals. Beyond the amphibians, CCK peptides are highly conserved but mammalian gastrin has diverged markedly from the gastrins of amphibians, reptiles, and birds. Prototherian mammals apparently do not produce either gastric acid or gastrin, and the distinct mammalian gastrin gene is demonstrable first among the marsupials.

The release of pepsinogen in *R. esculenta* can be induced by increasing parasympathetic activity. Two skin peptides, caerulein and BBS, have been associated with frog stomachs and may affect gastric secretion. Caerulin is known to stimulate acid secretion from stomach mucosa in a variety of vertebrates, and immunoreactive BBS has been reported in frog stomachs as well as in frog skin and brain. Recent chemical identification of gastrin releasing peptide (GRP) in the stomach of *Rana ridibunda* suggests that GRP may be an endogenous peptide stimulator of gastrin release.

Bayliss and Starling reported that extracts from frog intestines would evoke pancreatic secretion in dogs, providing evidence for the presence of secretin-like or CCK-like factors or both. Frog gallbladders will contract in the presence of porcine CCK *in vitro*, supporting the possible existence of a CCK-like factor in amphibians as well as a role for CCK in regulation of gastric processes. VIP also has been isolated from a frog stomach (see Chapter 12, Figure 12-14).

E. Reptiles

Bayliss and Starling reported that a factor or factors capable of causing pancreatic secretion in mammals is present in the intestine of a tortoise. Immunoreactive SST is present in the intestine of the lizard *Anolis carolinensis*, but motilin is not. In two chelonians, *Testudo graeca* and *Mauremys caspica*, immunoreactive BBS, NT, gastrin, glucagon-like peptides, SST, PYY, and insulin were demonstrated in the intestinal mucosa, but no functional roles were indicated. The same study failed to find immunoreactive motilin, secretin, VIP, CCK, GIP, and opioid enkephalins. However, alligator VIP has been characterized chemically and found to be identical to chicken VIP (see Chapter 12, Figure 12-14). It is remarkable that so few studies have been reported for reptiles, suggesting this is a group of vertebrates needing thorough endocrine examination.

F. Birds

Knowledge of the GI physiology of domesticated birds is more extensive than for any other non-mammalian group because of the importance of gastrointestinal research to poultry science. However, little information on wild species is available. Gastrin can stimulate acid secretion in birds, and large dosages of CCK cause release of enzymes from the avian exocrine pancreas. Extracts prepared from chicken intestines are strong stimulants of pancreatic secretion when assayed in turkeys, but these extracts are only weak stimulants in mammals (cat, rat) suggesting considerable molecular differences may exist in these avian factors. Glucagon and GIP appear to have no effects on pancreatic secretions in birds.

Other observations indicate there are some features in avian GI physiology that may be unique. For example, purified avian (chicken) or porcine secretin only weakly stimulates exocrine pancreatic secretion in turkeys, but purified mammalian VIP or peptide histidine isoleucine (PHI) are potent stimulators. VIP is a very conservative peptide in vertebrates, suggesting its functions have been conserved through evolution. Chicken VIP has been isolated and differs structurally from porcine VIP at only four positions (see Chapter 12, Figure 12-14). Immunoreactive SST and motilin have been demonstrated in the intestines of Japanese quail and chickens, but nothing is known about their possible functions.

III. Comparative Aspects of the Endocrine Pancreas

There are several general vertebrate patterns with respect to the proportions of these cellular types present in the endocrine pancreas (Table 13-1). However, careful analyses indicate that it is misleading to characterize classes of vertebrates as exhibiting a particular pattern (Table 13-2).

A. Anatomical Features

Five anatomical arrangements for pancreatic islet systems can be distinguished readily by examination of the major vertebrate groupings. The cyclostome type is composed of aggregations of islet cellular types with no obvious relationship to the homologous intra-intestinal equivalent of mammalian acinar cells. In hagfishes, islets surround the base of the common bile duct (Figure 13-2A), and in lampreys they are located on the surfaces of the intestine (epi-intestinal), within the intestinal mucosa (intra-intestinal; Figure 13-2B), and even within the liver (intrahepatic). Cyclostomes exhibit B-and D-cells but lack A-cells and PP-cells. GLPs have been identified in the gastric mucosa. The cyclostome pattern of islet distribution is considered to be the most primitive pattern in vertebrates. Exocrine pancreatic elements are embedded in the intestinal lining of these primitive fishes.

The primitive gnathostome type is found in the elasmobranchs (Figure 13-3), holocephalans, and coelacanth (*Latimeria* spp). In these fishes, the islet tissue occurs as layers surrounding the smaller ducts of a compact pancreas. In addition, some scattered cells are located throughout the exocrine pancreas. B- (insulin-secreting), A- (glucagon-secreting), D- (SST-secreting), and PP-cells occur in sharks and holocephalans similar to the condition for mammals (see Chapter 12).

Table 13-1. General Patterns of Islet Cellular Type Distributions in Vertebrates with Respect to A and B Cells[a]

Category	Dominant cytology	Representatives
I	Mostly B-cells	Cyclostomes
II	More than 50% B-cells	Teleosts, amphibians, mammals
III	Approximately 50% X-cells[b]	Holocephalans
IV	More than 50% A-cells	Most lizards, birds

[a] Based on Epple, A., and Brinn, J. E. (1987). "The Comparative Physiology of the Pancreatic Islets." Springer-Verlag, Berlin.
[b] X-cells contain glucagon-like peptides, but their function is unknown.

Table 13-2. Comparative Cytology of the Endocrine Pancreas with Respect to Relative Predominance of A-, B-, D-, and PP-Cells[a]

Class	A-cells	B-cells	D-cells	PP-cells
Agnathans				
Hagfish		++++	+	?
Chondrichthyeans				
Elasmobranchs	+++	++++	+	+
Osteichthyeans				
Teleosts	+++	++++	+	+
Amphibians				
Anurans and urodeles	+++	++++	+	+
Reptiles				
Saurians	++++	+	+	+
Crocodilians	+++	+++	+	?
Birds	+++++	+++	+	+
Mammals	++	+++++	+	+

[a] The number of + marks in each column represents only an attempt to show relative abundance and should not be construed as precise ratios.

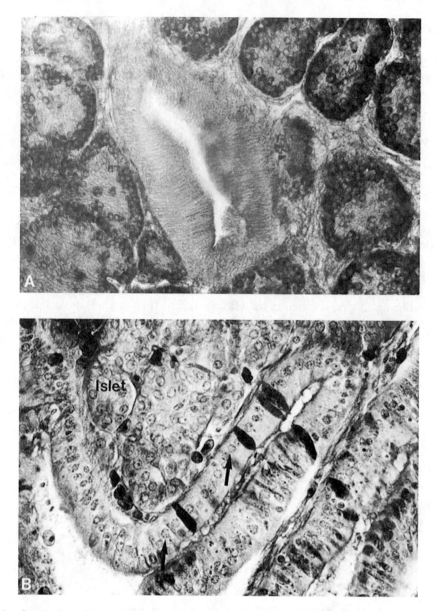

Figure 13-2. Islet tissues of hagfish and lamprey. (A) Follicles of islet tissue surrounding the lower bile duct from the hagfish *Eptatretus burgeri*. (B) Islet located in intestinal submucosa of the sea lamprey, *Petromyzon marinus*. (Photos courtesy of August Epple, Thomas Jefferson University.)

In contrast to the coelacanths (see below), we find the diffuse actinopterygian type among the other bony fishes where the exocrine pancreatic cells are scattered along the bile ducts, abdominal blood vessels, and on the outer surfaces of the gastrointestinal tract, gallbladder, and liver. However, an intrahepatic pancreas has been observed in several species. The islet tissue often accumulates as clumps near the common bile duct but is not usually separated from the acinar tissues. Most teleosts possess isolated masses of pancreatic islet tissue called Brockmann bodies. A given species may have a number of Brockmann bodies, or the islet tissue may be concentrated largely in one "principal islet" as in the Atlantic eel, *Anguilla anguilla*, or in bullheads, *Ictalurus* spp. Brockmann bodies of actinopterygian fishes contain A-, B-, and D-cells, but PP-cells occur only in those Brockmann bodies located in the pyloric region.

The pancreas of lungfishes forms a unique arrangement referred to as the lungfish type. It is a compact, intra-intestinal structure with a number of encapsulated islets. Only B-, A-, and D-cells have been identified in lungfish islets.

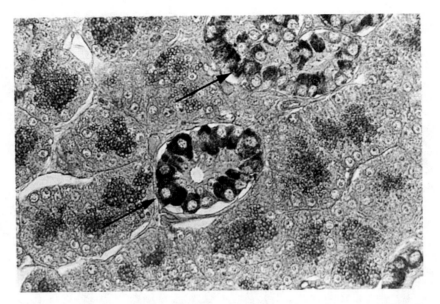

Figure 13-3. **Pancreas of dogfish,** *Scyliohrinus canicula*. These primitive islets consist of endocrine cells surrounding a small
unstained ductile of the exocrine pancreas. (Photo courtesy of August Epple, Thomas Jefferson University.)

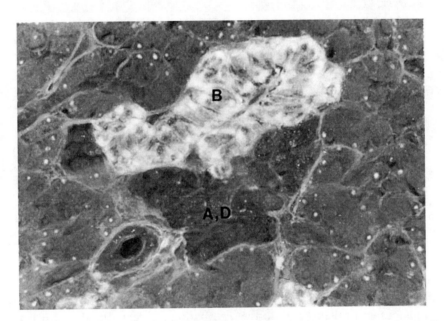

Figure 13-4. **B-cells in toad**. The presence of insulin is indicated by the light fluorescence. The dark area immediately surrounding the
B-cells consists mostly of A-cells with a few D-cells. (Photo courtesy of August Epple, Thomas Jefferson University.)

The tetrapod type of endocrine pancreas typically is a compact, extraintestinal structure containing scattered
islets and occasionally some scattered endocrine cells. In the toad *Bufo* (Figure 13-4) and in birds (Figure 13-5),
all four cell types known for mammals are present although their proportions often are very different from
mammals. Islets may be concentrated in particular lobes of the pancreas and often are not evenly distributed.

Immunoreactive insulin-like growth factors (IGFs) appear in the pancreatic islets or their homologues in
protochordates, fishes, amphibians, reptiles, birds, and mammals. In cephalochordates and urochordates, there
appears to be a single gene that produces a common insulin/IGF molecule associated with the enteroendocrine
cells. These observations support a common gene origin for both insulin and the IGFs. IGF-II is co-localized
with insulin in all vertebrates, but IGF-I may be co-localized in different pancreatic cells in amphibians,
reptiles, and birds (see Chapter 12, Table 12-3).

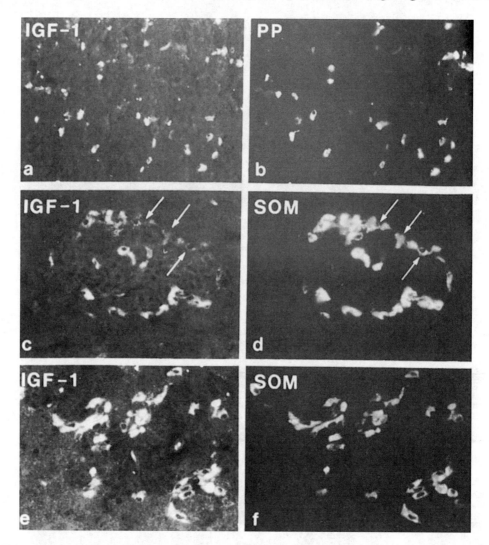

Figure 13-5. **Avian cell types in the pancreas.** (A–D) Co-localization of IGF-I in PP- and D-cells of the Japanese quail. (E–F) Co-localization of IGF-I and somatostatin (SOM) in D-cells of the domestic chicken. [From Reinecke, M. *et al.* (1995). Immunohistochemical localization of insulin-like growth factor I and II in the endocrine pancreas of birds, reptiles, and Amphibia. *Gen. Comp. Endocr.* **100**, 385–396.]

There are some generalizations we can make concerning the origin of the various components of the tetrapod pancreas and the relationship of their origin to the distribution of islets. The dorsal pancreatic bud gives rise to the tail and body of the pancreas (also known as the splenic portion) and the ventral buds give rise to the head or duodenal portion. Islets associated with the splenic lobe typically are larger and consist mainly of B-, A-, and D-cells. The islets of the duodenal pancreas are smaller and may contain many PP-cells.

B. Pancreatic Hormones in Non-Mammals

Insulin is a conservative protein in that few amino acid substitutions have occurred at the critical sites related to its structure and biological activity. Insulin A-chains and B-chains consist of 21 or 22 amino acids and from 31 to 38 amino acids, respectively. The number of amino acids in the B-chain especially varies when insulins from different vertebrate classes are compared. The C-peptide of proinsulin "tolerates" a greater number of substitutions, yet even portions of this peptide remain rather conservative; for example, the glycine-rich central core of the C-peptide. Single amino acid substitutions may have profound effects on the resultant molecule.

```
Source              Sequence

Mammals             H S Q G F T S D Y S K Y L D S R R A Q D F V Q W L M N T

Opossum (marsupial)                                                     S

Bullfrog (amphibian)                                                    S

Gila monster (reptile)                  T

Duck, Ostrich (birds)                   T

Common dogfish (shark)  E                 M   N       K

Coho salmon (teleost)   E     S   N       Q   E E   M                    S

Sculpin (teleost)       E     S   N           E T                   K   S

Sea lamprey (agnathan)  E                     E N K Q   K         R      S
```

Figure 13-6. **Amino acid sequences of vertebrate glucagons.** See Appendix C for explanation of letters used for amino acids. [Based on Hoyle, C. H. V. (1998). Neuropeptide families: Evolutionary perspectives. *Regulatory Peptides* **73**, 1–33.]

One substitution in hagfish insulin is believed responsible for the observation that hagfish insulin does not bind Zn^{2+} and therefore does not form the typical hexamer crystals characteristic of most vertebrate insulins.

Mammalian glucagons that have been characterized chemically exhibit no amino acid substitutions. Non-mammalian glucagons also are structurally conservative with the exception of teleosts (Figure 13-6). Turkey glucagon differs from mammalian glucagons only at position 28, where serine is substituted for asparagine. Chicken glucagon is identical to turkey glucagon, whereas duck glucagon has threonine at position 16 instead of serine. Glucagon extracted from eels *A. anguilla* also has 29 amino acids with only 4 differences from mammalian glucagons. A second form with 36 amino acids resembles mammalian GLP-2. However, glucagon has 31 amino acids in salmon, 29 and 31 amino acids in angler fish, and a GLP with 34 amino acids has been isolated from catfish. Glucagon from the flounder, *Platichthyes flesus*, is identical to the 29-amino acid form of the angler fish. Furthermore, the variation in amino acid sequence of glucagon among the teleosts is large. In contrast, glucagon isolated from the spiny dogfish shark *Squalus acanthias* and from *T. marmorata* are structurally more like mammalian glucagon than like teleosts.

B-cells and insulin activity have been identified in the guts or digestive organs of many non-chordate invertebrate animals, and a number of actions of insulin have been described. For example, mammalian insulin reduces blood sugar levels and promotes glycogen synthesis in a gastropod mollusk, *Strophocheilus oblongus*. Furthermore, insulin-like molecules have been found in distantly related taxonomic groups including protozoans, bacteria, and fungi. Insulin is therefore a widely distributed factor that appears to be capable of regulating carbohydrate metabolism in a great variety of organisms. The evolution of insulin must have involved a long and interesting process, most of which remains to be discovered.

Immunoreactive glucagon has been localized in the digestive glands of a crab, *Cancer pagurus*, and two gastropod mollusks, *Patella caerulae* and *Helix pomatia*. A glucagon-like molecule is present in extracts of a number of invertebrate chordates, including both tunicates and cephalochordates.

1. Agnathan Fishes: Cyclostomes

Insulin has been purified from hagfishes and three lampreys, *Lampetra fluviatilis*, *Petromyzon marinus*, and *Geotria australis*. The amino acid composition of hagfish and the northern hemisphere lampreys are more like mammalian insulins than like *Geotria* from the southern hemisphere, suggesting that *Geotria* diverged from the other lampreys very early in cyclostome evolution.

Hagfish insulin behaves similarly to other insulins in mammalian assays. The biological activity of purified hagfish insulin in mammals, however, is only about 4–7% of that reported for mammalian insulins in the same bioassay, indicating the evolution of greater specificity in target cells has occurred as well as some changes in the insulin molecule itself. When injected into hagfish, both mammalian and hagfish insulins cause hypoglycemia. Hagfish insulin stimulates both glycogen and protein synthesis in hagfish skeletal muscle but only stimulates protein synthesis in liver. Amino acids are known to stimulate insulin release in lampreys providing additional support for insulin's role as a regulator of protein metabolism. Known insulin antagonists, such as epinephrine, glucagon, T_4, corticotropin (ACTH), and prolactin (PRL) are all ineffective in altering blood sugar levels. Curiously, isletectomy of the hagfish *Myxine* does not cause hyperglycemia, and the response to a glucose load in isletectomized hagfish is normal. In contrast, total isletectomy of the lamprey *G. australis* resulted in a marked elevation in blood sugar within 24 hours. Hypophysectomy has no effect on islet cytology or blood sugar levels. There must be an explanation for the presence of insulin and the demonstration of its hypoglycemic action in the hagfish with the number of negative observations just mentioned, but it will require more research to reconcile these contradictory data.

Some large SSTs have been isolated from lampreys and their amino acid sequences determined. As described for insulin, SST_{33} from *Geotria* is very different from the SST_{34} molecules that characterize the other lampreys and which more closely resemble hagfish SST. Most of the variations occur among the first 18 amino acids, whereas little variation occurs in the rest of the molecules.

2. Chondrichthyean Fishes

Considerable variation in blood sugar levels occurs in chondrichthyean fishes. For example, values of 6 to 90 mg of glucose per 100 ml of blood have been reported for the dogfish shark. It appears that either blood sugar regulation is not very precise in these fishes or that blood sugar levels are very sensitive to capture and sampling procedures. Administration of mammalian insulin evokes hypoglycemia, and glucagon induces hyperglycemia in some species. Epinephrine also elevates blood glucose levels, and the effect of injected epinephrine occurs very rapidly. On a superficial basis, it appears that regulation of carbohydrate metabolism in these fishes is similar to the mammalian pattern.

There are many unusual features of metabolism in these fishes that require further study. Although liver glycogen levels in dogfish sharks conform with predicted responses to fasting and force feeding, the liver of holocephalans is either incapable of storing glycogen or is rapidly depleted of glycogen by the stress of capture and/or confinement. Injection of a glucose load does not alter tissue glycogen even though circulating glucose is increased. These observations may explain the inability of glucagon to increase blood glucose in the ratfish. Starvation forces sharks to rely on stored fats. Circulating levels of ketone bodies are elevated in fasting sharks as they are in mammals.

Protein and lipid metabolism with respect to the actions of pancreatic hormones have not been studied. Lipid metabolism in these fishes should be of special interest since hepatic fat content may be as high as 70% in the dogfish shark and 80% in the ratfish.

3. Bony Fishes

Insulins produced in several teleosts also are structurally similar to mammalian insulins. Like the chondrichthyean fishes, blood glucose levels of teleosts are very sensitive to handling and sampling stress, presumably due to the release and hyperglycemic action of epinephrine from chromaffin cells (see Chapter 8). Generally, both mammalian and teleost insulins produce hypoglycemia, and glucagon is hyperglycemic when tested in bony fishes. Injections of glucose or the amino acid leucine stimulate insulin secretion in the toadfish, *Opsanus tau*, and in the European silver eel, *A. anguilla*. Purified codfish insulin is a potent hypoglycemic agent in Northern pike, *Esox lucius*. Furthermore, mammalian insulin increases uptake and incorporation of labeled glucose and glycine into muscle lipids and protein in teleosts. Conversely, mammalian glucagon increases blood glucose, for example, in channel catfish. Glycogenolysis in isolated hepatocytes (liver cells) of goldfish is stimulated by either glucagon or epinephrine.

Teleost GLP-1 has been shown to have glycogenolytic and gluconeogeneic activity similar to glucagons, but GLP-1 is a weak stimulator of insulin release. Immunoreactive GIP has been demonstrated in pancreatic islets of rainbow trout and carp, although nothing is known about its gastrointestinal role or its ability to stimulate insulin release.

4. Amphibians

Mammalian insulin induces hypoglycemia in both anurans and urodeles, stimulates incorporation of amino acids into proteins, and lowers fatty acid levels. Following administration of a glucose load, blood sugar levels return to normal in about 24 hours. This response to a glucose load and the effects of pancreatectomy indicate an endogenous role for insulin. Mammalian glucagon causes hyperglycemia although it is ineffective in some amphibians. Epinephrine is hyperglycemic in tadpoles and adults of *Xenopus laevis*, and administration of epinephrine or norepinephrine causes reduction in liver and muscle glycogen.

Early research by Bernardo A. Houssay about 50 years ago on the amphibian pancreas led to a widely employed procedure for research into mammalian diabetes mellitus. It was in the toad *B. arenarum* that the antagonism of pituitary hormones and blood glucose of pancreatectomized or insulin-deficient animals was discovered. This discovery led to the widespread use of hypophysectomy to alleviate extreme diabetic conditions in experimental animals, and such doubly operated dogs, cats, and others became known commonly as Houssay animals. This action of hypophysectomy in the pancreatic-deficient animal is termed the Houssay effect.

Insulin has been extracted and characterized from several anurans, urodeles, and at least one apodan. Similarly, at least two forms of glucagons (29 or 36 amino acids) as well as several forms of GLPs have been analyzed. The amino acid sequences of some A chains of insulins, glucagons and GLPs are provided in Table 13-3 where they are compared to human sequences. Insulins and glucagons do not show nearly as much variation as do the GLPs, but all seem to be highly conserved. Data on PPs from amphibians are lacking.

5. Reptiles

Reptiles exhibit mammalian-like responses to injected insulin and glucagon and respond typically to a glucose load, returning to preloading levels in about 48 hours. Lizards, however, are particularly insensitive to insulin, and large quantities of mammalian insulin are required to invoke hypoglycemic responses. It is virtually impossible to induce insulin shock even with massive doses to lizards irrespective of their diets (Table 13-4). However, pancreatectomy induces a hyperglycemic state in lizards as it does in snakes and alligators. These observations suggest that in spite of the predominance of A-cells in lizard islets and their demonstrated

Table 13-4. Fatal Doses of Insulin for Various Vertebrates[a,b]

Animal	IU of insulin/kg body weight	Animal	IU of insulin/kg body weight
Nonmammals		**Mammals**	
Salamander	50	Rabbit	4–8
Lizard	>10,000[b]	Mouse	7–50
Canary	1000–4000	Rat	29–36
Pigeon	400–1200	Dog	16–300
Duck	50–500		

[a] Modified from Gorbman, A., and Bern, H. A. (1962). "A Textbook of Comparative Endocrinology." Wiley, New York.

[b] High doses of insulin cause intense hypoglycemia, followed by coma and death. Animals with fewer B-cells are less sensitive.

[b] A dose of 10,000 IU of insulin had no effect on survival of lizards.

insensitivity to mammalian insulin, endogenous insulin may play an important metabolic role in lizards as well as in other reptiles.

Insulin has been purified from a rattlesnake, *Crotalis atrox*, and its amino acid composition was found to be considerably different from bovine insulin with some uncommon substitutions occurring in the B-chain. In contrast, alligator insulin is structurally very much like chicken insulin, and the alligator responds equally with hypoglycemia to bovine, alligator, or turkey insulin. Comparative analyses of reptilian insulins may shed some light on pancreatic regulation of carbohydrate metabolism in reptiles, especially the apparent insensitivity of many species to mammalian insulins. Curiously, cyclostome insulin is structurally more like mammalian insulins than is rattlesnake insulin, which points out the difficulties of reconstructing evolutionary events using molecular data obtained from one or a few species as being representative of a major taxonomic group and/or relying only on the structure of the biologically active portion of a large gene product.

Although glucagon has been isolated from the alligator, its role in carbohydrate metabolism in reptiles has been inferred largely from observations following mammalian glucagon treatment. Glucagon is hyperglycemic in squamate reptiles as in birds, and circulating levels of glucagon often are high. For example, fasting lizards, *Varaus exanthematicus*, have high glucagon levels whereas glucagon is lowest during times of food intake.

Pancreatic polypeptide has been isolated from alligators. The amino acid composition of alligator PP is more like that of birds than like mammals (Figure 13-7).

Of particular interest is the absence of studies in which lipid and protein metabolism of reptiles were examined. Insulin and other "metabolic" hormones have not been examined for their roles in lipid or protein metabolism. Until all aspects of the hormonal regulation of metabolism in reptiles are integrated with the observations of effects of insulin and glucagon, a complete picture for the roles of reptilian hormones in metabolism will not emerge.

6. Birds

Hyperglycemia initially observed in birds following pancreatectomy is now believed to have been a result of overlooking the splenic lobe (rich in A-cells) during pancreatectomy. Total pancreatectomy results in

	1	11	21	31
Human	APLEP VYPGD	NATPE QMAQY	AADLR RYINM	LTRPR Y-NH$_2$
Porcine/Canine	APLEP VYPGD	DATPE QMAQY	AAELR RYINM	LTRPR Y-NH$_2$
Tapir	APLEP VYPGD	NATPE QMAQY	AAELR RYINM	LTRPR Y-NH$_2$
Rhino	ASLEP VYPGD	NATPE EMAQY	AADLR RYINM	LTRPR Y-NH$_2$
Horse/Zebra	APMEP VYPGD	NATPE QMAQY	AAELR RYINM	LTRPR Y-NH$_2$
Bovine	APLEP EYPGD	NATPE QMAQY	AADLR RYINM	LTRPR Y-NH$_2$
Rat	APLEP MYPGD	YATHE QRAQY	ETQLR RYIN T	LTRPR Y-NH$_2$
Turkey	GPSQP TYPGD	DAPVE DL IRF	YNDLQ QYLNV	VTRHR Y-NH$_2$
Goose	GPSQP TYPGN	DAPVE DL?RF	YDNLQ QYRLV	VFRHR Y-NH$_2$
Alligator	TPLQP KYPGD	GAPVE DL IQF	YNDLQ QYLNV	VTRHR P-NH$_2$

Figure 13-7. **Comparison of amino acid sequences for pancreatic polypeptide (PP).** There is considerable homology within a taxonomic group. Note the similarity between avian and alligator PPs that reflects their evolutionary closeness. See Appendix C for explanation of the amino acid symbols.

hypoglycemia rather than hyperglycemia and suggests that glucagon plays a major role in avian blood sugar regulation. This suggestion is supported further by observations that a high glucose load is required to induce insulin release in the duck and by the relative insensitivity of avian tissues to injected mammalian insulin (Table 13-4). Elevated glucose levels depress glucagon release, whereas high circulating levels of NEFAs induce glucagon release.

Avian tissues respond with hyperglycemia, glycogenolysis, and lipolysis following administration of mammalian glucagon. The avian pancreas contains about five to ten times the extractable glucagon per gram of pancreas as compared to mammals, emphasizing its probable importance to metabolic regulation in birds. In one of the few studies performed in wild birds, mammalian glucagon stimulated both plasma levels of free fatty acids and glucose in penguins, whereas insulin caused a reduction in blood glucose. Additional studies with wild avian species representing diverse taxonomic groupings would be welcome in order to confirm or alter generalizations based largely upon observations of inbred domesticated species.

Insulin has been extracted from the avian pancreas, and its structure has been examined. Chicken insulin is more effective in inducing hypoglycemia in birds than it is in mammals, and it is more potent in birds than is mammalian insulin. Glucagon has been extracted and its primary structure determined for duck, turkey, and chicken hormones. These hormones are almost identical structurally to mammalian glucagon.

Like mammalian PP, avian PP (aPP) consists of 36 amino acid residues and has a molecular weight of approximately 4200 Daltons (Figure 13-7). Avian PP, unlike its mammalian counterpart, appears to have a strong stimulatory influence on gastric acid secretion in chickens.

The biphasic release of aPP in chickens apparently is independent of protein, fat, or carbohydrate content of the diet. In fasting birds, PP plasma levels are about 40X greater than those observed in mammals. It is too early to decide whether these reports are related to the physiological roles of PP or not.

C. Non-Pancreatic Hormones and Metabolism in Non-Mammalian Vertebrates

In contrast to mammals, the endocrine regulation of metabolism has been neglected in vertebrate groups that have relatively little economic importance. The differences in body temperature, reliance on anaerobic metabolism, and great variety of activity levels make it difficult to generalize even within a reasonably defined taxonomic unit. A brief review of metabolism by non-pancreatic hormones in non-mammalian vertebrates is provided below.

1. Fishes

Lampreys exhibit hyperglycemia following treatment with either cortisol or epinephrine. Cortisol elevates liver glycogen, suggesting a gluconeogenic action. Insulin is hypoglycemic and a single injection can decrease plasma glucose levels significantly for several days. Hagfishes do not exhibit hyperglycemia to either cortisol or catecholamine treatment.

Chondrichthyean fishes have been studied less than have the jawless fishes, and few generalizations are possible. Blood sugar levels are relatively low in selachians but can be elevated with treatment by either ACTH or glucocorticoids, implying similar metabolic actions to those described in mammals.

Among teleosts, gluconeogenesis occurs mainly in the liver and kidney and is accelerated by high-protein diets or by starvation. Cortisol is the principal glucocorticoid secreted by the adrenocortical cells. In addition to its role as a mineralocorticoid, cortisol depletes lipid and protein stores and promotes gluconeogenesis as it does in mammals. High cortisol levels, for example, are associated with up to a 96% reduction in body fat and loss of more than half the body protein in spawning sockeye salmon. Catecholamines stimulate glycogenolysis, lipolysis, and gluconeogenesis. The possible role(s) of thyroid hormones (see Chapters 6, 7), is unclear at this time, but they do not appear to be important for regulating metabolism.

2. Amphibians

Corticosterone and, to a lesser extent, aldosterone are gluconeogenic and hyperglycemic in amphibians, but the primary role of these steroids as seen in fishes appears to be the regulation of ion and water balance. Specific gluconeogenic enzymes are activated by corticosteroids as well as are urea cycle enzymes associated with elimination of nitrogenous wastes generated from amino acid degradation. Epinephrine is a potent stimulator of glycogenolysis in both liver and muscle and therefore is hyperglycemic. Thyroid hormones can increase oxidative metabolism, but apparently only at higher temperatures; for example, 25°C (see Chapter 7), and any metabolic role is highly speculative.

3. Reptiles

The metabolism of reptiles and the roles of corticosteroids and catecholamines in regulating reptilian metabolism are poorly studied. Although there is little evidence to establish a gluconeogenic action in reptiles, there is some indirect evidence. Corticosteroids are hyperglycemic and favor deposition of glycogen in lizards, turtles, alligators, and snakes. Epinephrine is hyperglycemic in representatives of all major reptilian groups and promotes glycogenolysis in liver and glycogen deposition in alligator muscle. As reported for amphibians, thyroid hormones stimulate oxygen consumption in lizards at warmer temperatures (30°C) but not at lower temperatures (see Chapter 7).

4. Birds

Domestic birds exhibit all of the glycolytic, glycogenic, and glycogenolytic pathways for carbohydrate metabolism described for mammals. Because of the dependence of developing birds on lipid-rich yolk, the normal glycolytic and oxidative pathways are not important until after hatching.

Corticosterone is hyperglycemic and gluconeogenic primarily due to stimulation of protein catabolism. Corticosteroids also stimulate triacylglycerol (TAG) synthesis in the liver. These TAGs are transported to adipose tissue for storage, an important action during fattening prior to spring or fall migrations. This lipogenic action of corticosteroids is in marked contrast to the effects of glucocortioids in mammals and other vertebrates and may represent a special adaptation in long-distance migrators.

Epinephrine and norepinephrine are potent glycogenolytic and lipolytic hormones in birds. Catecholamines cause hepatic and muscle glycogenolysis that can lead to hyperglycemia. Thyroid hormones affect oxygen consumption and therefore have direct actions on metabolism and heat production.

IV. Summary

Regulation of feeding in non-mammals is similar to mammals although it has not been studied extensively in non-mammals. Orexigenic actions in fishes have been shown for ghrelin, NPY, galanin, and orexins. CCK_8, CRH, urotensin-I, CART, and PrRP are anorexic. Orexins stimulate feeding in anurans and leptin is present in newts as well as in reptiles. Urocortins are anorexic in amphibians. Ghrelin is present in gastric mucosa of a turtle. Leptin has been isolated from birds but orexins are ineffective, at least in chickens.

Comparative studies of GI hormones are limited primarily to demonstrations of the presence of immunoreactivity to antibodies prepared against various mammalian GI peptides. Some putative regulatory peptides have been isolated that are closely related to mammalian counterparts but their physiological roles are not clear. It appears that intestinal peptides with GI hormone activities occurred early in vertebrate evolution (class Agnatha) and some counterparts are in evidence among invertebrates as well.

Five patterns of pancreatic islet morphology can be distinguished in vertebrates: (1) cyclostome type; (2) primitive gnathostome type; (3) actinopterygian type; (4) lungfish type; and (5) tetrapod type. It is assumed that the most primitive anatomical arrangement for the endocrine pancreatic tissue occurs in lampreys as the follicles of Langerhans embedded in the gut lining. The equally if not more primitive hagfishes, however, have a definite endocrine pancreas. Bony fishes tend to have discrete islets but lack an acinar (exocrine) pancreas. Elasmobranchs, holocephalans, and *Latimeria* all exhibit the primitive gnathostome type of endocrine pancreas. Tetrapods have distinct pancreatic organs containing both acinar and islet tissues.

The most primitive function for insulin may be its effect on amino acid incorporation into protein. Glucose administration does not invoke insulin release in lampreys, lizards, or birds, and insulin stimulates only protein synthesis in hagfish liver. These observations suggest limited involvement of insulin in carbohydrate metabolism of non-mammals and that its hypoglycemic actions may be largely due to effects on protein and/or lipid metabolism. Furthermore, the effects of insulin on lipid metabolism may be largely a mammalian occurrence. Glucagon, glucagon-like peptides, pancreatic polypeptide, and SST are all present in nonmammals although their physiological roles are not clear.

Suggested Reading

Boorse, G. C., Crespi, E. J., Dautzenberg, F. M., and Denver, R. J. (2005). Urocortins of the South African clawed frog, *Xenopus laevis*: Conservation of structure and function in tetrapod evolution. *Endocrinology* **146**, 4851–4860.

Conlon, J. M., Reinecke, M., Thorndyke, M. C., and Falkmer, S. (1988). Insulin and other islet hormones (somatostatin, glucagon and PP) in the neuroendocrine system of some lower vertebrates and that of invertebrates—a minireview. *Horm. Metab. Res.* **20**, 406–410.

Conlon, J. M., Nielsen, P. F., Youson, J. H., and Potter, I. C. (1995). Proinsulin and somatostatin from the islet organ of the southern-hemisphere lamprey *Geotria australis*. *Gen. Comp. Endocr.* **100**, 413–422.

Conlon, J. M., Patterson, S., and Flatt, P. R. (2006). Major contributions of compoarative endocrinology to the development and exploitation of the incretin concept. *Journal of Experimental Zoology* **305A**, 781–786.

Galas, L., Vaudry, H., Braun, B., Van Den Pol, A. N., de Lecea, L., Sutcliffe, J. G., and Chartrel, N. (2001). Immunohistochemical localization and biochemical characterization of hypocretin/orexin-related peptides in the central nervous system of the frog, *Rana ridibunda*. *J. Comp. Neurol.* **429**, 242–252.

Gapp, D. A. (1987). Endocrine and related factors in the control of metabolism in nonmammalian vertebrates. *In* "Fundamentals of Comparative Vertebrate Endocrinology" (I. Chester-Jones, P. M. Ingleton, and J. G. Phillips, Eds.), pp. 509–660. Plenum, New York.

Kaiya, H., Sakata, I., Kojima, M., Hosoda, H., Sakai, T., and Kangawa, K. (2004). Structural determination and histochemical localization of ghrelin in the red-eared slider turtle, *Trachemys scripta elegans*. General and Compartive Endocrinology **138**, 50–57.

Kaiya, H., Sakata, I., Yamamoto, K., Koda, A., Sakai, T., Kangawa, K., and Kikuyama, S. (2006). Identification of immunoreactive plasma and stomach ghrelin and expression of stomach ghrelin mRNa in the bullfrog, Rana castesbeiana. *General and Comparative Endocrinology* **148**, 236–244.

Kawauchi, H. (2006). Functions of melanin-concentrating hormone in fish. *Journal of Experimental Zoology* **305A**, 751–760.

Ku, S.-K., Lee, H.-S., Koh, J.-K., Lee, J.-H. (2003). An immunohistochemical study on the neuropeptide-producing endocrine cells in the alimentary tract of the wrinkled frog, *Rana rugosa* (Ranidae). *Gen. Comp. Endocr.* **131**, 1–8.

Nelson, L. E. and Sheridan, M. A. (2006). Gastroenteropancreatic hormones and metabolism in fish. *General and Comparative Endocrinology* **148**, 116–124.

Reinecke, M., Hoog, A., Ostenson, C.-G., Efendic, S., Grimelius, L., and Falkmer, S. (1991). Phylogenetic aspects of pancreastatin- and chromogranin-like immunoreactive cells in the gastro-entero-pancreatic neuroendocrine system of vertebrates. *Gen. Comp. Endocr.* **83**, 167–182.

Reinecke, M., Broger, I., Brun, R., Zapf, J., and Maake, C. (1995). Immunohistochemical localization of insulin-like growth factor I and II in the endocrine pancreas of birds, reptiles, and Amphibia. *Gen. Comp. Endocr.* **100**, 385–396.

Sheridan, M. (1994). Mini review: Regulation of lipid metabolism in poikilothermic vertebrates. *Comp. Biochem. Physiol.* **107B**, 495–508.

Volkoff, H., Canosa, L. F., Unniappan, S., Cerda-Reverter, J. M., Bernier, N. J., Kelly, S. P. and Peter, R. E. (2005). Neuropeptides and the control of food intake in fish. *Gen.Comp. Endocr.* **142**, 3–19.

White, A. M., Secor, S. M., and Conlon, J. M. (1999). Insulin and proglucagon-dervied peptides from the horned frog. *Ceratophrys omata* (Anura: Leptodactylidae). *General and Comparative Endocrinology* **115**, 143–154.

Youson, J. H., Mahrouki, A. A., Amemiya, Y., Graham, L. C., Montpetit, C. J., and Irwin, D. M. (2006). The fish endocrine pancreas: Review, new data, and future research directions in ontogeny and phylogeny. *General and Comparative Endocrinology* **148**, 105–115.

14

Bioregulation of Calcium and Phosphate Homeostasis

Physiologists often focus on the regulation Na$^+$ and K$^+$ ion levels because of their importance in maintaining membrane potentials and their importance for neuronal and muscle function. However, calcium and phosphate also are extremely important for the regulation of many basic body functions including the release of neurotransmitters and other bioregulators from cells as well as the mechanics of muscle contraction. They are involved in the structure of bones and teeth that serve as the major reservoirs for maintaining plasma and interstitial fluid levels of these ions. Although inorganic calcium and phosphate are not related closely with respect to most of their essential roles in vertebrate physiology, they are regulated by some of the same hormones. Consequently, a discussion of the endocrine regulation of calcium homeostasis cannot be divorced entirely from the regulation of phosphate. A discussion of calcium and phosphate homeostasis in mammals will set the standard for making comparisons to other vertebrates.

I. Importance of Calcium and Phosphate

A. Calcium Homeostasis

Calcium levels in extracellular fluids and in the cytosol of cells must be regulated precisely if normal body functions are to be maintained. In addition to its role in bone and tooth construction, calcium ions have other important roles to play (Table 14-1). They are responsible for excitation and contraction of muscle cells and are important in the induction of spontaneous excitations of cardiac pacemaker cells. Calcium ions are essential for exocytosis of secretion granules in neurons and glandular cells and serve as second messengers in many target cells. Certain key metabolic enzymes are activated by calcium ions that can also serve as cofactors for several blood clotting proteins (factors VII, IX, X).

The calcium level in adult mammalian blood plasma is maintained at about 10 mg/dl or approximately 2.5 mM/liter. About half of this calcium is free in the plasma in ionic form (Ca^{2+}), and the remainder is bound to circulating proteins (40%) or occurs in other chemical complexes (10%). It is this free ionic calcium in the blood that is essential to so many important life processes because it can be exchanged readily with other extracellular fluids and cells. About 90% of the protein-bound calcium is linked to albumin, and this binding is pH-sensitive. Acute acidosis decreases binding and elevates ionic plasma calcium. Acute alkalosis increases binding and reduces free plasma calcium.

After birth, calcium is obtained in the diet, absorbed through the small intestine, deposited in bones and teeth, or excreted via urine or feces. Urinary excretion of calcium is directly proportional to plasma levels, and little calcium is excreted unless plasma calcium levels exceed normal. Calcium deposited in bone serves as a reservoir to provide adequate plasma Ca^{2+} for minute-to-minute regulation of body needs and during acute or chronic periods of dietary deprivation. Human body calcium levels vary according to size and age (Table 14-2).

B. Calcium Regulation

Blood calcium homeostasis is maintained by the cooperative actions of the bones and teeth and the intestine that together serve as internal and external sources of calcium (see Figure 14-1). The kidneys prevent loss

Table 14-1. Some Physiological Roles for Calcium and Phosphate

Roles for calcium	Roles for phosphate
Structural component (with phosphate) of bones, teeth	Structural component (with calcium) of bones, teeth
Necessary for contraction of skeletal, smooth, and cardiac muscle	Activator of enzymes from inactive form
Maintenance of membrane potentials in some neurons	Buffer in blood and other body fluids
Unique role in membrane potentials of pacemaker cells	Essential component for energy storage in chemical bonds of ATP, creatine phosphate, etc.
Second messenger in hormonal and neurocrine mechanisms of action	Essential component of nucleic acids
Role in exocytosis of secretory products from cells	Essential component of phospholipids in cell membranes
Necessary cofactor for certain enzymes	Involved in second messenger formation
Component of intercellular matrices (e.g., basement membrane)	Necessary for metabolism of glucose and other carbohydrates

Table 14-2. Calcium Content of Human Body[a]

Age (years)	Body weight (kg)	Calcium content (g)
1	10.6	100
5	19.1	219
10	33.3	396
15	55.0	806
20	67.0	1078

[a] Irving, J. T. (1973). "Calcium and Phosphorus Metabolism." Academic Press, New York.

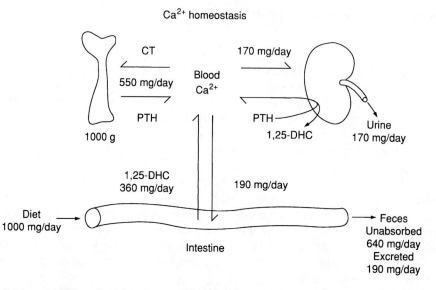

Figure 14-1. **Endocrine regulation of calcium homeostasis.** PTH and 1,25-DHC are hypercalcemic agents and CT is the only hypocalcemic agent protecting the skeleton during periods of griowth, pregnancy, or lactation. The skeleton represents the major reservoir of calcium ions in mammals. For humans, a daily intake of 1000 mg Ca^{2+}/day is necessary to offset what is lost normally through urine and feces.

of calcium to the urine or can allow excretion of excess calcium. The intestine also excretes calcium. Calcium homeostasis is maintained by three hormones in mammals. **Parathyroid hormone (PTH)** secreted by the **parathyroid glands** causes both calcium release from bones as well as deposition. It also favors calcium reabsorption by the kidneys. **Calcitonin (CT)** from C-cells embedded in the thyroid gland (see Chapter 6) or the parathyroids (dogs) promotes deposition of calcium into bone. A steroid derivative of vitamin D known as **1,25-dihydroxycholecalciferol (1,25-DHC)** or **Vitamin D₃** is secreted by the combined activities of skin, liver, and kidney (see below) and stimulates intestinal uptake of calcium.

C. Phosphate Homeostasis

Phosphate, like calcium, is an essential component of bones and teeth. Approximately 80% of the total body phosphate is sequestered in the skeleton as calcium phosphate. In addition, many essential molecules contain phosphate, including structural phospholipids in cellular membranes, nucleic acids, nucleotides, and hexose phosphates. Furthermore, phosphate is indispensable for energy storage within cells in the form of ATP or creatine phosphate. Hydrolysis of ATP or guanosine triphosphate (GTP) to form cyclic adenosine 3', 5'-monophosphate (cAMP) or cyclic guanosine 3', 5'-monophosphate (cGMP), respectively, is necessary for mediating the actions of many hormones, for neural transmission, and for many other cellular processes. The actions of protein kinases determine the presence or absence of phosphate that activates or inactivates key enzymes in metabolic pathways (see Chapter 12). Although phosphate ions play a minor role as buffers of hydrogen ions in most body fluids, they are the major buffer system in urine.

It is rare that phosphate becomes a limiting factor for an organism, and the usual phosphate disturbances in mammals are a result of excessive levels of phosphate. Inorganic phosphate (Pi) in mammalian plasma is generally about 3.1 mg/dl (about 1.0 mmol/L). Most of this phosphate (about 80%) is in the form of HPO_4^{-2} with almost 20% occurring as $H_2PO_4^{-1}$ and only a trace as PO_4^{-3}. Henceforth, the chemical formula HPO_4^{-2} will be used to represent all of the phosphate ions.

In normal plasma, about 90% of the Pi is free ionic (filterable) phosphate, and about 10% is bound to the plasma proteins. In addition to Pi, plasma contains considerable amounts of lipid-bound phosphate and esterified phosphate so that total plasma phosphate is actually about 12.5 mg/dl. Phosphate values vary considerably with diet, age, and metabolic state, however, and it is difficult to provide a "normal" value without specifying the conditions under which this "normal" occurs.

D. Interrelationship of Ca^{2+} and HPO_4^{-2}

Calcium and phosphate are regulated in such a way that the product of the free plasma concentrations of Ca^{2+} and HPO_4^{-2} ($[Ca^{2+}][HPO_4^{-2}]$) equals some constant called k. This constant, however, may change according to differing physiological states or pathological conditions. For example, k is greater in growing mammals than it is in adults. This relationship between Ca^{2+} and HPO_4^{-2} implies that if there is an increase in Ca^{2+}, a corresponding decrease in HPO_4^{-2} should follow. Likewise, an increase in HPO_4^{-2} should cause a decrease in Ca^{2+}. This generalization is useful to illustrate some of the relationships that exist between the regulatory mechanisms governing these ions. Minute-to-minute adjustments of Ca^{2+} and HPO_4^{-2} levels in extracellular fluids are accomplished primarily through a combination of bone destruction (resorption) or formation, absorption of dietary calcium by the small intestine, and renal excretion of phosphate.

E. Bone Formation and Resorption in Mammals

In bones and teeth, calcium phosphate occurs in the form of small submicroscopic crystals deposited upon an organic matrix composed primarily of **collagen fibers**. These crystals assume a uniform structural and complex chemical form known as **hydroxyapatite crystals**. Construction of bone through formation of calcium phosphate is not understood completely, but some of the major features are well accepted. Bone formation may involve **apatite formation** (deposition of new hydroxyapatite crystal) or simply **mineral accumulation** (the additional growth of existing crystals). Exchange of Ca^{2+}, HPO_4^{-2}, and water can occur between the surface of these crystals and the extracellular fluids. This exchange is inversely proportional to the size of the crystal. Thus, larger crystals contain considerable amounts of calcium phosphate that cannot engage in free exchange with the extracellular fluids. About 99% of bone calcium phosphate is found in these larger, nonexchangeable stable or **diffusion-locked crystals**.

The specific process of bone formation and growth also involves a number of local chemical factors that are responsible for collagen matrix formation, cartilage matrix deposition, and formation of hydroxyapatite crystals as well as cellular replication and differentiation. Cells known as **osteoblasts** (literally, bone-forming cells) are responsible for bone formation. (The homologous cell in teeth is termed an odontoblast.). The osteoblasts comprise the **endosteal membrane** that lines the cavities within bone, and they synthesize the collagen matrix upon which apatite formation occurs. The factors controlling osteoblast activities are poorly understood. Some osteoblasts give rise to **osteocytes** that become completely surrounded by bone except for minute channels through which the osteocytes communicate with one another. There seems to be little agreement on the role for osteocytes in calcium-phosphate metabolism, but they may be important targets for hormonal regulation.

Resorption of bone may involve either removal of the collagen matrix and/or solubilization of hydroxyapatite crystals with consequent release of Ca^{2+} and HPO_4^{-2} but both processes usually occur. Another bone cell, the **osteoclast** (literally, bone destroying) is primarily responsible for bone resorption. The osteoclast (Figures 14-2 and 14-3) is a large, multinucleate cell and is easy to distinguish from uninucleate osteoblasts or osteocytes. Osteoclasts arise from blood cell progenitors. These precursor cells interact with osteoblasts that induce them to differentiate into osteoclasts (Figure 14-4). Mature osteoclasts are characterized by possession of a number of unique biochemical features (e.g., presence of the enzymes carbonic anhydrase and cathepsin).

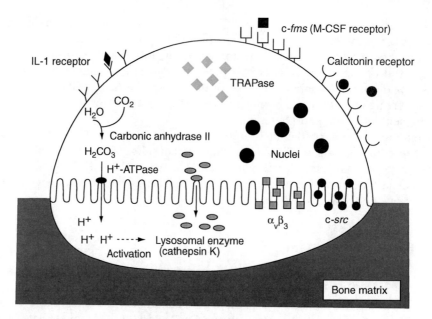

Figure 14-2. **An osteoclast (OC).** This multinucleate bone-destroying cell is a target for calcitonin that inhibits its activity. Osteoclast activity and the ratio of osteoclasts to osteoblasts is increased by PTH, but indirectly (see text). Note the ruffled border of the cell adjacent to the resorption space (stippled) that is involved in the active resorption of Ca^{2+}. [Reprinted with permission of the publisher from Martin, T. J., and Udagawa, N. Hormonal regulation of osteoclast function. *Trends Endocr. Metab.* **9**, 6–12. Copyright 1998 Elsevier Science Inc.]

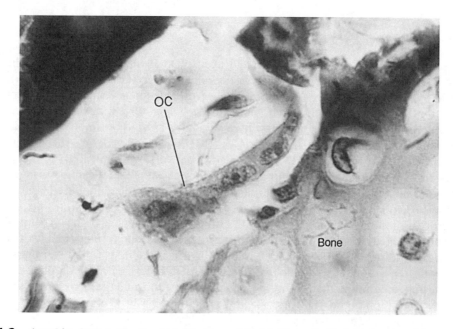

Figure 14-3. **A multinucleate turtle osteoclast.** (Courtesy of the late Nancy B. Clark, University of Connecticut, Storrs.)

II. Endocrine Regulation of Calcium and Phosphate Homeostasis in Mammals

Three hormones regulate calcium and phosphate homeostasis in mammals as mentioned earlier. Parathyroid hormone is a **hypercalcemic factor**; that is, its actions can cause an elevation in the level of plasma calcium.

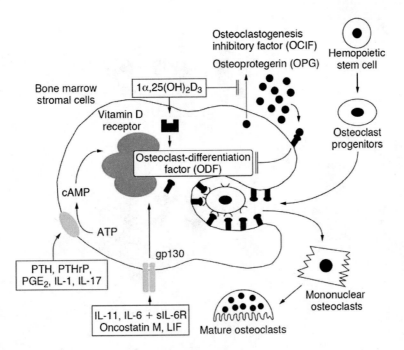

Figure 14-4. **An osteoblast.** Bone-forming osteoblasts are targets for PTH. Stimulated osteoblasts transform osteoclast progenitor cells into mature osteoclasts. [Reprinted with permission of the publisher from Martin, T. J., and Udagawa, N. Hormonal regulation of osteoclast function. *Trends. Endocr. Metab.* **9,** 6–12. Copyright 1998 Elsevier Science Inc.]

Its secretion is control by plasma calcium levels. Calcitonin is a **hypocalcemic factor**, and its release is related primarily to changes in plasma calcium. One major site of action for PTH is bone, where it may stimulate calcium release from bone (bone resorption) and release both calcium and phosphate ions into the circulation (see Figure 14-1). It also can stimulate calcium deposition in bone. Parathyroid hormone also increases calcium reabsorption by the nephron as well as the secretion of phosphate into the urine resulting in a decrease in plasma phosphate levels and a concomitant increase in urinary phosphate.

The effects of PTH on calcium homeostasis are linked closely to the actions of the third regulatory hormone, 1,25-DHC. Absorption of calcium from the gut lumen is stimulated by 1,25-DHC that also influences the actions of PTH on bone and kidney. Furthermore, as discussed later, PTH influences the production of 1,25-DHC by the kidney.

A. The Parathyroid Glands and PTH

Although the parathyroid glands had been observed previously, Sandstrom rediscovered and named them in 1880. In many species the parathyroids, which develop like the thyroid from pharyngeal tissues (Figure 14-5), are embedded within the thyroid glands, for example, in the mouse, cat, and man. In other mammals, such as goats and rabbits, they are separate glands located near the thyroid. Some mammals have more than four separate parathyroid glands, and accessory parathyroid tissue is not uncommon. Thyroidectomy may result in lowered plasma Ca^{2+} levels in some species because of simultaneous removal of the embedded parathyroid. Decreasing plasma calcium by artificial means can increase PTH secretion several fold. This can be accomplished by infusion of calcium-chelating (calcium-binding) agents such as EDTA.

The parathyroid glands developmentally arise from pharyngeal endoderm. However, the parathyroid **chief cells** that secrete PTH arise from the neuroectoderm as shown first in the frog *Rana temporaria*. Chief cells are part of the amine precursor uptake and decarboxylation (APUD) series of peptide-secreting cells (see Chapter 4). Indirect evidence also supports a similar origin for PTH-secreting cells in birds and mammals. Chief cells are cuboidal with no unique cytological features other than the presence of granules containing immunoreactive PTH. They are the dominant cellular type and comprise about 99% of the parathyroid's cellular population in most species. Chief cells exhibit β-adrenergic receptors suggesting some neural influence

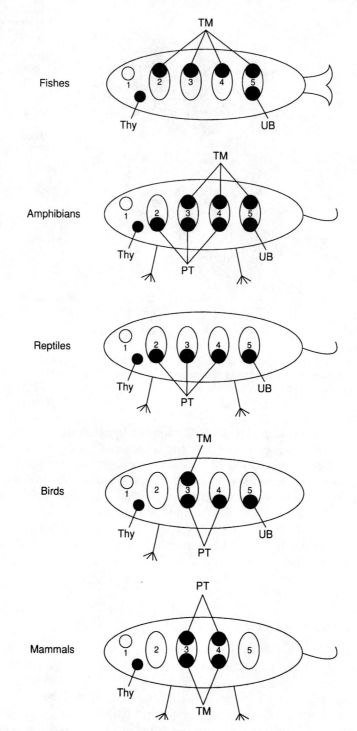

Figure 14-5. **Embryonic derivatives of the pharyngeal pouches in vertebrates**. The numbers refer to pouch number with anterior to the left. Pouch 1 remains only as the spiracle (elasmobranchs) or the eustachian tube. The thyroid (Thy) actually develops from the pharynx floor between the first and second pouches. Parathyroids (PT) appear first in amphibians. In reptiles, the origin of the thymus (TM) may be from pouches 2 and 3 (lizards), 3 and 4 (turtles), or 4 and 5 (snakes). In mammals, the origins of parathyroids and thymus are reversed. The ultimobranchial body (UB) is absent in mammal, and the calcitonin-secreting cells migrate to the thyroid instead of the UB.

on PTH release may exist. Glucocorticoid receptors also are present and when activated result in enhanced PTH release. Estrogens may diminish the response of the chief cells to lowered plasma calcium.

In a few species, such as deer, the parathyroids are composed exclusively of chief cells. However, in most species, a second cell type called an **oxyphil** is usually present in the parathyroids. Oxyphils are eosinophilic cells rich in mitochondria (hence their name). The function of the oxyphil and the significance for its large number of mitochondria are unknown. Oxyphils represent only about 1% of the total parathyroid cells.

B. Parathyroid Hormone

Mammalian PTH has been isolated and characterized from several species. It is a large polypeptide consisting of 84 amino acids (Figure 14-6). Apparently all of the biological activity resides in the first 34 amino acids. Synthesis of PTH occurs in two steps. **Preproparathyroid hormone (PreProPTH)** consisting of 115 amino acid residues is synthesized on the ribosomes of the rough endoplasmic reticulum (RER) but is rapidly cleaved at the NH_2-terminus to **proparathyroid hormone (ProPTH)** as it enters the cisterna of the endoplasmic reticulum. ProPTH consists of 90 amino acids and travels through the cisterna to the Golgi apparatus where the remaining 6 NH_2-terminal residues of the prohormone are removed. The resulting PTH is then packaged into storage vesicles to await release.

Numerous fragments of parathyroid hormone appear in the circulation. At first it was assumed they were formed from endopeptidase activity in the plasma, but we now know that these fragments are largely formed within the PTH cells. The biological half-life for PTH is about 20 minutes in cattle or rats.

C. Regulation of PTH Secretion

Earlier (Chapter 3), we emphasized the role of increased calcium in endocrine cell secretion of hormones through exocytosis. However, unlike most secretory cells, parathyroid cells release PTH when extracellular and intracellular calcium levels are minimal. Release of PTH normally occurs at a high rate but secretion of active hormone is decreased by elevated plasma calcium levels primarily through increased degradation of PTH prior to secretion. High levels of extracellular calcium causes the PTH cell to secrete a higher proportion of inactive fragments and less bioactive hormone (Figure 14-7).

Although the precise mechanisms for regulating PTH secretion have not been worked out completely, several cellular events are established. Low intracellular calcium is correlated with activated protein kinase C (PKC) that is a known participant in cellular regulation (see Chapter 3). High extracellular calcium induces formation of inositol trisphosphate (IP_3) that releases intracellular stores of calcium ions that activate neutral proteases called **calpains** and/or activate lysosomal hydrolytic enzymes. Degradation of intracellular PTH is accomplished by the actions of these enzymes. Furthermore, calpains can cause down-regulation of PKC that would prevent PTH secretion. Both calcium ions and 1,25-DHC have been shown to reduce PTH synthesis possibly through direct effects on transcription. Since PTH can elevate plasma levels of both calcium and 1,25-DHC, their effects on PTH release can be considered feedback.

	1	6	10	16	21	26	31
Bovine PTH	AVSEI	QFMHN	LGKHL	SSMER	VEWLR	KKLQD	VHNF---
Rat PTH	AVSEI	QLMHN	LGKHL	ASMER	VEWLR	KKLQD	VHNF---
Human PTH	SVSEI	QLMHN	LGKHL	NSMER	MQWLR	KKLQD	VHNF---
Human PTHrP	AVSEH	QLLHD	KGKSI	QDLRR	RFFLH	HHIAE	IHTA---

Figure 14-6. **Amino acid sequences of mammalian PTHs and PTHrP.** Only the first 34 amino acids are shown. Chicken PTHrP differs from human PTHrP at positions 23, 25–27, and 29–32. Explanation of the amino acid abbreviations is provided in Appendix C.

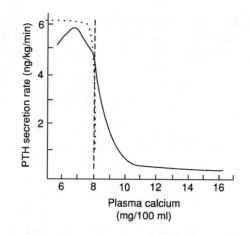

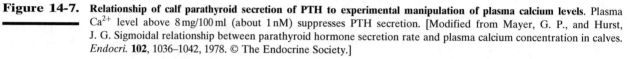

Figure 14-7. **Relationship of calf parathyroid secretion of PTH to experimental manipulation of plasma calcium levels.** Plasma Ca^{2+} level above 8 mg/100 ml (about 1 nM) suppresses PTH secretion. [Modified from Mayer, G. P., and Hurst, J. G. Sigmoidal relationship between parathyroid hormone secretion rate and plasma calcium concentration in calves. *Endocri.* **102**, 1036–1042, 1978. © The Endocrine Society.]

Extracellular calcium may open calcium channels in the chief cell membrane by binding to a G-protein-linked membrane receptor system. There is also evidence to support a direct action of calcium ions on membrane calcium channels. PTH release is not directly influenced by fluctuations in phosphate levels.

1. Parathyroidectomy Effects

In all cases, parathyroidectomy causes a reduction in plasma Ca^{2+} leading to detrimental muscular effects. As Ca^{2+} levels decrease, hyperexcitability of motor neurons and skeletal muscles occurs, resulting in twitches, spasms, and, in extreme cases, violent convulsions. This condition is known as **low-calcium-induced tetany**. If prolonged contractions (tetany) of the respiratory muscles occur, death due to asphyxiation may result. The severity of these neuromuscular effects, however, differs markedly with respect to species involved and under various physiological conditions. For example, exercise raises the body temperature and increases the breathing rate, causing a reduction of blood CO_2. Reduced blood CO_2 in turn alters blood pH (alkalosis) and retards ionization of Ca^{2+}. This further reduction in Ca^{2+} in a parathyroidectomized animal may precipitate a tetanic seizure. Animals on diets low in Ca^{2+} and high in HPO_4^{-2} exhibit tetany following parathyroidectomy more readily than do animals on normal diets. Hyperventilation reduces CO_2 levels and can induce tetany especially when calcium levels are already low.

2. Parathyroid Hormone-Related Peptide

A peptide with hypercalcemic activity first was isolated from patients exhibiting human hypercalcemia of malignancy (HHM) as a result of cancer. Because this protein had considerable N-terminal overlap with PTH (Figure 14-6), it was named **parathyroid hormone-related peptide (PTHrP)**. This peptide has proven to be a natural product of many cell types by a gene believed to have been derived from an ancestral gene that also gave rise to the PTH gene. This gene can be active in more than 20 tissues in humans including the heart, arterial smooth muscle, lactating mammary gland, the uterus, and the amnion and parathyroid glands of the fetus. It also stimulates growth in several cell lines including renal carcinoma, fibroblasts, osteoblasts, chondrocytes, and lymphocytes.

During fetal development, PTHrP is synthesized by the amnion and accumulates in amniotic fluid. It is also a major product of the fetal parathyroid. PTHrP may modulate transfer of Ca^{2+} across the fetal-placental unit and may be responsible for the high Ca^{2+} levels observed in fetal as compared to maternal plasma.

Table 14-3. Approximate Levels of PTHrP in Milk and Infant Formulas[a,b]

Type of milk/formula	PTHrP (ng eq/mL)
Fresh milk	
Human	50
Bovine	96
Commercial milk	
Whole milk	81
Nonfat milk	118
Buttermilk, chocolate milk	5–7
Milk-based formula	
Six brand names	1–30
Soy-based formula	Undetectable

[a] Using these contrived units, plasma PTHrP in an HHM patient would be 0.08 ng eq/L. This means that PTHrP in breast milk is about 1000× more concentrated than in plasma and about 10,000× greater than normal plasma PTHrP.

[b] Data from de Papp, A. E., and Stewart, A. F. (1993). *Trends Endocr. Metab.* **4**, 181–187.

PTHrP gene activity appears in the rat lactating mammary gland within 24 hours after birth and remains elevated during suckling. Removal of the pups causes a drop within 1–2 hours and PTHrP production ceases by 4 hours. Resumption of nursing reinstates lactating levels of PTHrP.

In humans, most but not all (12 of 19) breast-feeding women exhibit elevated plasma PTHrP (2–8 pmol/L), but PTHrP is absent from plasma of bottle-feeding mothers (0 of 16 examined). There are considerable amounts of PTHrP in human and bovine milk, suggesting it may be important for maintaining calcium homeostasis in newborns. Much lower levels of PTHrP are present in commercial, milk-based infant formulas, and PTHrP is absent from soy-based formulas (see Table 14-3).

PTHrP causes relaxation of both vascular (i.e., hypotensive) and nonvascular smooth muscle. During pregnancy, PTHrP may be an important relaxant of smooth muscle, and it decreases in the uterus prior to birth. It also has been shown to relax smooth muscle of vascular tissue, urinary bladder, and the stomach although a physiological role for PTHrP in these tissues is not established.

D. The C-Cells and CT

The **C-cells** (parafollicular) cells of the mammalian thyroid gland have been identified as the source of CT in most mammals. However, the actual origin of these cells is unclear. The most generally accepted origin is that proposed by Godwin suggesting that these cells originated from the ultimobranchial body that develops from the sixth pharyngeal pouch (endoderm, Figure 14-5). These ultimobranchial cells become incorporated into the thyroid gland of mammals just as parathyroids frequently do. The ultimobranchial body remains as a distinct separate structure in other vertebrate groups.

Like the chief cells of the parathyroids, the C-cells of the mammalian thyroid exhibit APUD characteristics. Some elegant studies employing cellular chimeras of chicken and quail embryonic tissues have confirmed the origin of the CT-secreting cells of the ultimobranchial body from neural crest cells. C-cells also contain somatostatin (SST) and ultrastructurally resemble the D-cells found in the intestinal lining. It has been suggested that SST released along with CT may play an autocrine or paracrine role.

1. Calcitonin

Production of a potent mammalian hypocalcemic factor by cells of the parathyroid gland was first reported by Copp and associates who named it calcitonin (CT). Other investigators provided evidence that the source of this hypocalcemic factor was the C-cells of the thyroid gland and suggested the alternative name of **thyrocalcitonin**

	1	6	11	16	21	26	31
Mammals							
Porcine	CSNLS	TCVLS	AYWRN	LNNFH	RFSGM	GFGPE	T P-NH$_2$
Bovine	CSNLS	TCVLS	AYWLD	LNNYH	RFSGM	GFGPE	T P-NH$_2$
Human	CGNLS	TCMLG	TYTQD	FNKFH	TFPQT	AIGVG	A P-NH$_2$
Rat	CGNLS	TCMLG	TYTQD	LNKFH	TFPQT	SIGVG	A P-NH$_2$
Teleosts							
Salmon-I	CSNLS	TCVLS	KLSQE	LHKLQ	TYPRT	NTGSG	T P-NH$_2$
Salmon-II	CSNLS	TCVLS	KLSQN	LHKLQ	TFPRT	NTGAG	V P-NH$_2$
Salmon-III	CSNLS	TCMLS	KLSQN	LHKLQ	TFPRT	NTGAG	V P-NH$_2$
Birds							
Chicken	CASLS	TCVLS	KLSQE	LHKLQ	TYPRT	DVGAG	T P-NH$_2$

Figure 14-8. **Amino acid sequences for calcitonins (CTs).** The sequence of the first 10 residues is highly conserved when comparing teleosts, birds, and mammals. The presence of valine (V) at position 8 increases the biological activity of the molecule 4 to 5X. Hence, salmon-I is more potent in humans than is human CT. Note also that human and rat CTs are more like each other than like bovine, porcine, or ovine (not shown), which are all similar. Explanation of the amino acid abbreviations is provided in Appendix C. [Modified from Matsumoto, A., and Ishii, S. (1992). "An Atlas of Endocrine Organs." Japanese Society for Comparative Endocrinology and Springer-Verlag, Berlin.]

to reflect its origin. It was soon discovered that ultimobranchial glands of sharks and chickens contained CT and that C-cells of the thyroid were of ultimobranchial origin.

Mammalian CT is a small, single-chain peptide of 32 amino acids with a disulfide bond linking residues 1 and 7. There are no active fragments of CT, and the entire molecule is necessary for biological activity. The amino acid sequence for some CT molecules is provided in Figure 14-8. It is cleaved from a prohormone of 136 amino acids. Circulating levels of CT in humans are reported from 5–100 pg/ml with a short biological half-life (5 min) related to the fact that all fragments of CT are inactive.

The CT gene product may be processed through several mRNA pathways. This results in formation of several peptides known as calcitonin gene-related peptides (CGRPs). CGRPs have no CT-like activity but may play other physiological roles (see Chapter 12).

E. Skin, Liver, Kidney, and 1,25-DHC

The actions of PTH on bone and possibly kidney require the steroid 1,25-DHC as does intestinal absorption of calcium. The first steps in the formation of 1,25-DHC involve the conversion of cholesterol to 7-dehydrocholesterol and then to **cholecalciferol (= vitamin D$_3$)** by the skin (see Figure 3-33). Conversion of cholesterol to 7-dehydrocholesterol occurs in the presence of adequate sunlight. This chemical transformation, 7-dehydrocholesterol to cholecalciferol, is a two-step process. The first step occurs quickly in the presence of ultraviolet (UV) light, and the second step is a temperature-dependent isomerization that requires several days. Penetration of the skin by certain wavelengths of UV light is strongly dependent on the angle of incidence of sunlight (influenced by time of day, season, and latitude) as well as by cloud cover and air pollution. Furthermore, window glass absorbs UV light effectively and reduces cholecalciferol synthesis. The brown skin pigment melanin also absorbs UV light and decreases cholecalciferol synthesis. Prolonged exposure of skin to sunlight not only increases melanin synthesis but causes cholesterol to be converted primarily to inert steroids known as lumisterol and tachysterol instead of to cholecalciferol. The lack of melanin pigment that evolved in northern Europeans may have served as an adaptation to increase UV penetration and hence enhancement of cholecalciferol synthesis as an adaptation for living in northern latitudes.

Transport of cholecalciferol to the liver is facilitated by a binding protein in the plasma that has a high affinity only for the isomerized cholecalciferol. Cholecalciferol is converted by the liver to **25-hydroxycholecalciferol (25-HC)** and then by the kidney to 1,25-DHC (see Chapter 3, Figure 3-32). Circulating levels of 25-HC reported for humans are between 7 and 42 ng/ml with an extensive biological half-life of about 15 days.

The kidney converts 25-HC primarily to 1,25-DHC. Some 24,25-DHC is made as well but is of little importance because 1,25-DHC is 100 to 1000X more potent. This final conversion to 1,25-DHC is stimulated by PTH. Circulating levels of 20–50 pg/ml of 1,25-DHC are reported for humans. These low levels are largely a product of its biological half-life of only 3 hr. During pregnancy, the placenta also will synthesize 1,25-DHC that augments uptake of dietary calcium for fetal growth.

In addition to its essential role in calcium absorption, 1,25-DHC has been implicated directly in muscle function and has been linked to a number of pathological conditions including autoimmune diseases. Older adults with 1,25-DHC insufficiency exhibit depressed muscular function associated with the lower limbs. Not only is locomotion impaired, but these people are more prone to falling that adults with higher 1,25-DHC levels. Lowered 1,25-DHC decreased some functions of lymphocytes and has been correlated with increased incidences of disease including cancer (prostrate, breast, colon), type 1 diabetes (see Chapter 12), multiple sclerosis, and others.

III. Interactions of PTH, CT, and 1,25-DHC

The major daily disturbance to calcium homeostasis is the influx of Ca^{2+} following ingestion of a meal. Periods of rapid growth cause an additional demand for dietary calcium as do pregnancy and lactation. The small intestine, kidney, and bone are the primary sites where these regulatory hormones (PTH, CT, and 1,25-DHC) produce their actions during times of calcium excess or deficiency to maintain calcium homeostasis (see Figure 14-1).

A. Calcium and Phosphate Regulation in Bone

Minute-to-minute regulation of plasma calcium and indirectly of plasma phosphate may reside in the activity of **osteocytes** embedded permanently in the bone matrix. PTH may cause **osteocytic osteolysis** (one form of bone resorption) through direct action on the osteocytes. This effect may be dependent on an interaction between PTH and 1,25-DHC. In contrast, major disturbances such as occur during growth, pregnancy, or lactation involve the interactions of PTH and CT on osteoclasts and osteoblasts.

Parathyroid hormone appears to stimulate osteoclast activity, and chronic elevation of PTH is correlated with an increase in the number of osteoclasts. However, these effects are indirect because the osteoclast has no receptors for PTH although it is well endowed with CT receptors. In fact, it is the osteoblast that is the target for PTH. In addition to PTH, PTHrP and 1,25-DHC also promote osteoclast formation. Differentiation of osteoclasts is then controlled by the physical interaction (cell-to-cell contact) between osteoblasts and osteoclast progenitor cells. Several paracrine regulators, such as interleukin-6 and interleukin-11, are necessary for the differentiation and proliferation of osteoclasts (see Figure 14-4). It is the production of hydrolytic lysosomal enzymes by osteoclasts that destroys both mineral and bone matrix components of bone and is responsible for bone resorption and release of Ca^{2+} and phosphate to the plasma.

Another hypothesis concerning PTH action on bone resorption is focused on PTH effects on the bone-forming osteoblasts. According to this hypothesis, the osteoblasts possess a pumping mechanism for calcium transport. PTH, through activation of adenylyl cyclase and cAMP formation, increases the flux of Ca^{2+} into the osteoblast from the bone surface and out of the osteoblast on the blood side of the endosteal membrane. There is evidence to suggest that, at normal physiological levels, PTH stimulates bone formation rather than bone resorption through an increase in osteoblast activity. Whereas constant infusion of PTH causes bone resorption, intermittent application of PTH can actually stimulate bone growth through osteoblast action.

Although CT may influence osteoblast functions to a limited extent, its major action appears to be a direct inhibition of the osteoclast. This role for CT is especially important during pregnancy, where CT protects the maternal skeleton while directing dietary calcium directly to the fetus.

B. Regulation of Calcium Uptake in the Intestine

Calcium uptake by the intestinal mucosal cell is dependent upon a **calcium-binding protein** within these cells that is linked to a calcium-activated ATPase. Calcium is actively absorbed by this binding protein-ATPase complex at the mucosal surface that is in contact with the lumen of the gut. Once in the cell, these calcium ions are transported to the opposite (serosal) border of the cell where calcium ions diffuse into the interstitial fluid and then into the blood capillaries. The negatively charged phosphate ions passively follow the movements of Ca^{2+}. Synthesis of both the calcium-binding protein and the calcium-activated ATPase are stimulated by 1,25-DHC.

No role has been hypothesized for CT in this intestinal mechanism for calcium uptake. Following the influx of Ca^{2+} ions, however, calcitonin may be released in response to the increase in plasma Ca^{2+}, but it may also be released by gastrin, a gastrointestinal hormone released from the gastric mucosa during the early phase of digestion of a meal (see Chapter 12). This increased level of CT inhibits the action of bone osteoclasts and favors addition of the absorbed dietary Ca^{2+} to the bone matrix that can be stimulated by PTH.

Calcitonin becomes indispensable during pregnancy and lactation with respect to Ca^{2+} mobilization. Its role is apparently to protect the maternal skeleton from excessive destruction in meeting the calcium requirements of fetus or neonate, respectively. The relative importance of CT in different species varies markedly according to the precise demands for maternal calcium.

C. Calcium and Phosphate Regulation in Kidney

The stimulation of calcium reabsorption by the kidney may be the most important physiological action of PTH, although some investigators believe the increased excretion of phosphate is equally or possibly more important. PTH also increases the enzymatic formation of 1,25-DHC in kidney and thus may enhance intestinal calcium absorption indirectly. Elevated 1,25-DHC feeds back and inhibits PTH secretion. Estrogens and prolactin (PRL) also enhance formation of 1,25-DHC, and these actions may be essential in pregnant and lactating mammals, respectively, for conserving calcium ions. Although CT antagonizes the action of PTH on bone resorption, it apparently does not influence renal processes in normal animals when present at physiological levels.

D. Other Hormones and Calcium-Phosphate Homeostasis

Estrogens, androgens, glucocorticoids, and thyroid hormones have direct and indirect effects on mineral homeostasis (see Table 14-4). In addition, GH has indirect effects through production of insulin-like growth factors (IGFs).

Although the effects of estrogens and androgens bring about cessation of long bone growth at puberty, these hormones also have important stimulatory effects on osteoblast activity, especially in adults. Estrogens not only protect the skeleton from resorption but enhance the reabsorption of calcium by the kidney and increase the production of 1,25-DHC that aids dietary uptake of calcium. Androgens are thought to play a similar role in males. The decrease in gonadal steroids with menopause or adrenopause (see Chapter 10) has serious implications of calcium homeostasis in aging adults.

Table 14-4. Hormones That Influence Calcium Metabolism in Mammals

Hormone	Action
Parathyroid hormone (PTH)	Stimulates bone resorption, renal calcium reabsorption, and synthesis of 1,25-DHC
Calcitonin (CT)	Antagonizes action of PTH on bone
1,25-Dihydroxycholecalciferol (1,25-DHC)	Facilitates calcium absorption from intestine
Growth hormone (GH)	Stimulates cartilage and bone growth
Thyroid hormones	Permissive effect on GH secretion and action
Insulin-like growth factors (IGFs)	Mediators of GH action on bone
Estrogens/androgens	Effects closure of epiphysial plate, blocking further long bone growth; protects adult skeleton from resorption; may reduce PTH release and prevent hypercalcemia
Glucocorticoids	High levels stimulate PTH release, causing increased bone resorption and resultant hypercalcemia

In addition to their ability to stimulate PTH secretion, chronic excesses of glucocorticoids, such as occur during prolonged stress, can reduce intestinal uptake and kidney reabsorption of calcium. This could result in a significant calcium loss and could lead to low-calcium-induced tetany.

Estrogens are hypothesized to alter the calcium setpoint in chief cells so that greater reduction in plasma calcium is required to elicit PTH release. This action might explain, at least in part, the effects of estrogen withdrawal on loss of skeletal calcium in females during and after menopause.

Growth hormone causes an increase in secretion of IGFs by the liver and stimulates IGF synthesis in bone. IGF-I stimulates bone proliferation as well as collagen synthesis by osteoblasts.

Hypothyroidism delays bone growth probably indirectly through its adverse effects on GH secretion and action. Delayed ossification of cartilage also is observed in hypothyroidism. In the hyperthyroid animal, excessive thyroid hormones augment bone resorption and can lead to weakening of the skeleton (see below).

E. Major Clinical Disorders Associated with Calcium Metabolism

In general, plasma calcium doesn't vary greatly, or else death results. Consequently, it is not easy to diagnose parathyroid abnormalities by examining plasma levels of calcium. **Hypercalcemia** (elevation of plasma calcium) is not excessive but often is accompanied by a reduction in bone density and possibly increased calcium in the urine. Similarly, **hypocalcemia** may show few overt symptoms.

F. Hypercalcemia

Excessive plasma calcium levels (greater than 10 mg/dl) can result from a variety of causes. **Primary hypercalcemia** is characterized by chronically elevated levels of PTH. The most common cause is a single parathyroid adenoma (90% of cases). Carcinomas of the parathyroids are very rare and may account for less than 1% of primary hypercalcemic cases. Primary hypercalcemia is difficult to diagnose since approximately one-third of these cases are without overt symptoms, and the remainder exhibit rather generalized and nonspecific symptoms such as weakness, nausea, and anorexia. Serum calcium levels are moderately elevated (10.2 to 11.0 mg/dl) and are usually accompanied by lowered phosphate levels. Often, elevated serum levels of calcium are not seen (i.e., there is no hypercalemia *per se*) because the kidney compensates with increased calcium excretion or **hypercalcuria**. Among the many causative factors that can induce **secondary hypercalcemia** are carcinomas that spontaneously secrete PTHrP. Breast carcinomas also may produce vitamin D-like sterols that increase calcium absorption. Chronic immobilization of an experimental animal or of humans can bring about extensive bone resorption and cause hypercalcemia.

G. Hypocalcemia

There are many different conditions that can lead to hypocalcemia. In most cases, there is a reduction in PTH secretion. This may be caused by abnormal development of the parathyroid glands, accidental damage, or removal by surgery. Hypomagnesemia impairs PTH secretion and indirectly can cause hypocalcemia. In some cases (e.g., pseudohypoparathyroidism), the target organs do not respond to PTH and in others an abnormal PTH is secreted that will not activate tissue receptors. Reductions in 1,25-DHC due to failure to convert 25-HC or to synthesize vitamin D also lead to hypocalcemia. Most cases are without serious overt symptoms. Tetany may be inducible under calcium stress but otherwise is absent.

H. Osteoporosis

This disease is characterized by decalcification and loss of bone matrix from the skeleton resulting in shrinkage, distortion, and increased brittleness of the bones. Milder decalcification is termed **osteopenia** but may be an early signal of developing osteoporosis. Bones that are extensively decalcified become subject to easy fracture as a result of falls, blows, or lifting (stress fractures). Approximately 1.2 million bone fractures each year in the US are attributed to osteoporosis. Of these, 530,000 vertebral and 227,000 hip fractures occur. Osteoporosis accompanies aging and is most common among postmenopausal women. It is eight times more common in women than men largely as a consequence of women having smaller bone calcium reserves and the fact that women tend to live longer. Maximal adult bone mass is achieved in women at about age 35 after which calcium losses exceed calcium gain. Beginning at menopause, there is a gradual reduction in estrogen levels that causes a disproportionate decrease in bone mass by allowing increased bone resorption to take place. Weight-bearing exercise and careful attention to dietary calcium and 1,25-DHC levels are important for postpubertal, premenopausal women to ensure maximal bone density prior to onset of menopause. Curiously, adult men exhibit estrogen levels comparable to those of postmenopausal women yet do not develop osteoporosis until much later in life. It has been suggested that the higher androgen levels in males provide ready substrates for local bone conversion by $P450_{aro}$ to estrogens that in turn can stimulate calcium deposition.

Type I osteoporosis may occur in women soon after the onset of menopause and is characterized by vertebral crush fractures or fracture of the arm just above the wrist. It is attributed to the marked reduction in estrogen levels accompanying menopause. **Type II osteoporosis** appears later in life and can affect both men and women. It is mainly a consequence of decreased ability to absorb sufficient dietary calcium with advancing age.

Drugs that stimulate calcium deposition, calcium supplements, and weight-bearing exercise are commonly prescribed for women at risk for osteoporosis. Calcium supplements usually are fortified with cholecalciferol or related compounds to facilitate synthesis of 1,25-DHC and ensure intestinal uptake of the ingested calcium. Recent studies demonstrate the efficacy of treatment with alendronate (Fosamax®) that is more effective than an alternative drug, risedronate (Actonel®) in stimulating calcium deposition and increasing bone density. Use of synthetic or natural estrogens (e.g., ethinylestradiol), although found to be beneficial for bone structure, has been discouraged due to recent studies demonstrating a slightly increased risk of reproductive cancers and cardiovascular disease in women treated with estrogens or estrogen-progestogen combinations.

Hormonal manipulations are ineffective without close attention to diet and exercise. Emphasis should be placed on weight-bearing activities (e.g., walking). Swimming, while an excellent aerobic exercise, does not stimulate bone deposition. Weightlessness, e.g., immobilization, accelerates bone resorption. Bone density in athletes is related directly to the type of exercise, with weight lifters having the densest bone, swimmers, the least dense, and runners in the middle. The racquet arms of tennis players are 35% and 28% more dense than the other arm, respectively, in men and women. Even mild activity for nursing home patients averaging 82 years of age not only prevented further bone loss but resulted in bone buildup over a 36-month period.

I. Paget's Disease

This disorder is caused by increased osteoclast activity resulting in accelerated bone resorption. It occurs in 3% of the population over age 40, and occurs with greatest frequency in North Americans of western European or Mediterranean descent. About one-third of the people afflicted with Paget's disease do not exhibit any overt symptoms, but the bones become brittle as the disease progresses, leading to fractures. Serum levels of calcium and phosphate are usually normal because the excess ions are excreted in the urine. Salmon CT has been used with some success to treat Paget's disease, because it is more effective compared to mammalian CT (Table 14-5), possibly due to its much longer biological half-life in mammals (Table 14-6). However, therapeutic treatment is thwarted in part by down-regulation of CT receptors on osteoclasts after a few days of treatment.

Table 14-5. Comparison of Relative Activity of Purified Human, Salmon, and Porcine Calcitonin as Determined by a Standard Bioassay

Source	Activity in MRC[a] units/mg hormone
Porcine	200
Human	120
Salmon	5000

[a] MRC, Medical Research Council of England.

Table 14-6. Effects of Calcitonin in Selected Non-Mammalian Vertebrates

Species	CT source	Effect
Agnathan fishes		
Myxine glutinosa	Mammalian	Decreased urine flow and electrolyte content of urine
Bony fishes		
Periophthalmus schosseri	Eel	Hypocalcemia
Carassius auratus	Goldfish	Hypocalcemia
Cyprinus carpio	Salmon	Hypocalcemia
Pacific salmon (*Oncorhynchus*)	Salmon	Decreased gill uptake of calcium
Amphibians		
Rana tigrina	Salmon	Transient hypocalcemia; increased calcium deposition in paravertebral calcium sacs
Ambystoma mexicanum	Eel	No effect on blood calcium; decreased calcium influx
Reptiles		
Dipsosaurus dorsalis	Salmon	No effect on kidney or basal salt gland handling of calcium

IV. Calcium and Phosphate Homeostasis in Non-Mammalian Vertebrates

An attempt to discuss the evolutionary aspects of this problem is complicated by major differences, indeed a distinct dichotomy, between the fishes and the tetrapods. Some fishes lack bone (agnathans, chondrichthyeans), and most of the bony fishes possess acellular bone (no osteocytes) rather than cellular bone. Scales may provide a major physiological reserve of stored calcium to bony fishes, and the surrounding waters (especially sea water) may be an important source of calcium as well. Furthermore, parathyroid glands are lacking in fishes although immunoreactive mammalian PTH has been shown in trout and goldfish plasma as well as in brain, pituitary, and the **corpuscles of Stannius** embedded in the kidneys of several species (Figure 14-9). Calcium metabolism in fishes appears to be regulated by one or more hypercalcemic factor from the pituitary and a hypocalcemic factor from the corpuscles of Stannius and/or the ultimobranchials. Definitive parathyroid glands and PTH first appear fully differentiated in the amphibians. The comparative approach also is hampered by the lack of detailed information concerning calcium and phosphate regulation in fishes, amphibians, and reptiles. The distribution of parathyroid and ultimobranchial glands in vertebrates is provided in Figures 14-10 and 14-11.

Estrogenic hormones elevate circulating calcium and phosphate levels indirectly in females of most non-mammalian species during the process of vitellogenesis associated with oocyte growth. Synthesis of phosphate-containing, calcium-binding, vitellogenic proteins by the liver is stimulated by estrogens. These proteins are released into the blood, through which they travel to the ovaries where they are incorporated into growing oocytes as yolk protein. Vitellogenic proteins readily bind Ca^{2+}, indirectly decrease free plasma Ca^{2+} levels, and consequently stimulate release of more Ca^{2+} from reservoirs such as bone. The presence of vitellogenic proteins elevates total plasma levels of Ca^{2+}, although free Ca^{2+} remains about the same. The relationship between reproductive hormones and vitellogenesis is discussed in more detail in Chapter 11.

A. Agnathan Fishes

Cyclostomes do not appear to have regulatory mechanisms specific for calcium and phosphate metabolism although mammalian CT does decrease urinary excretion (Table 14-7). Whatever regulatory mechanisms are employed, they appear to be not as efficient as those found in other vertebrates as evidenced by circulating levels of calcium. Marine species exhibit an intermediate level of plasma Ca^{2+} between that of sea water and plasma of tetrapods, whereas the plasma Ca^{2+} level in freshwater lampreys is intermediate between that found in plasma of freshwater teleosts and fresh water. These observations raise some interesting questions about the roles of calcium and its regulation in agnathans.

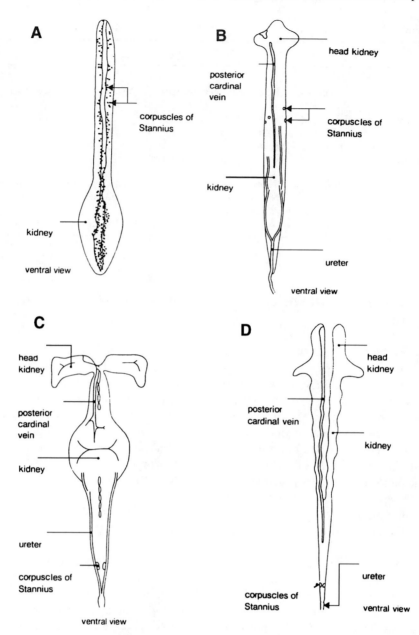

Figure 14-9. **Location of corpuscles of Stannius in selected bony fishes.** (A) The bowfin, *Amia calva*. (B) A salmonid, *Salvelinus pluvius*. (C) The Crucian carp. (D) *Mugil cephalus*. [Modified from Matsumoto, A., and Ishii, S. (1992). "An Atlas of Endocrine Organs." Japanese Society for Comparative Endocrinology and Springer-Verlag, Berlin.]

B. Chondrichthyean Fishes

Most elasmobranchs and other chondrichthyeans live in sea water where calcium availability is not as serious a problem as it is for freshwater species. Although these fishes lack true bone tissue, calcium salts are added to their cartilaginous skeletons for additional strength, especially in larger species. Elasmobranch ultimobranchial glands contain a potent hypocalcemic factor when assayed in mammals, but extracts of shark ultimobranchial glands, salmon CT, and porcine CT are all ineffective in sharks. Curiously, estrogens do not produce any appreciable alteration in plasma calcium as they do in bony fishes and non-mammalian tetrapods. No experimental evidence has been reported for an adenohypophysial factor that would directly affect plasma calcium. Studies of sharks that are either freshwater residents or that penetrate long distances up major rivers (such as the Mississippi) might provide some interesting insight into calcium homeostasis in these fishes.

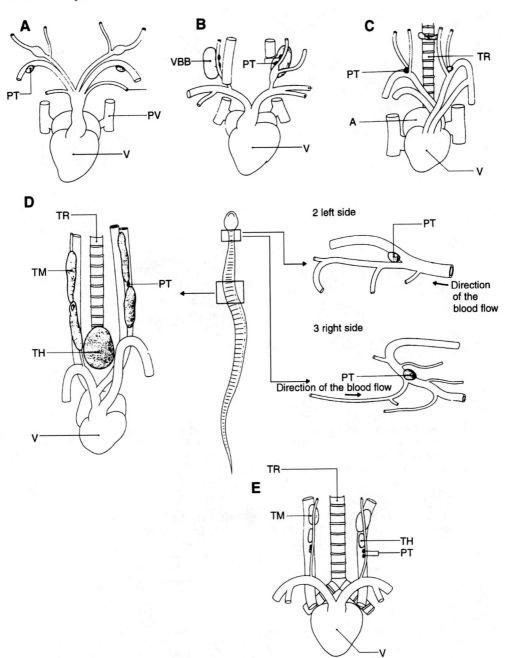

Figure 14-10. **Location of parathyroid glands in selected tetrapod vertebrates**. A, atrium; PT, parathyroid; Thy, thyroid; TM, thymus; TR, trachea; V, ventricle. (A) Newt, *Cynops pyrrhogaster*. Urodele amphibians typically have one pair. (B) Frogs and other anurans typically have two pair of parathyroids. (C) Lizards have one pair of parathyroids except for *Anolis* spp. that have two. (D) Snakes, such as *Agkistrodon halys*, have two pair of parathyroids with the posterior pair associated with the thymus gland. (E) Many birds such as the seagull (*Larus argentatus*), shown here, and domestic species have two pairs of parathyroids located near the thyroid although some (e.g., stork, quail) have one pair. [Modified from Matsumoto, A., and Ishii, S. (1992). "An Atlas of Endocrine Organs." Japanese Society for Comparative Endocrinology and Springer-Verlag, Berlin.]

C. Bony Fishes: Teleosts

Calcium regulation appears to be under the control of a hypercalcemic adenohypophysial factor and a hypocalcemic factor associated with the corpuscles of Stannius. Hypophysectomy of either *Anguilla* (which has cellular bone) or *Fundulus* (acellular bone) results in a decrease in serum calcium and induction of tetany. One

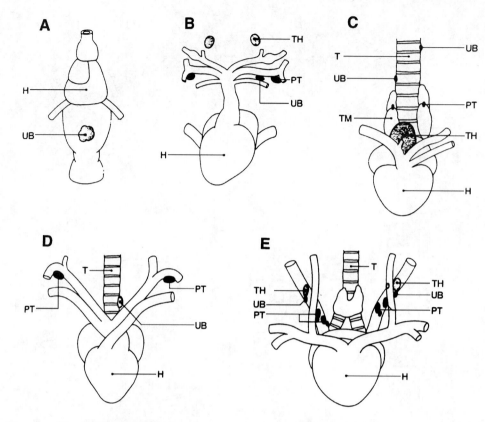

Figure 14-11. **Location of ultimobranchial tissue in non-mammalian vertebrates.** A, atrium; PT, parathyroid; Thy, thyroid; TM, thymus; TR, trachea; UB, ultimobranchial; V, ventricle. (A) Goldfish. (B) Newt. (C) Snake. (D) Lizard. (E) Bird. [Modified from Matsumoto, A., and Ishii, S. (1992). "An Atlas of Endocrine Organs." Japanese Society for Comparative Endocrinology and Springer-Verlag, Berlin.]

Table 14-7. Biological Half-Life for Purified Vertebrate Calcitonins When Incubated in Either Mammalian or Avian Blood Plasma

Source	Half-life (min)
Porcine	2
Salmon	20
Chicken	90

candidate for the pituitary hypercalcemic factor is PRL that would be similar to its action on Na^+ balance in freshwater fishes. Teleost pituitaries also produce **somatolactin (SL)** that can influence Ca^{2+} levels (see Chapter 5). In addition, PTHrP has been demonstrated in the brain, pituitary, and blood of several species. In the sea bream, *Sparus auratus*, two populations of pituitary cells are found that contain innumoreactive (IR) PTHrP. In the anterior group located in the rostral pars distalis, PTHrP is co-localized with β-thyrotropin (β-TSH). The second group of ir-PTHrP cells occurs at the borders of the proximal pars distalis and the pars intermedia. These cells do not react to antisera for β-TSH, CLIP, or ACTH. Although plasma levels of PTHrP in sea bream are 10X greater than in normal human plasma, no specific role for PTHrP is evident. The name **hypercalcin** has been applied to the pituitary hypercalcemic factor of teleosts, but this activity could be due to PTHrP, SL, and/or PRL.

The corpuscles of Stannius have been examined for their possible involvement in calcium homeostasis. Little experimental work has been performed with species other than teleosts, and only a few teleosts have been examined. Stanniectomy of the saltwater eel *Anguilla anguilla* results in an increase in serum calcium, and the administration of corpuscle extracts reduces calcium to normal levels. Stanniectomy of the closely related freshwater *Anguilla japonica* is followed by decreased urinary Ca^{2+} levels and increased urinary phosphate levels. It is possible that the corpuscles of Stannius are mainly active in reducing Ca^{2+} levels in fish adapted to high calcium environments such as sea water. The active hypocalcemic agent in the corpuscles may be called either **hypocalcin** or **stanniocalcin** (STC), and is a unique glycosylated protein consisting of two identical peptide subunits. STC blocks Ca^{2+} uptake by the gill and intestine and increases HPO_4^- reabsorption by the kidney.

Treatment with eel, salmon, or goldfish CTs lowers calcium influx across the gill, and the gill may be a major site where CT regulates Ca^{2+} transport. Salmon CT is a powerful hypocalcemic agent when tested in avian or mammalian systems (Tables 14-5 and 14-6), and it is now employed clinically to reduce pathological hypercalcemia (Paget's disease). This potency of salmon CT is related, at least in part, to its persistence in the circulation, that is, its long biological half-life as compared to mammalian CT (Table 14-7).

Some teleost kidneys are capable of hydroxylation of cholecalciferol to form 1,25-DHC. This hormone is apparently not necessary for Ca^{2+} uptake by the intestine, but large doses of 1,25-DHC enhance Ca^{2+} uptake. Treatment with 1,25-DHC increases plasma calcium and phosphate in the freshwater catfish, *Heteropneustes fossilis*. Calcium-binding proteins are present in the intestinal mucosa of teleosts (Table 14-8), and their synthesis may be controlled by 1,25-DHC as it is in mammals. In females, total plasma phosphate and calcium increase markedly during oogenesis due to the actions of estrogens on liver vitellogenic protein synthesis and secretion.

1. Thyroid State and Calcium Homeostasis in Teleosts

Serum calcium may be influenced by thyroid state, but the physiological importance of these observations has not been established. Serum calcium levels are decreased in juvenile steelhead trout (*Oncorhynchus mykiss*) that were radiothyroidectomized prior to complete resorption of the yolk sac (Table 14-9). It is not possible to distinguish between general effects of radiation that may have damaged some calcium-regulating mechanism and effects due to the absence of thyroid hormones, however. Growth of the skeleton is also abnormal following radiothyroidectomy, supporting an involvement of thyroid hormones at some level. Abnormal skeletal growth

Table 14-8. Calbindin Immunoreactivity in Vertebrate Tissues[a]

Species	Intestine	Kidney
Bony fishes		
Carassius auratus (goldfish)	+	
Salmo trutta (brown trout)	+	
Oncorhynchus mykiss (rainbow trout)		0
Amphibians		
Bufo bufo (toad)	+	0
Rana esculenta (frog)	+	0
Rana temporaria (frog)	+	
Xenopus laevis (frog)	+	
Triturus alpestris (newt)	+	
Reptiles		
Chrysemys (turtle)	+	
Psuedemys (turtle)		0
Gekko gecko (lizard)		0
Birds		
Japanese quail	+	
Chicken	+	+
Pigeon	+	
Mammals		
Rat	0	
Monkey	0	
Human	0	

[a] All tetrapods examined have two forms of brain calbindin, but the fish examined have only one. +, present; 0, absent; blank, no data.

Table 14-9. Serum Calcium Levels in Radiothyroidectomized Steelhead
Trout, *Oncorhynchus mykiss*

Treatment	Total serum calcium ± SEM (mg/100 ml)	Range (mg/100 ml)
Radiothyroidectomized as fingerlings	10	4–12
Intact controls	11	9–15
Radiothyroidectomized prior to yolk sac	11.8 ± 1.01	
Intact controls	14.9 ± 0.51	

observed in these fish could be related to ineffective action of growth hormone in the absence of thyroid hormones (see Chapter 7).

D. Bony Fishes: Lungfishes

The lungfishes lack parathyroid glands and are relatively insensitive to tetrapod calcium-regulating hormones. It is both surprising and somewhat disappointing that they do not exhibit some tetrapod-like feature. Parathyroid extracts, PTH, and salmon CT are all ineffective in altering Ca^{2+} levels in the South American lungfish *Lepidosiren paradoxa*. Surprisingly, however, CT and PTH are diuretic and antidiuretic, respectively, in these fishes. The physiological importance of these observations is not clear.

E. Amphibians

Studies of amphibians have shed little light on the origin of the parathyroid glands and the evolution of calcium regulation in tetrapods. Ultimobranchial and parathyroid glands are present in the apodans, anurans, and urodeles, and calcium regulation is similar to that observed in other tetrapods.

Parathyroid glands are not present in some urodeles until after metamorphosis, and parathyroids never develop in some permanently neotenic aquatic species such as *Necturus*. These glands are more important in calcium balance of early terrestrial urodeles and especially of anurans. Ultimobranchial bodies are well developed and produce a hypocalcemic CT-like factor. As in fishes, a hypercalcemic factor (probably PRL) is present in pituitaries of urodele amphibians, and it is of greater importance for calcium regulation in the more aquatic species.

Immunoreactivity to mammalian PTHrP has been reported in *Rana temporaria* at the time of emergence of metamorphosed animals from the water. Two PTH/PTHrP receptors have been detected in the genome of *Xenopus laevis* and have been shown in oocytes.

1. Amphibian Ultimobranchial Glands

The amphibian ultimobranchial glands develop as in all tetrapods from the fifth pharyngeal pouches. Most urodeles have only one ultimobranchial gland (usually on the left side). In apodans, anurans, and some urodeles (for example, *Necturus* and *Amphiuma*), the ultimobranchial glands are paired. Immunoreactive CT is present in the ultimobranchial glands of *Rana temporaria* and *R. pipiens*. Cytologically, the ultimobranchial gland consists of one or more simple follicles composed of C-cells, which may appear in either a "dark" form (relatively electron-dense) or in a less electron-dense "light" form, at least in anurans. In addition to the C-cells, the ultimobranchial gland of the apodan *Chthonerpeton indistinctum* contains cholinergic and purinergic neuronal endings. Although the presence of sympathetic neurons has been demonstrated in the frog *R. pipiens*, most anurans investigated do not exhibit innervation of the ultimobranchial glands. The condition of the urodele ultimobranchial gland with respect to innervation has not been described. Salmon CT produces a transient decrease in plasma calcium and phosphate in anurans. Eel CT decreases calcium influx in aquatic axolotls (*Ambystoma mexicanum*) as it does in fishes.

2. Amphibian Parathyroid Glands

As in mammals, parathyroidectomy results in lowered calcium and usually leads to tetany and death. The parathyroid glands appear to develop from the third and fourth pharyngeal pouches as they do in mammals. Chief cells responsible for PTH secretion actually arise from neuroectodermal pharyngeal components rather than from endoderm. In apodan parathyroids, only chief cells are present, whereas two cellular types have been described for anurans. However, these appear to be two forms of chief cells that occur in light and dark phases as described above for the ultimobranchial bodies. Two distinct cellular types have been reported in parathyroids of the urodele *Cynops pyrrhogaster*. One of these cells is considered to be only a "supportive" cell, however.

3. Endolymphatic Sacs

In addition to cellular bone, the endolymphatic sacs located at the base of the skull and/or along the vertebral column appear to be major targets for factors regulating calcium homeostasis. These sacs contain large amounts of calcium carbonate and may be important reservoirs of these ions, particularly during metamorphosis and subsequent ossification of bones. These structures also may provide bicarbonate ions for buffering the blood following the dissociation of calcium carbonate.

4. Amphibian Calcium and Phosphate Homeostasis

In general, the amphibians regulate plasma calcium and phosphate similarly to mammals. The parathyroids, pituitary gland, and ultimobranchial glands control calcium and phosphate metabolism, and the vitamin D complex seems to be related to at least some actions of PTH in amphibians. A calcium-binding protein occurs in the intestinal mucosa (Table 14-8), and this may be related to 1,25-DHC activity.

Removal of the ultimobranchial glands in frogs generally causes an increase in osteoclast activity and a consequent increase in blood calcium levels. The ultimobranchial gland secretions also prevent removal of calcium from the endolymphatic sacs and block uptake of calcium through the gut. Parathyroidectomy causes a decrease in plasma Ca^{2+} in anurans and in the newt *C. pyrrhogaster*. However, no changes in serum Ca^{2+} occur following parathyroidectomy of immature giant salamanders, *Megalobatrachus davidianus*. Administration of bovine PTH to frogs increases plasma Ca^{2+} and decreases plasma phosphate, implying that the kidney may also be a target for PTH.

F. Reptiles

The regulation of calcium and phosphate in lizards has been well studied, and in recent years these investigations have been extended to include snakes and turtles. Ultimobranchial glands and parathyroids have been described, and regulation of calcium is essentially like that in other tetrapods. The major sites for endocrine regulation of calcium metabolism are the kidney, the cellular bone, and the endolymphatic sacs, which in lizards, as in amphibians, are important reserves of calcium and carbonate ions. The presence of PTHrP and its possible roles in reptilian calcium metabolism have not been addressed.

1. Reptilian Ultimobranchial Glands

The ultimobranchial glands of reptiles are located near the thyroid and parathyroid glands. They are small glands consisting primarily of follicles. All the reptilian ultimobranchials are innervated, although the nature of these neuronal endings has not been examined extensively. In crocodilians, chelonians, and some snakes, the ultimobranchial glands are paired. In lizards, only the left gland persists. Seasonal changes in the cytology of ultimobranchial glands have been reported for a few species, but the relationship between these changes and physiological and environmental parameters has not been ascertained.

2. Reptilian Parathyroid Glands

Four reptilian parathyroids develop from the third and fourth pharyngeal pouches (Figure 14-5) as described for the amphibians, and they resemble mammalian parathyroids cytologically (Figure 14-12). Adult lizards and crocodilians have only one pair of parathyroid glands, whereas snakes and turtles have four glands. In addition to cellular cords, the presence of follicles containing PAS (+) material is a common feature of reptilian parathyroids although their functional significance is not known.

3. Calcium and Phosphate Homeostasis in Reptiles

Parathyroidectomy of lizards and snakes causes a marked decrease in plasma Ca^{2+} accompanied by tetany. However, there is little or no change in circulating Ca^{2+} in turtles following a similar operation, and tetany does not occur in turtles. This insensitivity of turtles to parathyroidectomy is apparently a consequence of the immense calcium reservoir represented by the shell. Treatment with mammalian PTH causes increased plasma Ca^{2+} and urinary phosphate as well as decreased urinary Ca^{2+} and plasma phosphate in both lizards and turtles.

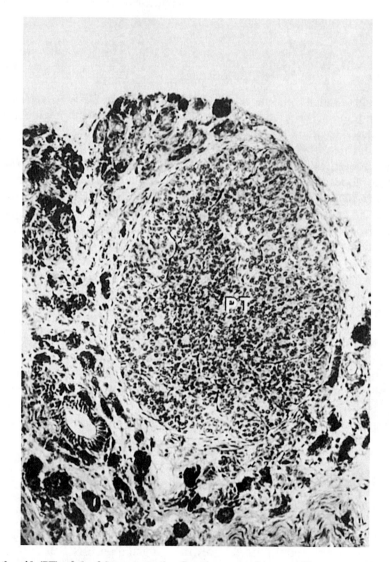

Figure 14-12. Parathyroid (PT) of the false map turtle, *Graptemys pseudogeographica*, surrounded by ultimobranchial tissue. (Courtesy of the late Nancy B. Clark, University of Connecticut, Storrs.)

The renal action of mammalian parathyroid extracts on phosphate excretion is marked in parathyroidectomized snakes (four species of *Natrix*) although calcium excretion is probably not affected significantly. Thus, it appears that reptiles possess basically the same regulatory control of calcium and phosphate homeostasis as exhibited by mammalian parathyroids.

The role of CT in reptiles is uncertain. Extracts of reptilian ultimobranchial glands produce hypocalcemia when injected into rats, and salmon CT has been shown to lower Ca^{2+} in the green iguana. As with fishes and amphibians, when reptilian ultimobranchial factors are tested in mammals, the presence of hypocalcemic factors is noted, but their endogenous physiological roles are not known.

No information is available on 1,25-DHC production or actions in reptiles. A calcium-binding protein has been demonstrated in the intestinal mucosa of three species (Table 14-8).

G. Birds

There are typically four parathyroid glands in birds, and separate ultimobranchial glands are present. Cytologically, the parathyroid glands resemble those of mammals, and the ultimobranchial cells are like the mammalian C-cell. The regulation of calcium and phosphate homeostasis is typically mammalian with only minor differences. It should be noted, however, that few avian species have been investigated thoroughly, and most of the physiological studies have been conducted with domestic birds (e.g., chickens, pigeons, Japanese quail).

1. Avian Parathyroid Glands

Avian parathyroid glands are separate and usually distinct, except for a few species, such as the domestic chicken, in which some fusion of the separate parathyroids may occur. Cytologically the parathyroid glands contain only chief cells; no oxyphils have been reported.

2. Avian Ultimobranchial Glands

The ultimobranchial glands are usually separate structures although some fusion with the thyroid gland occurs in the pigeon. There are both light and dark cells in chicken ultimobranchials. The light cell is more abundant and resembles the mammalian C-cell cytologically. A rich vagal innervation (parasympathetic) has been described for the chicken, but its importance has not been elucidated.

3. Calcium and Phosphate Homeostasis in Birds

Parathyroidectomy in birds usually causes marked hypocalcemia accompanied by tetanic seizures and death within 24 hours. This degree of sensitivity to parathyroidectomy is not manifest on this time scale in amphibians or reptiles and may be related to the much higher body temperature and metabolic rate of birds. Treatment with mammalian parathyroid extracts produces marked increases in plasma Ca^{2+}. Dietary deprivation of Ca^{2+} or vitamin D causes marked hypertrophy and hyperplasia of the parathyroid glands, whereas high Ca^{2+} diets result in regression of the parathyroids. As in mammals, estrogens and parathyroid extracts both increase levels of 1,25-DHC.

Mammalian parathyroid extract stimulates renal excretion of phosphate in normal starlings but does not seem to alter renal treatment of calcium. The effect of mammalian parathyroid extract or PTH on avian bone is similar to that described for mammals.

PTHrP has been isolated from chickens and is present in both embryos and adults. Numerous embryonic tissues express PTHrP, and it may be an important growth stimulator in bird embryos. Expression of the PTHrP gene in the isthmus and shell gland of the adult oviduct is related to entrance of the egg into the oviduct and the calcification of the shell. PTHrP relaxes vascular smooth muscle and increases blood flow to the shell gland during calcification. It is not known whether it alters Ca^{2+} transport as well. Relaxation of oviductal smooth muscle by PTHrP allows the entrance and passage of the egg though the oviduct.

Calcitonins that are structurally similar to mammalian CT have been isolated from chickens and turkeys and are potent hypocalcemic agents in both birds and mammals. Unlike the condition for fishes, amphibians, and reptiles, the avian kidney specifically binds CT, suggesting a renal action for CT in birds. Dietary levels of calcium are directly related to ultimobranchial activities, and high levels of Ca^{2+} cause marked stimulatory changes. An immunoreactive calcium-binding protein similar to that of other vertebrates is present in the intestinal mucosa of birds (Table 14-8).

V. Summary

Precise regulation of calcium and phosphate homeostasis is necessary for many processes in vertebrates. In birds and mammals, this regulation is accomplished through secretion of hypercalcemic PTH from the parathyroid glands and hypocalcemic CT produced by the C-cells embedded between the follicles of the thyroid gland (mammals) or by the ultimobranchial glands (birds). PTHrP may be an important regulator of calcium homeostasis and growth. Its presence in milk may help newborn mammals regulate calcium as well. PTHrP is involved in both avian embryonic development and shell formation in adults.

Parathyroid hormone increases plasma calcium levels through direct and indirect action on bone, kidney, and intestine. Parathyroidectomy invariably brings about tetany and usually death as a consequence of the decrease in circulating Ca^{2+} following this operation. This condition can be alleviated through administration of PTH or calcium. The actions of PTH on bone may be anabolic (bone formation mediated through the osteoblasts) or catabolic (bone reabsorption via the osteoclasts). In addition to the effect of PTH on calcium, PTH stimulates renal excretion of phosphate ions and reabsorption of Ca^{2+}. Both the resorption of bone and the kidney action of PTH may be dependent on a derivative of vitamin D, 1,25-DHC. The uptake of calcium through the intestinal wall requires 1,25-DHC. Synthesis of 1,25-DHC involves sequential intermediates produced in the skin, altered in the liver, and finally converted to 1,25-DHC in the cortical portion of the kidney. This enzymatic conversion in the kidney may be influenced by PTH as well as by estrogens and PRL.

Calcitonin has been isolated from mammalian parafollicular thyroid tissue and from bird ultimobranchial glands. The major site of action for CT is bone, where it antagonizes the action of PTH on osteoclasts.

The comparative aspects of calcium and phosphate regulation are complicated by the absence of parathyroid glands in fishes and the presence of the unique corpuscles of Stannius in teleosts. The pituitary of teleosts produces PRL, SL, and PTHrP that may be involved in calcium homeostasis. Cyclostomes and elasmobranchs have not been studied sufficiently and mineral regulation is not understood. Among bony fishes, calcium regulation appears to be accomplished by a hypercalcemic pituitary factor (PRL or hypercalcin) and a hyper-calcemic factor (staniocalcin or hypocalcin) from the corpuscles of Stannius embedded in the kidneys of some bony fishes. Scales are important calcium reservoirs in teleosts. The pituitary factors appear to be the more important regulators in freshwater fishes, and the corpuscles of Stannius appears to regulate calcium in sea water. Mammalian or fish CTs can decrease blood calcium, and the major target appears to be the gills. Salmon CT is a more potent hypocalcemic factor in mammals than is mammalian CT, and this greater potency may be a result of its relative resistance to clearance from the circulation. It is currently used for clinical treatment in some situations of CT insufficiency.

Parathyroid glands are distinct in amphibians and reptiles, and the effects of PTH and parathyroidectomy are similar to those observed in birds and mammals but occur with lessened intensity. The pituitary may have a hypercalcemic role in aquatic amphibians. Amphibians and some reptiles possess endolymphatic sacs, which may be important sites for calcium carbonate storage. CT has been demonstrated in amphibians, and extracts of their ultimobranchial glands have hypocalcemic activity when tested in birds or mammals. Treatment with CTs alter calcium and phosphate metabolism as in other vertebrates.

One feature that appears to be dominant throughout the tetrapods examined to date is the strong tendency for innervation of the ultimobranchial glands, although the nature of this innervation (e.g., cholinergic, adrenergic) and biological significance are not clear. Mammalian C-cells contain both CT and SST, implying a paracrine role for these cells.

A second consistent relationship appears in all oviparous species except the cyclostomes and possibly the elasmobranchs. Estrogens increase the production of vitellogenic phosphoproteins by the liver that bind Ca^{2+} when they are secreted into the blood. Consequently, there is an elevation in total plasma calcium and phosphate associated with vitellogenesis in females that appears to be a mechanism whereby increased Ca^{2+} become available for production of egg shells (birds and reptiles) and/or for incorporation into the eggs. Egg stores of Ca^{2+} are used for early developmental processes prior to hatching and feeding by the offspring. A similar mechanism operates in mammals whereby maternal dietary calcium is directed during development or during lactation to the offspring by actions of PTH with protection of the maternal skeleton afforded through the actions of CT. Estrogens also stimulate production of 1,25-DHC in both birds and mammals.

Suggested Reading

Books

Azria, M. (1989). "The Calcitonins." Karger, Basel.
Bikle, D. D., and Negro-Vilar, A. (1995). "Hormonal Regulation of Bone Mineral Metabolism." The Endocrine Society Press, Bethesda, MD.
Bilezikan, J. (2001). The Parathyroids. Academic Press, San Diego.
Bilezikian, J. P. (1994). "The Parathyroids: Basic and Clinical Concepts." Raven, New York.
Crass, III, M. F., and Avioli, L. V. (1995). "Calcium-Regulating Hormones and Cardiovascular Function." CRC Press, Boca Raton, FL.
Dacke, C. G. (1979). "Calcium Regulation in Sub-Mammalian Vertebrates." Academic Press, New York.
Favus, M. J. (1993). "Primer on the Metabolic Bone Diseases and Disorders of Mineral Metabolism." Lippincott-Raven, New York.

General Articles

Chirgwin, J. M., and Guise, T. A. (2003). Cancer metastasis to bone. *Sci. Med.* **9**, 140–151.
Dempster, D. W., Cosman, F., Parisien, M., Shen, V., and Lindsay, R. (1993). Anabolic actions of parathyroid hormone on bone. *Endocr. Rev.* **14**, 690–709.
Mallette, L. E. (1991). The parathyroid polyhormones: New concepts in the spectrum of peptide hormone action. *Endocr. Rev.* **12**, 110–117.
Martin, T. J., and Udagawa, N. (1998). Hormonal regulation of osteoclast function. *Trends Endocr. Metab.* **9**, 6–12.
Orloff, J. J., Reddy, D., de Papp, A. E., Yang, K. H., Soifer, N. E., and Stewart, A. F. (1994). Parathyroid hormone-related protein as a prohormone: Posttranslational processing and receptor interaction. *Endocr. Rev.* **15**, 40–60.
Suda, T., Takahashi, N., and Martin, T. J. (1992). Modulation of osteoclast differentiation. *Endocr. Rev.* **13**, 66–80.
Wagner, G. F., and DiMattia, G. E. (2006). The stanniocalcin family of proteins. *Journal of Experimental Zoology* **305A**, 769–780.
Watson, P. H., and Hanley, D. A. (1993). Parathyroid hormone: Regulation of synthesis and secretion. *Clin. Invest. Med.* **16**, 58–77.

Clinical Articles

Marie, P. J., Hott, M., Launay, J. M., Graulet, A. M., and Gueris, J. (1993). *In vitro* production of cytokines by bone surface-derived osteoblastic cells in normal and osteoporotic postmenopausal women: Relationship with cell proliferation. *J. Clin. Endocrinol. Metab.* **77**, 824–830.
Schneider, D. L., Barrett-Connor, E. L., and Morton, D. J. (1994). Thyroid hormone use and bone mineral density in elderly women. *J. Am. Med. Assoc.* **271**, 1245–1249.
Siris, E. S., and Canfield, R. E. (1991). Paget's disease of bone. *Trends Endocr. Metab.* **2**, 207–212.

APPENDIX A

Abbreviations of Endocrine Terms

Alphabetical by Abbreviation

1,25-DHC	1,25-Dihydroxycholecalciferol
17,20β,21P	17,20β,21-Trihydroxy-4-pregnen-3-one
17β-HSD	17β-Hydroxysteroid dehydrogenase
1α-OHB	1α-Hydroxycorticosterone
3β-diol	DHT metabolite
3β-HSD	3β-Hydroxy-Δ_5-steroid dehydrogenase
5-HIAA	5-Hydroxyindole acetic acid
5-HT	Serotonin
5-HTP	5-Hydroxytryptophol
5-MP	5-Methoxytryptophol
AAAD	Adrenal ascobic acid depletion
ABP	Androgen-binding protein
ACE	Angiotensin-converting enzyme
ACE2	Angiotensin converting enzyme 2
ACELA	Angiotensin-converting enzyme-like activity
AcetylCoA	Acetyl coenzyme A
ACh	Acetylcholine
AChE	Acetylcholine esterase
ACTH	Corticotropin
ADH	Antidiuretic hormone
ADHD	Attention-deficit hyperactivity disorder
AgRP	Agouti-related protein
AHN	Anterior hypothalamic nucleus
ahR	Aryl hydrocarbon receptor
AMH	Antimüllerian hormone (same as MIS)
α-MSH	α-Melanotropin
ANG-I	Angiotensin I
ANG-II	Angiotensin II
ANG-III	Angiotensin III
ANP	Atrial natriuretic peptide
AOB	Accessory olfactory bulb
APUD	Amine precursor uptake and decarboxylation
AR	Androgen receptor
ARC	Arcuate nucleus
ARNT	Aryl hydrocarbon nuclear translocator protein
ASP	Agouti signaling protein
AspT	Aspargtocin
AsvT	Asvatocin
AVP	Arginine vasopressin
AVT	Arginine vasotocin
B	Corticosterone
βARK	β-Adrenergic receptor kinase
BBS	Bombesin
βERKO	ERβ knockout mice
βFGF	Basic fibroblastic growth factor
β-LPH	β-Lipotropin
BMI	Body mass index
BMP	Bone morphometric protein
BNP	Brain natriuretic peptide
BPA	Bisphenol A
BSD	Behavioral sex determination
CAH	Congenital adrenal hyperplasia
cAMP	Cyclic adenosine monophosphate
CART	Cocaine and amphetamine regulated transcript
CAT	Choline acetyltransferase
CAT	Computer axial tomography
CBG	Corticosteroid-binding globulin
CC	Chorionic corticotropin
CCK	Cholecystokinin

512

cDNA	Copy DNA		FSH-RH	FSH releasing hormone
CG	Chorionic gonadotropin		FXR	Farnesoid X receptor
cGMP	Cyclic guanosine monophosphate		GABA	γ-Aminobutyric acid
CGRP	Calcitonin gene-related peptide		GAD	Glutamate decarboyxlase
CLIP	Corticotropin-like peptide		GAL	Galanin
CNP	C natriuretic peptide		GAP	Gonadotropin-releasing hormone-associated peptide
CNS	Central nervous system			
CO	Carbon monoxide		GDF	Growth differentiation factor
COH	Compensatory ovarian hypertrophy		GFP	Green fluorescent protein
COMT	Catechol O-methyltransferase		GH	Growth hormone
CREB	cAMP regulatory element-binding protein		GHRH	Growth homone-releasing hormone, somatocrinin
CREB	Cyclic AMP regulatory element binding protein		GHRIH	Growth hormone release-inhibiting hormone, somatostatin
CRF-R	CRF receptor		GIP	Glucose-dependent insulinotropic peptide, gastric inhibitory peptide
CRH	Corticotropin-releasing hormone			
CRH-R	CRH receptor		GLP	Glucagon-like peptide
CS	Chorionic somatomammotropin		γ-LPH	γ-Lipotropin
CSF	Cerebral spinal fluid		GLT	Glumitocin
CT	Calcitonin		GLUC	Glucagon
CT	Chorionic thyrotropin		GLUT	Glucose transporter
DA	Dopamine		Gn	Gonadotropin
DAG	Diacylglycerol		GnIH	Gonadotropin release-inhibiting hormone
DDE	1,1-Dichloro-2,2-bis(p-chlorophenyl) ethylene			
			GnRH	Gonadotropin-releasing hormone
DDT	1,1-Dichloro-2,2-bis(p-chlorophenyl) ethane		GRBP	Growth factor receptor-binding protein
			GRP	Gastrin-releasing peptide
DES	Diethylstilbestrol		GRPP	Glucagon-related polypeptide
DHEA	Dehydroepiandrosterone		GSD	Genotypic sex determination
DHEAS	Dehydroepiandrosterone sulfate		GTH	Gonadotropin
DHP	17,20β-Dihydroxy-4-pregnen-3-one		GTP	Guanosine triphosphate
DHT	5α-Dihydrotestosterone		HDL	High-density lipoprotein
DIT	Diiodotyrosine		HIOMT	Hydroxyindole-O-methyltransferase
DIV	Dorsal infundibular nucleus		HMG-CoA	Hydroxymethylglutaryl coenzyme A
DMN	Dorsomedial nucleus		HP	Hypothalamus-pituitary
DNA	Deoxyribonucleic acid		HPA	Hypothalamus-pituitary-adrenal axis
DOC	Deoxycorticosterone		HPG	Hypothalamus-pituitary-gonad axis
DOPA	Dihydroxyphenylalanine		HPH	Hypothalamus-pituitary-hepatic axis
DSIP	Delta sleep-inducing protein		hPL	Human placental lactogen
E	Epinephrine		HPLC	High-performance liquid chromatography
EbyNP	Hagfish natriuretic peptide			
EDC	Endocrine disrupting chemical		HPT	Hypothalamus-pituitary-thyroid axis
EDRF	Endothelium-derived relaxing factor		HRE	Hormone response element
EDTA	Ethylenediaminetetraacetate		ICSH	Interstitial cell-stimulating hormone (same as LH)
EE$_2$	Ethinylestradiol			
EGF	Epidermal growth factor		IDDM	Insulin-dependent diabetes mellitus = Type 1 diabetes
ELISA	Enzyme-linked immunoabsorbent assay			
EOP	Endogenous opioid peptide		IDL	Intermediate-density lipoprotein
EPTH	Extrapancreatic tumor hypoglycemia		IFN	Infundibular nucleus
ER	Estrogen receptor		IGF	Insulin-like growth factor
ERR	Estrogen-related receptor		IL	Interleukin
F	Cortisol		IP$_3$	Inositol trisphosphate
FSH	Follicle-stimulating hormone		IRMA	Immunoradiometric assay

IRS	Insulin response proteins
IST	Isotocin
JAK-STAT	Janus kinase-signal transducer and activator of transcription
KO	Knockout
LAF	Luteinization of atretic follicles
LatH	Lateral hypothalamus
LATS	Long-acting thyroid stimulator
LDL	Low-density lipoprotein
LH	Luteinizing hormone
LHRH	Luteinizing hormone-releasing hormone (same as GnRH)
LPH	Lipotropin
LVP	Lysine vasopressin
MAG	Monoacylglyceride
MAO	Monoamine oxidase
MAPK	Mitogen-activated protein kinase
MCH	Melanin-concentrating hormone
MG	Menopausal gonadotropin
MIS	Müllerian-inhibiting substance (same as AMH)
MIT	Monoiodotyrosine
MMC	Migrating motor complex
MR	Mineralocorticoid receptor
MRH	Melanotropin-releasing hormone
MRIH	Melanotropin release-inhibiting hormone
mRNA	Messenger RNA
MRT	Magentic resonance tomography
MSH	Melanotropin
MST	Mesotocin
NADPH	Nictoinamide adenine dinucleotide phosphate
NAT	N-Acetyltransferase
NE	Norepinephrine
NEFA	Nonesterified fatty acids
NGF	Nerve growth factor
NHF	Nasohypophysial factor
NID	Dorsal infundibular nucleus
NIDDM	Non-insulin-dependent diabetes mellitus; Type 2 diabetes
NIS	Sodium iodide symporter
NIV	Ventral infundibular nucleus
NLT	Nucleus lateralis tuberis
NMRI	Nuclear magentic resonance imaging
NO	Nitric oxide
NOS	Nitric oxide synthetase
NP	Natriuretic peptide
NPY	Neuropeptide Y
NRIH	Melanotropin release-inhibiting hormone
NT	Neurotensin
OAAD	Ovarian ascorbic acid depletion
oatps	Organic anion transporter polypeptides
OVLT	Organum vasculosum lateralis terminae
OXY	Oxytocin
PACAP	Pituitary adenylyl cyclase activating peptide
PAG	Pineal antigonadotropic peptide
PC	Convertase enzyme
PCB	Polychloinated biphenyl
PCOS	Polycystic ovarian syndrome
PCR	Polymerase chain reaction
PDE	Phosphodiesterase
PDGF	Platelet-derived growth factor
PEP	Phosphoenolpyruvate
PEPCK	Phosphoenolpyruvate carboxykinase
PERIV	Periventricular nucleus
PET	Positron emission tomography
PFK	Phosphofructokinase
PG	Prostaglandin
PGA	PG series A
PGE	PG series E
PGF	PG series F
PGI	PG series I
PhaT	Phasvatocin
PHI	Peptide histidine isoleucine
PHM	Peptide histidine methionine
PIP$_2$	Phosphoinositol diphosphate
PIPAS cell	Calcium-sensitive cell
Pit-1	Pituitary transcription factor
PK	Pyruvate kinase
PKA	Phosphokinase A
PKC	Protein kinase C
PL	Placental lactogen
PLC	Phospholipase C
PMSG	Pregnant mare serum gonadotropin
PNMT	Phenylethanolamine-N-methyltransferase
POA	Preoptic area
POMC	Proopiomelanocortin
PON	Preoptic nucleus
PP	Pancreatic polypeptide
PPAR	Peroxisomal proliferator activated receptor
PR	Progestogen receptor
PRH	PRL releasing hormone
PRIH	PRL release-inhibiting hormone
PRL	Prolactin
PRP	PACAP-related peptide
PrRP	Prolactin-releasing peptide
Pst	Pancreostatin
PTH	Parathyroid hormone
PTHrP	Parathyroid hormone-related protein
PTU	Propylthiouracil
PVN	Paraventricular nucleus

PVP	Phenypressin		TBPA	Thyroid-binding prealbumin
PYY	Peptide YY		TCDD	2,3,7,8-tetrachlorodibenzo-p-dioxin
RAR	Retinoic acid receptor		TEM	Transmission electron microscope
RER	Rough endoplasmic reticulum		TETRAC	Tetraiodothyroacetic acid
RIA	Radioimmunoassay		TF	Transcription factor
RNA	Ribonucleic acid		Tgb	Thyroglobulin
rT_3	Reverse T_3		TGF-α	Transforming growth factor α
RXR	Retinoid X receptor		TGFβ	Transforming growth factorβ
SAD	Seasonal affective disorder		tGLP-I	Truncated GLP-I
SCG	Superior cervical ganglion		THC	Tetrahydrocanabinol
SCN	Suprachiasmatic nucleus		TNF	Tissue necrosis factor
SCO	Subcommissural organ		TPO	Thyroid peroxidase
SDN	Sexually dimorphic nucleus		TR	Thyroid receptor
SEM	Scaning electron microscope		TRAP	Thyroid receptor auxiliary protein
SERM	Selective estrogen receptor modulator		TRE	Thyroid response element
SF-1	Steroidogenic factor-1		TRH	Thyrotropin-releasing hormone
SIAD	Syndrome of inappropriate diuresis		TRIAC	Triiodothyroacetic acid
SL	Somatolactin		TSD	Temperature-dependent sex determination
SON	Supraoptic nucleus			
SOS	Son of sevenless protein		TSH	Thyrotropin
SP	Substance P		TTR	Transthyretin
SS	Somatostatin = SST		TU	Thiourea
SST	Somatostatin; also SS_{14}, SS_{28}, SS_{34}		Ucn	Urocortin
StAR	Steroidogenic acute regulatory protein		UCP	Uncoupling protein
STC	Stanniocalcin		ValT	Valitocin
STH	Somatotropin = GH		VDR	Vitamin D receptor
STP	Steroidogenic stimulating protein		VEGF	Vascular endothelial cell growth factor
SU4885	Metyrapone		VIP	Vasoactive intestinal peptide
T_3	Triiodothyronine		VLDL	Very-low-density lipoprotein
T_4	Thyroxine (tetraiodothyronine)		VMN	Ventromedial nucleus
TAG	Triacylglyceride		VNO	Vomeronasal organ
TBA	Thyroid-binding albumin		VNP	Ventricular natriuretic peptide
TBG	Thyroid-binding globulin		VSCC	Voltage-sensitive calcium channels

Alphabetical by Term

1,1-Dichloro-2,2-bis (p-chlorophenyl)ethane	DDT		Acetylcholine esterase	AChE
			Adrenal ascorbic acid depletion	AAAD
1,1-Dichloro-2,2-bis (p-chlorophenyl)ethylene	DDE		Agouti signaling protein	ASP
			Agouti-related protein	AgRP
1,25-Dihydroxycholecalciferol	1,25-DHC		Aldosterone synthase	$P-450_{c18}$
1α-Hydroxycorticosterone	1α-OHB		α-Melanotropin	α-MSH
2,3,7,8-Tetrachlorodibenzo-p-dioxin	TCDD		Amine precursor uptake and decarboxylation	APUD
3β-Hydroxy-Δ$_5$-steroid dehydrogenase	3β-HSD			
5α-Dihydrotestosterone	DHT		Androgen receptor	AR
5-Hydroxyindole acetic acid	5-HIAA		Androgen-binding protein	ABP
5-Hydroxytryptophol	5-HTP		Angiotensin converting enzyme 2	ACE2
5-Methoxytryptophol	5-MP		Angiotensin I	ANG-I
17,20β,21-Trihydroxy-4-pregnen-3-one	17,20β,21P		Angiotensin II	ANG-II
17,20β-Dihydroxy-4-pregnen-3-one	17,20βP		Angiotensin III	ANG-III
17β-Hydroxysteroid dehydrogenase	17β-HSD		Angiotensin-converting enzyme	ACE
Accessory olfactory bulb	AOB		Angiotensin-converting enzyme-like action	ACELA
Acetyl coenzyme A	AcetylCoA			
Acetylcholine	ACh		Anterior hypothalamic nucleus	AHN
			Antidiuretic hormone	ADH

Antimüllerian hormone (same as MIS)	AMH	Cyclic adenosine monophosphate	cAMP
Arcuate nucleus	ARC	Cyclic AMP regulatory element binding protein	CREB
Arginine vasopressin	AVP	Cyclic guanosine monophosphate	cGMP
Arginine vasotocin	AVT	Dehydroepiandrosterone	DHEA
Aryl hydrocarbon nuclear translocator protein	ARNT	Dehydroepiandrosterone sulfate	DHEAS
		Delta sleep-inducing peptide	DSIP
Aryl hydrocarbon receptor	ahR	Deoxycorticosterone	DOC
Aspargtocin	AspT	Deoxyribonucleic acid	DNA
Asvatocin	AsvT	DHT metabolite	3β-diol
Atrial natriuretic peptide	AN	Diacylglycerol	DA
Attention-deficit hyperactivity disorder	ADHD	Diethylstilbestrol	DES
		Dihydroxyphenylalanine	DOPA
β-Adrenergic receptor kinase	βARK	Diiodotyrosine	DIT
Basic fibroblastic growth factor	bFGF	Dopamine	DAG
Behavioral sex determination	BSD	Dorsal infundibular nucleus	DIV
Bisphenol A	BPA	Dorsomedial nucleus	DMN
β-Lipotropin	β-LPH	Endocrine disrupting chemical	EDC
Body mass index	BMI	Endogenous opioid peptide	EOP
Bombesin	BBS	Endothelium-derived relaxing factor	EDRF
Bone morphometric protein	BMP	Enzyme-linked immunoabsorbent assay	ELISA
Brain natriuretic peptide	BNP	Epidermal growth factor	EGF
C natriuretic peptide	CNP	Epinephrine	E
Calcitonin	CT	ER knockout mice	βERKO
Calcitonin gene-related peptide	CGRP	Estrogen receptor	ER
Calcium-sensitive cell	PIPAS cell	Estrogen-related receptor	ERR
cAMP regulatory element binding protein	CREB	Ethinylestradiol	EE$_2$
		Ethylenediaminetetraacetate	EDTA
Carbon monoxide	CO	Extrapancreatic tumor hypoglycemia	EPTH
Catechol O-methyltransferase	COMT	Farnesoid X receptor	FXR
Central nervous system	CNS	Follicle-stimulating hormone	FSH
Cerebral spinal fluid	CSF	FSH releasing hormone	FSH-RH
Cholecystokinin	CCK	Galanin	GAL
Choline acetyltransferase	CAT	γ-Aminobutyric acid	GABA
Chorionic corticotropin	CC	Gastric inhibitory peptide	GIP
Chorionic gonadotropin	CG	Gastrin-releasing peptide	GRP
Chorionic somato-mammotropin	CS	Genotypic sex determination	GSD
Chorionic thyrotropin	CT	γ-Lipotropin	γ-LPH
Cocaine and amphetamine regulated transcript	CART	Glucagon	GLUC
		Glucagon-like peptide	GLP
Compensatory ovarion hypertrophy	COH	Glucagon-related polypeptide	GRPP
Computer axial tomography	CAT	Glucose transporter	GLUT
Congenital adrenal hyperplasia	CAH	Glucose-dependent insulino-tropic peptide	GIP
Convertase enzyme	PC		
Copy DNA	cDNA	Glumitocin	GLT
Corticosteroid-binding globulin	CBG	Glutamate decarboyxlase	GAD
Corticosterone	B	Gonadotropin	Gn
Corticotropin	ACTH	Gonadotropin	GTH
Corticotropin-like peptide	CLIP	Gonadotropin release-inhibiting hormone	GRIH
Corticotropin-releasing hormone	CRH		
Cortisol	F	Gonadotropin-releasing hormone	GnRH
CRF receptor	CRF-R	Gonadotropin-releasing hormone-associated peptide	GAP
CRH receptor	CRH-R		

Green fluorescent protein	GFP	Melanotropin release-inhibiting hormone	MRIH
Growth differentiation factor	GDF	Melanotropin-releasing hormone	MRH
Growth factor receptor-binding protein	GRBP	Menopausal gonadotropin	MG
Growth hormone	GH	Mesotocin	MST
Growth hormone release-inhibiting hormone, somatostatin	GHRIH	Messenger RNA	mRNA
		Metyrapone	SU4885
Growth hormone-releasing hormone, somatocrinin	GHRH	Migrating motor complex	MMC
		Mineralocorticoid receptor	MR
Guanosine triphosphate	GTP	Mitogen-activated protein kinase	MAPK
Hagfish natriuretic peptide	EbyNP	Monoacylglyceride	MAG
High-density lipoprotein	HDL	Monoamine oxidase	MAO
High-performance liquid chromatography	HPLC	Monoiodotyrosine	MIT
		Müllerian-inhibiting substance	MIS
Hormone response element	HRE		(same as
Human placental lactogen	hPL		AMH)
Hydroxyindole-O-methyltransferase	HIOMT	N-Acetyltransferase	NAT
Hydroxymethylglutaryl coenzyme A	HMG-CoA	Nasohypophysial factor	NHF
		Natriuretic peptide	NP
Hypothalamus-pituitary	HP	Nerve growth factor	NGF
Hypothalamus-pituitary-adrenal axis	HPA	Neuropeptide Y	NPY
Hypothalamus-pituitary-gonad axis	HPG	Neurotensin	NT
Hypothalamus-pituitary-hepatic axis	HPH	Nictoinamide adenine dinucleotide phosphate	NADPH
Hypothalamus-pituitary-thyroid axis	HPT	Nitric oxide	NO
Immunoradiometric assay	IRMA	Nitric oxide synthetase	NOS
Infundibular nucleus	IFN	Nonesterified fatty acids	NEFA
Inositol trisphosphate	IP_3	Non-insulin-dependent diabetes mellitus = Type 2 diabetes	NIDDM
Insulin response proteins	IRS		
Insulin-dependent diabetes mellitus = Type 1 diabetes	IDDM	Norepinephrine	NE
		Nuclear magentic resonance imaging	NMRI
Insulin-like growth factor	IGF	Nucleus lateralis tuberis	NLT
Interleukin 1	IL-1	Organic anion transporter polypeptides	oatps
Interleukin 2	IL-2		
Interleukin 6	IL-6	Organum vasculosum lateralis terminae	OVLT
Intermediate-density lipoprotein	IDL		
Interstitial cell-stimulating hormone	ICSH	Ovarian ascorbic acid depletion	OAAD
Isotocin	IST	Oxytocin	OXY
Janus kinase–signal transducer and activator of transcription	JAK-STAT	PACAP-related peptide	PRP
		Pancreatic polypeptide	PP
Knockout	KO	Pancreostatin	Pst
Lateral hypothalamus	LatH	Parathyroid hormone	PTH
Lipoprotein	LPH	Parathyroid hormone-related protein	PTHrP
Long-acting thyroid stimulator	LATS	Paraventricular nucleus	PVN
Low-density lipoprotein	LDL	Peptide histidine isoleucine	PHI
Luteinization of atretic follicles	LAF	Peptide histidine methionine	PHM
Luteinizing hormone	LH	Peptide YY	PYY
Luteinizing hormone-releasing hormone	LHRH (same as GnRH)	Periventricular nucleus	PERIV
		Peroxisomal roliferators activated receptor	PPAR
Lysine vasopressin	LVP		
Magentic resonance tomography	MRT	PG series A	PGA
Melanophore-concentrating hormone	MCH	PG series E	PGE
Melanotropin	MSH	PG series F	PGF

PG series I	PGI	Son of sevenless protein	SOS
Phasvatocin	PhaT	Stanniocalcin	STC
Phenylethanolamine-N-methyltransferase	PNMT	Steroidogenesis-stimulating protein	STP
		Steroidogenic acute regulatory protein	StAR
Phenypressin	PVP	Steroidogenic factor-1	SF-1
Phosphodiesterase	PDE	Subcommissural organ	SCO
Phosphoenolpyruvate	PEP	Substance P	SP
Phosphoenolpyruvate carboxykinase	PEPCK	Superior cervical ganglion	SCG
Phosphofructokinase	PFK	Suprachiasmatic nucleus	SCN
Phosphoinositol diphosphate	PIP$_2$	Supraoptic nucleus	SON
Phosphokinase A	PKA	Syndrome of inappropriate diuresis	SIAD
Phospholipase C	PLC	Temperature-dependent sex determination	TSD
Pineal antigonadotropic peptide	PAG		
Pituitary adenylyl cyclase activating peptide	PACAP	Tetrahydrocanabinol	THC
		Tetraiodothyroacetic acid	TETRAC
Pituitary transcription factor	Pit-1	Thiourea	TU
Placental lactogen	PL	Thyroglobulin	Tgb
Platelet-derived growth factor	PDGF	Thyroid peroxidase	TPO
Polychloinated biphenyl	PCB	Thyroid receptor	TR
Polycystic ovarian syndrome	PCOS	Thyroid receptor auxiliary protein	TRAP
Polymerase chain reaction	PCR	Thyroid response element	TRE
Positron emission tomography	PET	Thyroid-binding albumin	TBA
Pregnant mare serum gonadotropin	PMSG	Thyroid-binding globulin	TBG
Preoptic area	POA	Thyroid-binding prealbumin	TBPA
Preoptic nucleus	PON	Thyrotropin	TSH
PRL release-inhibiting hormone	PRIH	Thyrotropin-releasing hormone	TRH
PRL releasing hormone	PRH	Thyroxine (tetraiodothyronine)	T$_4$
Progestogen receptor	PR	Tissue necrosis factor	TNF
Prolactin	PRL	Transcription factor	TF
Prolactin-releasing peptide	PrRP	Transforming growth factor	TGF
Proopiomelanocortin	POMC	Transforming growth factor α	TGF-α
Propylthiouracil	PTU	Transmission electron microscope	TEM
Prostaglandin	PG	Transthyretin	TTR
Protein kinase C	PKC	Triacylglyceride	TAG
Pyruvate kinase	PK	Triiodothyroacetic acid	TRIAC
Radioimmunoassay	RIA	Triiodothyronine	T$_3$
Retinoic acid receptor	RAR	Truncated GLP-I	tGLP-I
Retinoid X receptor	RXR	Uncoupling protein	UCP
Reverse T$_3$	rT$_3$	Urocortin	Ucn
Ribonucleic acid	RNA	Valitocin	ValT
Rough endoplasmic reticulum	RER	Vascular endothelial cell growth factor	VEGF
Scaning electron microscope	SEM		
Seasonal affective disorder	SAD	Vasoactive intestinal peptide	VIP
Selective estrogen receptor modulator	SERM	Ventral infundibular nucleus	NIV
		Ventricular natriuretic peptide	VNP
Serotonin	5-HT	Ventromedial nucleus	VMN
Sexually dimorphic nucleus	SDN	Very-low-density lipoprotein	VLDL
Sodium iodide symporter	NIS	Vitamin D receptor	VDR
Somatolactin	SL	Voltage-sensitive calcium channels	VSCC
Somatostatin = SST	SS	Vomeronasal organ	VNO
Somatostatin; also SS$_{14}$, SS$_{28}$, SS$_{34}$	SST		
Somatotropin = GH	STH		

APPENDIX B

Vertebrate Tissue Types

I. The Origin of Vertebrate Tissues

During embryonic development the process of gastrulation defines the three **primary germ layers**: ectoderm, mesoderm, and endoderm. The **ectoderm** gives rise to the nervous system, including the neural crest and its derivatives, the epidermis, the lining of the oral cavity, and parts of certain sense organs. The **endoderm** gives rise to the mucosal lining of the gut and a number of derivatives of the gut, including the lungs, thyroid gland, liver, and pancreas. **Mesoderm** is the source of muscle, dermis, linings of the coelomic cavity (peritoneum, pleura, pericardium), and blood vessels (endothelium), and special organs such as the kidneys, adrenal cortex, and the gonads. The skeleton is formed from mesoderm as well as from neural crest (certain skull bones).

The primary germ layers give rise to four primary tissues: epithelium, connective tissues, muscle, and nervous tissue. These tissue types are defined below. Ectoderm gives rise to nervous tissue, and certain epithelia. Endoderm gives rise to both covering epithelia and glandular epithelia. Mesoderm gives rise to special epithelia (mesothelia, endothelia), in addition to glandular epithelia, the elements of the various connective tissues, and all muscle. The origin of primordial germ cells that eventually reside in the gonads in at least some vertebrates has been traced to endoderm, although it is possible that mesoderm may be involved in some species.

A. Epithelium

An epithelium consists of closely associated cells organized into sheets that develop into coverings of either outer and inner surfaces or is modified into a glandular structure. Little intracellular material is found between the cells of epithelia, but they are typically associated with a distinct basement membrane associated with the basal portion of the cells. The basement membrane is secreted by cells of the epithelium. Epithelia also may occur as tubes (**ducts, cords**) or spheres (**follicles, acini**). Individual cells may differ markedly in shape, and some cells may exhibit specialized adornments such as cilia or microvilli (brush border). Cilia may be responsible for producing currents to aid the flow of materials through a duct or other passageway as a result of coordinated rhythmic beating. Sometimes cilia are sensory structures, too. Microvilli greatly increase the total surface area of cells. Presence of microvilli is a clue to an epithelium's involvement in transport of molecules between the cells and extracellular fluids. Epithelia may consist of a single layer or sheet of cells (**simple**) or several layers of one (**stratified**) or several (**compound**) types of simple epithelia appearing in layers. Some examples of epithelia are listed below:

- Simple squamous epithelium: thin, flat cells organized in sheets such as the peritoneum
- Simple cuboidal epithelium: cube-shaped cells comprising the lining of certain ducts such as portions of the nephron

- Simple columnar epithelium: tall, rectangular cells that may also be found lining certain ducts as well as the intestinal lumina
- Stratified squamous epithelium; epidermis of skin
- Glandular epithelium: cords of cells as in the adrenal cortex, acini (solid balls of cells with a central duct) as found in the exocrine pancreas, follicles or hollow balls of endocrine cells as those comprising the thyroid gland

B. Connective Tissues

The cells of connective tissue are generally separated from one another by extensive intracellular material (matrix) that they have secreted. Mesenchyme derived from mesoderm gives rise to four basic kinds of connective tissue: blood and lymph-forming tissues, connective tissue proper, cartilage, and bone.

1. Blood-Forming Tissues

The blood-forming elements give rise to circulating **erythrocytes** or red blood cells (RBCs) and **leukocytes** (leucocytes) or white blood cells (WBCs) in adult vertebrates. The RBCs of mammals are unique among the vertebrates in that the mature circulating cell lacks a nucleus. The WBCs are further subdivided into cells with granular cytoplasm, the **granulocytes (eosinophils, basophils, neutrophils)** and **agranulocytes (lymphocytes, monocytes, plasma cells)**. Circulating eosinphils are identical to those associated with many organs such as the uterus and the lung. Basophils may be identical to **tissue mast cells** that secrete histamine. The extracellular matrix of blood is called **plasma**.

2. Connective Tissue Proper

A large number of tissue types are lumped under the title of **connective tissue proper**, including **loose fibrous connective tissue**, **dense fibrous connective tissue** (e.g., tendons), **elastic tissue**, and **reticular connective tissue**. The fibrous components are proteins (collagen, elastin, reticular fibers) and are found in the different connective tissue types to various extents.

3. Adipose Tissue

Adipose (fat) tissue consists of cells (adipocytes) that contain large amounts of fat restricted to a central vacuole which confines the cytoplasm to a thin rim adjacent to the plasmalemma. In rodents, there are two readily distinguishable types of adipose tissue termed white and brown. **White adipose tissue** shows regular variations in the amount of stored fat with nutritional state.

Brown fat is more vascular than white adipose tissue, and the cells have numerous small vacuoles filled with fat whereas a single vacuole is present in the white adipose cell. It does not vary with nutritional state but has been correlated with hibernating behavior. In most mammals it is not possible to differentiate brown and white types of adipose tissue.

4. Cartilage

Cartilage cells or **chondrocytes** secrete a matrix consisting of a glycoprotein, **chondromucoid**, that contains the sulfonated polysaccharide chondroitin sulfate. The extensive matrix between the chondrocytes may have few fibrous components (**hyaline cartilage**) or may contain collagen (**fibrocartilage**) or elastin fibers (**elastic cartilage**). Cartilage may also be strengthened by addition of calcium salts.

5. Bone

Bone is the strongest connective tissue and the densest. The extensive matrix of bone is comprised of crystalline calcium salts, primarily calcium phosphate, and very little water. Bone occurs in a uniformly dense, compact form (**compact bone**) and in a less dense, more easily modified form (**cancellous** or spongy **bone**). The bone-forming cells are known as **osteoblasts** and are rich in phosphatase. Osteoblasts that have become embedded within the bone matrix are termed **osteocytes**. Giant multinucleated cells, the **osteoclasts**, produce hydrolytic enzymes and are responsible for bone destruction (resorption). The osteoblasts and osteoclasts are responsible for bone forming, resorbing, and reforming in accordance with physical stresses placed on bone, with physiological demands, and with external sources of calcium and phosphate.

6. Muscle

Mesoderm gives rise to three basic muscle types: smooth, striated, and cardiac. **Smooth muscle** frequently is termed involuntary muscle since it is under control of the autonomic nervous system. It is associated with internal organs and is found in such places as the gut wall, blood vessels, various ducts, and the wall of the uterus. Individual muscle cells are smaller than striated cells, and the contractile elements (myofibrils) are not highly organized within the cell. Smooth muscle is characterized by slow, rhythmic contractions.

Striated or **skeletal muscle** is the so-called voluntary muscle tissue that is under conscious control, although it also may be influenced by the autonomic system. Striated muscle cells are large cells with myofibrils so highly organized as to produce regular bands or striations when the cells are viewed with the aid of a microscope. Movements of the skeleton are controlled by striated muscles that are attached to the bone by dense fibrous connective tissue. In addition, a few sphincter muscles are also of this type and hence are under conscious control (e.g., the external urinary bladder sphincter).

Cardiac muscle possesses properties of both skeletal muscle (striations due to highly organized myofibrils) and smooth muscle (rhythmic contractions that are innate properties of cardiac muscle cells). Instead of inserting on bones, the cardiac cells connect directly to one another through specialized tendinous attachments known as intercalated disks.

7. Nervous Tissue

Nervous tissue is specialized for integrative functions and conduction of information throughout the body. **Neurons** are specialized cells for conducting electrochemical neural impulses to coordinate body processes. Most neurons release chemical neurotransmitters to control the activity of other neurons, muscle cells, and glands. **Neurosecretory neurons** produce neurohormones that are secreted into the blood vascular system and constitute a second type of control mechanism. The central nervous system also contains several types of **glial cells** (neuroglia), which perform many supportive functions for the neurons including production of paracrine regulators. One important role of glial cells is the secretion of myelin that forms the white matter of the central nervous system. The ependymal cells that line the brain ventricles are another form. The **Schwann cell**, a type of glial cell in the peripheral nervous system, secretes the myelin sheath characteristic of many peripheral neurons.

C. General Tissue Responses

In response to various stimuli a given tissue may exhibit no morphologically observable response, degeneration (atrophy, resorption), or growth. The last response may be due simply to an increase in cell size (**hypertrophy**) or to increased cellular divisions with an actual increase in cell numbers (**hyperplasia**) or both. Tumors or neoplasms are abnormal proliferations of tissues (**neoplasia**) having no normal physiological function. Such growths may be classified as either **benign** (harmless) or **malignant** (very harmful or likely to cause death; i.e., a cancer). The term **adenoma** refers to a benign tumor of glandular origin that may or may not synthesize and release abnormal amounts of hormones. Connective tissue tumors are called **sarcomas**, whereas a lymphatic tumor is a **lymphoma**. Malignant growths of any epithelial tissue, including glandular epithelia, are termed **carcinomas**. Some adenomas or carcinomas also produce excessive quantities of hormones or hormone-like substances, as in the production of excessive amounts of growth hormone by pituitary adenomas or secretion of gastrin (a hormone that stimulates hydrochloric acid secretion in the stomach) by a pancreatic carcinoma.

APPENDIX C

Amino Acids and Their Symbols

Amino acid	Old system	New system	Basic AA	Acidic AA
Alanine	Ala	A		
Arginine	Arg	R	+	
Asparagine	Asn	N	+	
Aspartate	Asp	D		+
Cysteine	Cys	C		
Glutamate	Glu	E		+
Glutamine	Gln	Q	+	
Glycine	Gly	G		
Histidine	His	H		
Isoleucine	Ile	I		
Leucine	Leu	L		
Lysine	Lys	K	+	
Methionine	Met	M		
Phenylalanine	Phe	F		
Proline	Pro	P		
Serine	Ser	S		
Threonine	The	T		
Tryptophan	Trp	W		
Tyrosine	Tyr	Y		
Valine	Val	V		

APPENDIX D

Bioassays

The bioassays described below represent the more common ones for the major peptide and protein hormones. Although largely of historical interest, these bioassays sometimes are useful when precise radioimmunoassay or chemical identification is not possible.

I. Gonadotropins

Specific bioassays have been developed in a variety of vertebrates for distinguishing between follicle-stiumulating hormone (FSH) and luteinizing hormone (LH) biological acitivity. A summary of some typical responses is provided in Tables D-1 and D-2.

A. Luteinizing Hormone (LH)

One of the first bioassays was the **spermiation test** observed following injection of pituitary extracts or purified LH into frogs or toads. At one time, this bioassay was widely employed by doctors to detect the presence of CG in urine of women and confirm early pregnancy. The structural and functional similarity of hCG and

Table D-1. Relative Potencies of Follicle-Stimulating Hormone and Luteinizing Hormone Purified from Different Vertebrates and Tested in the *Anolis* and *Xenopus* Gonadotropin Bioassays[a]

Hormone	Relative potency	
	Anolis bioassay	*Xenopus* bioassay
Ovine FSH	100.0[b]	< 0.005
Ovine LH	0.04	2.0[c]
Snapping turtle FSH	3.0[b]	0.002
Snapping turtle LH	0.13	1.8[c]
Chicken FSH	4.3[b]	< 0.0015
Chicken LH	0.85	0.08[c]
Bullfrog FSH	7.0[b]	0.004
Bullfrog LH	1.2	0.33[c]

[a] Based on Licht, P., Papkoff, H., Farmer, S. W., Muller, C. H., Tsui, H. W., and Crews, D. (1977). Evolution of gonadotropin structure and function. *Recent Prog. Horm. Res.* **33**, 169–248.
[b] *Anolis* bioassay for FSH: maintenance of testis weight in hypophysectomized lizard.
[c] *Xenopus* bioassay for LH: *in-vitro* ovulation.

Table D-2. Relative Effectiveness of Purified Ovine Gonadotropin (FSH and LH) in Some Gonadotropin Bioassays

| | Minimal effective dose (μg/ml or μg/injections[a]) | | |
Bioassay	FSH	LH	Relative potency
A. Testis weight maintenance in hypox lizard (*Anolis carolinensis*)	0.01	20.0	FSH >> LH
B. *In-vitro* ovulation of frog ovary (*Xenopus laevis*)	> 200.0	0.5	LH >>> FSH
C. Spermiation response by frog (*Hyla regilla*)	0.5	1.0	FSH $\cong$ LH

[a] Injection for bioassays A and C.

hLH to amphibian gonadotropins is the basis for this clinical test. A spermiation test, however, responds to highly purified FSH, too, and cannot be considered a specific bioassay for LH-like hormones. Pregnancy is now determined from urine samples with a simple and highly sensitive immunoassay involving an antibody produced specifically against hCG.

A popular early bioassay for LH was the **ovarian ascorbic acid depletion test (OAAD)**, which was based upon a quantitative reduction of ascorbic acid in ovarian tissue following administration of LH. The degree of depletion is proportional to the dose of LH, and this bioassay is not affected by FSH. The relationship of ascorbic acid to hormone secretion is not understood, however, and this rather cumbersome assay is seldom used.

The pigment response to LH by feathers of the African weaver finch, *Euplectes franciscanus*, was another highly specific bioassay for LH or CG, but it too is cumbersome.

The **frog ovulatory response** *in vitro* to LH or CG (ovulation) has resulted in development of several similar bioassays. Administration of pituitary LH or progesterone stimulates ovulation in isolated fragments of anuran or urodele amphibian ovaries. Luteinizing hormone causes progesterone synthesis in follicular cells surrounding the oocyte, and it was believed that the local progesterone binding to oocyte receptors induces the ovulatory event. This *in-vitro* ovarian bioassay also has been used for detection of progesterone. However, recent studies suggest that the progesterone is further metabolized to testosterone and the latter is responsible for final oocyte maturation. Although the system is somewhat responsive to a few other steroids, it is relatively unresponsive to FSH and other tropic hormones.

B. Follicle-Stimulating Hormone (FSH)

The major bioassay for FSH prior to development of RIAs was the increase in testis or ovarian weight in hypophysectomized rats following injection of pituitary extracts or purified preparations of tropic hormones. Development of any of the androgen-sensitive sex accessory structures in the test animals would be evidence of LH contamination. Another specific bioassay for FSH is the maintenance of testis weight in male *Anolis carolinensis* lizards following hypophysectomy. The lizard testis regresses rapidly following hypophysectomy and normally is unresponsive to LH. Hence, this bioassay is very specific for small quantities of highly purified FSH.

II. Thyrotropin (TSH)

Stimulation of thyroid gland function can be quantified cytologically by means of the TSH dose-dependent stimulation of **epithelial cell height** of the thyroid follicles in hypophysectomized animals. However, this bioassay requires several days to obtain results of these tissue changes, and a more rapid bioassay measures the amount of **radioiodide uptake** by thyroid follicles following administration of purified TSH or pituitary extracts (see Chapter 6, Table 6-4). This bioassay can be performed *in vitro* as well as *in vivo*. Epithelial cell height and radioiodide accumulation indicate the degree of TSH stimulation and are also proportional to circulating TSH levels.

III. Category 2 Tropic Hormones

A. Growth Hormone (GH)

The classical bioassay for GH is the histological measurement of the thickness of the **epiphysial cartilage** in the tibia of the hypophysectomized rat or mouse following treatment with pituitary extracts or purified molecules. Some typical results are provided in Table D-3.

B. Insulinlike Growth Factors (IGFs)

A bioassay for IGFs has been developed using costal cartilage from pigs *in vitro*. The rate of incorporation of radioactive sulphate ions is measured and is directly proportional to the amount of IGF.

C. Prolactin (PRL)

Several specific bioassays for PRL have been reported utilizing animals representing four major vertebrate classes (teleosts, amphibians, birds, and mammals). Not all vertebrate PRLs are effective in every assay as indicated in Table D-4. The bioassays are

1. The sodium-retaining bioassay in the cichlid teleost *Sarotherodon (Tilapia) mossambicus*
2. The xanthophore-expanding bioassay in the teleost *Gillichthyes mirabilis*
3. The red-eft water drive performed in the newt *Notophthalmus viridescens*
4. The crop-sac assay performed in the domestic pigeon
5. The *in-vitro* mouse mammary gland assay

1. Fish Bioassays for PRL

The **sodium-retaining bioassay** in fishes stresses the osmoregulatory actions of PRL in teleost fishes, and particularly its effect on sodium uptake across the gill and resultant alterations in plasma sodium levels. Only some pituitaries from teleosts, however, will produce a measurable response in this bioassay, and all other piscine and other non-mammalian preparations are inactive. Purified mammalian PRLs, curiously, work very well in this bioassay. This observation supports the hypothesis that the osmoregulatory portion of the piscine PRL molecule has been retained in the structure of mammalian PRL with the addition of new structural

Table D-3. Potencies of Growth Hormone Determined in the Rat Tibia Assay[a]

Species	Potency[b]
Sturgeon	0.40
Tilapia	0.05
Bullfrog	1.15
Leopard frog	0.36
Snapping turtle	0.24
Sea turtle	0.12
Ostrich	0.94
Duck	0.16
Marsupial	0.03
Mammal	1.00

[a] From Chester-Jones, I., Ingleton, P. M., and Phillips, J. G. (1987). "Fundamentals of Comparative Vertebrate Endocrinology." Plenum Press, New York.
[b] Bovine GH standard = 1.0. Marsupial GHs were nonparallel.

Table D-4. Bioassayable Prolactin in Vertebrate Pituitaries

Vertebrate group	*Gillichthyes*[a] xanthophore-yellowing response	Tilapia Na$^+$-retaining response	Red-eft water drive	Pigeon crop-sac assay	Mouse mammary *in vitro*
Agnatha	+	−	−	−	−
Chondrichthyes	+	−	+	−	−
Chondrostei	+	−	?	−	−
Holostei	+	−	?	−	−
Teleostei	+	+, −	+	−	−[b]
Dipnoi	+	−	+	+	+
Amphibia	+	−	+	+	+
Reptilia	+	?	+	+	+
Aves	+	?	+	+	+
Mammalia	+	+, −	+	+	+

[a] This assay system may not be specific for prolactin (see text).
[b] Purified tilapia PRL stimulates casein synthesis in the rabbit mammary gland.

modifications that are responsible for crop-sac and mammary gland actions. This bioassay was developed for fish PRL first in hypophysectomized guppies, *Poecilia latipinna*. Later, it was modified to use intact, seawater-adapted tilapia. Adaptation of these fishes to seawater almost eliminates PRL from the circulation and alleviates the need for hypophysectomy.

The **xanthophore-expanding bioassay** is performed in the gobiid fish *Gillichthyes mirabilis*, the longjawed mudsucker. It is an all-or-none bioassay for determination of the smallest dose of purified hormone or the greatest dilution of pituitary homogenate or extract that will cause local yellowing in 50% of the fish tested following injection of the test material beneath the preopercular skin. The bioassay does have the distinct advantage, however, of being extremely sensitive to piscine (including agnathan) and amphibian pituitary homogenates. For example, teleost pituitaries are more than 100,000 times more effective in the assay than is oPRL that is used as a standard. As little as 1/100th of a tiger salamander pituitary gives a positive response in the xanthophore-expanding bioassay, whereas an entire salamander pituitary of the same size is required to produce a minimal response in the pigeon crop-sac bioassay.

2. The Red Eft Water-Drive Bioassay for PRL

Prolactin induces a second metamorphosis or **"water drive"** in newts that is characterized by migration of the juvenile terrestrial form, the eft, back to water where breeding will occur (Figure D-1). Water-drive behavior, which also occurs in salamanders, is accompanied by a series of physiological and morphological changes as well, but these are not related to the bioassay *per se*. Following injection of PRL, the adults leave the dry areas of their laboratory containers and enter the water where they remain for breeding. No other hormone has been found to induce water-drive behavior. This bioassay has the disadvantage of being an all-or-none response. Pituitary preparations for all classes of vertebrates except the class Agnatha possess water-drive-inducing activity (Table D-4). Treatment with mammalian PRL stimulates locomotor activity in tiger salamanders that may be a component of water-drive behavior. Curiously, terrestrial anuran amphibians that migrate to water for breeding do not exhibit elevated PRL levels. The failure for PRL to elicit water-drive behavior in anurans suggests that the PRL-based water drive is a phenomenon limited to caudate amphibians.

The antithesis of water drive is the return to land by newts and salamanders as well as by frogs and toads after breeding (Figure D-1). This **land-drive** behavior appears to be a consequence of elevated thyroid hormones, and experimentally elevated thyroid hormones prevent breeding migrations of anurans to water. Antibodies against PRL as well as treatment with thyroxine can influence substrate preference in urodeles.

3. The Pigeon Crop-Sac Bioassay for PRL

The pigeon crop-sac bioassay is a precise quantitative, dose-related bioassay that yields a standard curve from which relative activities of unknown preparations can be assessed. The bioassay is performed on 6-week-old

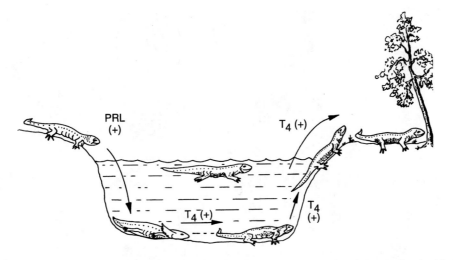

Figure D-1. **Land- and water-drives in urodele amphibian life histories.** Prolactin (PRL) is associated with increased locomotor behavior and a preference for seeking out water associated usually with reproductive behaviors. Increased thyroid activity is associated with a terrestrial preference that probably causes the newly metamorphosed animal or post-reproductive animal to leave the water. Similar relationships may occur in anurans (see Chapter 7). T_4, thyroxine.

pigeons that have not reached sexual maturity. The pigeon crop-sac is a bilateral extension of the esophagus that in brooding birds produces a cytogenous secretion that is fed to the hatchlings. For this bioassay, the crop-sac first is "primed" by injection of the birds with a small amount of mPRL (usually ovine). Then, on one side of the crop, the test solution containing either a known or unknown amount of mPRL or pituitary extracts is applied by subcutaneous injection directly over the crop surface. On the opposite side, a control solution (usually the same saline vehicle used for the test solution) is similarly applied. After removal of the crop-sac several days later, a given area of the crop epithelium is scraped off around each control or test application site, dried, and weighed. The weight of the dried crop-sac epithelial area is plotted against the known dose of mPRL used so that a standard curve is produced. The PRL content of unknowns can be identified by extrapolation from the standard curve.

Positive results have been obtained in the crop-sac bioassay with lungfish pituitaries as well as pituitaries from all tetrapod groups, but most piscine PRLs will produce only an atypical response or no response at all. Although this bioassay is very consistent and sensitive, it has the major disadvantage of the time involved in performing it.

4. Mammary Gland *In-Vitro* Bioassay for PRL

For this bioassay, mammary gland explants from pseudopregnant or midpregnant mice (or rabbits) are cultured in a precise medium that includes some other hormones (e.g., glucocorticoids, insulin). The addition of PRL or pituitary homogenates to the culture medium causes cytological changes that can be quantified according to a numerical index (Figure D-2). These cytological changes are correlated with the ability of PRL to stimulate milk synthesis. Like the crop-sac bioassay, mammotropic (lactogenic) activity is present in the pituitaries of all tetrapod species tested in the mouse mammary bioassay, but piscine pituitary preparations yield minimal responses, if any. Like the crop-sac bioassay, the mammary gland response is not a rapid assessment.

IV. POMC-Related Hormones

A. Adrenocorticotropin (ACTH)

The classical bioassay for ACTH has been the **adrenal ascorbic acid depletion test (AAAD)**, which is similar to the OAAD bioassay described for LH. The lowest effective dose of purified ACTH in this bioassay is

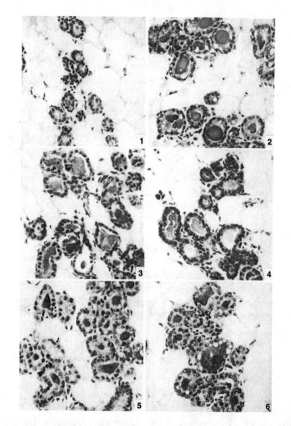

Figure D-2. *In-vitro* **mouse mammary gland bioassay for prolactin (PRL).** Secretion rating (SR) is accomplished using a visual scale (SR = 1, lowest activity, to 5, highest activity). (1) Control explant, alveoli (lumen) not distended and containing little secretion; SR = 1. (2) Effect of extract from amphibian pituitary; SR = 5. (3) Effect of retile pituitary extract; SR = 4. (4) Effect of avian pituitary extract; SR = 3. (5) Effect of guinea pig pituitary extract; SR = 4. (6) Purified ovine PRL; SR = 5. [From Nicoll, C. S., Bern, H. A., and Brown, D. (1966). Occurrence of mammotrophic activity (prolactin) in the vertebrae adenohypophysis. *J. Endocr.* **34**, 343–354.]

0.2 mU or about $1.2 \times 10 - 9$ g (about 1 ng). The adrenal cortex secretes certain corticosteroids in response to ACTH stimulation. The AAAD test is rarely used today and has been replaced by measurement of either circulating ACTH or corticosteroids with RIA.

B. Melanotropin (MSH)

The standard bioassays for MSH have been developed in amphibians and reptiles utilizing their ability to adapt to dark or light backgrounds. One bioassay involves measurement (using a reflectometer) of the quantity of light reflected from an isolated piece of skin removed from a light-adapted frog. A similar bioassay employs isolated pieces of skin from the light background-adapted *Anolis carolinensis*, the American chameleon. A rapid all-or-none response (darkening) occurs *in vitro* in the presence of MSH.

The Hogben Index was a subjective analysis developed to measure the effects of MSH on the amphibian melanophore. It ranked the degree of melanosome dispersion within the melanophore on a scale of 1 to 5 (see Figure D-3).

C. Lipotropin (LPH)

A standardized bioassay for LPH activity involves culturing mouse or rabbit epididymal fat pads (isolated from testes) and measuring the release of glycerol or free fatty acids or both into the culture medium. Another bioassay technique for LPH employs measurement of the inhibition of incorporation of ^{14}C-labeled acetate

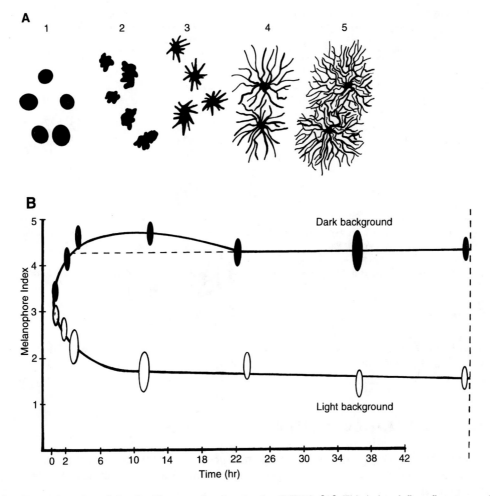

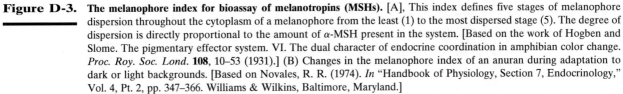

Figure D-3. **The melanophore index for bioassay of melanotropins (MSHs).** [A], This index defines five stages of melanophore dispersion throughout the cytoplasm of a melanophore from the least (1) to the most dispersed stage (5). The degree of dispersion is directly proportional to the amount of α-MSH present in the system. [Based on the work of Hogben and Slome. The pigmentary effector system. VI. The dual character of endocrine coordination in amphibian color change. *Proc. Roy. Soc. Lond.* **108**, 10–53 (1931).] (B) Changes in the melanophore index of an anuran during adaptation to dark or light backgrounds. [Based on Novales, R. R. (1974). *In* "Handbook of Physiology, Section 7, Endocrinology," Vol. 4, Pt. 2, pp. 347–366. Williams & Wilkins, Baltimore, Maryland.]

into lipid following addition of LPH to the culture medium. This procedure is, in effect, a measurement of lipogenesis, which is inversely related to lipolysis. The value of the bioassay is questionable since LPH does not seem to play a significant physiological role in lipid metabolism.

V. Nonapeptides of Pars Nervosa

A variety of bioassays have been developed in vertebrates to quantify the amount of oxytocin-like or vasopressin-like activity. Sample responses in each assay for various nonapeptides are found in Table D-5. These bioassays include

1. Antidiuretic bioassay for vasopressin (rat)
2. Pressor bioassay for vasopressin (rat)
3. Uterotonic bioassay for oxytocin (rat)
4. Depressor activity for oxytocin (chicken)
5. Milk ejection reflex (rabbit)

Table D-5. Biological Activity of Neurohypophysial Peptides[a,b] in Various Bioassays

Hormone	Activity units[c]				
	Uterotonic (rat)	Depressor (chicken)	Milk ejection (rabbit)	Pressor (rat)	Antidiuretic (rat)
Oxytocin	450	450	450	5	5
Mesotocin	291	502	330	6	1
Isotocin	145	310	290	0.06	0.18
Glumitocin	10	—	53	0.35	0.41
Valitocin	199	278	308	9	0.8
Aspargtocin	107	201	298	0.13	0.04
Arginine vasotocin	120	300	220	255	260
Arginine vasopressin	17	62	69	412	465
Lysine vasopressin	5	42	63	285	260

[a] Based on data from Acher, R. (1974). Chemistry of the neurohypophysial hormones: An example of molecular evolution. *In* "Handbook of Physiology, Sec. 7, Endocrinology, Vol. 4, Part 1," pp. 119–130. Williams & Wilkins, Baltimore, MD.

[b] For distribution of these hormones among the vertebrates, see Table 5-14.

[c] Units are expressed in international units per micromole of pure synthetic substance; 1 mg of synthetic oxytocin = 500 USP units.

VI. Bioassay of Glucagon

Related to its role in fasting mammals, glucagon is often bioassayed in the fasting cat in which it induces hyperglycemia. As in the case of insulin, however, rapid RIAs have been developed for measuring blood glucagon levels, and these are employed routinely.

VII. Parathyroid Hormone (PTH)

The classical bioassay for PTH was an increase in plasma calcium following administration of parathyroid gland extracts or PTH to normal or parathyroidectomized dogs. Later bioassays employed parathyroidectomized rats maintained on a calcium-deficient diet.

INDEX

Entries followed by f and t denote figures and tables, respectively.

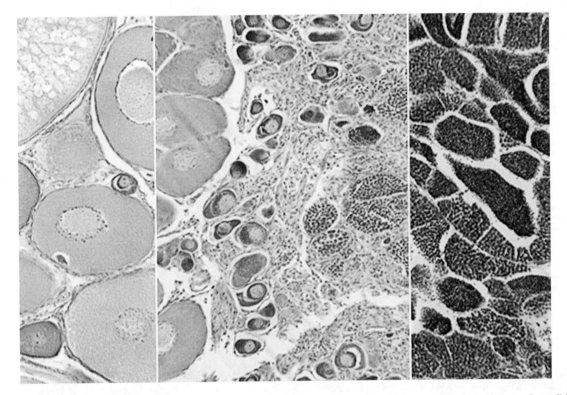

Plate 1 **Intersex gonad from white sucker *(Catostomus commersoni)*.** The left panel illustrates the normal ovary from fish at a reference site. The middle panel shows ovarian tissue to the left and spermatogenetic tissue to the right in an intersex gonad of a fish collected downstream of the discharge from a wastewater treatment plant (WWTP). To the right is a section through a normal testis from the reference site. Courtesy of Alan Vajda, University of Colorado.

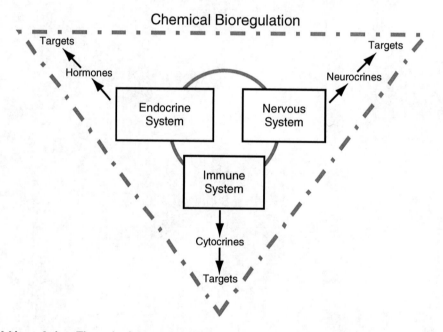

Plate 2 Chemical bioregulation. The endocrine system, nervous system, and immune system each secretes its own bioregulators: hormones, neurocrines, and cytocrines, respectively. However, all of these systems influence each other and from a homeostatic viewpoint, we can assume they function as one great bioregulatory system.

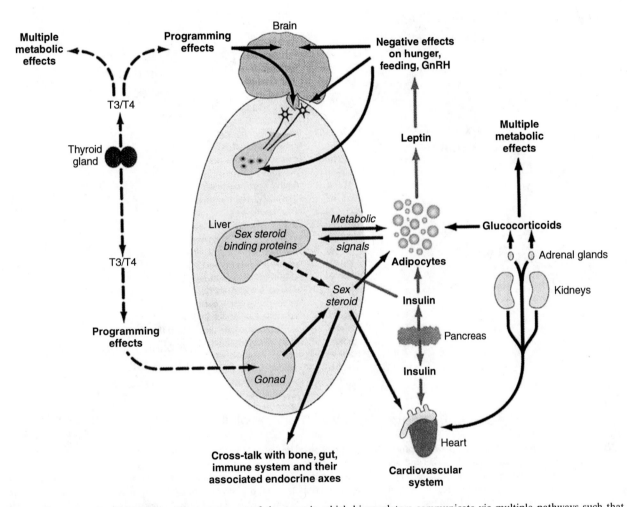

Plate 3 Cross-talk. This diagram illustrates some of the ways in which bioregulators communicate via multiple pathways such that one bioregulator may influence the effectiveness of another. [From Demstra, IPCS Global Assessment of EDCs, 2002, p. 20. Damstra, T., Barlow, S., Bergman, A., Kavlkock, R., and Van der Kraak, G. (2002). Global Assessment of the State-of-the-Science of Endocrine Disruptors. World Health Organization.]

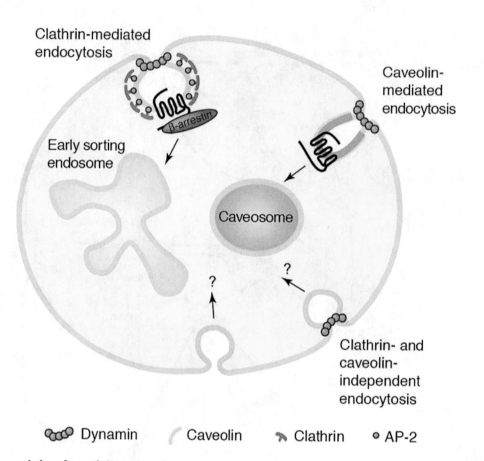

Clathrin-mediated endocytosis

Caveolin-mediated endocytosis

Early sorting endosome

β-arrestin

Caveosome

?

?

Clathrin- and caveolin-independent endocytosis

Dynamin Caveolin Clathrin AP-2

Plate 4 **Down-regulation of occupied receptors**. Occupied receptors migrate along the cell membrane to locations where endosomes form. These sites may be associated with the special proteins such as clathrin or caveolin as well as dynamin. Clathrin- and caveolin-independent endocytosis may occur where only dynamin is present. Fusion of endosomes with lysosomes to form endolysosomes results in degradation of both ligand and most or all of the receptors. Formation of small vesicles containing some receptors allows for possible recycling of receptors directly to the cell surface or indirectly via the Golgi apparatus. (Reprinted from Gaborik, Z., and Hunyady, L. Intracellular trafficking of hormone receptors. *Trends in Endocrin. and Metabolism* **15**, 286–293, 1994. Elsevier Publishers.)

(A) Fish brain

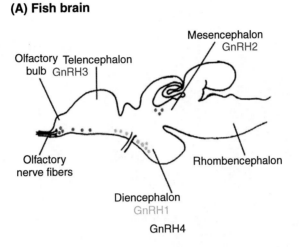

Mesencephalon
GnRH2

Olfactory Telencephalon
bulb GnRH3

Olfactory
nerve fibers

Rhombencephalon

Diencephalon
GnRH1

GnRH4

(B) Mouse brain

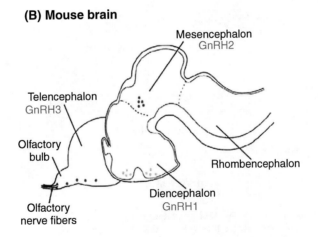

Mesencephalon
GnRH2

Telencephalon
GnRH3

Olfactory
bulb

Rhombencephalon

Olfactory
nerve fibers

Diencephalon
GnRH1

Plate 5 **Distribution of the forms of GnRH in the brain**. See text for explanation of abbreviations. [Reprinted with permission from Whitlock, K. E. (2005). Origin and development of GnRH neurons. *Trends Endocr. Metab.* **16**, 145–151. Elsevier Science Inc.]

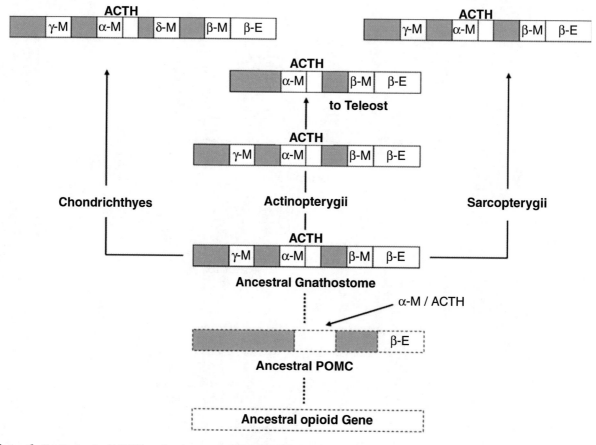

Plate 6 Corticotropin (ACTH) and melanotropin (MSHs) evolution. Four forms of MSH (α-M, β-M, γ-M, δ-M) are depicted in this scheme. The sarcopterygian branch would be similar to the tetrapod condition. [From Dores, R. M., and Lecaude, S. (2005). *Gen. Comp. Endocri.* **142**, 81–93.]

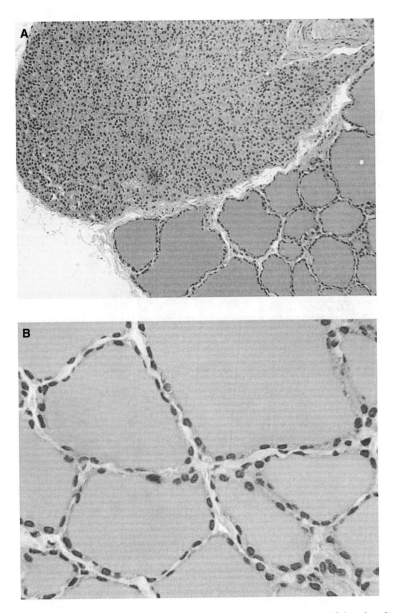

Plate 7 **Thyroid and parathyroid glands**. (A) Low magnification of compact parathyroid gland (above) embedded in the thyroid gland consisting of colloid-filled follicles (below). (B) High magnification of thyroid follicles with squamous epithelium surrounding colloid.

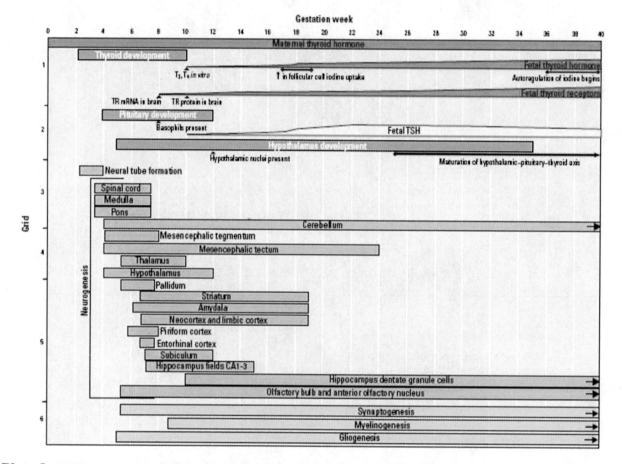

Plate 8 **Thyroid hormones and development of the nervous system in humans**. Note that many critical events in the nervous system are correlated with periods of thyroid hormones secretion. [Reprinted from Howdeshell, K. L. (2002). A model of the development of the brain as a construct of the thyroid system. *Environ. Health Persp.* **110** (Suppl 3), 337–348. Used with permission.]

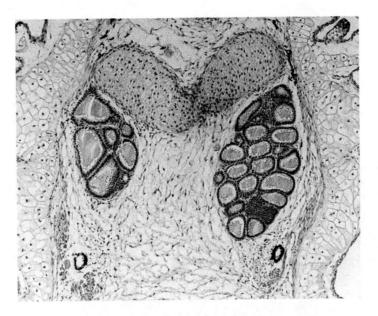

Control

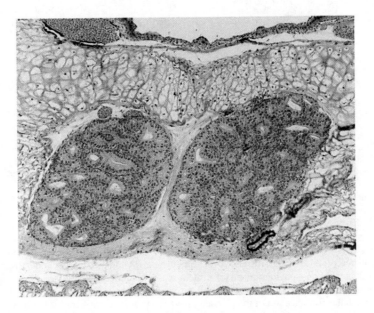

14 ppm AP

Plate 9 **Effect of perchlorate exposure in the laboratory.** The paired thyroid glands of a control frog can be seen at the top in marked contrast to the goitrous thyroids in the frog exposed to 14 ppm of ammonium perchlorate. This goitrous response is typical of the anti-thyroid action of perchlorate resulting in excessive production of thyrotropin and resultant stimulation of the thyroid gland. (Photomicrograph courtesy of Dr. James A. Carr, Texas Tech University.)

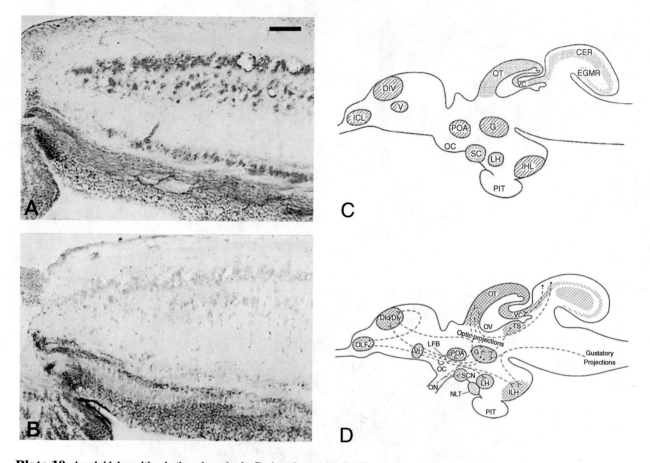

Plate 10 Amyloid deposition in the salmon brain. Brains of spawning Pacific salmon are characterized by extensive neurodegeneration and the deposition of immunoreactive β-amyloid as shown in the optic tectum (A) compared to an adjacent section of the same brain that was pretreated with immune serum (B) Staining in the optic tectum of a prespawning animal would resemble the immune control. (C) Distribution of immunoreactive glucocorticoid receptors in the brain of kokanee salmon. Compare to D. (D) Distribution of immunoreactive β-amyloid in the brain of kokanee salmon. Compare to the distribution of glucocorticoid receptors in C. [A, B, and D reprinted from Maldonado, T.A., Jones, R.E., and Norris, D.O. (2000). Distribution of β-amyloid and amyloid precursor protein in the brain of spawning (senescent) salmon: a natural brain-aging model. *Brain Research* **858**, 237–251. C reprinted with permission from Carruth, L.L., Jones, R.E., and Norris, D.O. 2000. Cell density and intracellular translocation of the glucocorticoid receptor in the kokanee salmon (*Oncorhynchus nerka kennerlyi*) brain, with an emphasis on the olfactory system. *Gen. Comp. Endocr.* **117**, 66–76.]

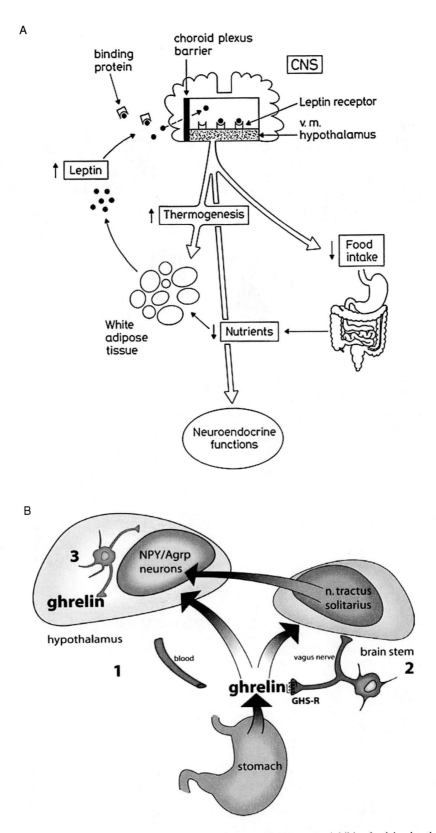

Plate 11 **Actions of leptin and grehlin on food intake**. (A) Leptin from adipocytes inhibits food intake through actions at the hypothalamus. [Reprinted with permission of the publisher from Sahu, A. Leptin signaling in the hypothalamus: Emphasis on energy homeostasis and leptin resistance. *Frontiers in Neuroendocr.* **24,** 225–253. Copyright 2003 Elsevier Science Inc.] (B) Ghrelin produced in the stomach also operates at the hypothalamus to alter food intake. See text for details. [Reprinted with permission of the publisher from Korbonits, M., Goldstone, A. P., Gueorguiev, M., and Grossman, A. B. Ghrelin—a hormone with multiple functions. *Frontiers Neuroendocr.* **25,** 27–68. Copyright 2004 Elsevier Science Inc.]

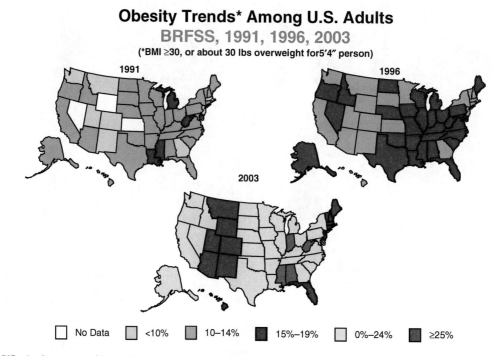

Obesity Trends* Among U.S. Adults
BRFSS, 1991, 1996, 2003
(*BMI ≥30, or about 30 lbs overweight for5'4″ person)

1991   1996   2003

☐ No Data   ☐ <10%   ■ 10–14%   ■ 15%–19%   ☐ 0%–24%   ■ ≥25%

Plate 12 **US obesity trends.** (These figures are from the Centers for Disease Control website, http://www.cdc.gov/needphp/dnpa/obesity/trend/index.htm)

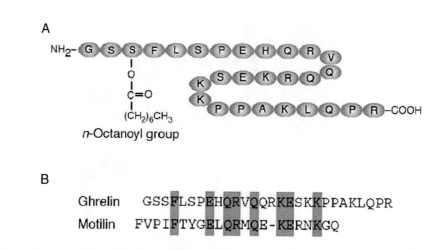

A

NH_2– G S S F L S P E H Q R V
KSEKRQQ
KPPAKLQPR–COOH

O
|
C=O
|
$(CH_2)_6CH_3$
n-Octanoyl group

B

Ghrelin   GSSFLSPEHQRVQQRKESKKPPAKLQPR
Motilin   FVPIFTYGELQRMQE-KERNKGQ

Plate 13 **Structure of human ghrelin.** (A) This molecule consists of 28 amino acids. Modification of the serine at position 3 with the addition of *n*-octanoic acid is an essential modification for ghrelin activity. (B) Comparison of the structure of ghrelin with another gastrointestinal hormone, motilin. [Reprinted with permission from Kojima, M., Hosoda, H., Matsuo, H., and Kangawa, K. 2001. Ghrelin: discovery of the natural endogenous ligand for the growth hormone secretogogue receptor. *Trends Endocr. Metab.* **12**, 118–126].

Edwards Brothers Malloy
Ann Arbor MI. USA
August 27, 2012